Paediatric Neurology

To the memory of
Paul Sandifer and *Ronnie MacKeith*
who taught us so much,
and to the children and their parents
who continue to do so.

Paediatric Neurology

Edited by

Edward M. Brett MA DM FRCP

Consultant Neurologist, The Hospital for Sick Children,
and The National Hospitals for Nervous Diseases, London and
Queen Mary's Hospital, Carshalton, Surrey

CHURCHILL LIVINGSTONE
EDINBURGH LONDON MELBOURNE AND NEW YORK 1983

CHURCHILL LIVINGSTONE
Medical Division of Longman Group Limited

Distributed in the United States of America by Churchill
Livingstone Inc., 1560 Broadway, New York, N.Y.
10036, and by associated companies, branches and
representatives throughout the world.

First published 1983

ISBN 0 443 01373 X

British Library Cataloguing in Publication Data
Paediatric neurology.
   1. Pediatric neurology
   I. Brett, Edward M.
   618.92'8   RJ486

Library of Congress Cataloging in Publication Data
Main entry under title:
Paediatric neurology.
   Includes index.
   1. Pediatric neurology.   I. Brett, Edward M. [DNLM: 1.
Nervous system diseases — In infancy and childhood.   WS
340 P1261]
RJ486. P25   1983   618.92'8   82–4526 AACR2

Printed and bound in Great Britain by
William Clowes (Beccles) Limited, Beccles and London

Preface

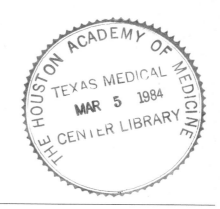
'Disease is very old, and nothing about it has changed. It is we who change, as we learn to recognize what was formerly imperceptible.'

Jean Martin Charcot,
De l'expectation en médecine.

Paediatric neurology has travelled far since the time of Charcot and of his successors, Freud, Tay, Sachs and Batten. The change to which Charcot referred was one which neurologists were undergoing in the 19th and early 20th centuries, and an equally remarkable metamorphosis has since affected the practitioners of child neurology. Advances in the understanding of neurometabolic disorders of childhood have been dramatic, leading in many cases to an unravelling of the biochemical and enzymatic aberrations underlying these diseases, which would have amazed the founding fathers of the subject. The implications of Folling's work on phenylketonuria for the prevention of mental handicap are immeasurable. Striking progress has been made in the prevention of some forms of cerebral palsy and there is scope for further improvement.

There has been, is still and probably always will be, debate and disagreement about the relative importance of paediatrics and neurology in the parentage and practice of child neurology, particularly as it affects the training of the would-be specialist. Successful practitioners are drawn from the ranks of neurology and of paediatrics. Both these disciplines are hard taskmasters. Since the art is long and life is short, the period of training spent in one of them is usually longer than that spent in the other. The relative emphasis on the two fields and on their offspring child neurology itself, varies in different countries, with more rigid requirements laid down in some than in others. While it must be admitted that too narrow a base in *either* of the parent disciplines can be disastrous (and one can sympathize with the eminent neurologist who felt that the trouble with paediatric neurologists was that they were not really interested in neurology, but only in children) the greatest errors are likely to result when an adequate knowledge of young children, and their normal and abnormal development, is lacking. Happily this situation is becoming rarer and the idea that the child is simply a miniature adult, a concept sanctified by centuries of adult-oriented thinking in medicine and in education, is now widely recognized as grotesque.

Despite the scientific advances in recent decades, the basic approach to all problems of paediatric neurology must still be a *clinical* one, with an accurate history an essential ingredient. Trite though this statement must sound, the principle must be stressed. More errors stem from an inadequate history, from failure to discover or acknowledge a mother's concerns about her child, failure to understand exactly what she is describing, or failure to pay sufficient attention to the developmental history, than from any other source. Examples of these errors are referred to repeatedly in the chapters which follow. The neurological examination, though it may present difficulties, is a less frequent source of error. The clinical assessment of the child and his symptoms will dictate the plan of investigation and should usually point to a limited list of tests appropriate to the situation rather than a 'blunderbuss' approach. The CT scan has revolutionized paediatric neurology in recent years, but it has not reduced the importance of clinical assessment — nor is it likely to do so.

Diagnostic accuracy is important as the foundation for treatment, prognosis and genetic counselling. Sadly, for many of the disorders encountered by the paediatric neurologist there is, as yet, no basic effective treatment. The diagnoses made are sometimes death-sentences, in the case of the progressive diseases, and in the case of the chronic neurological handicaps, especially mental subnormality, life-sentences. With so few treatable disorders it is particularly important that these few should not be missed. It is a tragedy when bacterial meningitis or spinal cord compression are diagnosed late or treated inadequately and persistent deficits result, or when status epilepticus is allowed to continue unchecked for hours with consequent brain damage. It is also a tragedy when the diagnosis of Duchenne muscular dystrophy is made late or when correct genetic advice is not given and as a result further affected boys are born.

The paediatric neurologist is involved with many incurable disorders and must be prepared to play a supportive role towards the child and his family, sometimes for many years. Head and heart are both required. The initial diagnostic exercise may have been brief or prolonged, but the diagnosis is not the end of the story, merely the start of another chapter. Those who are unfamiliar with our work will sometimes comment that it 'must be very rewarding'. There are in fact few rewards of the dramatic kind enjoyed by many other physicians or surgeons working with children. Such rewards as there are are simpler and humbler. 'Small profits, slow returns' might be a realistic description of the aims in many cases. Some improvement in fit control, the achievement of continence by a retarded child, the provision of suitable education for an intelligent child with athetoid cerebral palsy represent triumphs for the child and his family. The necessarily close contact with the parents of the child may be very demanding, but the predominant feeling of most doctors who are closely involved in the care of a handicapped or deteriorating child is one of admiration for the parents, and of privilege at assisting.

No one could claim that 'all is for the best, in the best of all possible worlds' in this field. Much of what is available in terms of medical expertise and facilities, education and support for the handicapped falls far short of what is desirable. There can be no panglossian complacency; Dr Pangloss was not a paediatrician. Much remains to be done in educating the public and the 'caring' professions in the problems of child neurology; in epilepsy alone judicious enlightenment of teachers and others can greatly improve the lot of the child patient, as the work of the British Epilepsy Association has proved. The concept of teaching is implicit in the word doctor, and there is unlimited scope for this role.

In a book of this kind common and rare conditions alike must be discussed. In most sections I have drawn on my own experience and that of others. Some subjects of a more specialized nature have been covered by colleagues whose experience is far wider than mine. Some disorders of great rarity I have not knowingly encountered. The gibe of 'neuro-philately' (pre-occupation with the neurological equivalent of the Cape Triangular) has been levelled at child neurologists as well as at their adult brethren, yet the rare must be covered as well as the common. This must result in an occasional imbalance in the space given to various disorders of differing frequency. Though undesirable I do not believe this is avoidable.

The subject of paediatric neurology is a growth area. Though young, it is advancing at an increasingly rapid rate; metaphorically it now lies between adolescence and young adult life. This is one of the many factors which combine to make it, to my mind, the most interesting branch of medicine, but it has as a corollary the implication that what is written today is out-of-date, if not tomorrow, then by next year. Inevitably also there are many areas of disagreement in this, as in any field of medicine. In these areas I have stated my personal opinion and have attempted also to present the opposing view.

London, 1983   E.M.B.

Acknowledgements

To work in any Teaching Hospital, and particularly a Children's Hospital, is a learning experience of great value. The further education gained is a continuing and mutual process. The exchange of information goes on in the more formal settings of ward round, lecture and conference, in the leisurely discussions over lunch or coffee, and in the snatched few moments of conversation in the corridors. Thus my thanks are due to countless colleagues at all levels, in many disciplines and over many years.

Many colleagues, quite apart from those who have kindly contributed chapters to this book, have helped me with advice and comments. In guiding my errant feet through their own particular fields and (it is to be hoped) obviating disastrous falls, the following must be singled out for mention: Dr Judith Chessells, Dr Robert Dinwiddie, Mr Norman Grant, Dr Ann Harden and Dr Isobel Smith. Dr S. Lingam and Dr Nicholas Cavanagh have also given helpful advice.

Dr Josef Egger has been a cornucopia of references, ancient and modern.

I am grateful to Dr R. D. Hoare for generous help with radiological illustrations and captions.

Many have helped with the typing of the manuscript, especially Miss Julia Hodges, my own secretary, Penelope and Redwood Fryxell, Miss Susan Langridge and Mrs Vivienne Holiday, and I am most grateful to them.

Many members of the Photographic Department, The Hospital for Sick Children, and Department of Medical Illustration, the Institute of Child Health, have worked hard and long to produce photographic and other illustrations. Miss Carole Reeves, Mr Martin Johns and Miss Pauline Henry have been especially helpful. Mrs Isobel Ellis has provided many line drawings for the first two chapters; many of these are based on photographs from *The Development of the Infant and Young Child, Normal and Abnormal*, by Professor Ronald Illingworth, to whom I am grateful for his kind agreement to this plagiarism.

My thanks are due to the following for permission to reproduce their tables and figures:

Figure. 2.1. Dr Peter Robson and the Editor, *Developmental Medicine and Child Neurology*.

Table 8.1. Dr Anita Harding, the Oxford University Press and the Editor of *Brain*.

Figure 11.9 Professor Bengt Hagberg and the Managing Editor, *Acta Paediatrica Scandinavica*.

Table 13.1 Dr Eva Alberman and Miss Maeve O'Connor, Senior Editor, The Ciba Foundation and *Excerpta Medica*, Amsterdam.

I am most grateful to the poet, Mr Thom Gunn and to Faber and Faber Ltd and the University of Chicago Press, for permission to reproduce two verses from his work, *Positives*, in Chapters 1 and 2.

Mr Denis Watkins-Pitchford (BB) has very kindly given me permission to reproduce, in Chapter 3, the lines which form the 'signature tune' of all his books, and which are derived from a tombstone discovered by his father in a North Country Churchyard.

The death, in 1980, of Dr Ruth Harris robbed Clinical Neurophysiology of one of its few practitioners skilled in the investigation of children, as well as depriving many of us of a valued colleague and friend. Her chapter had been completed earlier, and I felt it would be wrong to alter it, though I was anxious to include an authoritative account of some more modern techniques for the investigation of neuromuscular disease. The suggestion of Dr Robin Willison that Dr Diane Smyth should write a short contribution on recent advances in paediatric electromyography provided the happy solution. I am most grateful to her for helping in this way.

Contributors

Edward M. Brett MA DM FRCP
Consultant Neurologist, The Hospital for Sick
Children, Great Ormond Street and The National
Hospitals for Nervous Diseases, London, and
Queen Mary's Hospital for Children, Carshalton,
Surrey

C. O. Carter MA DM FRCP
Director, MRC Clinical Genetics Unit and
Professor in Clinical Genetics, Institute of Child
Health, University of London, London

H. B. Eckstein MA MD MChir FRCS
Consultant Surgeon, The Hospital for Sick
Children, Great Ormond Street, London, and
Queen Mary's Hospital for Children, Carshalton
Surrey

Neil Gordon MD FRCP
Consultant Paediatric Neurologist, Royal
Manchester Children's Hospital, Pendlebury, and
Booth Hall Children's Hospital, Manchester

The late **Ruth Harris** MD FRCP DCH
Consultant Neurophysiologist to the Bethlem
Royal and Maudsley Hospitals, London and to
Queen Mary's Hospital for Children, Carshalton,
Surrey

Brian D. Lake BSc PhD MRCPath
Reader in Histochemistry, Department of
Histopathology, Institute of Child Health,
University of London, and The Hospital for Sick
Children, Great Ormond Street, London

J. V. Leonard PhD MRCP
Senior Lecturer, Institute of Child Health,
University of London, and Honorary Consultant
Physician, The Hospital for Sick Children, Great
Ormond Street, London

Mary E. Lobascher MA MPhil
Principal Clinical Psychologist, The Hospital for
Sick Children, Great Ormond Street, and
Psychologist to the Medical Research
Council/Department of Health and Social Security
Phenylketonuria Register, London

W. C. Marshall MD PhD FRACP MRCP DCH
Consultant Physician in Infectious Diseases, The
Hospital for Sick Children, Great Ormond Street;
Consultant Paediatrician, St Ann's Hospital,
Tottenham; Senior Lecturer, Department of
Microbiology, Institute of Child Health,
University of London, London

Diane P. L. Smyth MD MRCP DCH
Senior Registrar in Paediatrics, Honorary Senior
Registrar in Paediatric Neurology, The John
Radcliffe Hospital, Oxford

Contents

Neurology of the newborn

E. M. Brett

She has been a germ, a fish,
and an animal; even now
she is almost without hair
or sex. But the body
is feeling its way
                    feeling
the minute hands grip, the big
baldish head beams, the feet
press out in the strange element

there is a perception of
warm water, warm, but cooling

Thom Gunn, *Positives* (1973)

'The fetal infant becomes a kind of open-sesame for
defining the nature of this development, for he is not
walled off from direct observation as is his unborn
counterpart.' (Gesell and Amatruda 1945)

HISTORICAL INTRODUCTION: DEVELOPMENT OF KNOWLEDGE OF FETAL BEHAVIOUR IN MAN

Premature delivery of the fetus gives valuable
opportunities for the study of fetal behaviour in
man and of the dramatic process of neurological
development which takes place during the later
months of pregnancy.

The first recorded scientific observations of a living human fetus were probably those of Erbkam
(1837) who described movements of the head and
extremities of a fetus of four months. Strassman
(1903) was possibly the first to record the movements of a human fetus removed at operation, in
a case of tubal pregnancy in which, through a rupture of a tube wall, slow movements of the limbs
of the 22 mm fetus were seen. More detailed observations were made by the Danish neurologist

Krabbe when in 1912 he found himself at the bed-
side of a woman, four months pregnant, who
aborted; he took the opportunity to examine the
fetus, a female of 24 mm, which showed a lively
heartbeat and slow movements of the limbs. He
found that the tendon reflexes at knee and ankle
could not be obtained, but that the abdominal
reflexes were brisk, and he was particularly interested to find that the plantar responses were repeatedly flexor, but without movement of the great
toes. The plantar response and other reactions in
prematurely born babies were also studied by Bersot (1920), who was the first to emphasize the continuity of development in intra-uterine and extra-
uterine life. He believed that as the prematurely
born baby approached (what he called) 'the conceptional age' of forty weeks, so his reactivity came
more and more to resemble that of the child born
at term.

Far more detailed observations of fetal development were made by Minkowski, in a series of publications from 1920 onwards, (e.g. 1921), by
Hooker (1952), Peiper (1963) and Humphrey
(1964). In Hooker's Pittsburg studies 131 fetuses
were observed. They ranged from $6\frac{1}{2}$ weeks of menstrual age to a postmature of 45 weeks. Hooker
found that reflex activity was first obtained at about
the middle of the seventh week of menstrual age
(about 5 weeks of fertilisation age) when light
stroking of the upper or lower lip or alae nasi
resulted in contralateral flexion of the neck and
uppermost trunk. Increasing complexity of
response was seen in fetuses of increasing menstrual age. From $7\frac{1}{2}$ to 10 weeks' menstrual age the
only skin area sensitive to light stroking with a hair
was in the perioral distribution of the maxillary and
mandibular divisions of the fifth cranial nerve. At

about $10\frac{1}{2}$ weeks the palms of the hands became sensitive, the fingers partially closing when stroked. With increasing menstrual age the sensitive areas gradually increased. By $12\frac{1}{2}$ weeks the response to stimulation changed from a 'total pattern' type of activity to an increasing number of specific responses or 'partial patterns', such as downward rotation of the eyeballs in response to stimulation over one eyelid, and lip closure to stimulation of the lips. By $13\frac{1}{2}$ to 14 weeks a stereotyped total pattern activity had almost completely disappeared, and the whole body surface, except for the back and top of the head, appeared sensitive to stroking: at this age Hooker believed the framework for the gradual development of the reflexes of postnatal life was present. Over the remaining months of gestation existing reflexes matured and new ones were gradually acquired. Between $18\frac{1}{2}$ and $23\frac{1}{2}$ weeks' 'menstrual age' he first elicited tendon reflexes, at knee and ankle, when respiration was briefly established; these became more complete at 25 weeks, at which age he inadvertently elicited a Moro reflex.

Fetuses delivered at 27 weeks (an age at which many fetuses, though formerly regarded as non-viable, have survived) were found by Hooker to have matured still further. The palmar grasp reflex, first adumbrated at $10\frac{1}{2}$ weeks, was so strong in one case that almost the entire weight of the fetus was briefly suspended with the grasp of one hand.

ANATOMICAL, BIOCHEMICAL AND ELECTRICAL CORRELATES OF FETAL DEVELOPMENT

The correlation between the appearance of early human fetal activity and the development of the nervous system has been studied by many workers (Langworthy 1933, Windle & Fitzgerald 1937, Minkowski 1938, Hooker 1952, Hooker & Humphrey 1959, Humphrey 1964). Langworthy (1933) described the sequence of myelination of pathways in the order in which they develop phylogenetically in man (as in the opossum and cat) and also the evidence that tracts become myelinated at the time when they first become functional. Windle & FitzGerald (1937) showed that the first spinal reflex arcs are completed during the eighth week, a time

when the first embryonic movements have been seen. The increasing responses to trigeminal stimulation described by Hooker were correlated by Humphrey (1964) with the development of the peripheral receptors and of the spinal tract of the trigeminal nerve from $6\frac{1}{2}$ weeks of menstrual age, when no responses are obtainable and only a few scattered axones reach the first cervical level of the spinal cord, to $8\frac{1}{2}$ weeks when contralateral flexion follows perioral stimulation and descending fibres reach the fourth cervical segment.

Myelination occurs in various tracts of the spinal cord in man from the twenty-second week of fetal life onwards, and a little later in some tracts in the brain. It continues postnatally and may not be complete until adult life, but its maximum rate of progress seems to be from about the seventh intra-uterine month to the first few months of post-natal life. Dobbing, who has studied myelination in man and other species (in which its pattern is very different) suggests (Davison & Dobbing 1966) that there may be a vulnerable period for myelination during which the human infant is at special risk from external factors such as maternal toxaemia and placental insufficiency. This would imply that, despite the relative 'sparing' of the brain in intra-uterine growth retardation compared with other organs (Gruenwald 1963), its function may nonetheless be seriously compromised. Opportunities for studying these correlations are limited and the situation is still unclear.

Larroche (1962) has studied the morphology, 'myelinogenesis' and cyto-architecture of the central nervous system from two months of conceptional age to term. In relation to total body weight the brain becomes relatively smaller with increasing age, and has achieved most of its growth potential by the age of 6 years. Thus at two months of fetal age the brain makes up about 25% of total body weight, at birth 10% and in the adult only 2%. These changes are reflected in increasing head circumference. Cerebral sulci first appear over the surfaces of the hemispheres at about 3 months of menstrual age, becoming more numerous and complex towards term when the convoluted adult pattern of sulci and gyri is established. Disturbances of formation of sulci can occur at various stages of gestation and give rise to different appearances of the surface of the brain (Ch. 17). In lissencephaly or agyria the cerebral hemispheres are smooth and resemble those of the two to four month fetus. In pachygyria the gyral patterns are coarse and scanty. This anomaly and micropolygyria, in which there is an excess of sulci and of very small gyri, results from insults to the developing nervous system occurring up to the fifth month of gestation, when the primary sulci have already been formed.

It has been shown (e.g. Gruenwald 1963) that in placental insufficiency and intrauterine growth retardation the human brain is much less affected than any other part of the body. The head is relatively large in the dysmature infant who is the victim of 'placental deprivation' of supply. At autopsy not only the weight but also the development of convolutions of the brain is often strikingly more advanced than might be expected for the low birth weight. Relevant experimental animal work has been reviewed by Winick (1976). Rats subjected to either prenatal or postnatal mulnutrition show a 15% reduction in total brain cell number at birth and at weaning respectively, but those who have been malnourished in both periods suffer a 60% reduction in brain cells by the time of weaning.

Opportunities for correlating early human fetal activity with enzymatic and metabolic studies on fresh post-mortem material have understandably been very limited. The carbonic anhydrase content of the nervous system in six human fetuses of from 6 to 9 months' gestation was studied by Ashby and Butler (1948). The enzyme was found to be absent in the cerebrum. In the more premature fetuses the spinal cord showed the highest content and the more rostral areas contained least. In the most mature fetus the content of the medulla had reached adult levels. In a more ambitious and detailed project Diebler et al (1979) studied developmental changes in enzymes associated with energy metabolism and in the synthesis of some neurotransmitters in discrete areas of human neocortex. Eight enzymes were studied in material from the motor, visual and associative cortex and their changes with age were analysed from 8 fetal weeks to adult life. The patterns of change for the various enzymes were different. Those associated with glycolytic pathways show a high activity in early fetal life, decline until the end of the active phase of neurogenesis and then rise continuously till the end of the first year of life. Glucose-6-phosphate dehydrogenase shows a high activity at 8 fetal weeks and gradually declines till the end of active neurogenesis, after which it either remains unchanged or increases slightly. Enzymes related to the tricarboxylic pathway have low levels of activity throughout the first half of gestation and then rise markedly during the last fetal months and first year after birth. Other enzymes show individual patterns of development.

The oxygen uptake of various parts of the nervous system was studied by Himwich et al (1956) in human fetuses and stillborn babies. At the twentieth week of gestation the oxygen uptake of the medulla was found to be higher than that of the cerebral cortex, caudate nucleus or thalamus. By the fortieth week the cortical uptake had risen to that of the medulla. The relative inactivity of the cerebral cortex in fetal life correlates well with these results.

Electroencephalographic studies on premature babies have been made by Dreyfus-Brisac and her colleagues (Dreyfus-Brisac et al 1962, Dreyfus-Brisac 1964), by Ellingson (1964) and by Engel & Benson (1968). Dreyfus-Brisac and her fellow-workers, from studies of the EEG, from five months of conceptional age to one year of post-natal age, concluded that certain bio-electric characteristics are seen at different ages, and that the 'EEG age' may sometimes be used to determine the conceptional age when other criteria are unreliable. Measurement of the latency of cortical evoked electrical responses to photic stimulation was used by Engel and Benson (1968) in an attempt to assess the conceptional age of newborn babies. This latency decreased with increasing gestational age and appeared to provide a reliable estimate of gestation although slight differences were found at term between the sexes, latency being shorter in females.

NEUROLOGICAL MATURATION OF THE NEWBORN IN THE LAST TRIMESTER OF PREGNANCY

The contribution of André Thomas and his school

In 1944, the French neurologist André Thomas, after many years of work in adult neurology, became interested in the neurology of newborn infants and devoted his remaining years to the problems peculiar to this age-group. He developed specialised techniques of neurological examination of the newborn and built up a body of knowledge of the normal and abnormal in a field where previously speculation had overshadowed scientific observation. His work and that of his colleague, Saint-Anne Dargassies, who has continued and expanded it, is well summarised in their joint publication, 'Etudes neurologiques sur le nouveau-né et le jeune nourrisson' (1952) and in Saint-Anne Dargassies' 'Le développement neurologique du nouveau-né à terme et prématuré (1974). Saint-Anne Dargassies has applied the methods of André Thomas particularly to the examination of premature babies and has shown the neurological maturation of the prematurely born infant as he nears the date of expected delivery, and defined criteria to which he conforms at certain stages of maturation. From these she believes the conceptional age of the newborn can be accurately estimated. Descriptions in English of these methods are given by many authors (Polani 1959, André Thomas Chesni & Saint-Anne Dargassies 1962, Brett 1966, Amiel-Tison 1968), but they are so important in the examination of the newborn and older infant, and as the basis of early 'developmental neurology', that they will be described in some detail.

The three aspects of the neurological neonatal examination

The neurological examination of the newborn can be considered under three main headings; the exploration of 'tonus', the study of the primary or 'automatic' reactions, and the more conventional aspects common to the examination of older subjects, such as deep tendon reflexes and sensory testing. The first two of these will be described in detail, and discussion of the third will be deferred until after a consideration of their value in neonatal assessment.

1. 'TONUS'

The concept of 'tonus' implies much more than the word 'tone' does to the English-speaking physician and the two words are not synonymous. For French and other continental European neurologists tonus has two main aspects, *active* and *passive, permanent or sustained* tonus, ('tonus actif' and 'tonus passif'). Active tonus comprises, *and determines*, posture at rest, and spontaneous and provoked movement. Passive or permanent tonus has three aspects; first, the *consistency* of the muscles on palpation; second, 'extensibilité', and third, 'passivité'. (There are no entirely satisfactory English equivalents to these words.) 'Extensibilité' is defined as the lengthening capacity of limb muscles as shown by the range through which certain joints can be passively moved. [This test was used by Babinski (1896)]. 'Passivité', or the degree of lack of reaction to passive stretching, comes nearer to the English concept of tone. It probably depends on the excitability and strength of the stretch reflexes and may be assessed by the degree of passive movement, flapping or 'ballant' imparted to a limb or part of a limb (hand, arm, foot or leg) on shaking it, and also by the return of a limb joint (elbow or knee) to the position of flexion after passive extension. *Extensibilité* may be measured at the wrist ('window sign'), elbow or shoulder ('signe de foulard' or 'scarf sign' and 'posterior scarf sign') in the upper limb, at the ankle, hip or knee [popliteal angle (see Fig. 1.10)] in the lower, and in the trunk where flexion, extension and lateral flexion are tested.

The distinction between active and passive tonus is illustrated by the dissociation often seen in these two aspects of tonus. Thus in cerebral depression in the newborn period an increase in 'extensibilité', indicating hypotonia, may co-exist with a decrease in 'passivité', with prompt arrest of the flapping hand, due to a brisk stretch reflex. The hypotonia of infants with Down's syndrome (mongolism) may show itself as abnormal passive tonus contrasting with normal active tonus, the child having normal posture and movements, whereas a newborn baby with respiratory distress or heart disease may sometimes show reduced active but normal passive tonus.

2. PRIMARY OR AUTOMATIC REACTIONS

The normal newborn infant shows a repertoire of primary or automatic reactions which can be exploited to examine not only the functional integrity of his nervous system, but also his degree of maturity. Most of these are mediated at a sub-cortical level (Paine 1960), and some are even obtainable in anencephalics (Gamper 1926).

The method of eliciting these reactions has been well described by Paine (1960), André Thomas et al (1962) and Peiper (1963). Paine and his colleagues (1964) have described their evolution in normal infants and in 'chronic brain syndromes', with their normally relatively predictable times of disappearance. They have a limited predictive value in assessing the probability of abnormality on re-examination at one year of age (Donovan et al 1962). Their value and interest lies mainly in their correlation in the newborn with gestational age, regardless of birth weight, and the opportunity they offer for comparing one side of the body with the other, since most are bilateral reactions.

Automatic walking or primary stepping (marche automatique)

When the normal newborn, in the necessary state of wakefulness, is held upright under the axillae, inclined forward and slowly advanced, one foot being first brought firmly in contact with a flat surface such as a table, automatic walking is seen (Fig. 1.1). This can also be obtained on a wall or up an inclined plane. While the traction response is elicited the baby, having reached the sitting position, will sometimes respond to further traction on his arms by starting to climb up the examiner's chest. Automatic walking usually disappears by four weeks of age, but if the neck is extended by the examiner it can often be elicited in older infants up to 11 months of age (MacKeith 1965).

Placing reaction of the feet (réaction d'enjambement: stehbereitshaft)

This is elicited (Fig. 1.2) by holding the infant upright so that the dorsum of one foot is brought up against the under-surface of a table edge or other projection. The foot so stimulated is then actively raised by the child and placed squarely on the surface. The placing reaction often has the effect of facilitating automatic walking. A similar placing reaction of the hands is seen when the same

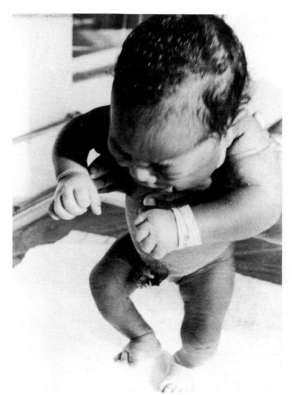

Fig. 1.1 Full-term newborn baby showing mature pattern of automatic walking

procedure is applied to them. These reactions may sometimes be difficult to elicit in sleepy or crying babies and in those who are generally depressed by respiratory or cardiac disease, severe jaundice or birth shock. They are said to be absent in anencephalic infants (André Thomas et al 1944).

The positive supporting reaction

This is the response of the newborn to being held upright with the feet firmly in contact with a flat surface; it consists of a movement of extension of both legs at the knees, which in babies at or near term is often followed by a straightening up of the trunk.

Extension of the trunk may also be elicited when the child is suspended horizontally with his head pointing forwards, buttocks against the examiner's chest and legs hanging down. Firm pressure on the soles of the feet is then followed by extension of the trunk and neck, so that he appears to 'sit up'.

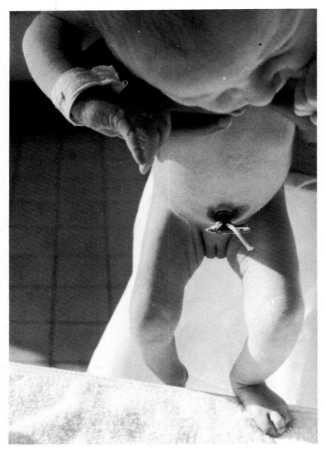

Fig. 1.2 Placing reaction in feet

The crossed extension response

This describes the response obtained in the opposite leg by stimulating the sole of one foot while the stimulated leg is prevented from moving by pressure on its knee. In its complete form it consists of flexion, followed by extension and adduction of the free leg, the foot being brought towards the stimulated foot as if to push away the stimulus. The latter should not be painful, since this may provoke an ipsilateral withdrawal reaction, or an attempt at it. The normal neonatal crossed extension response must be distinguished from the abnormal reaction seen with spinal cord lesions, when the stimulated foot withdraws in an automatic and often clonic way, followed by vigorous extension of the opposite leg, the face usually showing no evidence of pain.

The Moro reflex

This reflex, probably the most familiar of the neonatal responses, can be elicited in various ways. A loud noise, a sudden blow to the surface on which the child lies, holding the infant's hands, extending and then suddenly releasing them, or lifting his head and shoulders slightly off the surface and then letting the head drop back about 30 degrees in relation to the axis of the trunk, all provoke the reaction via different pathways. In its mature form the Moro reflex consists of arm extension followed by flexion with extension of the fingers, and usually flexion of the thighs at the hips, often with a cry (Fig. 1.3). It is absent or incomplete in the more premature babies but should be consistently present in the normal mature newborn. It may be

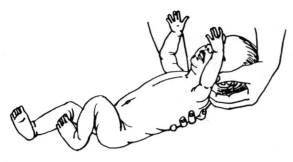

Fig. 1.3 Moro reflex

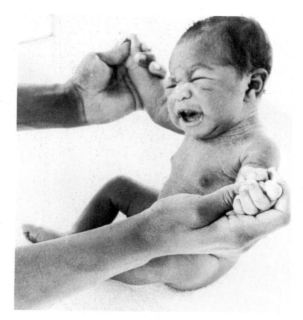

Fig. 1.4 Traction response with good head control

absent or depressed with severe illness of any kind, especially kernicterus, and general depression of the central nervous system. An asymmetrical Moro is seen with brachial plexus palsy and with trauma to the clavicle, humerus or shoulder joint, as well as congenital hemiplegia, (which is rarely detected, however, in the newborn period.) The response begins to fade by four to eight weeks but can be reinforced by pressure on the knees and then obtained at later ages.

The palmar and plantar grasp reflexes

These reactions are elicited by placing a finger or thumb firmly in the infant's palm or at the base of his toes. The palmar grasp is conveniently combined with testing the traction response. The baby's hand firmly grasps the examiner's finger.

The traction response

The infant, as he lies on his back and grasps the examiner's fingers in both hands, can be slowly pulled upright into a sitting position. The shoulder girdle muscles usually come into play in the more mature newborns to assist in the process. The degree of head control seen in traction varies; some degree of head lag is usual, but most often in mature infants the head is brought forward actively from a point near the vertical. Figures 1.4 and 1.5 show the traction response with good and poor degrees of head control. Often the head falls suddenly forward on to the chest on reaching the upright position, but is usually then brought back to the vertical, particularly if the nose or mouth are stimulated.

Automatic reactions in the prone position

With the infant in the prone position, with his arms extended alongside his trunk, one or both arms are spontaneously brought forward so that the hands lie level with the shoulder or face. This *passage des bras* usually occurs first, or only, on the side to which the face is turned (Fig. 1.6). It may be facilitated by pressure on the baby's opposite buttock.

In the prone position also, the normal newborn is seen to turn his head to one side, and sometimes to raise it briefly from the surface, even in some cases turning it from one side to the other.

In the same position *alternating crawling* or creeping movements of the legs are usually seen (Fig. 1.6). These may be stimulated by gentle pressure on the soles of the feet, and may be vigorous enough to propel the baby forward for some distance.

Trunk incurvation (Galant's reflex)

This may be elicited with the infant suspended horizontally or prone on a flat surface, when the examiner runs his finger down the paravertebral area on one side. The response is a swinging of the pelvis

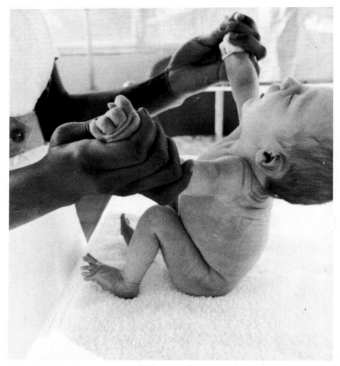

Fig. 1.5 Traction response with poor head control in less mature baby

towards the stimulated side, but may vary, like the other reactions described, from time to time, so that failure to elicit it on one occasion cannot be taken as proof of its absence. It is said to occur in anencephalics and in even the most premature of newborn infants (André Thomas et al 1944, André Thomas & Saint-Anne Dargassies 1952). Although it is said to disappear in the first year of life, it can be obtained in minor degree in many normal children up to 10 years of age. In some neurologically abnormal infants it can be obtained from an unusually wide afferent area, including the arms, and even from the ventral surface of the trunk. The reflex may be of some value in mapping a sensory level on the trunk, being absent in spina bifida or other spinal cord conditions below the level of the lesion.

Rooting reflex (réaction des points cardinaux) and reflex sucking

When the examiner's finger toughes the mouth of the normal newborn at the four points of the compass (top, bottom, left and right), his head turns to bring his mouth towards the finger, which he may then suck. Sucking tends to reinforce rooting, and a recent feed to suppress it. Rooting and sucking should be present in normal neonates except for the more premature infants, but may be absent with depression of the CNS by anoxia or maternal anaesthesia, or with congenital brain defects. Rooting persists until three or four months of age, and later in sleep. Visual cues become involved in older children who may root for a bottle but not for a finger. The rooting reflex may persist abnormally long in neurologically abnormal children, and occasionally reappears in those with progressive degenerative brain diseases.

Head-turning towards diffuse light (réaction de la fenêtre)

From 32 weeks of gestation onwards the newborn baby, when held upright in a dark room with a sin-

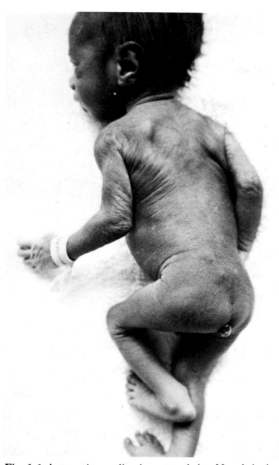

Fig. 1.6 Automatic crawling in mature baby. Note bringing up of left arm

gle source of light such as a window, will tend to turn his head so as to look towards the light and, as he is turned away from the light by the examiner, will continue to turn towards it. This reaction has been shown to depend on the presence of normally functioning visual cortex (Goldie & Hopkins 1964) and thus differs from many of the reactions described above which are mediated at a sub-cortical level.

Asymmetric tonic neck response (ATNR)

This response differs from those described above in being less prominent in the newborn period but appearing and becoming more marked at a few weeks of age. When the infant's head is turned, spontaneously or passively, to one side, the arm on the side which he faces is seen to extend and that on the other side to flex, while a similar posture of the legs is often adopted, so that his position resembles that of a fencer (Fig. 1.7). The response is at its height between 2 and 4 months of age when the infant's limbs are in ATNR postures for about 50% of the time. It is usually not imposable by 7 months, though very minor degrees of the reflex can be elicited in normal children up to 9 years of age when placed on all-fours (Parr et al 1974). It should never be completely obligatory, in the sense that the child cannot escape from the posture imposed on him by head turning, and its abnormal persistence in older children with cerebral palsy and severe developmental retardation is of diagnostic and prognostic significance (Ch. 11).

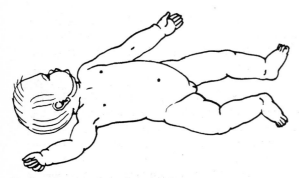

Fig. 1.7 Asymmetric tonic neck reflex

CORRELATION OF THE NEUROLOGICAL FINDINGS WITH GESTATIONAL MATURITY IN THE LAST TRIMESTER

The French workers have shown that in later fetal life increasing conceptional age is associated with an evolving pattern of neurological findings. This evolution is seen particularly in tonus and in the complexity and constancy of primary or automatic reactions in the last three months of pregnancy.

The changes occurring in tonus with maturation are in the direction of an increase in *flexor* tonus, which starts in the legs and spreads to the arms. The posture of the most premature infant of about twenty eight weeks' gestation is commonly one of extension of all limbs or 'deflexion'. With increasing maturity flexor tonus increases in the legs so that at about 35 weeks of conceptional age the child lies mainly with legs flexed and arms extended in the so-called 'frog-position'. Thereafter progressive increase in flexor tonus in the arms brings them also into a predominantly flexed position as term is neared. With increasing tonus the limbs become more and more limited in their range of spontaneous movement. The free windmill-like movements of the very premature infant gradually decrease and contrast strongly with the relative immobility of the term infant, who may be described as 'a prisoner of his own tone', or as Gesell & Amatruda (1945) have described it, 'muscle-bound'.

Figure 1.8 shows the bizarre transient posture of a premature baby of 32 weeks' gestation which would be impossible in an infant at term. It con-

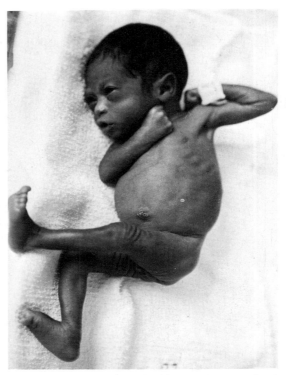

Fig. 1.8 Premature baby showing bizarre posture associated with physiological hypotonia and mobility

trasts with the persisting flexed posture of the postmature baby shown in Figure 1.9.

The posture of the head of the newborn baby is also influenced by changes in tonus. The most premature infant in the supine position has his head usually inclined to one side, whereas the term baby often lies with his head in the midline, with little freedom of lateral movement.

In the prone position the normal term newborn infant has his pelvis high and his knees drawn up under his belly. He will usually turn his head to one side and sometimes raise it slightly. Often crawling movements of the legs are seen, and one or both arms may be brought forward, usually first on the side towards which the head is turned.

Extensibilité may be assessed, as mentioned, at many joints, but is conveniently studied at the knee. With the baby lying on his back on a firm surface, his hips are flexed and knees extended so that the popliteal angle is opened up to the maximum extent without undue force (Fig. 1.10). The

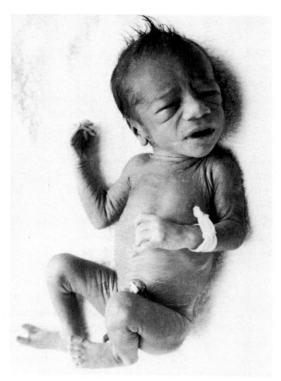

Fig. 1.9 Postmature baby showing flexed and immobile posture

angle measures 160° or more in the most premature infants and becomes progressively smaller with maturity, so that it is usually about 90° or less near term. *Extensibilité* can also be assessed at the ankle, where passive dorsiflexion becomes increasingly freer so that the dorsum of the foot touches the shin shortly before term, whereas this is usually not possible in more premature babies. The angle between hand and forearm may also be measured on passive flexion of the wrist ('window-sign') and tends to become larger as term is approached. Simultaneous changes are seen in *passivité*, the other aspect of passive tonus; 'flappability' imparted to the limbs decreases with maturation.

The automatic responses of the newborn increase progressively in strength, consistency and complexity from 28 weeks of gestation to term. In some of these the various stages of their development correlate closely with gestational age in the well infant, and, together with the evolution of tonus mentioned above, allow a fairly accurate assessment of gestational maturity whether maturation has occurred *in utero* or outside the womb.

Thus, automatic walking, an activity which usually delights and amuses the baby's mother (as well as the nursing and medical staff), shows develop-

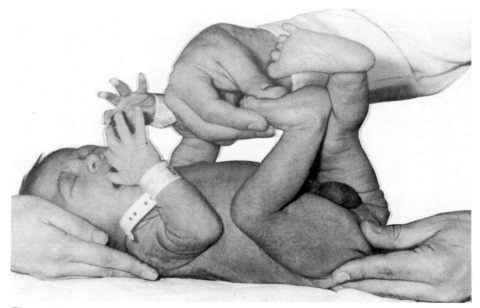

Fig. 1.10 Popliteal angle in mature baby

ment from an 'equinus' type of gait in the more premature infant, who steps on the anterior parts of his feet with heels high, like an older individual with a spastic paraplegia, to a plantigrade gait at or near term, often with the heels coming down first as in true voluntary walking (Fig. 1.1).

The crossed extension response also shows increasing complexity with advancing maturity and I have found it, used in conjunction with assessment of tonus, to correlate well with this and to allow fairly accurate assessment of gestational age. In the infant at, or very near, term a complex response to stimulating the sole of one foot is seen in the contralateral free leg. First flexion occurs at hip and knee, followed soon afterwards by extension, and finally by a movement of adduction which brings the free foot towards the stimulus. The toes of the mobile foot extend. Sometimes the adducting movement brings the free foot into contact with the opposite leg at knee level and extension continues with the foot pushed downwards against the lower leg, as if trying to perform the heel-knee-shin test. In the most premature infants the reaction may be completely absent. At 28 weeks' gestation the response is usually limited to flexion of the opposite leg. At about 32 weeks flexion is generally followed, after a latent period, by extension. At about 37 weeks extension quickly follows flexion, and only at or near term is the third stage of adduction added. From the neurological point of view absence of this third stage of the response is regarded as evidence of prematurity.

Increasing strength and complexity are also seen, as gestational age advances, in the Moro reflex, palmar and plantar grasp, head control in traction, straightening reactions of the lower limbs and trunk, placing reactions of the feet, and rooting reactions.

My experience with the French method of neurological examination of the newborn has led me to believe that it allows a fairly accurate assessment of gestational age in white babies, but that it tended to over-estimate with statistically significant frequency that of coloured babies (mainly West Indian) in the newborn population studied (Brett 1966). This finding seems to accord with the common observation of nursing staff that West Indian neonates seem more advanced than white babies of the same maturity, and with the work of Geber & Dean (1964) on newborn African infants in Uganda, using a modified form of the French method.

Many of the observations in the neurological examination described above can be applied to very premature babies in incubators and do not involve a harmful degree of handling. The general condition of the infant must be taken into account, and pathological conditions such as the effects of birth trauma, anoxia, maternal analgesics and hyperbilirubinaemia tend to depress the results to a less mature level. Between 6 and 9 days of post-natal age is probably the best time for a single examination for the criteria of maturity, since most babies have by then recovered from the effects of delivery.

Physiological variation in the infant also affects the findings on examination so that definite conclusions as to prematurity should not be drawn from the results of a single examination if the child, for example, appears very sleepy. Examination needs to be adjusted to feeding schedules, so that the baby is neither too hungry and active, nor too sated and soporific. Often he can be aroused or pacified so as to bring him to the most appropriate state. The 'state' of the newborn infant has been classified on a five point scale by Beintema (1968) using criteria of eyes closed or open, respiration regular or irregular, movements absent, moderate or gross, and presence or absence of crying.

State 1: eyes closed, regular respiration, no movements

State 2: eyes closed, irregular respiration, no gross movements

State 3: eyes open, no gross movements

State 4: eyes open, gross movements, no crying

State 5: eyes open or closed, crying.

A rather different approach to the neurological neonatal examination in assessing gestational age from that of the French workers was adopted by Robinson (1966). He placed most reliance on a number of *discontinuous* variables, which change from negative to positive over a relatively short period, rather than on continuous variables, such as tonus, posture and strength of responses which increase or change steadily during the whole of the last trimester. Robinson found that five responses appeared at definite times in the gestational period, which were the same in normal and 'small-for-dates' babies. These were the pupil reaction to light (appearing between 30 and 31 weeks), the glabellar tap reflex (32 to 34 weeks), the traction response (33 to 36 weeks), the neck-righting reflex — rotation of the trunk in the same direction as that to which the head is passively turned — (36 to 37 weeks) and head-turning to light (32 to 36 weeks). He believed that these five responses give a useful indication of gestational age, but without the degree of accuracy claimed for the French method of examination. Dubowitz and his colleagues (1970) and Dubowitz & Dubowitz (1981) have devised a score combining neurological and other criteria for the assessment of fetal maturity. The 10 neurological observations used involve various aspects of 'tonus', rather than primary or automatic reactions. This selection was designed to use criteria which are reproducible by different observers and least influenced by the 'state' of the baby or the presence of neurological abnormality. The criteria are: posture in supine, 'square window' (flexion of hand on forearm), ankle dorsiflexion, arm recoil after elbow extension, leg recoil after hip and knee extension, popliteal angle, heel to ear manoeuvre, scarf sign, head lag when pulled to sitting position and ventral suspension. The external criteria involve observations of oedema of the extremities, texture, colour and opacity of the skin, lanugo over the back, plantar creases, nipple formation, breast size, form and firmness of the ears, and development of the genitalia. Scores from zero to 35 are assigned to the two groups of criteria. The authors applied this scoring system to 167 newborn infants, and found that the external score gave a better correlation with gestation than did the neurological score, but that the combined total score was better than either alone.

MORE CONVENTIONAL ASPECTS OF NEUROLOGICAL EXAMINATION

Observation of the spontaneous and provoked behaviour of the newborn infant with exploitation of the primitive responses described above will give much information about the functioning state of his nervous system. It will demonstrate paralysis of limbs and may allow detection of a congenital hemiplegia, paraplegia or tetraplegia and of a brachial plexus palsy.

More conventional methods of neurological examination are needed to gain further information. tion.

Some modification of the methods used for older children is needed, and the examiner must (as in all paediatric examinations) be adaptable and be ready to make observations as the opportunity allows. The more disturbing procedures (tendon reflexes, examination of tongue and palate, and sensory testing) should be left until the end.

Examination of the head and neck

Examination can usefully begin with inspection of the head. The maximum occipitofrontal circumference (OFC) should be measured with a metal or paper tape (rather than linen, since linen can stretch) and *recorded*; this most vital of the vital statistics is also the most often neglected, and absence of this measurement in the newborn period can make interpretation of abnormal head circumference at later ages extremely difficult when dealing with problems of hydrocephalus and microcephaly. The shape of the head may suggest craniostenosis affecting various sutures (Ch. 17). A large head with bulging forehead and fullness in the temporal regions may suggest hydrocephalus. Suture separation, bulging or tension of the anterior fontanelle, a setting sun sign (Ch. 17) and an abnormal 'cracked pot' sound on percussion of the skull are other signs of raised intracranial pressure which may be seen in hydrocephalus and some other conditions. Bilateral subdural effusions often produce a large head which is abnormally wide from side to side and rather square in appearance. Signs of trauma such as bruising, cephalhaematoma and depressed fractures should be looked for. The skull sutures are often over-riding in the newborn. They may also be palpably separated in some cases. Transillumination of the head may be helpful in neurologically abnormal infants. It requires a strong torch with a rubber seal for applying to the head and a dark room. Hydrocephalus, hydranencephaly, porencephalic cysts and subdural collections may be suspected from the finding of abnormal degrees of transillumination.

The neck should be examined in conjunction with the head. Opisthotonos and neck retraction are important signs of meningeal irritation, which may be due to intracranial haemorrhage, meningitis, kernicterus or, rarely, tumours in the posterior fossa or cervical spine. Neck stiffness, a classical sign of meningitis in older patients, is often absent in newborns, and its absence should never be taken to exclude this diagnosis. The same is true of other signs of meningeal irritation. Neonatal meningitis (Ch. 22) is notoriously difficult to diagnose and whenever it is suspected lumbar puncture must be performed.

The entire length of the spine should be carefully examined, including the sacral segment, for evidence of spina bifida, overt or occult, or of dermal sinuses (Ch. 17).

Examination of the eyes

The position of the eyes at rest should be noted. Abnormalities include squints, real or 'apparent,' and the setting sun sign. This could equally well be called the rising sun sign since it consists of downward rotation of the eyes with upper eyelid retraction, sometimes with raising of the brows, so that the lower edges of the pupils may be level with or below the lower lids, and a rim of sclera is visible above each iris (Ch. 17). The sign may occur as a transient feature in some otherwise normal premature babies, but in more mature infants often indicates raised intracranial pressure and is seen in many cases of hydrocephalus, when it is often combined with strabismus and undulating eye movements. It may not be constantly present and can sometimes be provoked by changes of posture or removal of light as by switching off a torch. The sign is also seen in newborn babies with kernicterus.

Spontaneous and provoked eye movements should be studied. Although it is often stated that infants do not fix and follow visually until about six weeks of age, healthy newborn babies can easily be shown to follow visual lures in the first days of life when in the appropriate state of alertness. Doll's head movements of the eyes can be seen when the child's head is turned passively. Rotational vesti-bular nystagmus is also easily elicited in many newborns and allows horizontal movements of the eyes to be assessed; it is most easily seen when the baby is held facing upwards in front of the examiner with his head towards the latter and inclined slightly downwards (Paine 1961). Optokinetic nystagmus can be studied with the aid of a striped revolving drum and provides a useful criterion of vision. The pupil reaction to light can be shown in normal babies of 30 weeks' gestation or more, and blinking will occur in response to a bright light. Blindness may be suspected from absence of pupillary light responses and from the presence of wandering, disorganized eye movements. Eyelid myotonia can sometimes be seen when the child tries to open his eyes after closure in dystrophia myotonica (Ch. 3).

Ophthalmoscopic examination is an important part of the neonatal neurological examination. In some cases it may be difficult and require dilatation of the pupils with mydriatics, but it can often be achieved with patience while the baby is feeding. The optic discs may show pallor, hypoplasia, or abnormalities to suggest septo-optic dysplasia (Ch. 17), the retinae may show choroidoretinitis indicating intrauterine infections (toxoplasmosis or cytomegalovirus), pigmentary changes to suggest congenital rubella, haemorrhages, phakomas and anomalies of the retinal arteries. Swelling of the optic discs is rare in the young child, since raised intracranial pressure usually causes separation of the cranial sutures. Raised pressure is often associated with retinal haemorrhages which are also common after trauma.

The pupils of the newborn are usually equal but occasional inequality may be of no pathological significance. Horner's syndrome may be seen with a smaller pupil on one side, sometimes associated with ptosis and enophthalmos. Hippus, with rhythmically alternating constriction and dilatation of the pupils, is common and usually has no diagnostic significance.

Ptosis is usually easily recognized and may occur as part of Horner's syndrome, in the rare cases of neonatal myasthenia gravis and as an isolated congenital anomaly. In some case of congenital ptosis, usually unilateral, the Marcus Gunn phenomenon of jaw-winking is seen, in which movements of the jaw in feeding or crying cause reflex elevation of the ptosed upper lid.

Other cranial nerves

Facial nerve paralysis due to obstetric injury is usually unilateral and easily detected in the crying infant. It may be transient or persistent. Minor degrees of bilateral facial weakness may be less easy to detect but severe degrees, such as occur in Möbius syndrome, myasthenia gravis and certain congenital myopathies, are usually obvious. Congenital hypoplasia of the depressor anguli oris muscle occurs in 0.5 to 1% of newborn babies and may be misinterpreted as a facial palsy on the *opposite* side. It may be associated with congenital defects in the cardiovascular and other systems. Some assessment of the hearing can usually be made in the healthy neonate by observing his reaction of blinking and startle to a loud noise, his quieting to a soft continuous noise such as humming, and sometimes turning his eyes towards the source of the sound.

Movement of the palate can be observed during crying or gagging in response to a stimulus.

Observation of head control and the degree of head lag seen when the infant is pulled up to the sitting position allows assessment of the sternomastoid muscles.

Examination of the tongue may be difficult. It should be examined when possible at rest inside the mouth. Wasting and fasciculation may be seen in some cases of Werdnig-Hoffman disease, but may be difficult to detect in a crying child. It is often helpful to examine the tongue through an auriscope from which the speculum has been detached.

Examination of the limbs

Observations of spontaneous and provoked movements of the limbs will usually have given evidence of any gross paralysis. Formal examination of tone by handling the limbs and of the tendon reflexes will often add only limited information. The patellar hammer is less important in the newborn period than at other ages. It is essential to use a *small* hammer, since the adult-size instrument will often fail to elicit a reflex as the area in contact with the limb is too large to apply an adequate stretching force to the tendon. The head of the hammer, whatever its shape, should be of sufficiently soft rubber or other material not to hurt the infant.

If the baby's head is inclined to one side the asymmetric tonic neck reflex often causes an increase in tone and reflexes on that side. The effect of the reflex should be excluded by keeping the head in the midline, if necessary with the help of an assistant. Persistent asymmetry of reflexes is likely to be significant.

In the normal newborn at term the mainly flexed position of the arms often makes the arm reflexes, particularly the triceps jerks, difficult to elicit. The knee jerks are usually easily obtained, but the ankle jerks may be somewhat difficult, and are often most easily elicited, as in older children, in the prone position. In infants and young children in general there is often marked variability in the briskness of the tendon reflexes from one time to another, and also from one subject to another. It is common to find the reflexes in the legs brisker than those in the arms. The knee jerks can often be obtained from a wider area than is usual in older people, and this finding in itself should not be taken as abnormal if unaccompanied by other signs of pyramidal dysfunction. Crossed adduction of the contralateral thigh is commonly seen when the knee jerk is elicited in the newborn and older infants and indeed often in older children, and this sign in isolation should also not be regarded as abnormal. Sustained ankle clonus in the newborn is common particularly in babies who are crying, hungry or 'jittery'. This finding in itself is seldom of serious import.

The normal plantar response in the newborn is often said, following the statement of Babinski (1896) himself, to be extensor. It is also described as being very variable. The latter statement is probably true, since it can be readily affected by the state of sleep or wakefulness of the infant, by the position of the head through the asymmetric tonic neck reflex, and by other factors. Withdrawal of the foot may also make its assessment difficult and care must be taken not to elicit the plantar grasp reflex. Hogan & Milligan (1971) attempted to define the newborn plantar response more clearly by controlling these variables and judging the response by the first movement of the great toe; they found that 93 to 100 newborn infants had bilateral flexor responses, while 4 had bilateral and 3 unilateral extensor responses.

Sensory testing in the newborn is difficult since the examiner must depend on the infant's response, of crying or moving, to touch or pinprick. Painful stimuli are more likely to provoke a consistent and reliable response, but examination is often interrupted by crying and may be distressing to mother and doctor as well as to the child. In spinal cord lesions the trunk incurvation reflex may be absent below the level of the lesion.

No paediatrician can afford to ignore other systems than the one of chief interest to him. Particularly in the newborn period clues must be sought elsewhere which may be relevant to neurological disease. Careful examination of the skin is important to detect naevi which may be stigmata of the neurocutaneous syndromes (Ch. 20). Enlargement of liver and spleen may be found in certain infections and neurometabolic disorders. Congenital cardiac and renal anomalies may increase the chances of congenital cerebral defect.

THE IMPLICATIONS FOR FUTURE DEVELOPMENT OF THE NEWBORN OF THE FINDINGS ON NEUROLOGICAL EXAMINATION

Desirable, in some ways, though it might be to be able to make accurate predictions for the future from the neurological findings in the neonate, it does not seem possible at present to do so. The study by Donovan et al (1962) of 192 full-term infants illustrated the poor correlation between the findings on double neurological examination at about 72 hours of age and those at one year. Seventy-eight of 80 infants thought to be normal by both examiners in the newborn period were also normal by the criteria applicable at 1 year, but about 80% of those regarded as abnormal by one or both examiners were also passed as normal at one year. The conventional neurological signs and infantile postural automatisms in the newborn period all seemed individually and in combination to be of only very limited value in predicting abnormality at one year. The single most ominous combination was that of depressed automatic responses, especially the traction response and Moro reflex, with exaggerated tremulousness.

When dealing with *asphyxiated* newborn infants Brown et al (1974) found that clinical observations could be correlated with later outcome. They selected a series of 94 infants from among 760 asphyxiated newborn babies on the basis of seven criteria — feeding difficulties, apnoeic and cyanotic attacks, apathy, convulsions, hypothermia, persistent vomiting and a high-pitched cerebral cry. These criteria were found to be prognostic for subsequent handicap. The 94 infants were also classified on the basis of muscle tone, graded as hypotonia, extensor hypertonus, or normal flexor tone, or in transition from hypotonia to extensor hypertonus. 93 of the infants were followed up to a mean age of 21 months. There were 20 deaths and 24 infants had a functionally significant handicap (mental retardation, microcephaly, cerebral palsy, and epilepsy in varying combinations). The severity of the handicap was related to the earlier classification according to muscle tone. It was found that infants with hypotonia or with hypotonia progressing to extensor hypertonus had a very bad prognosis, while the outlook for those with normal flexor tone was very good. The Apgar score has also been used to try to relate the degree of hypoxic-ischaemic insult to the prognosis. In several large series an Apgar score of 6 or less at 5 minutes was associated with neurological sequelae in approximately 5 to 17% of cases, while low scores at one minute carried half this risk (Volpe 1975).

Visual function and its possible predictive value in the newborn

It is understandable that the neonatal findings, which depend largely on reflex responses and maturation of the nervous system, should not correlate well, in infants who are not obviously neurologically abnormal, with later intellectual status. Certain perceptual performances resemble more closely later intellectual behaviours and might therefore seem more relevant to these. Visual perception in the newborn has been studied by Fantz and others following his development of an objective test of pattern perception. Pattern vision was studied in newborn infants (Fantz 1963) who were found to show strong visual preferences for stripes or other black and white patterns over plain gray, white or coloured surfaces. Further work has shown that the newborn can discriminate between more specific variations in patterns. In the course of testing hundreds of infants, it was noted that some of them did not respond in the usual way and these were usually found to be among those regarded as being at high risk for neurological or mental handicap. An attempt was therefore made to assess the predictive value of neonatal visual responses in a group of 33 high-risk infants (Miranda et al 1977), compared with that of neurological examination. At follow-up at ages up to 60 months the children were graded as normal, abnormal or borderline on neurological and developmental assessment. The predictions made from the visual fixation test were correct in 27 of the 33 infants whereas the neonatal neurological examination gave only 21 correct predictions. Of 23 infants considered normal by the neonatal visual test, only one was abnormal on follow-up and three were borderline. Of the 8 rated as abnormal none was normal on follow-up, 7 being frankly abnormal and one borderline. The sample studied included a high proportion of potentially abnormal infants, and the value of visual-perceptual neonatal screening needs to be assessed in more normal populations with fewer damaged infants. Nonetheless the technique may well provide a more reliable guide to prognosis than any other.

Dubowitz et al (1980) have studied visual function in preterm and full term newborn infants by the Fantz technique of pattern preference and fixation and also by the visual orientation (tracking) technique of the Brazelton infant behaviour test. Both these methods showed that discriminative visual function had developed by 31 to 32 weeks' gestation, and had reached a level of maturity comparable to that of full term infants by 34 weeks.

Visual following and pattern discrimination were also studied in the newborn by Goren et al (1975) who showed that 40 normal newborn infants at a mean age of 9 minutes turned their heads and eyes significantly more often to follow a stimulus resembling a human face than either of two equally complex stimuli composed of the same facial features 'scrambled' or a blank. An unlearned perceptual organization may be present at birth which allows the infant to respond selectively to the human face.

Auditory brainstem responses

The auditory brainstem responses (ABR) of premature and more mature newborn infants can be studied by neurophysiological techniques (Despland & Galambos 1980). These responses gave information on both neurological and audiological

status in 120 premature infants in intensive care units and may be of value for long-term prediction.

Neonatal seizures

The important topic of neonatal seizures is discussed for convenience in the chapter on epilepsy and convulsions (Ch. 12). Their causes are many, and at this point I would only stress the need to consider and exclude or treat the treatable and potentially serious conditions, particularly hypoglycaemia, hypocalcaemia, meningitis and pyridoxine-dependency.

Neonatal screening

Neonatal population screening for phenylketonuria (Ch. 6) is almost universal in the developed nations.

National screening programmes for congenital hypothyroidism exist in many countries. A progress report on neonatal thyroid screening in Europe (Delange et al 1981) showed that the screening rate varied in different nations and was 23.3% in the United Kingdom. The cases detected numbered 1 per 3600 newborns screened for the entire series. The value of such screening in the prevention of mental handicap is great and it should be applied to all newborns.

Screening of male infants for Duchenne muscular dystrophy (Ch. 3) is also effective but more controversial since there is no effective treatment.

Neonatal screening for deafness is now possible with the auditory response cradle, an automatic micro-processor-controlled hearing screening device (Tucker 1982). The importance of such screening, especially in at-risk babies, is shown by the frequency of hearing loss in very low birthweight infants treated with neonatal intensive care (Abramovich et al 1979). Sensory neural hearing loss was found in 9% of 111 perinatal intensive care survivors with birth weights 1500 g or less, when assessed at a mean age of $6\frac{1}{2}$ years.

PERINATAL HYPOXIC-ISCHAEMIC BRAIN INJURY

As Volpe (1976) has pointed out, hypoxic-ischaemic brain injury is the single most important neurological problem occurring in the perinatal period, accounting for more of the non-progressive neurological deficits of childhood than any other type of brain injury. Mental retardation, epilepsy and the various forms of cerebral palsy are its main sequelae. This has been known clinically since the time of Little (1862), and indeed earlier, but has come to be more fully understood in recent years as a result of animal work and clinical and pathological studies in many centres. The subject is well reviewed by Volpe (1976, 1979, 1980), Pape & Wigglesworth (1979), and Fenichel (1980), among others.

The common denominator of hypoxic-ischaemic injury to the newborn is deprivation of the supply of oxygen to the CNS. Volpe (1976) has reviewed the pathophysiological aspects of these insults, the clinical features in the newborn period, and the neuropathological lesions with their neurological sequelae.

Pathophysiology

The neonatal brain may be deprived of oxygen by two main pathogenetic mechanisms, hypoxaemia (reduced amount of oxygen in the blood supply) or ischaemia (reduced amount of blood perfusing the brain.)

Hypoxaemia is associated with acceleration in the uptake of glucose, rate of glycolysis and production of lactate, and with diminution in the concentration of various intermediates of the tricarboxylic acid cycle and in the production of adenosine triphosphate (ATP) and phosphocreatine (P-creatine). Conversion of pyruvate to lactate, in the absence of oxygen and of the function of the mitochondrial electron transport system, results in raised levels of lactate which at first have a helpful effect by lowering pH and causing local vasodilatation and an increase in supplies of substrate. Any associated hypercapnia may also contribute to this vasodilatation. At higher levels of lactate more serious tissue acidosis occurs and leads to inhibition of glycolysis at the phosphofructokinase step, local oedema and loss of vascular autoregulation. Brain dysfunction may develop *before* a fall in energy reserves has occurred in severe hypoxia, so that coma in this situation may represent a protective mechanism by leading to a marked reduction

in energy expenditure (Duffy et al 1972).

Ischaemia has very similar biochemical effects on the CNS to those of hypoxaemia. Glycolysis is increased but uptake of glucose cannot be augmented since the blood supply is impaired. The concentrations of glucose, ATP and P-creatine in the brain fall. The increased lactate resulting from accelerated glycolysis cannot be removed from the tissue and an added complication is seen with ischaemic but not with hypoxaemia injury, the 'no reflow' phenomenon (Ames et al 1968). This refers to small vessel lesions which prevent the reflow of blood into the ischaemic zones when perfusion pressure is restored. Severe but brief ischaemic episodes may thus have irreversible results. The importance of cerebral oedema in further compromising cerebral blood flow is suggested by work with asphyxiated perinatal monkeys.

Clinical features

Perinatal asphyxia is the commonest association of hypoxaemia. In the large Edinburgh series of Brown et al (1974) the asphyxia was antepartum in 50%, intrapartum in 40% and postpartum in 10% of cases. Recurrent apnoeic attacks and severe respiratory disease were relatively rare causes. Perinatal asphyxia and recurrent apnoeic spells also lead to ischaemia by causing severe bradycardia or cardiac arrest. Cardiac failure and sepsis resulting in vascular collapse are other causes of ischaemia.

Volpe (1976) has described the neurological syndrome of neonatal hypoxic-ischaemic encephalopathy. In the first 12 hours signs of bilateral cerebral hemisphere dysfunction predominate, with deep stupor or coma, periodic breathing, intact pupillary and oculomotor reflexes, hypotonia with little movement and seizures in about half the affected infants. There may be irritability and a high-pitched cry. By 12 to 24 hours the baby's conscious level improves but seizures become more frequent and severe apnoeic spells are common, and jitteriness may be marked. Focal muscle weakness may be seen in infants with ischaemic damage, most marked in the hip and shoulder muscles in term babies and in the legs in prematures. In the third stage between 24 and 72 hours of age further deterioration may occur with a return to deep stupor or coma and respiratory arrest. Brainstem disturbances with pupillary abnormalities and disorders of eye movement may be seen. Fixed, dilated pupils and absence of eye movements with the doll's head manoeuvre or cold caloric stimulation suggest irreversible brainstem damage and a very poor prognosis for survival. Signs of raised intracranial pressure may be present with a bulging anterior fontanelle and separated cranial sutures. Death in hypoxic-ischaemic encephalopathy is commonest at this stage. The survivors usually show improvement over a variable period which may span many months. A rapid improvement suggests a better prognosis than a slow one.

Treatment

Volpe has stressed the importance of preventing hypoxic-ischaemic encephalopathy by careful monitoring of the fetus and intervention when signs of fetal distress appear. Vigorous supportive care to correct acidosis is essential, particularly via adequate ventilation to reduce carbon dioxide levels and prevent the recurrence of hypoxaemia. Cautious administration of sodium bicarbonate may also help to correct metabolic acidosis. Circulatory failure may also result from associated hypoxic injury to the myocardium and this too should be watched for and treated energetically. Seizures can aggravate the infant's condition by increasing cerebral oxygen consumption and intracranial pressure and must be treated vigorously. Phenobarbitone is now favoured as an anticonvulsant in this situation since it may lower the cerebral metabolic rate. Adequate glucose is needed and may have a protective effect against the hazards of asphyxia. Babies with intrauterine growth retardation already have limited glycogen stores. Cerebral oedema must be combated since it may compromise cerebral blood flow and favour infarction. Fluids should be restricted to minimal maintenance levels and dexamethasone may be helpful in selected cases.

Svenningsen et al (1982) have stressed the value of what they call brain-orientated intensive care treatment in severe neonatal asphyxia. They found that in severely asphyxiated term infants such treatment, which included protective phenobarbitone with assisted ventilation and other measures, reduced the 0 to 1 year mortality rate to 14% and the incidence of neurodevelopmental handicap at 18 months to 17% from a previous figure of 50% for both.

Neuropathological lesions and their clinical correlates

Four main types of lesion result from hypoxic-ischaemic encephalopathy. Neuronal necrosis and status marmoratus of the basal ganglia and thalamus are associated with hypoxaemia. Watershed infarcts and periventricular leukomalacia are seen particularly with ischaemia in full-term and premature infants respectively. The lesions may occur in combination.

Neuronal necrosis

Neurons of the cerebral and cerebellar cortex are affected with severity varying from mild loss of hippocampal and Purkinje cells to gross shrinkage of gyri. Neurons in the brain stem and thalamus may also be affected. These changes are usually bilateral but may show a unilateral predominance. The clinical correlates in the children who survive with these lesions are mental retardation, epilepsy and cerebral palsy of spastic tetraplegic and hemiplegic distribution or ataxia.

Status marmoratus

This refers to a bilaterally symmetrical marbled appearance of the basal ganglia, especially the putamen and caudate nucleus, and of the thalamus which occurs only in the perinatal period and primarily in full-term infants. Neuronal loss, gliosis and hypermyelination are seen. The neurological sequelae are gross extrapyramidal movement disorders, especially choreoathetosis and rigidity, which do not usually appear until near the end of the first year of life or later. Intellectual defect occurs in about half the patients but is usually not severe.

Watershed infarcts

These necrotic areas in the cerebral cortex and subcortical white matter are typically distributed over the superomedial aspects of the cerebral convexities, bilaterally but sometimes asymmetrically. They occur, particularly in full-term infants, as a result of a generalized decrease in cerebral blood flow. The infarcts occur in the boundary zones between the territories supplied by the major cerebral arteries, regions which are most vulnerable to a fall in systemic blood pressure. Similar lesions have been produced in monkeys rendered profoundly hypotensive by drugs while normal arterial oxygen saturation was maintained mechanically. Watershed infarcts are rare in premature babies. They probably provide the pathological basis for some cases of spastic cerebral palsy, visual, auditory, and learning problems. Neuronal necrosis may co-exist as a result of hypoxaemia associated with the hypotension.

Periventricular leukomalacia

This term refers to necrotic areas in the periventricular white matter especially in the regions just adjacent to the outer angles of the lateral ventricles. These lesions result from a generalized reduction in cerebral blood flow and occur typically in premature infants. Their incidence seems to have decreased since they were first described by Banker & Larroche (1962) in 20% of infants who died under one month of age. The lesions occur in three periventricular arterial border or end zones defined by De Reuck et al (1972) and appear to be of ischaemic origin. The premature baby with ischaemia may be spared the larger watershed infarcts seen in the full-term infant by the presence of many meningeal anastomoses between the anterior, middle and posterior cerebral arteries in fetal but not in postnatal brain. Clinically periventricular leukomalacia correlates strikingly with the spastic diplegic type of cerebral palsy which is the most important, though increasingly rare, motor deficit of prematurely born infants. The lesions involve the area of white matter through which the long descending tracts pass from the motor cortex. Fibres from the leg area of the motor strip are closest to the ventricles and hence most likely to be damaged. The arms may be affected by lesions which extend more laterally, but to a lesser degree than the legs. The past 15 years have seen a decrease both in the incidence of spastic diplegia after premature birth (Hagberg et al 1975) (see

Ch. 11) and in that of periventricular leukomalacia, which may be related to improved neonatal care over the same period.

INTRAVENTRICULAR HAEMORRHAGE

Intraventricular haemorrhage (IVH) affects primarily liveborn premature infants. The subject is discussed by Volpe (1977), Pape & Wigglesworth (1979) and Fenichel (1980), among many others. In one series of 46 liveborn infants with birth weights under 1500 g, 43% had evidence of IVH on the CT scan (Papile et al 1978). The use of CT scanning and ultrasound in the newborn have made recognition and management of the problem much easier, but it still constitutes a very serious problem for the neonatologist (Fig. 1.11).

IVH usually occurs on the second or third day after delivery, usually in association with hypoxia and often with the respiratory distress syndrome. In premature babies the bleeding occurs in the germinal matrix beneath the ependyma of the lateral

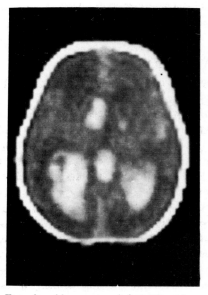

Fig. 1.11 Four-day-old premature infant (28 weeks gestation) with subarachnoid and intraventricular haemorrhage. CT. Blood is present in the ventricular system especially in the occipital horns of the lateral ventricles, and also in the subarachnoid space in the right sylvian fissure. The lateral ventricles are enlarged. There is diffuse low attenuation throughout the cerebral hemispheres which probably represents the premature brain.

ventricles. It usually overlies the caudate nucleus, the germinal matrix in this region having a very rich capillary network. It has been suggested that bleeding is provoked by venous congestion secondary to systemic circulatory failure, but an arterial mechanism may be more plausible. A sudden rise in arterial and arteriolar blood pressure may cause leaking from the capillary bed which cannot be limited in the normal way since autoregulation of cerebral blood flow is impaired by hypoxia (Lou et al 1979).

The severity of IVH can be classified by CT and autopsy findings into four grades of increasing severity, grade I with an isolated subependymal haemorrhage, grade II an intraventricular haemorrhage without ventricular dilatation, grade III similar haemorrhage but with ventricular dilatation, and grade IV with both ventricular dilatation and haemorrhage into the cerebral parenchyma. The prognosis for survival correlates well with this grading system. However, recent ultrasound studies have indicated that IVH, especially in babies weighing less than 1500 g, is much commoner than may be suspected clinically. (Thorburn et al 1981). The long-term outcome for infants with asymptomatic IVH is not yet known.

Clinical features

In a few infants showing CT evidence of IVH there may be no clinical signs of bleeding. In most cases neurological deterioration is obvious and two clinical syndromes are recognized: catastrophic and 'saltatory' (Volpe 1977). Catastrophic deterioration evolves rapidly over a short space of time with the conscious level decreasing, severe hypotonia and respiratory insufficiency. Convulsions are common. Increased intracranial pressure leads to a bulging fontanelle and to signs of progressive brainstem compression, with loss of pupil and oculomotor reflexes, decerebrate postures and respiratory arrest. A substantial fall in haematocrit level may be found if a large volume of blood has been lost. This severe syndrome is usually associated with a grade III or IV haemorrhage and carries a poor prognosis. 'Saltatory' deterioration shows a more prolonged evolution over some hours or days during which periods of stabilization or improvement may be seen. The earliest features may be

subtle with no change in the vital signs and with clear CSF so that the diagnosis can only be made by CT. This stage, beyond which the condition may not progress, correlates with grade I haemorrhage (subependymal only). Clinical deterioration occurs when blood enters the ventricles, and further worsening follows when the ventricles become dilated and bleeding occurs into the cerebral substance, with decreasing consciousness, hypotonia and convulsions.

IVH in premature babies of 1500 g or less carries a high mortality rate and morbidity. The survivors have a high incidence of neurological dysfunction. There is also a high risk of developing communicating hydrocephalus. The growth of the head circumference should be followed and plotted carefully. If hydrocephalus is suspected CT should be performed and repeated at one and six months of age.

Treatment

The management of severe IVH is difficult and involves active support of respiration and blood pressure, reduction of cerebral oedema and control of convulsions. Dexamethasone may be valuable. In those who survive the acute illness the prevention of hydrocephalus or the staving off of the time when a shunting procedure must be done are important. Shunt procedures in very young infants, whose CSF may still contain blood and increased amounts of protein, carry a high rate of complications. Isosorbide has been used with some success in this situation (Lorber 1972); with this the serum electrolytes should be measured daily to avoid hypernatraemia.

PRIMARY SUBARACHNOID HAEMORRHAGE (PSH)

This refers to haemorrhage originating within the subarachnoid space, by contrast with bleeding into the subarachnoid space secondary to intracranial haemorrhage elsewhere. It occurs typically on the second day after delivery and affects premature more often than term babies. PSH is associated with hypoxia, and probably results from rupture of congested thin-walled veins in the subarachnoid space or from tearing of these by shearing forces during a difficult delivery. The condition is not usually diagnosed clinically but is detected when a diagnostic lumbar puncture is performed in the investigation of convulsions or suspected sepsis. If PSH is massive, however, catastrophic deterioration of the kind seen in severe IVH may occur.

REFERENCES

Abramovich S J, Gregory S, Slemick M, Stewart A 1979 Hearing loss in very low birthweight infants treated with neonatal intensive care. Archives of Disease in Childhood 54: 421–426

Ames A, Wright R L, Kowada M 1968 Cerebral ischemia. The no-reflow phenomenon. American Journal of Pathology 52: 437–453

Amiel-Tison C 1968 Neurological evaluation of the maturity of newborn infants. Archives of Disease in Childhood 43: 89–93

André-Thomas, Lepage F, Sorrel-Déjèrine 1944 Examen anatomo-clinique de deux anencéphales protubérantiels. Revue neurologique 76: 173–193

André-Thomas, Saint Anne-Dargassies S 1952 Etudes neurologiques sur le nouveau-né et le jeune nourrisson. Masson, Paris

André-Thomas, Chesni Y, Saint Anne-Dargassies S 1960 In: The neurological examination of the infant, MacKeith R, Polani P E, Clayton-Jones E (eds) Little Club Clinics in Developmental Medicine 1, National Spastics Society

Ashby W, Butler E 1948 Carbonic anhydrase in the central nervous system of the developing fetus. Journal of Biological Chemistry 175: 425–432

Babinski I 1896 Relâchement des muscles dans l 'hémiplégie organique. Compte rendu de la Société de Biologie 9 Mai:i: 47

Banker B Q, Larroche J C 1962 Periventricular leukomalacia of infancy. Archives of Neurology 7: 386–410

Beintema D J 1968 A neurological study of newborn infants. Clinics in Developmental Medicine No. 28, Spastics International Medical Publications and William Heinemann Medical Books Ltd.

Bersot H 1920 Développement réactionnel et réflexe plantaire du bébé né avant terme à celui de deux ans. Schweizer Archiv für Neurologie und Psychiatrie 7: 212–231 and 8: 47–48

Brett E M 1966 The estimation of foetal maturity by the neurological examination of the neonate. Gestational Age, Size and Maturity, Clinics in Developmental Medicine: 19, National Spastics Society: 105–115

Brown J K, Purvis R J, Forfar J O, Cockburn F 1974 Neurological aspects of perinatal asphyxia. Developmental Medicine and Child Neurology 16: 567–580

Davison A N, Dobbing J 1966 Myelination as a vulnerable period in brain development. British Medical Bulletin 21: 40–44

Delange F, Illig R, Rochiccioli P, Brock-Jacobsen B 1981 Progress Report 1980 on neonatal thyroid screening in Europe. Acta paediatrica scandinavica 70: 1–2

De Reuck J, Chattha H A, Richardson E P 1972 Pathogenesis and evolution of periventricular leukomalacia. Archives of Neurology 27: 229–236

Despland P A, Galambos R 1980 Use of the auditory brainstem responses by premature and newborn infants. Neuropädiatrie 11: 99–107

Diebler M F, Farkas-Bargeton E, Wehrlé R 1979 Developmental changes of enzymes associated with energy metobalism and the synthesis of some neurotransmitters in discrete areas of human neocortex. Journal of Neurochemistry 32: 429–435

Donovan D E, Coues P E, Paine R S 1962 The prognostic implications of neurologic abnormalities in the neonatal period. Neurology (Minneapolis) 12: 910–914

Dreyfus-Brisac C, Flescher J, Plassart E 1962 L'électro-encéphalogramme: critère à terme et prématuré. Biologia neonatorum (Basel) 4: 154–172

Dreyfus-Brisac C 1964 The EEG of the premature infant and full-term newborn. In: Kellaway P, Petersen I (eds) Neurological and EEG correlative studies in infancy, Grune and Stratton, New York

Dubowitz L M S, Dubowitz V 1970 Clinical assessment of gestational age in the newborn. Journal of Pediatrics 77: 1–10

Dubowitz L M S, Dubowitz V, Morante A, Verghote M 1980 Visual function in the preterm and fullterm newborn infant. Developmental Medicine and Child Neurology 22: 465–475

Dubowitz L, Dubowitz V 1981 The neurological assessment of the preterm and full-term newborn infant. Clinics in Developmental Medicine 79: Spastics International Medical Publications, William Heinemann Medical Books, London, J B Lipincott, Philadelphia

Duffy J E, Nelson S R, Lowry O H 1972 Cerebral carbohydrate metabolism during acute hypoxia and recovery. Journal of Neurochemistry 19: 959–977

Ellingson R J 1964 Studies of the electrical activity of the developing human brain. Progress in Brain Research 9: 26–53

Engel R, Butler B V 1963 Appraisal of conceptual age of newborn infants by electroencephalographic methods. Journal of Pediatrics 63: 386–393

Erbkam 1837 Lebhafte Bewegung eines Viermonatlichen Fötus. Neue Zeitschrift für Geburtskunds 5: 324–326

Fantz R L 1963 Pattern vision in newborn infants. Science 140: 296–297

Fenichel G M 1980 Neonatal neurology. Churchill Livingstone, Edinburgh

Gamper E 1926 Bau und Leistungen eines Menschlichen Mittelhirnwesens (Arhinencephalie mit Encephalocele) zugleich ein Beitrag zur Teratologie und Fasersystematik. Zeitschrift für die Gesamte Neurologie und Psychiatrie 102: 154–235 and 104: 49–120

Geber M, Dean R F A 1964 Le développement psychomoteur et somatique des jeunes Africains en Ouganda. Courrier 14: 425–437

Gesell A, Amatruda C S 1945 The embryology of behavior — the beginnings of the human mind. Hamish Hamilton, London

Goldie L, Hopkins I J 1964 Head turning towards diffuse light in the neurological examination of the newborn infant. Brain 87: 665–672

Goren C C, Sarty M, Wu P Y K 1975 Visual following and

pattern discrimination in newborn infants. Pediatrics 56: 544–549

Gruenwald P 1963 Chronic fetal distress and placental insufficiency. Biologia neonatorum (Basel) 5: 215–265

Gunn T 1973 Positives. Verses by Thom Gunn, Photographs by Ander Gunn. Faber and Faber, London

Hagberg B, Hagberg O, Olow I 1975 The changing panorama of cerebral palsy in Sweden 1954–1970. Acta paediatrica scandinavica 64: 187–192

Himwich W A, Benaron H B W, Tucker B E 1956 Metabolism of premature and full-term infant brain. Federation Proceedings, Baltimore 15: 93

Hogan G R, Milligan J E 1971 The plantar reflex of the newborn. New England Journal of Medicine 285: 502–503

Hooker D 1952 The prenatal origin of behavior. University of Kansas Press, Lawrence, Kansas

Humphrey T 1964 Some correlations between the appearance of human fetal reflexes and the development of the nervous system. Progress in Brain Research, Growth and Maturation of the Brain 4: 93–135

Krabbe K 1912 Les réflexes chez le foetus. Revue neurologique 24: 434–435

Langworthy O 1933 Development of behaviour patterns and myelination of the nervous system in the human fetus and infant. Contributions to Embryology, Carnegie Institution XXIV No. 193: 1–57

Larroche J C 1962 Quelques aspects anatomiques du développement cérébral. Biologia neonatorum (Basel) 4: 126–153

Lorber J 1972 The use of isosorbide in the treatment of hydrocephalus. Developmental Medicine and Child Neurology 14: Suppl. 27: 87–93

Lou H C, Lassen N A, Friis-Hansen B 1979 Impaired autoregulation of cerebral blood flow in the distressed newborn infant. Journal of Pediatrics 94: 118–124

MacKeith R C 1965 The placing response and primary walking. Guy's Hospital Gazette 79: 394–399

Minkowski M 1921 Sur les mouvements, les réflexes et les réactions musculaires du foetus humain de 2 a 5 mois et leurs relations avec le système nerveux foetal. Revue neurologique 2: 1105–1118 and 1235–1250

Minkowski M 1938 L'élaboration du système nerveux. In: Wallon H (ed) Encyclopédie Français. Librairie Larrousse, Paris

Miranda S B, Hack M, Fantz R L, Fanaroff A A, Klaus M H 1977 Neonatal pattern vision: a predictor of future mental performance? Journal of Pediatrics 91: 642–647

Pape K E, Wigglesworth J S 1979 Haemorrhage, ischaemia and the perinatal brain. Clinics in Developmental Medicine 69/70. Spastics International Medical Publications, William Heinemann Medical Books, London, J B Lippincott, Philadelphia

Papile L A, Burstein J, Burstein R, Koffler H 1978 Incidence and evolution of subependymal and intraventricular haemorrhage: a study of infants with birth weights less than 1500 gm. Journal of Pediatrics 92: 529–534

Paine R S 1960 Neurologic examination of infants and children. Pediatric Clinics of North America 7: 471–510

Paine R S, Brazelton T B, Donovan D E, Drorbaugh J E, Hubbell J P Sears E M 1964 Evolution of postural reflexes in normal infants and in the presence of chronic brain syndromes. Neurology (Minneapolis) 14: 1036–1048

Parr C, Routh D K, Byrd M T, McMillan J 1974 A developmental study of the asymmetrical tonic neck reflex. Developmental Medicine and Child Neurology 16: 329–335

Peiper A 1963 Cerebral function in infancy and childhood. Translation of 3rd revised German edition by B Nagler and H Nagler. Pitman Medical Publishing, London (Consultants Bureau Enterprises Inc, New York)

Polani P 1959 Neurological examination of the newborn according to the work of Professor André-Thomas. Cerebral Palsy Bulletin 5: 19–22

Robinson R J 1966 The assessment of gestational age by neurological examination. Archives of Disease in Childhood 41: 437–447

Saint Anne-Dargassies S 1974 Le développement neurologique du nouveau-né à terme et prématuré. Masson et Cie, Paris

Strassman P 1903 Das Leben vor der Geburt. Sammlung Klinischer Vorträge No. 353 (Gynäkologie No. 132): 947–968

Svenningsen N W, Blennow G, Lindroth M, Gäddlin P O, Ahlström H 1982 Brain-oriented intensive care treatment in severe neonatal asphyxia. Archives of Disease in Childhood 57: 176–183

Thornburn R, Lipscomb A P, Stewart A, Reynolds E O R, Pope P L, Pape K 1981 Prediction of death and major handicap in very preterm infants by brain ultrasound. Lancet 1: 1119–1121

Tucker S M 1982 Screening for hearing in the newborn using the auditory response cradle. In: Wharton B (ed) Topics in Perinatal Medicine 2. Pitman Books, Tunbridge Wells, p 126–135

Volpe J J 1975 Neurological disorders. In: Avery G B (ed) Neonatology. Pathophysiology and Management of the newborn. J B Lippincott, Philadelphia

Volpe J J 1976 Perinatal hypoxic-ischemic brain injury. Pediatric Clinics of North America 23: 383–397

Volpe J J 1977 Neonatal intracranial haemorrhage. Pathophysiology, neuropathology and clinical features. Clinics in Perinatology 4: 77–102

Volpe J J 1979 Cerebral blood flow in the newborn infant: relation to hypoxic-ischemic brain injury and periventricular hemorrhage. (Editorial) Journal of Pediatrics 94: 170–173

Volpe J J 1981 Neurology of the newborn. Volume XXII in the series Major problems in clinical pediatrics. W B Saunders, Philadelphia

Windle W F, Fitzgerald J C 1937 Development of the spinal reflex mechanism in human embryos. Journal of Comparative Neurology 67: 493–506

Winick M 1976 Malnutrition and brain development. Oxford University Press, London

2

Normal development and neurological examination beyond the newborn period

E. M. Brett

The body blunders forward
into the next second, in
its awkward bold half-aware
fashion, and getting there too
— doing things for the first time.

Precarious exploration
from coast to interior:
by which a workable route is
opened, for the later transport
of lathes, heavy crosses and
crates through the undergrowth.

Meanwhile, before the next push,
a triumph, a triumph.

Thom Gunn, *Positives* (1973)

INTRODUCTION

The distinction which has grown up between 'disease paediatrics' and 'developmental paediatrics' is a somewhat artificial one, but it has the merit of emphasising the importance of developmental considerations in all that relates to child health and disease. Few physicians today would regard children as miniature adults, as was common until relatively recently. No one working with children in any capacity can fail to be impressed by the great differences between those of different ages, the breadth of the spectrum ranging from the scarcely viable fetus struggling for survival in an incubator to the husky or nubile adolescent struggling for self-expression, extremes increasingly catered for by the subspecialities of neonatology and adolescent medicine. The differences between the paediatric age-groups are far greater than those which the physician of adults will encounter between his youngest and oldest patients.

The concept of development is central to most paediatric problems, but is particularly important in neurological conditions, since abnormal brain function and structure are commonly reflected in abnormal development. No paediatrician or paediatric neurologist can look at a child without asking himself whether his development is normal or not and, if not, whether it has been abnormal from the beginning, or has become abnormal after a period of normality. On the answers to these questions depend the important decisions whether one is dealing with a *static* problem (such as mental retardation and/or cerebral palsy), with a *progressive* condition (whether cerebral — degenerative or neoplastic — or neuromuscular), or with an acute process causing rapid deterioration followed by resumption of development.

The developmental assessment is based on the twin foundations of the history given by the child's mother or other informant, (its Pinteresque associations make me prefer to avoid the term 'caretaker', popular though it has become in recent years) and the findings on examination. Thus a knowledge of normal child development from the newborn period onwards is essential. In general the younger the child, the more important are the developmental aspects of the assessment and the less important the more conventional features of the neurological examination. In the newborn period in particular, as already described, the formal tools of neurology contribute relatively little, and a pair of warm and steady hands is far more useful than a patellar hammer.

There are many excellent reviews of normal child development (Egan et al 1969, Sheridan 1973, Illingworth 1973, 1980, Drillien 1977). In this field 'every picture tells a story' and the more profusely illustrated accounts such as those of Illingworth are particularly useful. The necessary observations can usually be made in a fairly short space of time, though they should not be hurried and a child may sometimes need to be seen on a second occasion to confirm a point. The state of the child at the time of examination must be taken into account, since factors such as fatigue, hunger, thirst, fear of strangers and maternal anxiety may profoundly affect his performance.

The development of children is normally a continuous, if not always steady, process and the principles described in the account of the newborn apply in the assessment and examination of older children. Beyond the newborn period, however, the mother's account of her infant's abilities becomes more important. It must be borne out by observation. Pitfalls abound both in the taking of the developmental history and in the observations made by the doctor. Some of these are mentioned below.

SOME PITFALLS FOR THE UNWARY

1. Communication between mother and doctor

If a mother does not understand exactly what the doctor means by his question, her answer will be misleading. It is wise to ask, for example, not 'How old was he when he crawled?', but 'Does he crawl?', and if the answer is clearly 'Yes', to establish the age at which it began. Unquestioning acceptance of maternal reports of speech skills can be particularly misleading. The double syllable babble of the 8-month infant (mum-mum, baba, dada) is often mistaken by fond parents for real words. The older child's utterance of 'ereyare' may be quoted as evidence of sentence production ('here you are').

Understanding of language may be overestimated by failure to notice that a mother is giving her child non-linguistic clues, such as gestures, eye-pointing etc. (akin to the dog who reacts, not to the word 'Walks', but to the familiar routine of producing his collar and lead).

2. Mothers are usually (but not always) right

Mothers are usually (but not always) right when they suspect that their child is abnormal in some way. Their suspicions should be treated with respect; to ignore them is to court disaster. Harrison in his *Familiar Letters on the Diseases of Children: Addressed to a Young Practitioner* (1862) wrote, 'It is a good rule always to be very attentive to what mothers say; for, however foolish they are in their way of treatment, you may rely on it that they are good observers where their own children are concerned. They are full of prejudices, conceits and absurdities, but still they are no bad observers; and let me tell you never to neglect to notice what they say. If you *do*, you will assuredly some day repent not having given more notice to their tales.' We may be more sophisticated and less patronizing today about the attitudes of mothers, but the warning is as much needed today as it was when published. Paediatricians regularly see children with mental retardation, cerebral palsy, visual and hearing defects and with progressive cerebral and neuromuscular diseases whose mothers have previously been 'reassured'.

It should be mentioned, however, that on occasion an alert mother may be unaware of a handicap in her child. For example, an intelligent deaf baby's use of his peripheral vision may deceive his mother and unwary doctors. The more experienced a mother, the more astute and reliable she generally is in her observations.

3. Normal variation in development

The ages of acquiring various skills can vary widely in normal children. Families are seen in which all or many children walk or speak late, but do so entirely normally in time. However, one must avoid the mistake of assuming that delay in a particular milestone is familial and benign, without excluding a causal abnormality (e.g. deafness in delayed speech).

Bottom-shuffling, hitching, scooting and sliding are names given to a normal variant which replaces crawling in the locomotor development of many children. This is often a familial trait present in siblings, parents and cousins. It is associated with delay in unsupported sitting and walking. Robson, (1970) in a study of 30 shuffling children, found that as infants they showed mild to moderate hypotonia with delayed motor development and a

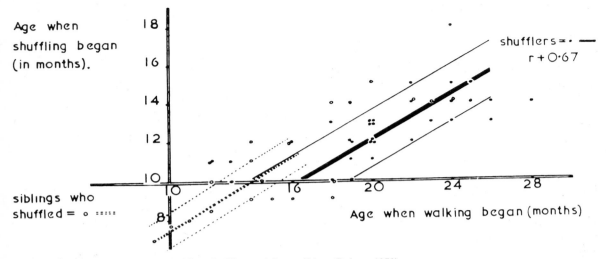

Fig. 2.1 Relationship between ages of first shuffling and first walking. (Robson 1970)

posture of hip flexion with knee extension in vertical suspension ('sitting on air') so that it was difficult to demonstrate weight bearing capacity in the legs. This posture disappeared with the start of voluntary weight bearing. Robson showed that it is possible to relate the ages of first shuffling and first walking. This relationship is shown in Figure 2.1 from which it is possible to predict the approximate age of walking from the age of first shuffling.

Another normal locomotor variation is that in which the child suddenly progresses from sitting to walking, missing out the usual intermediate stages of crawling or shuffling.

4. Adverse testing conditions

A. Environment

Peaceful surroundings are needed for reliable assessment. Some outpatient clinics resemble a Persian market and are quite unsuited for any paediatric purpose, let alone the delicate interplay between three people which is needed for developmental and neurological assessment of the young child.

B. The child

A hungry, angry, tired or frightened child presents a challenge to the doctor, who must be concerned about the validity of observations made in such adverse conditions and how much allowance to make for them. Failure to perform a particular task may be explained by a mother as due to 'naughtiness', but if the child's reaction to a simpler task is similar, the explanation may be 'can't' rather than 'won't'.

C. The mother

Some mothers find it difficult or impossible not to intervene and assist their child when he seems unable to perform a task. Others are so anxious that their tension is communicated to the child and even to the doctor. Great patience is needed.

D. The doctor

Not all doctors possess great patience. Their own contribution to the complex situation may at times be harmful, especially when working under pressure with insufficient time, a recipe for disaster often brought about by a combination of tight schedules and problems of transport — even with the most careful planning.

5. Social, cultural and ethnic factors

Parents differ widely, and so do their children. Patterns of life-style, rearing and expectations vary greatly in our society. The child of an immigrant manual worker often has less opportunities for self-expression and play activities than that of a middle-class professional native of Britain. Exposure to nursery school can enrich a child's experience and advance his performance, while eight hours a day spent lying in a cot or bed at a 'baby minder's' provide a poor basis on which to build. These factors are discussed more fully in Chapters 13 and 14.

NORMAL DEVELOPMENT

In the abbreviated account of normal development which follows I have drawn heavily on the work of Illingworth (1973, 1980) based in turn on that of Gesell. (The norms refer to those born at term, since children born prematurely may be developmentally less advanced than those of the same postnatal age who were born at term.)

Illingworth stresses several points which, though well known, may be overlooked and merit repeated emphasis. Development is continuous from conception to maturity and its sequence is the same in all children though its rate varies from one child to another. There is normally a fairly close parallelism between development in the different fields. 'Dissociation' or lack of parallelism may suggest specific deficits such as cerebral palsy or deafness. Maturation of the nervous system determines development, so that no child can be made to walk or to speak until he and his nervous system are ready for it. The evolution of movement in development is from generalized mass activity to specific individual responses, as in early fetal development. Development proceeds in a cephalocaudal direction, so that head control and considerable use of the hands precede walking. Certain primitive automatic responses, such as the grasp reflex and automatic walking, must be lost before the equivalent voluntary movement can be acquired.

Development of locomotion

This may be considered under the headings of ventral suspension, prone position, sitting and upright posture.

a. Ventral suspension (Figs 2.2 to 2.4)

The full-term newborn baby, when held face downwards with the examiner's hands under his abdomen and chest usually lacks head control. By

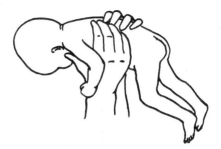

Fig. 2.2 Ventral suspension — normal 6-week-old baby

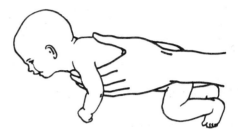

Fig. 2.3 Ventral suspension — normal 8-week-old baby

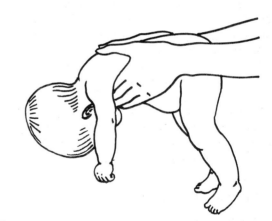

Fig. 2.4 Ventral suspension — abnormal 6-week-old baby developing cerebral palsy

6 weeks of age he can momentarily hold his head in the same plane as the rest of his body (Fig. 2.2) and by 8 weeks can maintain this position and can hold the head up well beyond the plane of the body (Fig. 2.3). The abnormal posture of a 6 week old baby with developing cerebral palsy is shown in Fig. 2.4, with head and extended limbs dangling downwards and without extension of the hips.

b. Prone position (Figs 2.5 to 2.9)

The behaviour of the normal term newborn in

prone has been described, with head turned to one side, pelvis high and knees drawn up under the abdomen, (Fig. 2.5) often with automatic crawling. With increasing maturity the pelvis becomes lower and the hips and knees extend so that the knees are not so far beneath the belly at 3 or 4 weeks of age (Fig. 2.6). At 4 weeks the chin can be held momentarily off the couch. A little later at 4 to 6 weeks the pelvis is still rather high and the hips extend intermittently (Fig. 2.7). By 12 weeks the chin and shoulders are held up off the couch with the plane of the face at right angles to it (Fig. 2.8) and weight born on the forearms, while the legs are fully extended. Later at 24 weeks the baby holds the chest and upper abdomen off the couch, supporting his weight on his hands with elbows extended (Fig. 2.9) He rolls from prone to supine and about a month later in the reverse direction. By 28 weeks he can bear weight on one hand,

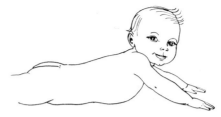
Fig. 2.9 Prone position — normal 24-week-old baby

and by 9 months can usually crawl, though often backwards initially. Creeping on hands and knees follows at about 44 weeks and a bear-like walking on hands and feet at about one year.

c. Sitting (Figs 2.10 to 2.14)

The traction response as the newborn baby is pulled forward by his hands into a sitting position has been described. There is a degree of head lag initially, after which the head is often brought forward as it nears the vertical. Once the sitting position is reached the baby's back is rounded, forming a continuous curve from neck to sacrum (Fig. 2.10). By 4–6 weeks (Fig. 2.11) the back is less rounded and by 16 weeks (Fig. 2.12) still less so. Meanwhile head control has improved greatly. By 26 or 28 weeks the child sits with his hands forward for support (Fig. 2.13) and by 11 months is sitting so steadily that he can pivot round to pick up a toy without losing his balance (Fig. 2.14).

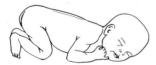
Fig. 2.5 Prone position — normal newborn

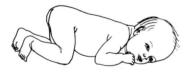
Fig. 2.6 Prone position — normal 3–4 week old baby

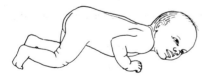
Fig. 2.7 Prone position — normal 4–6 week old baby

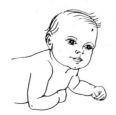
Fig. 2.8 Prone position — normal 12-week-old baby

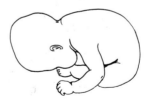
Fig. 2.10 Sitting — first 4 weeks of life — rounded back

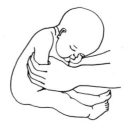
Fig. 2.11 Sitting — 4–6 weeks

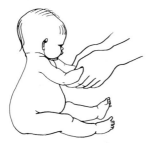

Fig. 2.12 Sitting — 16 weeks

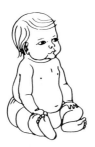

Fig. 2.13 Sitting — 26 weeks

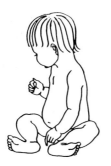

Fig. 2.14 Sitting — 11 months, pivoting and turning round

d. Standing and walking (Figs 2.15 to 2.19)

The automatic walking shown by the normal new-born decreases and has usually disappeared by a few weeks of age. In the early weeks when held up the baby sags at the hips and knees, but by 12 weeks takes a good deal of weight on his legs (Fig. 2.15) by 24 weeks most of his weight, (Fig. 2.16) and by 28 weeks his full weight

(Fig. 2.17) At 36 weeks he can stand holding on to the furniture and can pull himself to stand but not lower himself to the floor again. At 44 weeks he can raise one foot off the ground, at 48 weeks walk holding on to the furniture and at 52 weeks walk with one hand held (Fig. 2.18). At 13 months he walks without support with a broad-based gait and uneven steps, tending to hold his shoulders abducted and elbows flexed (Fig. 2.19). Walking

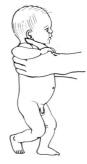

Fig. 2.15 Standing — about 12 weeks, bearing much weight

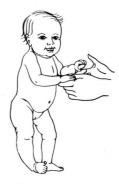

Fig. 2.16 Standing — 24 weeks, bearing most of the weight

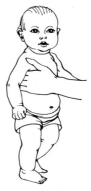

Fig. 2.17 Standing — 28 weeks, bearing full weight

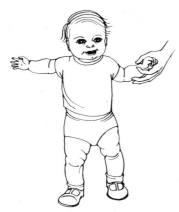

Fig. 2.18 52 weeks, walking with one hand held

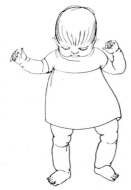

Fig. 2.19 13 months, walking without support, arms abducted, elbows flexed, broad base, steps varying in length and direction

becomes steadier and more mature and he learns to manage stairs, at first creeping, later at 2 years with two feet on each step, and later still, at 3, going upstairs with one foot on each step and downstairs with two. Coming downstairs with one foot on each step is achieved at 4. Running is usually achieved at 2, jumping with both feet at 2½ and jumping off the bottom step of the stairs at 3 years. The ability to skip develops between 4 and 5 years, first on one foot and later on both.

MANIPULATION AND ITS DEVELOPMENT

The primitive grasp reflex prevails for the first 8 to 12 weeks of life. At 4 weeks the hands are mainly closed but at 8 weeks are often open. The grasp reflex has usually disappeared by 12 weeks (it may persist in some abnormal babies and return after disappearing in some children with acquired brain disease). At 12 weeks the normal baby looks at an object as if wanting to grasp it, and will hold a toy placed in his hand. At 16 weeks his hands come together in the midline as he plays. He will try to reach for an object but will overshoot the mark, and will play with and shake a rattle put in his hand. At 20 weeks he is able to grasp an object voluntarily, convey it to his mouth and play with his toes.

The complexity of the grasp increases from a grasp on the ulnar side of the palm in the first 6 months (Fig. 2.20) to a more radial palmar grasp

A

B

C

D

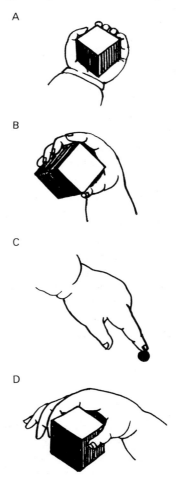

Fig. 2.20 Evolution of grasp:
A. Immature palmar grasp of cube
B. Intermediate stage grasp
C. Index approach at 40 weeks
D. Mature grasp at one year

at 24 to 32 weeks, to an intermediate grasp with the index, ring and little fingers pressing the object against the thumb, and to the final mature grasp between finger and thumb at about 40 weeks. The speed and smoothness of reaching and grasping improve progressively with age. At 6 months the baby can transfer objects from one hand to another and can usually feed himself with a biscuit. He shows much 'oral behaviour', putting everything to his mouth. At 40 weeks he shows an index approach to objects, pointing at them as he moves his hand to pick them up (Fig. 2.20). Illingworth believes that the development of manipulation is a better guide to the level of intelligence than is gross motor development, and that good finger-thumb apposition and a definite index approach at 10 months make mental deficiency very unlikely. Unusually advanced manipulative skills may presage a high eventual IQ level. At 40 weeks the child can readily release objects and soon learns to hand a toy to his mother and to enjoy putting things into a basket or other container and taking them out again. By about one year the normal child stops taking everything to his mouth but this behaviour continues in some retarded children.

Constructive play with cubes begins with building a tower of 2 one-inch cubes at 13 months, increasing to one of 10 cubes at three years of age.

At 15 months the child can usually pick up and drink from a cup and lay it down again. At 18 months he can turn over the pages of a book, 2 or 3 at a time, and can turn them singly by 2 years. At $2\frac{1}{2}$ he can thread beads and hold a pencil in his hand rather than in his fist. By 3 years he can largely dress and undress himself and manage many buttons. In drawing he can copy a circle.

EYES AND EARS

The visual responses of the neonate have been referred to in Chapter 1, with the use of pattern vision studies (Miranda et al 1977) to predict later development. There is no doubt that the newborn baby shows visual fixing and following of objects from an earlier age than was recognized until recently. The perceptual world of the child has been well described by Bower (1977) including the newborn baby's use of vision. The fascinating communication between infants and their mothers by facial expression and vocalization and the complex 'infant-elicited social behaviours' which are so important for normal social development were reviewed by Stern (1977).

At an early age the infant watches his mother's face intently as she speaks to him and as she displays a wide range of facial expressions towards him. The earliest infant smiles, in the first two weeks of life, are seen during rapid eye movement or dreaming sleep and during drowsiness, and rarely in the waking state. Between 6 weeks and 3 months the smile becomes 'exogenous', being elicited by external events, various sights and sounds of which the human face and gaze, the voice and tickling are the most potent stimuli. It is now a social response and soon evolves into an instrument of behaviour, used by the infant or 'care-giver'. Fixation, convergence and focussing improve progressively and the infant's gaze is directed more accurately at objects and at the sources of sounds.

Between 12 and 24 weeks of age the child often gazes at his hands as he lies on his back (Fig. 2.21). (This 'hand regard' can also occur in blind children.) Its persistence much beyond 24 weeks of age is cause for concern since this is often associated with mental retardation.

At 20 weeks the normal child will usually smile at his reflexion in a mirror and at 28 weeks will pat it in friendly fashion.

The localization of sound by turning of the head towards its source becomes progressively more accurate from 3 months of age.

GENERAL UNDERSTANDING

The early signs of understanding are shown by the infant's visual behaviour and vocalising. From 1 to

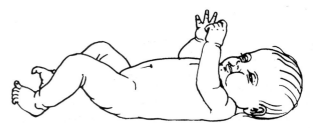

Fig. 2.21 Hand regard — 12–24 weeks

4 weeks of age he starts to watch his mother when she speaks to him, becoming quiet, opening and shutting his mouth and bobbing his head up and down. From 6 weeks he develops a social smile and at about 8 weeks starts to vocalize. At 12 weeks he is interested in watching people and things around him, and is excited when shown a toy. By 12 to 16 weeks he opens his mouth for breast or bottle, anticipating a feed. At 20 weeks he smiles at his mirror image. A little later he shows that he understands the permanence of objects by looking for a toy when it has dropped out of his sight. At 24 weeks he stretches out his arms when his mother is about to pick him up, and he smiles and vocalises at his image in a mirror. Imitation of actions such as a cough or tongue protrusion develops at about 6 months. He may use a cough as a social signal to claim attention. He enjoys playing 'peep-bo'. At 32 weeks he responds to 'No' and tries to touch objects beyond his reach.

At 40 weeks he may tug at his mother's clothes to gain her attention and imitates playing 'patacake' and waving 'bye-bye', being pleased when his performance is appreciated and sometimes giving an encore. At 44 weeks he helps in dressing, putting out his arm or foot for a coat or shoe. He soon develops an interest in picture books and shows an understanding of words which rapidly increases over the next year. He plays in a more complex and imaginative way, develops an appreciation of form and colour and can manage simple jig-saw puzzles by $2\frac{1}{2}$ years.

From one year of age much may be learned from the child's performance with 10 one-inch cubes, simple formboards and pencil and paper. He will build progressively taller towers with the cubes, from 2 at 15 months to 6 or 7 at 2 years and 9 at 3. A 'train' of 9 cubes in a row is constructed in front of him and he is asked to imitate it. This is usually possible at 2 years, while a more complex train with the tenth cube added as chimney can be imitated at $2\frac{1}{2}$. A bridge made of 3 cubes can be imitated at 3 years and copied (i.e. built after he has seen the completed model without watching its construction) at $3\frac{1}{2}$. A gate of 5 cubes can be imitated at 4 and copied at $4\frac{1}{2}$. By 6 years the child can often build a set of steps with the 10 cubes.

A simple formboard with 3 pieces (circle, triangle and square) can be used from 21 months of age.

From 2 years all 3 pieces are usually correctly placed. When the board is rotated the child usually places them correctly again after 4 errors.

The child's performance in drawing a person (the Goodenough Draw-a-man test) gives helpful information about his intellectual level. Children usually enjoy drawing their parents or teachers. Some will draw the whole family and the way the various members are depicted sometimes illuminates relationships within the family. The manner in which the child handles the pencil, and indeed all test materials, gives opportunities to observe any neurological deficit such as ataxia, involuntary movements or a spastic approach to an object with splaying out of the fingers.

The copying of simple shapes with a pencil is also useful. The normal child can usually copy a circle at 3 years, a cross at 4, a square at $4\frac{1}{2}$, a triangle at 5 and a diamond at 6. More complex shapes are achieved at later ages. The proviso must be made, with regard to all activities using pencil and paper, that the child's previous exposure to these articles is important: there are families in which a child may never see a pencil, paper, book or toy, and others in which he is exposed to educational and artistic material from the cradle.

DEVELOPMENT OF FEEDING

The milestones of feeding begin with the newborn sucking on the teat of breast or bottle with increasing efficiency. The very premature baby and the sick infant may be unable to do this adequately and may need tube-feeding for a time. At 24 weeks the child can drink from a cup held to his lips, and soon afterwards chew and eat a biscuit. At 15 months he can manage a cup, picking it up, drinking from it and putting it down without spilling, and can usually feed himself unaided with a spoon. He can often manage a knife and fork by $2\frac{1}{2}$ to 3 years.

DRESSING

In the average child dressing skills start with the ability to take off his shoes at 15 months and his socks a little later. He can put on and take off these items and his pants at 2 years and manage most of his buttons by 3 years. Shoelaces can be tied from 5 years, though some normal children will take longer to master this.

SPEECH

Vocalising begins at about 7 weeks or earlier mainly with vowel sounds, and at 12–16 weeks the baby 'converses' with his mother, uttering a few consonants towards the end of this period. He will laugh, gurgle and coo. At 20 weeks he says 'Ah, goo'. At 28 weeks he makes sounds like 'ba', 'da', and 'ka' and at 32 weeks combines syllables like 'dada'. More consonants are added. Words with meaning are not usually spoken until 44 to 48 weeks of age. Comprehension precedes this, the child understanding 'no', and obeying simple commands at 40 weeks. At 1 year 2 or 3 words are spoken with meaning. Jargon speech is common between 15 and 18 months with great expressiveness and vivacity but usually incomprehensible to all except sometimes to slightly older siblings. Two and three word phrases and the pronouns 'I', 'me' and 'you' are spoken by 21 to 24 months. Infantile pronunciations abound with substitution of letters and lisping. Speech becomes more copious with sentences by the age of 3 and matures progressively over the ensuing years.

SPHINCTER CONTROL

Micturition in the newborn baby occurs reflexly, the bladder and bowels often being emptied immediately after a feed. From about a month of age the infant can be conditioned to empty his bladder when placed on a pottie, but voluntary control does not develop until 15 or 18 months of age when the child first tells his mother when he has wet his pants. Next he tells her just before he wets himself, too late to save the situation, and soon afterwards is able to tell her in time when he 'wants to go'. At first there is great urgency of micturition so that he must be given the opportunity as soon as he feels the need since otherwise he will wet himself. With maturity the urgency decreases. By two to two and a half years he can largely manage his own affairs

when he goes to the toilet, pulling his pants down and getting up on to the lavatory seat unaided, though he needs help in wiping himself. Often, when engrossed in play, he will forget to go to the toilet and this can cause accidents and distress. Usually he learns to remember these bodily needs and to minister to them. By 2 years of age 50% of children are dry by night if lifted out in the evening, and by 5 years about 90%.

NEUROLOGICAL EXAMINATION OF THE OLDER CHILD

My son, be gentle in carrying out your business, and you will be better loved than a lavish giver.
Ecclesiasticus 3:17

A similar, but milder, modification of the conventional neurological examination to that applied to the newborn is needed in examining the older infant and child. Certainly a formal approach to the neurological examination is inappropriate and with most young children counter-productive. Rapport must first be established with the child, and his mother, if he is to co-operate in the many tasks expected of him. The initial history and observations will often give a fair idea of the child's developmental level and this impression will partly determine the approach. Unrealistic demands should not be made of a child who is clearly developmentally retarded, distressed or in pain. Many normal young children, however, co-operate in a more mature way than their age would suggest. Patience and flexibility are needed by the examiner. His aim should be to keep the exercise as pleasant and enjoyable as possible for the child and his parent. Ingenious use of toys, adaptation of instruments and a flow of reassuring patter will usually achieve good results. The role of the strong, silent man (or woman) does not suit most paediatricians.

Observation of spontaneous and elicited manipulation and gait gives much helpful information about the integrity of the child's nervous system. This is true even of the child who is unco-operative either because he is in a bad mood or is emotionally immature in keeping with a degree of mental retardation. Thus, to quote an extreme case, the speed and accuracy with which a retarded child snatches the doctor's spectacles from his nose can make it clear that there is no motor defect such as weakness, inco-ordination or involuntary movements, even though a more formal demonstration of this is impossible. The strength with which a fractious child fights off the doctor's attempts to handle his limbs in order to assess tone and elicit tendon reflexes may indicate that power, at least, is normal, or it may suggest that there is a degree of weakness, either global or perhaps more focal. The child's use of play material such as toy furniture, beads for threading, bricks for building, and pencil and paper for drawing will yield more precise clues to the nature of a deficit, showing ataxia, weakness, involuntary movements, or a spastic approach and grasp.

The 'parachute' reaction in the arms is a postural reaction which normally appears at about seven months of age. The examiner holds the infant facing downwards firmly round the chest with both hands. By extending his arms he then plunges the child downwards. The normal response is an immediate, symmetrical extension of the infant's arms with spreading of the fingers as if he were attempting to break his fall (Fig. 2.22) (the reaction does not depend on vision and can be obtained in blind or blindfolded babies). The response is valuable in giving evidence of upper limb involvement in spastic diplegia or suggesting a hemiplegia when it is asymmetrical.

The gait should be studied in all its aspects. In the younger child the mode of crawling or shuffling can be observed. The performance of the co-operative older child in walking, running, jumping, hopping, walking on toes and heels and tandem-walking gives valuable information as to normality or otherwise of the pattern and as to the type of deficit. The 'scissoring' spastic diplegic gait, the limp of a hemiplegia, the wide-based gait of cerebellar ataxia, the waddle of proximal lower limb weakness, most often seen in Duchenne muscular dystrophy, and the foot-drop of peroneal muscular atrophy are obvious examples. These gaits can often be *heard* as well as seen, as the child approaches the consulting room. The varied gaits seen in extrapyramidal disorders such as athetoid cerebral palsy, juvenile Parkinsonism and Wilson's disease may be more difficult to analyse, and the bizarre gait seen in some cases of torsion dystonia

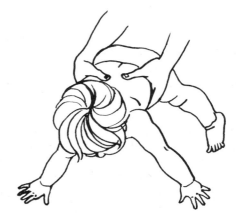

Fig. 2.22 Parachute reaction in the arms

is sometimes easier to imitate than to describe and often raises suspicions of conversion hysteria. Although hysterical gaits are occasionally seen in children, the suspicion should make one think very hard about a diagnosis of torsion dystonia or Wilson's disease since most patients with these disorders have been at one time regarded as hysterical (Ch. 8).

Whenever the history suggests weakness the child should be observed climbing up and down stairs, if he is able to do so. Minor degrees of weakness of the hip girdle muscles may be detected in this way. When possible, more than one flight of stairs should be climbed as this will allow the phenomenon of fatiguability to be detected. The examiner should accompany the child as he climbs. He can thus not only act as a control of sorts, but can also ask the child whether he feels tired or has cramp, pain or other symptoms, and note whether he seems to show undue breathlessness. If the patient sprints up the stairs ahead of the doctor and parents, a significant motor abnormality is unlikely.

When appropriate the child should also be asked to rise from lying supine on the floor to see whether he adopts Gowers' manoeuvre (Ch. 3).

These informal observations will often point clearly to the nature of the neurological deficit or alternatively suggest that no such deficit is present. When possible a more formal approach should be made to examining the nervous system under the conventional headings of cranial nerves, tone, power, co-ordination, and sensory testing.

The head circumference should always be recorded. Though many children tolerate the measuring process well, especially if they have seen their parents' or siblings' heads measured first (these figures may be relevant especially with large heads), the attempt may provoke a battle and should usually be made at a later stage of the examination. A little make-believe, such as 'Let's measure Mummy and Teddy and you for a hat', and the production of a paper hat, will often facilitate the process.

Many aspects of the neurological examination are discussed in the chapter on neurology of the newborn and in later chapters on particular disorders. An excellent account is given by Paine & Oppé (1966). In this chapter no attempt will be made to give an exhaustive account but certain aspects will be considered.

THE CRANIAL NERVES

1st (olfactory) nerve

The sense of smell can be tested in co-operative children in the same way as in adults, but test substances familiar to the child, such as chocolate, oranges and chewing gum, are more suitable than the more esoteric odours of adult neurology (Paine & Oppé 1966). Though unable to name an odour a small child nonetheless can say that he smells something and the facial expression of a non-vocal child may indicate that he has smelled the test substance.

Anosmia is less important as a physical sign in children than in adults, in whom it can provide a valuable pointer to an olfactory groove meningioma or a frontal lobe glioma.

2nd (optic) nerve and visual assessment

Vision

Evidence of the presence and integrity of vision in the older, more co-operative child can be found by the standard methods used with adults, but in the case of the younger or mentally retarded child, or with reduced visual acuity other criteria must be used. The pupil reaction to light, present from 30 weeks of gestation onwards, depends on a functioning reflex arc and is absent with complete but not with partial optic atrophy. From 4 to 6 weeks of age the blink reflex to menace, when a finger is thrust towards the eye, provides a crude test of vision; the open hand should not be used since it creates a breeze which may elicit the corneal reflex. The baby will glance intermittently at his mother's face from birth and consistently watch it while feeding from about 2 weeks of age.

Sheridan (1977) has described the tests of vision appropriate for different age groups. The 4 to 6-month-old infant shows smooth following eye movements for a dangling ball, watches the movements of his own hands, and feet, and reaches out accurately for toys, which he grasps and regards closely.

The Stycar series of tests (Sheridan Tests for Young Children and Retardates, Sheridan 1976) includes the Stycar graded balls tests which are applicable from 6 months to $2\frac{1}{2}$ years of age. These are used to test three visual functions, the ability to follow the movement of very small objects (rolling balls), the ability to fixate, and peripheral vision (mounted balls).

From 2 to 5 years of age the Sheridan miniature toys vision test can be used. In this the child is asked to name and/or match with a duplicate 7 toys. The letter matching test can be used with children of normal intelligence aged 4 years.

For normal children of school entry age (usually 5 years in the United Kingdom), the Stycar letter test using the nine most favoured letters (T, L, H, O, C, X, V, U, A) has given good results.

Abnormal eye movements

Abnormal eye movements at rest are seen in almost all children with congenital blindness, ocular or cortical, or with blindness acquired in early life. Roving eye movements of large amplitude and often disconjugate character are seen when blindness is present early in life. The appearance of unilateral nystagmus may be the first sign of severe asymmetrical visual impairment in cases of optic nerve or pathway lesions such as glioma or craniopharyngioma. Unilateral blindness or severe visual impairment may be unrecognized and difficult to demonstrate in a young child, but extreme resistance to having one eye, but not the other, covered should alert the examiner to this possibility.

Visual fields

The visual fields can be tested crudely as soon as the infant starts to pay attention to his surroundings. Much can be learned by simple observation from which a field defect can be suspected. For more formal testing the examiner faces the child, who sits on his mother's lap, and dangles an object to maintain fixation while another object is silently introduced into the quadrants of the visual field. The examiner watches for accurate re-fixation by the child. A homonymous hemianopia can be shown in this way, but the detection of a bitemporal hemianopia requires one eye to be covered at a time. More accurate mapping of the visual fields is possible in older children by confrontation. The child points to whichever of the examiner's hands moves when the latter has his arms extended sideways and the child fixates on his nose (a coloured spot on the end of the nose or even a false paper nose may help to rivet the child's gaze on the desired target). More formal mapping of the fields is possible by perimetry in older children in whom the blind spot can be examined (enlargement is seen in papilloedema and optic neuritis).

Pupils

The state of the pupils and their reactions to light and convergence should be studied. (It is important to check that mydriatics have not been used recently. Confusion can result when a child is transferred from one hospital to another without any mention of mydriatics in the referring letter.) The pupil size is affected by many drugs and also, inconsistently, by emotion. When assessing the pupil reaction to light it is important to ensure constant fixation and to use a bright light source. Checking pupillary size and light reaction is a vital part of the periodic neurological observations made in cases of head injury, raised intracranial pressure and other acute neurological disorders.

A minor degree of pupillary inequality (anisocoria) is not unusual in normal children. In Adie's syndrome, commoner in girls than boys, there is absence of pupil reaction to light, often unilateral, associated with absence of tendon reflexes. The Argyll-Robertson pupil of acquired syphilis is now very rare; this is a small irregular pupil which reacts to near fixation but not to light. Many lesions in the mid-brain cause impairment of the pupil reaction to light while the 'near' response is preserved; this is part of the sylvian aqueduct syndrome. Miosis is seen as part of Horner's syndrome.

The direct and consensual pupil reaction to a light shone into the ipsilateral and opposite eye respectively, should be examined. With 3rd nerve lesions both are absent in the affected eye but present in the normal. A blind eye shows no direct pupil reaction to light while the opposite eye shows no consensual reaction, but light shone into the normal eye may cause the pupil of the blind eye to constrict.

Examination of the eyes

Examination of the eyes themselves may show stigmata of specific neurological diseases, Down's syndrome, Wilson's disease and ataxia-telangiectasia showing respectively Brushfield spots, a Kayser-Fleischer ring, and conjunctival telangiectasia. Cataracts are less specific abnormalities, seen in metabolic disorders such as galactosaemia, congenital rubella, Lowe's syndrome, and, at a later stage, dystrophia myotonica and Down's syndrome. Diagnostic scintillating crystalline lens opacities may be seen on slit-lamp microscopy in dystrophia myotonica many years before they become symptomatic.

Ptosis should be looked for. It occurs in 3rd nerve lesions when it may be severe and is often associated with external ophthalmoplegia and a dilated pupil. It is also seen in Horner's syndrome with paralysis of the cervical sympathetic associated with miosis, enophthalmos and lack of sweating on the same side of the face. It is also a feature of many myopathies, including myasthenia and myasthenic syndromes, in which it tends to fluctuate (Ch. 3). Many cases of isolated ptosis are congenital. The Marcus Gunn phenomenon of 'jaw-winking' associated with a congenital ptosis has been mentioned in Chapter 1.

Exopthalmos, when unilateral, is often due to localized intraorbital or intracranial disease such as orbital cellulitis, retrobulbar orbital masses, cavernous sinus thrombosis and tumours in the anterior cranial fossa. Pulsating exophthalmos may be seen with a carotico-cavernous fistula between the internal carotid artery and the cavernous sinus but also with an intracranial aneurysm. In such cases a bruit may be heard on listening over the eye and its neighbourhood with a stethoscope

A unilateral pulsating exophthalmos is sometimes seen in neurofibromatosis (Ch. 20) very early in life. It is due to a bony defect in the sphenoid bone and anterior clinoid process and is associated with enlargement of the middle cranial fossa. A retro-orbital plexiform neurofibroma is occasionally seen as a cause of proptosis in neurofibromatosis. Proptosis is rarely caused by an optic nerve glioma, which is another association of von Reckinghausen's disease but also occurs without it.

Ophthalmoscopy

Ophthalmoscopic examination of the eye grounds can be achieved in most children with patience and ingenuity. Some method of darkening the room is needed: bright sunshine makes the procedure very difficult. Sedation should not usually be needed. Infants often allow a good view while they are sucking on a bottle: most examiners find that breast feeding is not so effective for this purpose! Forceful restraint of an angry or frightened child is sometimes needed, but this unhappy situation should be avoided whenever possible. An interesting toy such

as a glove puppet or a pin-wheel which emits sparks will attract the child's attention and facilitate a good view. Mydriatic eye drops are often used to dilate the pupils but their use cannot be recommended in all cases and is contra-indicated in some. If raised intracranial pressure is suspected the patient is at risk of herniation of the temporal lobe through the tentorial opening with stretching of the third nerve, and it is hazardous to rob oneself of potentially valuable eye signs by producing artificially fixed and dilated pupils. The mydriatic effect of atropine is prolonged, but other drugs, such as tropicamide 1%, and mydrilate 1%, have a shorter effect and are therefore preferable.

The optic discs are examined for papilloedema (Fig. 2.23), optic neuritis or pallor suggesting optic atrophy. Papilloedema, often first seen as blurring of the nasal and upper edges of the disc, is a valuable sign of raised intracranial pressure, but is often absent in children since separation of their skull sutures may act as a form of safety valve. The disc swelling of optic neuritis (papillitis) must be distinguished from that of papilloedema: in the former the visual loss is more severe than in papilloedema. Persistent embryonic myelinated nerve fibres radiating from the optic disc should not be confused with papilloedema or papillitis (Fig. 2.24).

Optic atrophy is shown by abnormal pallor of the disc (Fig. 2.25), Gross degrees of atrophy with a

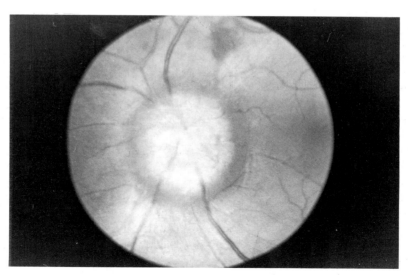

Fig. 2.23 Papilloedema, moderate, shown by elevation of optic disc. Note small retinal haemorrhage above the disc

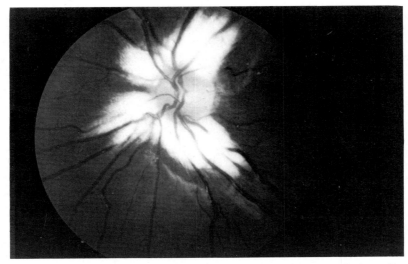

Fig. 2.24 Myelinated nerve fibres. The striking whiteness of the myelinated fibres has a feathered edge and contrasts with the surrounding normal nerve fibres

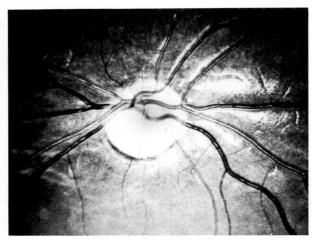

Fig. 2.25 Optic atrophy, with atrophy of retinal nerve fibre layer

'paper-white' disc are unmistakable, and a difference between the two discs usually indicates abnormality. Minor degrees of atrophy may be more difficult to assess in young children whose discs tend to be paler than in older people. In doubtful cases attention to the blood vessels on the surface of the disc may be helpful since the number and prominence of the capillaries may be reduced. Thinning of the retinal nerve fibre layer, whose axons form the optic nerve, helps in the recognition of retinal neuronal loss.

Examination of the macula shows characteristic changes in some of the degenerative brain disorders (Ch. 5). The cherry-red spot is typical of Tay-Sachs disease, but a similar appearance is seen in some cases of Niemann-Pick disease and metachromatic leucodystrophy. Pigmentary macular changes may be seen in the various forms of Batten's disease ('neuronal ceroid lipifuscinosis') in which the peripheral retinae may show obvious diffuse pigmentation. Choroidoretinopathy is suggestive of intrauterine infection with toxoplasma (Fig. 2.26) and a more diffuse pigmentary retinopathy is seen in the rubella syndrome (Fig. 2.27). Pigmentary degeneration of the retina is a feature of some familial syndromes (α-betalipoproteinaemia, Tangier disease, Refsum's syndrome, Laurence-Moon-Biedl syndrome) associated with various neurological deficits.

In Aicardi's syndrome (Ch. 17) an unusual form of choroidoretinopathy with a lacunar appearance is seen in girls with infantile spasms and agenesis of the corpus callosum.

Retinal haemorrhages are seen in young children with acutely raised intracranial pressure, with trauma, often associated with subdural haematoma, with hypertensive encephalopathy and with haemorrhagic disorders such as leukaemia.

Retinal phakomas occur in many children with tuberose sclerosis, increasing in frequency with age. Angiomatosis of the retina is seen in Von Hippel-Lindau disease.

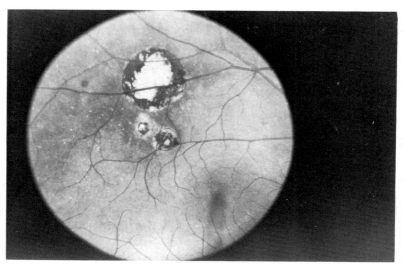

Fig. 2.26 Toxoplasma choroidoretinopathy. The multiple white lesions with a black edge are caused by a combination of atrophy and hyperplasia of the retinal pigment epithelium

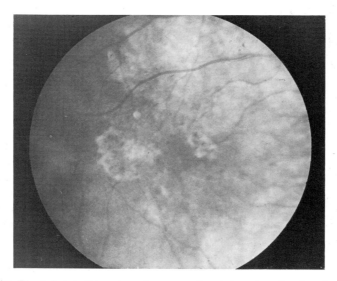

Fig. 2.27 Rubella retinopathy. The defects in this retinopathy are usually subtle and consist of small areas of retinal pigment epithelial thinning together with hyperplasia, giving rise to the granular appearance shown here

3rd, 4th and 6th (oculomotor, trochlear, and abducens) cranial nerves

The examiner should note the position of the eyes at rest, the presence or absence of a squint, spontaneous movements of the eyes and eye movements on following a visual lure, and, when possible and appropriate, on command and reflexly, with the doll's head manoeuvre.

Resting position of the eyes

With paralysis of the individual nerves the affected eye adopts various positions of deviation. In 3rd nerve palsy it deviates laterally and slightly downwards. There may be associated ptosis and a large pupil. With 4th nerve palsy there is little change in the position of the eye at rest, but slight elevation may be seen which increases as the eye is adducted.

6th nerve palsy leads to an internal strabismus. This is common as a false localizing sign with raised intracranial pressure and associated with ipsilateral facial palsy in pontine glioma. With unilateral lesions of recent onset the head is often held rotated slightly towards the affected side in an attempt to suppress the double vision.

Striking deviation of the eyes is seen in certain pathological conditions. The 'setting sun sign', with downward deviation of the eyes at rest and paralysis of upward gaze, is seen in many children with raised intracranial pressure and is common in hydrocephalus (Ch. 17). It is also seen in babies with kernicterus and in some normal infants, especially prematures. In some cerebellar and posterior fossa disorders skew deviation of the eyes is seen, with one eye turned downwards and inwards and the other upwards and outwards. Conjugate deviation of the eyes to one side is sometimes seen with an irritative lesion in the opposite frontal lobe.

Eye movements

The movements of the eyes are usually easily studied by persuading the child to follow a visual lure. Attractive toys such as glove puppets or pin-wheels are useful for this purpose. The shining metal end of the classical 'Queen Square' reflex hammer intrigues many young children who will follow it closely. Some infants prefer to focus on the examiner's spectacles rather than on the proferred lure, and in these cases the doctor can often assess the eye movements by inclining his head to the four points of the compass (if he has a supple neck). Conjugate gaze is studied first and later the movements of the eyes separately if necessary and if tolerated. In the co-operative child the question of diplopia can be explored during conjugate movements.

The many functions of the 3rd nerve will often allow a distinction to be made between a nuclear and an infranuclear lesion. The former may pick out one or more of the 4 eye muscles (medial, superior and inferior recti and inferior oblique) while sparing levator palpebrae superioris and the constrictor pupillae. Infranuclear lesions tend to affect all 4 eye muscles unless situated in the orbit itself. Nuclear 6th nerve lesions usually affect the adjacent 7th nerve also so that ipsilateral facial paralysis accompanies the squint. This is not the case with infranuclear lesions.

More complex disorders of eye movements

Conjugate gaze in a vertical or horizontal plane may be affected by supranuclear disturbances with individual eye movements remaining unaffected. Following conjugate eye movements are reduced or lost, but movements in the same direction can be elicited by the 'doll's eye manoeuvre' in which the child maintains his gaze on a point while his head is rotated or tilted. An example is Parinaud's syndrome in which paralysis of conjugate upward gaze is associated with lesions, such as pineal tumours, vascular lesions, encephalitis and disseminated sclerosis, in the region of the superior colliculi. A supranuclear ophthalmoplegia in the vertical and in the horizontal direction respectively are recognized in two rare neurometabolic degenerative brain diseases (Ch. 5).

Duane's retraction syndrome, often mistaken for a lateral rectus palsy, is a rare condition in which the lateral rectus muscle on one or both sides is largely fibrosed and a complex disorder of eye movements is seen on attempted lateral gaze. This movement is limited and the palpebral fissure widens as the child tries to abduct the eye and narrows on adduction, during which the globe is also retracted and elevated. The cause of the condition is unknown.

These features may occur alone or — much more rarely — as part of a more complex congenital disorder with a cluster of other anomalies, the cervico-oculo-acoustic or Wildervanck's syndrome (Wildervanck 1961, Fraser & MacGillivray 1968). The associated features are the Klippel-Feil syndrome of cervical vertebral abnormalities, and deaf-mutism.

Another complex disturbance of eye movements on attempted conjugate horizontal gaze is seen when there is an internuclear ophthalmoplegia due to a lesion of the medial longitudinal bundle which links the 6th nerve nucleus on one side with that part of the contralateral 3rd nerve nucleus which innervates the medial rectus muscle. There is paralysis of adduction of the eye furthest from the visual target with nystagmus in the abducting eye only, sometimes with some limitation of abduction.

Various lesions in the brain stem can produce this form of ophthalmoplegia which is not common in children. In adults the commonest cause is disseminated sclerosis.

Cogan's oculomotor apraxia (Cogan & Adams 1953) is a rare condition of unknown cause, commoner in boys, with a defect of rapid horizontal eye movements and of 'attraction' movements with normal random eye movements. The normal eye movements by which the reader scans the page from left to right are affected and the patient tends instead to move his head to follow the lines. He may also show jerking sideways movements of the head to bring his eyes into the desired position. Some cases of reading difficulty have this defect as their basis. Difficulty and unsteadiness in changing direction rapidly when walking, running or riding may be associated with a tendency to fall when turning. This condition is occasionally found among those classed as 'clumsy boys', and this underlines the need for careful neurological examination in all such children. A rather similar defect of eye movements is seen in ataxia-telangiectasia (Ch. 20).

Nystagmus

The involuntary eye movements of nystagmus may be rhythmic or non-rhythmic and may be physiological (as in the opticokinetic nystagmus provoked by watching the stripes of a revolving drum or the passing landscape from a moving vehicle) or pathological. Pathological forms of nystagmus occur with eye disorders and disease of the CNS. Ocular nystagmus, pendular in type with coarse, slow 'searching' movements, is seen with blindness of early onset. The term 'congenital nystagmus' is sometimes used for a specific condition of unknown origin with rapid rhythmic or non-rhythmic eye movements, usually with normal vision. It is usually recognized at a few months of age, may be associated with rhythmic nodding or shaking movements of the head (which are slower than those of the eyes) and often improves with age. It is usually bilateral but sometimes asymmetrical and occasionally unilateral. (When unilateral, however, nystagmus should always raise the suspicion of a structural cause such as a lesion affecting the optic nerve or pathways). In some cases congenital nystagmus shows a familial tendency.

Cerebellar nystagmus is the most important neurological form of nystagmus in childhood. It is seen when the patient looks to left or right, and shows a quick component in the direction of gaze and a slow component towards the neutral position. These directions are reversed when he looks towards the other side. Cerebellar nystagmus is increased on looking towards the side of the cerebellar lesion.

Vestibular nystagmus differs from the cerebellar variety in showing the slow phase towards the side of the lesion. It may be seen with disorders of the semicircular canals, vestibular nerves or nuclei. Brain stem tumours, demyelinating or vascular disease may produce it, often with a vertical or rotary quality. Vertigo may be complained of with central lesions affecting the vestibular system and occasionally vestibular nystagmus is associated with a non-rotational sensation of movement, known as oscillopsia, in which objects seem to oscillate in the direction of the nystagmus.

5th (trigeminal) nerve

The motor targets of the 5th nerve, the muscles of mastication, can be tested in older children formally as in adults. The masseter and temporalis muscles can be palpated as the child clenches his teeth. The bulk of the masseters may be increased in boys with Duchenne muscular dystrophy (Ch. 3). The jaw is opened with and without resistance and any deviation or weakness are noted. Younger children will happily bite on a biscuit or a jelly-baby. They may be asked to bite on a wooden spatula and to resist the doctor's efforts to remove it; asymmetry of their tooth marks may suggest unilateral weakness.

The jaw jerk is tested with the child's mouth slightly open and relaxed. The examiner taps his own finger, placed lightly over the centre of the child's chin, with the reflex hammer. The extent of the raising of the lower jaw which results varies from one time to another, as does the briskness of the tendon reflexes. It may be very brisk when the child is upset. The reflex arc runs through the sensory and motor roots of the trigeminal nerve. An exaggerated jaw jerk, which may be accompanied by clonus, indicates an upper motor neurone lesion above the level of the pons.

Sensation may be tested over the three divisions of the 5th nerve in the usual way, to light touch, pin-prick and other modalities, but this is only of importance in a minority of children and may be difficult and upsetting. The same is true of the corneal reflex, usually elicited with a wisp of cotton wool; a cruder, but better tolerated, approach is by blowing gently into the child's eye.

7th (facial) nerve

The motor branches of the facial nerve supply all the muscles of the face and ear, stapedius, the platysma, the stylohyoid muscles and posterior belly of the digastric. The facial muscles are easily studied in all children by observation during spontaneous movements, while in young, retarded and unco-operative children it may only be possible to study them in this way. Older, more biddable children will perform to request when asked to smile, frown, raise their eyebrows, puff out their cheeks, whistle, close their eyes and keep them closed against resistance. Movements of the upper and lower parts of the face should be studied separately since lower motor neurone weakness, such as that due to facial nerve lesions, affects both parts whereas the upper face is usually spared in upper motor neurone lesions.

With involvement of the nerve to the stapedius muscle the patient may complain of an unpleasant, exaggerated perception of sound in the affected ear, known as hyperacusis. This symptom is difficult to assess in children.

When the chorda tympani nerve is affected there is impairment of salivation and of taste over the anterior two thirds of the tongue. Lacrimation is impaired in the ipsilateral eye with lesions affecting the pathways involved (petrosal nerve, geniculate ganglion or facial nerve proximal to the ganglion). In doubtful cases a difference between the two sides may be shown by Schirmer's test with strips of filter paper hooked over the edges of the lower lids and comparison made between the lengths of paper moistened in 5 minutes.

Congenital hypoplasia of the depressor anguli oris muscle, often familial, should be distinguished from facial palsy.

8th (auditory) nerve

The 8th nerve has two functionally different components, the cochlear division conveying auditory impulses, and the vestibular carrying postural sensation from the labyrinth.

The testing of hearing

For the clinical testing of hearing various sources of sound and techniques are used depending on the age of the child and his developmental level. In the vocal child his vocalizations give valuable clues to his ability to appreciate the elements of spoken language so that his utterances should be observed and his mother's report of them noted.

Hearing loss may be of sensorineural or conductive type, due to lesions in the middle or outer ear. The latter are commoner in older children. When hearing is tested the ears should be examined for disorders which may cause conductive deafness, such as wax or foreign bodies in the canal, otitis media or glue ears.

Sheridan (1976b, 1977) has given a useful review of the principles involved in testing hearing and of the methods appropriate at different ages. Infants aged 6–12 months are fairly easy to test and look enquiringly for the source of a sound. The sound sources used are a high-pitched rattle, a spoon in a cup, tissue paper, a hand bell and selected speech sound, (the low-tone vowel, 'oo-oo', repeated and high-tone consonants 's-s, t-t, ps-ps-ps, pth-pth-pth', repeated rapidly several times.) A clear-cut response to 4 of the 5 test-sounds, including rattle and high-tone speech sounds, suggests that the child has adequate hearing for speech but cannot be taken fully to exclude partial deafness (particularly high-tone loss) so that infants with doubtful responses and those regarded as 'at risk' should be followed up carefully.

The 12–14-month-old child may be more difficult to test, since he is active, resents interference and may show only limited interest in the test sounds.

At 14 months to 2 years the child will often co-operate in tests involving the recognition and naming of 4 and 5 familiar toys. From 2 to 3 years he may take part in a 'game' involving a cued action (putting a wooden 1-inch brick into a cup and taking it out) whenever the test words, 'in' and 'lift' are heard. These are spoken increasingly quietly and progressively truncated — 'in-in-n-n-n' and 'lift-lift-ift, -f, th' (as in 'thin'). The test is used with each ear and is very sensitive.

From 3 to 4 years (and with mentally retarded children up to 16) a test with 7 toys, another with 8 wooden cubes to be picked up on the cue of a high-tone consonant and a picture vocabulary test can be used.

The 5–7 year old child will usually co-operate in various audiometric tests and in clinical speech tests with pictures, word lists and sentences.

With the mentally retarded, tests suitable for younger children must be chosen.

Vestibular function

Vestibular function is not usually tested in children unless there are specific indications such as vertigo, nystagmus, ataxic gait and deviation of the eyes. The tests are complex and are well described by Paine & Oppé (1966). Vestibular nystagmus is described earlier.

9th (glossopharyngeal) and 10th (vagus) nerves

These two lower cranial nerves are conventionally considered in tandem since their close anatomical and functional association causes them often to be affected together by pathological processes. Since both nerves leave the skull through the jugular foramen together with the 11th nerve, all three nerves may be affected by lesions at the base of the skull.

Their motor fibres arise in the nucleus ambiguus in the medulla. Those of the 9th nerve supply only the stylopharyngeus muscle, paralysis of which may be very difficult to detect. Those of the 10th nerve (vagus) supply all the voluntary muscles of the soft palate, pharynx and the larynx, except the stylopharyngeus. Unilateral lesions cause drooping of the palatal arch on the affected side with the uvula and median raphe deviating towards the normal side. This deviation increases on phonation. With bilateral vagal paralysis the palatal arch may be fairly well maintained, but the palate does not elevate normally on phonation. The palatal reflex can be elicited by touching the lower surface of the

uvula or soft palate with a throat swab. The response is elevation of the soft palate and retraction of the uvula. The sensory arc of the reflex is via the 9th and the motor arc via the 10th nerve. The same pathways are involved in the gag reflex, which is obtained by stimulating the pharyngeal wall, pillars of the tonsils or base of the tongue on either side. Both these procedures are deeply resented by most children. They should not be performed as a routine and should be left until a late stage of the examination.

With acute vagal lesions there may be dysphagia, especially for fluids, and some nasal regurgitation of liquids when swallowing. There may also be a nasal quality to the voice, resembling that heard with cleft palate; this is more marked with bilateral than unilateral lesions. Direct or indirect examination of the larynx may be needed. This is better carried out by an expert rather than by an 'occasional practitioner'.

Glossopharyngeal sensation is tested to touch and pinprick (when indicated by the clinical features) on the pharyngeal walls around the tonsils and posterior third of the tongue. The 9th nerve also supplies the sense of taste over the same area of the tongue. Sensation to the eardrum, external auditory meatus and part of the pinna of the ear are supplied by the vagus, but with some overlap from other nerves. Testing these areas in a young child is difficult.

11th (spinal accessory) nerve

This is a motor nerve which supplies the upper fibres of the trapezii and the sternomastoid muscles. It has cranial fibres which arise in the nucleus ambiguus, like those of the 9th and 10th nerves, and spinal fibres from the upper cervical segments.

The bulk of the trapezius may be assessed by inspection and palpation and its strength by asking the child to raise his shoulders against resistance, in a shrugging action. Fasciculation is occasionally seen in denervating diseases, such as spinal muscular atrophy, but is more difficult to detect in children than in adults because of their relatively thicker layer of overlying fat.

The bulk of the sternomastoid muscles can be assessed at rest and in action, by inspection and palpation, and their strength by persuading the child to turn his head to one side against resistance from a hand applied to his chin. With younger children a request to turn to look at their mother or an attractive toy will usually produce the desired movement.

12th (hypoglossal) nerve

This nerve supplies the muscles of the tongue, its nucleus being the homologue in the medulla of the anterior horn cells in the spinal cord. In the various forms of spinal muscular atrophy the tongue is often affected, when it appears atrophic and weak and shows fasciculation with fine worm-like wriggling movements (Ch. 3). In infants and young children with these disorders the tongue may be the only muscle in which fasciculation can be recognized, so that it should be examined with care.

With unilateral lesions of the 12th nerve or its nucleus the tongue is deviated towards the side of the lesion and may show unilateral atrophy and fas-

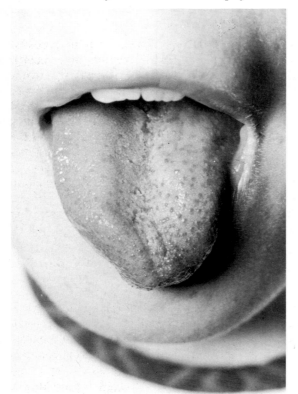

Fig. 2.28 Unilateral tongue wasting in 9-year-old girl with Moebius' syndrome

ciculation (Fig. 2.28). In pyramidal disorders the tongue may be spastic. In the very rare disorder 'congenital suprabulbar paresis' (Ch. 17) the tongue, palate and muscles of the lower part of the face are affected and there is great difficulty in protruding or moving the tongue, chewing and swallowing, although the muscles of the upper face function normally.

In myotonia congenita and other disorders with myotonia, this phenomenon can sometimes be shown in the tongue. With the tongue protruded a wooden tongue-depressor is held resting on and at right angles to it. When this is tapped sharply with a small reflex hammer a dimple develops at the site and persists much longer than usual. This is not a test which children enjoy (indeed adults have been known to express vociferous resentment) and the examiner should ask himself in each case whether it is really necessary.

EXAMINATION OF THE LIMBS

In examining the limbs observations should be made of muscle bulk, tone, power, co-ordination, involuntary movements, reflexes and sensory findings. Skeletal deformities, contractures and asymmetry in the size of the limbs should also be noted. Many older children will co-operate well in a formal examination on classical neurological lines. In younger and in retarded, and therefore less co-operative, children a good deal of adaptation is needed. Many of the comments made on the examination of the newborn apply also to older children, some of whom may prove very negativistic and present the examining doctor with a real challenge.

The Medical Research Council (MRC) Memorandum on *Aids to the examination of the peripheral nervous system* (1976) is a valuable illustrated guide particularly useful in the motor and sensory testing of older, more co-operative children. In younger children assessment may be more difficult, but can often be achieved by patience, coaxing and the use of toys. The examiner must clearly know what movement he wants to elicit and is well advised to carry a copy of the booklet in his bag. It lists the MRC scale for recording muscle power which is widely used in the United Kingdom:

0. No contraction

1. Flicker or trace of contraction
2. Active movement, with gravity eliminated
3. Active movement against gravity
4. Active movement against gravity and resistance
5. Normal power.

Muscle bulk

Assessment of muscle bulk by inspection and palpation may be helpful in neuromuscular diseases in which there may be wasting, hypertrophy or both. Enlargement of calf and other muscles is seen in Duchenne and some other forms of muscular dystrophy. Wasting, like weakness, may be focal. Both these features tend to be more marked proximally in many muscular dystrophies and other myopathies and distally in many neuropathies. In Duchenne dystrophy certain muscles are singled out and show marked wasting at an early stage. Brachioradialis and the sternal fibres of pectoralis major are most affected. Minor degrees of wasting may be difficult to detect because of the relatively large layer of fat in the child. The same is true of fasciculation, but in some patients with spinal muscular atrophy small range jerky movements of the fingers are seen as evidence of denervation in the small muscles of the hands.

Tone

This may be assessed in the conventional way by passive movement of the limbs in older children. Many of the aspects of 'tonus' described in the newborn may also be helpful in older children. Thus abnormal postures dictated by severe hypotonia are seen in some patients with neuromuscular disease and an abnormal range of movement is shown at various joints both on passive movement and on 'flapping' the extremity ('ballant'). In a very hypotonic child the testing should not be performed too vigorously since iatrogenic fractures have been known to result. Increased tone may be of spastic or rigid plastic type and in sometimes intermediate between the two. A cogwheel type of rigidity is found in some extrapyramidal disorders. Tone may vary from one time to another under the influence of physiological factors (emotion, exercise, fatigue, sleep or physiotherapy) and of drugs,

being reduced by benzodiazepines and Lioresal. It is increased under the influence of the asymmetric tonic neck reflex in the limbs on the side to which the head is turned. This effect should be prevented by keeping the head in a central position.

Power

Observation of spontaneous and provoked movement, gait and manipulation allows the grosser degress of weakness to be detected, though trick movements may be deceptive. Weakness can be graded according to the Medical Research Scale in older children. In younger patients a fairly accurate idea of strength can often be gained by an informal approach involving play material, the pulling down or pushing away of a glove puppet or other toy, squeezing of gloved fingers and other manoeuvres. Other methods of assessing muscle strength including the use of an ergometer are discussed in Chapter 3.

Co-ordination

The assessment of co-ordination is fully discussed in Chapters 9 and 10 in relation to cerebellar ataxia and various kinds of involuntary movements. As with other motor functions a spectrum of testing methods is available ranging from simple observation of movements through play activity (threading beads, peg boards etc.) to the formal tests of adult neurology (finger-nose, heel-knee-shin test, heel-to-toe walking.) A wide range of unwanted movements may impair co-ordination in childhood (ataxia, chorea, athetosis, dystonia, tremor.) Their differentiation is discussed in Chapters 9 and 10.

Deep tendon reflexes (Table 2.1)

Eliciting the tendon reflexes requires more co-operation from the child than some other parts of the neurological examination, since their assessment in a patient who is struggling to evade the hammer can be very difficult. (As partial compensation for this, a child who struggles and fights vigorously and successfully during this procedure is unlikely to have an important degree of motor deficit.)

Table 2.1 The spinal levels involved in the more important deep tendon reflexes

Reflex	Spinal segment	Peripheral nerve
Biceps jerk	Cervical 5 and 6	Musculocutaneous
Supinator or Brachioradialis jerk	Cervical 5 and 6	Radial
Triceps jerk	Cervical 6 and 7	Radial (Musculospiral)
Knee jerk	Lumbar 2,3 and 4	Femoral
Ankle jerk	Sacral 1	Tibial

It should be realized that the patellar hammer may seem a very threatening object to a small child who may regard its use on him an assault. The type of hammer used is of some importance. The traditional round-headed 'Queen Square' model is effective and is better tolerated than other types; in particular the triangular headed variety, with its resemblance to a tomahawk or a stone-age axe, has little to recommend it, especially since the solid head is usually harder than the rubber circle of the round-headed model. The doctor's approach is also important. With younger and potentially more unco-operative children the tendon reflexes are better left until a later stage of the examination. Some idea of the child's likely reaction can be gained by his response to the preceding manoeuvres. Sometimes an observant child will be intrigued by the instrument and demand to know what it is for. There will be little difficulty in such cases (if the child has a toy doctor's set the hammer should hold no terrors for him.) With young children and apprehensive older ones it is helpful to show the use of the hammer by tapping one's own limbs and then doing the same to the child's mother and father, explaining what one is doing. The child, like many adults, is often fascinated by the knee jerk and will want to have it demonstrated on himself. A game can easily be made of this: the doctor says to the child, 'you won't kick me, will you?', placing his own leg in such a position that the patient's foot will inevitably kick it as the knee jerk is elicited. Many young children will happily offer their opposite arm or leg when they have seen the reflexes obtained on the other side. An enthusiastic child may make the task difficult for the examiner by insisting on grabbing the hammer and hitting his own knees or those of the doctor and a spare

instrument can be useful in this situation. From the age of two years many intelligent children can elicit their own knee jerks, though (as far as I know) 'norms' have not yet been worked out for this skill!

It is not necessary for the child to be supine on a couch to elicit the reflexes, and it is preferable for younger children to sit on their mother's lap or a chair. It is often helpful, when eliciting the knee and ankle reflexes, to have the child's foot resting on the examiner's knee.

Infants and young children show greater variability in the briskness of tendon reflexes and a greater tendency to crossed adduction i.e. adduction of the opposite leg with the knee jerks, than older patients. These can normally be obtained from a wider area of the lower leg than in older people. The young tend to have brisker reflexes in the legs than in the arms and many normal children have upper limb reflexes which are sluggish by adult standards. Finger flexion is a common accompaniment of the supinator and biceps jerks in children, decreasing with age.

Difficulty in obtaining tendon reflexes must be assessed in relation to symptoms and to other signs. Various methods of reinforcement of reflexes may be needed. Squeezing a parent's hand or a doll are helpful. Older children will perform the classical Jendrassik's manoeuvre, pulling with the flexed fingers of one hand against those of the other.

The ankle jerks may be difficult to elicit in the conventional supine or sitting position in children, but can often be obtained readily in the prone or kneeling position. Older children will co-operate by kneeling up on a chair while their Achilles tendons are tapped from above. If the foot is held gently by the examiner as he taps the tendon any movement of plantar flexion can be felt. Since absence of the ankle jerk may be useful, or indeed the only, evidence for a peripheral neuropathy, it is important to be certain whether they are truly absent. Preservation of the ankle jerks with reduction or loss of other tendon reflexes is a common finding in myopathies. The tendon reflexes on the two sides of the body are compared in order to detect any asymmetry. Minor degrees of asymmetry in the absence of other signs may be of no significance. A central position of the head should be maintained in order to eliminate the effect of the asymmetric tonic neck reflex on the briskness of the tendon jerks (increased on the side to which the face is turned).

Apart from the presence, absence and briskness of the tendon reflexes, *qualitative* changes in their character may be noted in certain conditions. Thus the knee jerks have a pendular character with cerebellar lesions, the lower leg if hanging downwards, swinging in an arc three or more times. In chorea a sustained or 'hung-up' knee jerk is sometimes seen, with the leg maintained in extension owing to prolonged contraction of the quadriceps. In hypothyroidism the ankle jerk may be delayed and slower than normal. A clonic character to the ankle jerk is sometimes seen in pyramidal disease, the reflex not only being exaggerated but also accompanied by clonus. In such cases ankle clonus is obtainable by the conventional method of rapidly dorsiflexing the ankle. Patellar clonus may also be shown with pyramidal dysfunction by rapidly stretching the patellar tendon, either by pushing it downwards or by tapping a finger placed on the upper border of the patella. The knee jerks are usually exaggerated when patellar clonus is present.

Superficial (cutaneous) reflexes (Table 2.2)
Abdominal reflexes

These are best elicited with a thin wooden stick. Any instrument which causes pain should be avoided. The upper reflexes are tested first by drawing the stick sharply from one side towards the midline, repeating the procedure on the other side, and then eliciting the lower reflexes. Most children show a brisk contraction of the abdominal muscles and a movement of the umbilicus towards the side stimulated. The reflexes may be absent in very young infants, obese children and those with a distended abdomen or with absent or paralysed abdominal wall muscles. Some children find the

Table 2.2 The spinal levels involved in some cutaneous reflexes

Reflex	Spinal segment
Superficial abdominal reflexes	Thoracic 7 to 12
Cremasteric reflex	Lumbar 1
Plantar response	Sacral 1
Anal reflex	Sacral 4 and 5

test so ticklish that they double up with laughter after the first touch of the stick and prevent any further approach despite parental remonstration.

Reduction or asymmetry of the reflexes may be significant. They are depressed with recent pyramidal tract lesions, when they are often associated with exaggerated tendon reflexes. With longer-standing lesions, as in most cases of cerebral palsy, they are usually normal. Absence of the abdominal reflexes on one side in a child with hemiplegia suggests that this is of fairly recent origin. The level of a spinal cord lesion can sometimes be suspected by the finding of differential reduction of the abdominal reflexes with preservation of the upper but loss of the lower responses. In some cases the reflexes are present on initial testing, but with repeated eliciting may diminish at one level or on one side as evidence of milder or incipient dysfunction.

Cremasteric reflex

This is tested in boys by stroking the skin of the upper and medial aspect of the thigh. The cremaster muscle on the same side contracts and the testis is raised. The reflex may be reduced or absent in the presence of a pyramidal lesion or in a nervous child. It need not be elicited routinely.

Ano-cutaneous reflex

The stimulus for this test is a rapid pinprick to the perianal skin and the normal response is a contraction or 'winking' of the external anal sphincter. It should not be tested routinely, but should be looked for particularly when there are sphincter problems or any suspicion of a spinal lesion. Spinal segments S2, 3, 4 and sometimes 5 are involved in the innervation of the anal and of the external sphincter of the bladder, so that an intact ano-cutaneous reflex is an encouraging sign in a child with a myelomeningocoele or with a congenital imperforate anus.

Trunk incurvation (Galant) reflex

This has been described in the chapter on the newborn but the reflex, elicited by stroking down the paravertebral region on either side with the response a curving of the spine to the side stimulated, persists into later childhood so that it can be helpful in finding the level in lesions of the spinal cord.

Plantar reflex

Already referred to in connection with the neonatal examination, this reflex may be more difficult to assess in older children because of withdrawal or resistance. It is often helpful to test it gently and almost surreptitiously, concealing the wooden stick or other instrument to be used. (Car-keys, though often used in adults, are best avoided in children.) In many cases no instrument is needed and the plantar reflex can be elicited with the thumbnail. The sole of the foot should be stroked from the heel forwards along the outer side of the foot. It is usually recommended that the stimulus should then move medially across the ends of the metatarsal bones, but in many cases a frankly flexor or extensor response is obtained when it has travelled only a short distance. It may be more difficult to decide on the nature of the response and a firmer and longer stimulus may be needed. Comparison between the responses on the two sides is helpful in detecting asymmetry which may be significant. With severe weakness of the distal leg muscles there may be no movement of the hallux.

It is inadvisable to attribute great significance to an 'equivocal' plantar response. Like all other neurological findings, it must be construed in the context of the clinical picture and of other findings.

Toe flexion reflexes ('toe jerks')

These abnormal reflexes are found in some children, especially younger patients, with pyramidal tract dysfunction, in response to various manoeuvres. They may be elicited by tapping the base of the toes or the dorsum of the foot and are associated with several eponyms including that of Rossolimo. They are quite distinct from the plantar reflex and from plantar grasping. They may be seen in some children with cerebral palsy but seem to be commoner in children with progressive degenerative brain disease. In metachromatic and in Krabbe's leucodystrophy toe jerks may be present when the deep tendon reflexes are reduced or even absent as a result of the associated peripheral neuropathy. In this situation they are a valuable sign of pyramidal tract disorder.

'SOFT SIGNS' IN CHILD NEUROLOGY

This rather unfortunate term is often used, *faute de mieux*, to indicate a state of mind in the examiner, rather than an objective finding in the patient (Ingram 1973). This does not necessarily imply a criticism of the examiner, since uncertainty as to the presence of abnormal findings and their significance in terms of neurological dysfunction is not uncommon in dealing with children. The contrast implied is with *hard* signs, meaning those which are unmistakably abnormal and are taken to indicate disorder of a particular part of the nervous system, such as an extensor plantar response or exaggerated tendon reflex pointing to 'pyramidal' dysfunction, or ataxia in the finger-nose test to cerebellar disorder.

As has been stressed already, it may sometimes be difficult to be certain whether a finding is abnormal or not. For example in a struggling child, asymmetry in tone or tendon reflexes may be difficult to judge, and the direction in which his hallux moves on plantar stimulation may sometimes be impossible to determine rapidly. With patience and various subterfuges it is often possible to come to a firm decision. When it proves impossible to do so the situation must be judged in its clinical context, i.e. the presenting symptom and the way in which the child can be seen to function when observed informally. Clearly a dubious plantar response is more likely to be significant if a limp of recent onset is complained of and is clinically obvious than if the complaint is of occasional headache and the child walks normally and evades the examiner with agility.

Allowance must be made for the variability of findings, particularly the briskness of tendon reflexes, in young children from one time to another in relation to factors such as emotional state; degree of alertness or sleepiness etc. The influence of the asymmetric tonic neck reflex must be guarded against with its tendency to produce an increase in tone and reflexes on the 'face' side if the head is not kept in the midline.

Minor degrees of reflex asymmetry unaccompanied by other signs are rarely significant of serious neurological disease, but may occasionally reflect a hemiparesis of minimal degree, especially if associated with some asymmetry in the size of the hands or feet.

More problematical is the interpretation of minor degrees of inco-ordination and involuntary movements. These must be judged in relation to the child's age. Poor manipulative ability acceptable as within normal limits at three years of age is unacceptable at 5 or 6. The child's intellectual level must also be taken into account since poor co-ordination and unwanted movements are common in the mentally retarded patient without the classical physical signs which allow a diagnosis of cerebral palsy of one or other kind. The retarded child often shows a marked degree of immaturity in neurological function with poor co-ordination in the hands, and in an older child a gait more appropriate for a normal toddler. Thus it often happens that a retarded child is wrongly labelled as ataxic until the passing years have brought his co-ordination to an acceptable level.

In addition a similar pattern of motor immaturity is seen in many children of normal intelligence who lack the conventional signs to justify a diagnosis of cerebral palsy. These children, more often boys than girls, are labelled 'clumsy' and labour under the accurate but pejorative description 'clumsy boys' or sometimes the more controversial epithets 'minimal brain damage' (MBD) or 'minimal cerebral dysfunction' (MCD) (Ch. 15). Apart from difficulty with discrete finger movements, as in successively touching each finger to the thumb, and with rapid alternating movements as in tapping one hand with the other or tapping the floor with the feet, these children often show movements of the outstretched hands of choreiform type. Their performance at jumping, hopping, walking on toes and heels, and walking heel to toe is primitive and elephantine. There may be a history of a similar poor motor performance in one of the child's parents. This should be enquired for and when appropriate the parent shoud be examined. In rare cases a tremor of a benign familial type may be detected.

REFERENCES

Aids to the examination of the peripheral nervous system 1976 Medical Research Council Memorandum 45. Her Majesty's Stationery Office, London

Bower T 1977 The perceptual world of the child. Fontana/Open Books, London

Cogan D G, Adams R D 1953 A type of paralysis of conjugate gaze (ocular motor apraxia). Archives of Ophthalmology 50: 434

Drillien C M 1977 Developmental assessment and development screening. In: Drillien C M, Drummond M B (eds) Neurodevelopmental problems in early childhood, Assessment and Management. ed. Blackwell Scientific Publications Oxford

Egan D, Illingworth R S, MacKeith R C 1969 Developmental screening 0–5 years. Clinics in Developmental Medicine 30. Heinemann, London

Fraser W I, MacGillivray R C 1968 Cervico-oculo-acoustic dysplasia (The syndrome of Wildervanck). Journal of Mental Deficiency Research 12: 322–329

Gunn T 1973 Positives. Verses by Thom Gunn. Photographs by Ander Gunn. Faber and Faber, London

Harrison J B 1862 Familiar letters on the diseases of children: addressed to a young practitioner. Churchill, London, p. 16

Illingworth R S 1977 Basic developmental screening. 0–2 years. Blackwell Scientific Publications, Oxford

Illingworth R S 1980, The development of the infant and young child, normal and abnormal, 9th edn. Churchill Livingstone, Edinburgh

Ingram T T S 1973 Soft signs. Developmental Medicine and Child Neurology 15: 527–529

Miranda S B, Hack M, Fantz R L, Fanaroff A A, Klaus M H 1977 Neonatal pattern vision: a predictor of future mental performance. Journal of Pediatrics 91: 642–647

Paine R S, Oppé T E 1966 Neurological examination of children. Clinics in Developmental Medicine 20/21. Heinemann, London

Robson P 1970 Shuffling, hitching, scooting or sliding: some observations in 30 otherwise normal children. Developmental Medicine and Child Neurology 12: 608–617

Sheridan M D 1973 Children's developmental progress from birth to five years. The Stycar sequences. NFER Publishing

Sheridan M D, 1976 a Manual for the Stycar vision tests, 3rd edn. National Foundation for Educational Research, London

Sheridan M D 1976b Manual for the Stycar hearing tests, 3rd edn. National Foundation for Educational Research, London

Sheridan M D 1977 Development and assessment of vision and hearing. In: Drillien C M, Drummond M B (eds) Neurodevelopmental problems in early childhood, assessment and management. Blackwell Scientific Publications, Oxford

Stern D 1977 The first relationships: infant and mother. Fontana/Open Books, London

Wildervanck L S 1961 Proceedings of the second International Congress of Paedo-Audiology, Groningen

3

Neuromuscular disorders: I. Primary muscle disease and anterior horn cell disorders

E. M. Brett and B. D. Lake

INTRODUCTION

The voluntary striated muscles depend for the maintenance of their normal functioning and structure on their links with the central nervous system via the peripheral motor nerves which originate from the anterior horn cells of the spinal cord and from homologous cells in the brain-stem. This two-stage link constitutes the lower motor neuron and is the final common path through which nervous impulses from the brain reach the voluntary muscles. Disorder of the lower motor neuron from whatever cause and at either level (spinal cord or peripheral nerve) produces a clinical picture of weakness and hypotonia (flaccid paralysis) with absence or reduction of tendon reflexes, and progressive muscular atrophy. Within a few weeks of an acute lesion of the lower motor neuron, particularly with disease of the anterior horn cell, increased irritability of the denervated muscle fibres develops shown by the electrical phenomenon of fibrillation (spontaneous contractions of individual muscle fibres detected with the electromyography needle) and the clinical phenomenon of fasciculation in which spontaneous muscle fibre contractions can be seen with the naked eye. Fasciculation in young children is usually more difficult to detect than in adults since the former usually have more subcutaneous fat, and it is often visible only or principally in the tongue.

The clinical effects of primary disease of voluntary muscle or of the neuromuscular junction are very similar to those of lower motor neuron disorder, hypotonia and weakness being prominent. The tendon reflexes are less likely to be affected and muscle atrophy is usually less severe, while fibrillation and fasciculation are not seen as in the disorders causing denervation.

In young children and infants the clinical distinction between disease of the spinal cord, peripheral nerve, neuromuscular junction and muscle fibres is often difficult because the clinical picture, dominated by weakness and hypotonia, is very similar. In infancy also the clinical picture resulting from disorder of the central nervous system at higher levels and from general medical illnesses affecting other systems may show close similarities to that due to disorder of the lower motor neuron and muscle. Thus what has come to be called 'the floppy infant syndrome' may be due not only to the various types of neuromuscular disease mentioned above, but also to uncomplicated mental retardation or to noxious effects on the brain in the perinatal period of a kind which may give rise later in development to that persisting disorder of movement and posture which constitutes cerebral palsy. The same clinical picture can result from certain metabolic, endocrine, cardiac and prolonged debilitating illnesses and from some disorders of connective tissue.

The floppy infant syndrome and its differential diagnosis has been well reviewed by Dubowitz (1969, 1980) in a monograph which is essential reading for all paediatricians. Historically much of the confusion surrounding the subject in the past had semantic causes. Just as outmoded terms lingered on in the field of progressive degenerative brain disease (the term 'amaurotic family idiocy' continuing to be used to cover what have since been recognised as the gangliosidoses, various forms of Batten's disease and other neuronal storage disorders) so an archaic and confusing nomenclature survived, and has still not completely disappeared, as a legacy from some of the founding fathers of neurology. Although infantile progressive spinal muscular atrophy (Werdnig-Hoffmann disease, as it came to be known) was well described by the eponymous authors in a series of papers in the 1890s, various neologisms were later coined which were applied not only to such cases but also to other diseases with a similar clinical picture. The term *myatonia congenita* was proposed by Oppenheim (1900) for a condition with early hypotonia but without deterioration, but the similarity of this name to *myotonia congenita* (Thomsen's disease) led Collier & Wilson (1908) to suggest the alternative term *amyotonia congenita*. This gained wide currency in the English literature and circulated extensively over the next four or five decades. Critical reviews of cases so labelled (Brandt 1950, Walton 1956) have shown that many varied conditions were concealed within this collective term which has clearly outlived any usefulness it may have had.

Walton's (1956) review of 109 patients from a series of 115 previously diagnosed as amyotonia congenita at the National Hospital for Nervous Diseases, Queen Square, and the Hospital for Sick Children, Great Ormond Street, between 1930 and 1953, showed that 56 had died and 55 of these had infantile spinal muscular atrophy. In 12 survivors the same diagnosis was made. The second largest diagnostic group was of 17 surviving patients with a similar clinical picture of initial hypotonia and gradual improvement; 8 of these had recovered completely while 9 had some residual weakness. Walton proposed the term 'benign hypotonia' for this group, and the name *benign congenital hypotonia* came into use for such cases with a favourable course over the next 12 or 15 years. History has repeated itself, however, since increasing refinement of diagnostic methods has caused this category also to shrink progressively, as various forms of histologically and histochemically identifiable congenital myopathy have been identified. Dubowitz (1969) found that many children who had been diagnosed by him as 'benign hypotonia' later turned out to be examples of the Prader-Willi syndrome (hypotonia-obesity). He believed the term would eventually disappear from our nomenclature, and suggested the alternative 'essential hypotonia' to indicate our ignorance of the basic cause.

CLINICAL ASSESSMENT OF THE HYPOTONIC INFANT AND YOUNGER CHILD

In the infant and younger child the methods of examination described for the newborn baby (Ch. 1) can be used with slight modifications. The assessment of tone by studying its effect on posture at rest, on spontaneous and provoked movement, and on posture under different conditions of gravity is usually at least as valuable as its assessment by the more conventional method of passively moving the limbs through a range of movement. The infant or child who is very hypotonic will often lie in the supine position in the so-called 'frog posture', with his hips abducted and externally rotated. He has also been aptly compared to a rag doll, in that he tends to flop and to lie in whatever position he is placed. Ventral suspension, with the child supported by a hand beneath his chest, allows the degree of head and limb control and curvature of the trunk to be easily assessed. A grossly hypotonic infant will dangle limply like an inverted U, whereas the normal term infant will hold his head at an angle of 45 degrees or less above the horizontal, and hold his back straight or only slightly flexed and his elbows and knees flexed. Even the premature infant will show some degree of postural tone which will depend on the length of gestation. In the supine position the traction response (Ch. 1) allows the degree of head lag to be assessed, and also the extent to which the pectoral girdle muscles fix the shoulders.

The basic question to be decided when dealing with a hypotonic infant is whether he is weak as well as hypotonic, or merely hypotonic. In the first category, of paralytic conditions with incidental hypotonia, are the many neuromuscular disorders affecting the lower motor neuron, neuromuscular junction or muscle fibre which concern us in this chapter. In the second or non-paralytic category the causes lie in other systems or in other parts of the central nervous system. They include mental retardation and cerebral palsy at an early, pre-hypertonic stage of its evolution.

An assessment of the strength of the infant's limbs can usually be made while observing his posture at rest and in different positions. Often the child will spontaneously move his limbs against gravity. If he does not he can usually be encouraged to do so by a gentle stimulus, which usually does not need to be painful, to his feet or hands. If a stronger stimulus is needed, a slightly sharpened orange stick is usually adequate and a pin should not be needed. In the older child who has achieved such milestones as sitting, crawling, taking weight on his feet or walking, the manner in which he performs these functions will give some indication of the degree of weakness. Formal assessment of strength involving active co-operation from the child can be obtained only in an older age-group, and even then more information is usually gained by observing spontaneous performance rather than manoeuvres carried out to order.

The value of the tendon reflexes is limited. Their variability in infants and young children often makes it difficult to be certain whether they are increased. In denervating diseases such as Werdnig-Hoffmann disease and peripheral neuropathy the reflexes are likely to be absent or reduced. In primary disorders of muscle, they are more likely to be preserved, but may be absent. If they are clearly exaggerated the possibility that the child is in a hypotonic stage of the evolution of cerebral palsy is increased, and this may be further strengthened by the finding of an abnormally obligatory degree of the asymmetric tonic neck reflex or an exaggerated or symmetrical Moro reflex. Fasciculation should be looked for carefully in the tongue with a bright light. It must be distinguished from the normal tremulous tongue movements of the crying child. If present it is evidence of a denervating process, usually Werdnig-Hoffmann disease. As always the spine should be examined for evidence of spina bifida and the skin for signs of neurocutaneous syndromes. Evidence of a motor or sensory level, with a flaccid paraplegia and normal or partially paralysed arms, or of a flaccid tetraplegia with normal motor cranial nerve function will suggest the possibility of spinal cord injury or of cord compression.

General examination will often give obvious clues to the situation in the non-paralytic, hypotonic infant who is mentally retarded. Down's syndrome is suggested by the characteristic facies, various dysmorphic features may suggest other syndromes of mental retardation, with or without chromosomal anomalies, and microcephaly or hydrocephalus may suggest the role of fetal infection. Choroido-retinitis, hepatosplenomegaly, rashes or cataracts may increase this suspicion.

MEASUREMENT OF MUSCLE STRENGTH IN OLDER CHILDREN

In infants and young children the assessment of muscle power is made by observing spontaneous and provoked movements. Young children who are not co-operative enough for formal assessment will often happily engage in play activities, sometimes rather aggressively, as in squeezing the doctor's fingers, pushing him away, resisting force applied to a limb by a hand in a glove puppet or similar activities.

In older, more co-operative children more formal, structured assessment is usually possible by determining the ability of muscles to act against gravity and the examiner's resistance. The Medical Research Council (MRC) Scale (Medical Research Council 1946) provides a grading system, widely used in adults, for expressing muscle strength on a zero to 5-point scale, from no contraction to normal power. Inter-observer differences are common due to the subjectiveness of the examiner's impression of the force exerted by the patient.

An attempt to overcome these problems has been made by Hosking et al (1976), who assessed muscle power in children with normal and with diseased muscle by two simple methods. In one the length of time for which the leg and the head could be held at 45° above the horizontal was measured with the child supine. In the other a myometer was used to measure the isometric strength of six muscle groups (neck flexors, shoulder abductors, wrist extensors, hip flexors, knee extensors, foot dorsiflexors). The myometer measurements were found to give reproducible results, whereas the timed performance tests, though distinguishing normal children from those with muscle disease, were not sufficiently reproducible to make the test reliable for sequential measurements.

INVESTIGATIONS IN THE VARIOUS CATEGORIES OF NEUROMUSCULAR DISEASE

Despite great advances in recent years, it must be admitted that the methods at present available for investigating neuromuscular disease are somewhat crude. There is also the problem that — as with all kinds of investigation — the facilities for and reliability of certain tests vary from one centre to another. Thus the methods of neurophysiological examination of young children, described by Dr Harris in Chapter 24, are often difficult to apply in a young and unco-operative patient, and reliable results cannot be expected from an examiner who only encounters a handful of children each year. With muscle biopsy close co-operation is needed between surgeon and laboratory, and many biopsies have been wasted through inadequate communication. There are certain advantages to the biopsy being examined by the doctor who takes it. This is perhaps simpler when a needle biopsy is performed, rather than an open biopsy.

Although various muscle enzymes may be measured, the serum creatine kinase (CK) is generally regarded as the most helpful. It tends to be elevated in primary muscle disease, particularly in the Duchenne and Becker types of muscular dystrophy, and sometimes in polymyositis and other myopathies. In many myopathies, however, it may be normal or only slightly raised, and a normal figure cannot be taken to exclude a myopathy. Occasionally raised levels are found in denervating diseases. Trauma to muscle (such as by a biopsy or injection) or vigorous exercise can result in temporary elevation of the CK and these pitfalls should obviously be avoided.

PRIMARY DISORDERS OF MUSCLE (PRIMARY MYOPATHIES)

The term 'myopathy' is applied to conditions with clinical features attributable to pathological, clinical or electrical changes in the muscle fibres or interstitial tissues of voluntary muscle, in which the abnormal muscle function is not the result of disorder of the central or peripheral nervous system. Disease of inflammatory, metabolic and endocrine origin are included in the definition.

The muscular dystrophies form a subgroup of the myopathies, but the two terms are not synonymous; all muscular dystrophies are myopathies, but the reverse is not true.

PROGRESSIVE MUSCULAR DYSTROPHY

This category includes those forms of genetically determined myopathy in which a degenerative process develops primarily in the muscle fibres themselves. The basic cause of this is still unknown. Although a metabolic defect seems likely, vascular causes and abnormalities of innervation have also been suggested.

Clinically these diseases show weakness and wasting which is usually progressive, and contractures may also occur. In some forms there may be enlargement (pseudohypertrophy) of certain muscles. The central nervous system is not usually considered to be involved, and most affected children show normal intelligence.

The muscular dystrophies can be classified as the 'pure' forms, which make up the majority, and those with associated myotonia. The former group can be subdivided according to their distribution and patterns of inheritance, which may be X-linked, autosomal recessive, or autosomal dominant, while sporadic cases are also seen.

CONGENITAL MUSCULAR DYSTROPHY

Very rarely muscular dystrophy with an autosomal recessive pattern of inheritance may have its onset in fetal life. The resulting clinical picture is one of severe weakness and hypotonia at birth (the limp and floppy baby syndrome) (Fig. 3.1) often with joint contractures. These may be mild and limited to talipes or so gross as to constitute a severe form of arthrogryposis multiplex congenita. (In its literal sense this term implies only the presence of congenital contractures at two or more joints, but it is often used for the most severe cases.) There is nothing specific about such congenital contractures which can occur in a wide variety of neuromuscular disorders, particularly myopathies, including congenital myotonic dystrophy, central core disease, and in one case of congenital myasthenia, but some

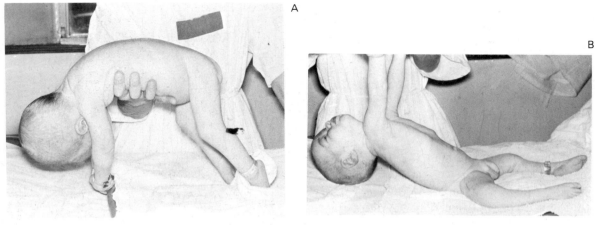

Fig. 3.1 4-week-old boy with congenital muscular dystrophy.
A. Ventral suspension.
B. Pulled to sitting. Note gross head lag and hypotonic posture of legs with external rotation.

of the grossest examples seem to have occurred in children with congenital muscular dystrophy, such as those reported by Banker et al (1957). In some cases the intrauterine onset of weakness is further attested by a history of feeble fetal movements. The weakness at birth may sometimes lead to delay in establishing independent respiration and so threaten the child's survival. Cerebral anoxia from this cause can complicate the clinical picture by adding the features of cerebral dysfunction, acute and chronic, to the neuromuscular problems. The child who survives neonatal anoxia may later show evidence of mental retardation and cerebral palsy. Contractures and spinal deformity are often troublesome (Fig. 3.2).

It has been suggested by Zellweger and his colleagues (Zellweger et al 1967a, 1967b) that congenital muscular dystrophy exists in a severe and a more benign form. These workers reported 3 personal cases of the severe variety with 28 from the literature; many of these had died in infancy and half of them by 13 years of age. The survivors, of whom the oldest was aged 10 years at the time of reporting, showed a stationary course or even slight improvement. The CK was usually normal or only slightly raised. These features contrasted with the same authors' benign group of 13 cases. In these hypotonia and slight to moderate weakness were present at birth and tended to remain stationary or to improve. In their 3 personal cases the patients all walked before the age of 2 years and

were later able to play competitive games, so that the condition did not produce a major handicap. CK levels were more often raised than in the severe form. It was reasonably suggested that the severe form at birth must represent the end-stage of an active dystrophic process starting in fetal life and not progressing further.

A Finnish series (Donner et al 1975) of 15 children with congenital muscular dystrophy suggests that the condition may be commoner in Finland than elsewhere, since these patients made up 9% of 160 cases of neuromuscular disorders seen over a 10 year period. The severity of the weakness varied. Two children died, and seven achieved independent walking at ages between three and fifteen years. All were hypotonic in the newborn period, when nine had contractures and seven had difficulty with breathing or sucking, or both. The limb weakness was more marked proximally than distally. 14 of the 15 children had a myopathic face. Five had weakness of the muscles of mastication but none had ophthalmoplegia. All were of normal intelligence. The evolution of the disease was studied by follow-up over a mean period of 4 years (1 to 15 years). It was noted that the tendon reflexes were present at first but were usually lost later. The contractures present at birth improved but there was a tendency for new contractures to appear from the second or third year onwards, especially at the hips, knees, elbows and ankles. Scoliosis developed in five patients. The CK was raised in the first one

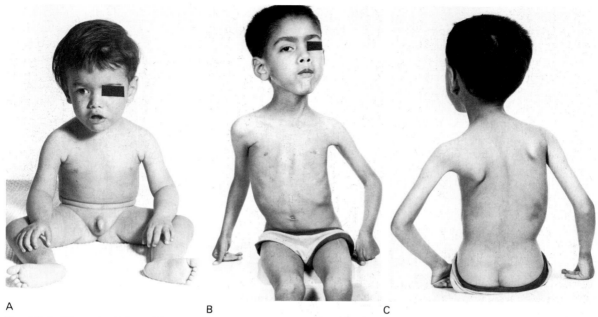

A   B   C

Fig. 3.2 A. 15-month-old boy with congenital muscular dystrophy.
B & C. Same boy, aged 6 years, showing spinal deformity and contractures.

or two years but gradually fell thereafter to normal or near normal levels.

From Finland also has come a report of a new syndrome of congenital muscular dystrophy combined with severe eye problems (retinal and/or optic hypoplasia and optic colobomas) and cerebral involvement. Santavuori et al (1977) have called this syndrome 'muscle, eye and brain disease'.

A further variety of congenital muscular dystrophy has been reported from the Middle East, in 23 members of an Arab kindred associated in 6 cases with congenital heart disease of various types (Lebenthal et al 1970).

Investigations

The electromyogram shows the changes of primary muscle disease of variable severity. The CK level may be normal or raised: in some cases it is raised initially and later falls.

Muscle biopsy, which is needed to exclude the congenital myopathies of histochemically identifiable type, such as central core disease, nemaline myopathy, etc., typically shows islands of muscle fibres surrounded by fat. The fibres are rounded and have increased endomysial connective tissue.

The changes vary in severity. In the series of Donner et al, for example, the changes were very mild in three patients while in others the appearances were of a 'burnt-out' stage, with a few atrophic and hypertrophic muscle fibres scattered in a large mass of adipose and fibrous tissue. In two patients who had a second biopsy two to three years after the first the active myopathic changes seen originally had changed to inactive type lesions, dominated by increased adipose tissue.

The differential diagnosis includes other forms of congenital myopathy and denervating diseases. The histological appearances of muscular dystrophy in the setting of a congenital myopathy make the diagnosis difficult to avoid, but occasional cases of the even rarer congenital polymyositis may cause confusion.

Congenital muscular dystrophy with cerebral involvement

Most children with congenital muscular dystrophy are free from other neurological defects, but an autosomal-recessive disease has been recognised in Japan combining the features of congenital muscular dystrophy with severe 'dysgenetic' brain pathology (Fukuyama et al 1960, Yoshioka et al 1980). In Japan the condition is known as cerebro-muscular dystrophy, Fukuyama type. At autopsy the brains of the affected children show pachygyria and microgyria of the neocortex, 'fused' frontal lobes, cerebellar microgyria and sometimes hydrocephalus.

Two siblings with this disorder have recently been reported in a Dutch family (Krijgsman et al 1980), so that it is not restricted to the Japanese.

Cases of congenital muscular dystrophy with CNS involvement have also been reported from other parts of the world. Three personal cases showing this association (Egger et al 1983) included two siblings with mild muscle disease and progressive neurological deterioration including dementia and epilepsy, and a girl with severe muscle weakness who died in her fifth year. CT showed low attenuation in the deep white matter of the cerebral hemispheres in all three cases while autopsy in the child who died showed widespread patchy demyelination of the white matter of the centrum semiovale, foci of micropolygyria and heterotopia.

DUCHENNE MUSCULAR DYSTROPHY

Duchenne de Boulogne was largely responsible for the initial separation and classification of various muscle diseases. In 1868 he described the pseudohypertrophic form of muscular dystrophy which usually affects boys. Gowers (1879) collected 220 cases and gave a clear description of the disorder with superb drawings including the procedure adopted by the patients in rising from the floor by 'climbing up their own legs', now known as Gowers' sign or manoeuvre.

The essential clinical features of the disease are an X-linked recessive mode of inheritance, onset of symptoms usually in the first three years of life, a distribution of weakness more proximal than distal and apparent earlier in the pelvic girdle than shoulder girdle muscles, and a progressive course with inability to walk by the age of 12 years and death late in the second or early in the third decade. Enlargement of calf and other muscles is usually seen, and the disease is therefore sometimes called pseudohypertrophic muscular dystrophy.

Independent walking may be achieved at the normal age or slightly later, but is almost invariably abnormal from the start. The gait is slow and awkward and the child never learns to run normally and has difficulty in climbing stairs. These problems are often regarded as unimportant and ignored for a time. They may be explained away by parents and initially by doctors as due to the normal toddler pattern of walking or to a mild orthopaedic abnormality. Many mothers, however, are quite certain there is something seriously wrong with their affected sons, but may have been reassured repeatedly that all is well since the signs, though invariably present, are at first mild enough to escape notice by the inexperienced. As he grows older the boy at a certain stage of his development is learning new motor skills at a rate which outpaces the increase in his weakness, and he is therefore thought to be improving. His parents, and sometimes his doctors, will feel reassured at this stage of spurious improvement that all will turn out well. Later increasing difficulty shown mainly by his worsening gait forces this view to be revised.

The boy walks with a waddling gait, leaning towards one side to compensate for a tendency to fall towards the side on which the foot is off the ground. He shows an exaggerated lumbar lordosis and stands straddled with feet apart to increase stability. He has difficulty in jumping and hopping and when standing on one leg, he may show Trendelenburg's sign, the hip dipping down on the side on which the foot is raised. Attempts to run produce a fast walk, reminiscent of an exhausted London to Brighton walker. Contractures of the heel cords appear early and the heels may fail to touch the floor. Rising from sitting or lying on the floor is effected by means of the manoeuvre described by Gowers; first the boy gets onto his hands and knees, and then pushes himself upright with his hands on his knees and progressively advanced upwards. (Fig. 3.3) If tables or chairs are nearby he may prefer to pull himself up with the help of these.

This pattern of stance, gait and rising is highly suggestive of Duchenne muscular dystrophy, although it can occur in any disease causing severe proximal weakness of the legs, including denervating disorders; 'all that waddles is not Duchenne', as Dubowitz has put it.

Examination of the cranial nerves is usually nor-

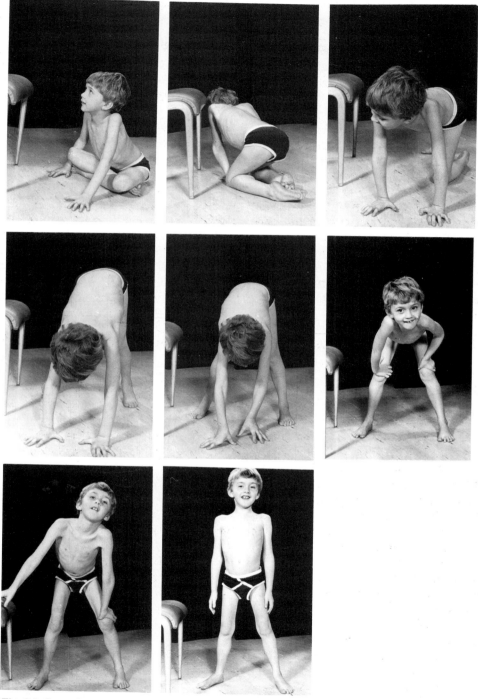

Fig. 3.3 Gowers' manoeuvre in 7½ year old boy with Duchenne dystrophy.

mal, although the muscles of mastication and the tongue may be enlarged and facial weakness may be seen at a late stage. Selective involvement of certain muscles in the upper limbs is characteristic of this form of muscular dystrophy, serratus anterior, latissimus dorsi and pectoralis major being affected early, and showing weakness and wasting before symptoms in the arms are complained of. Scapular winging may be present on pushing against resistance and the scapulae at rest may be carried more laterally than normally. The sternal heads of pectoralis major are more affected than the clavicular heads, and thus the normal lower margins of the axillary folds may be altered and appear horizontal or even show a reversal of their normal slope downwards and medially. Brachioradialis and biceps are affected slightly later; the former muscle is easily felt in the forearm when the elbow is flexed against resistance with the dorsum of the thumb upwards, and reduction in its bulk is readily detected. There may be enlargement of the deltoids and sometimes of other shoulder girdle muscles. Tendon reflexes

in the arms are often reduced early but can frequently be elicited until the weakness becomes severe.

In the legs the most striking feature is enlargement of the calf muscles. (Fig. 3.4) In the earlier stages this has an element of true muscular hypertrophy, but later is a pseudohypertrophy with fatty replacement of muscle tissue. These muscles often have a firm and rubbery feel when palpated. The large calves contrast with the thinning of the quadriceps muscles. Weakness of ankle dorsiflexion occurs early in contrast with plantar flexion which is preserved much longer, and this imbalance explains the early appearance of heel cord contractures. (Fig. 3.5) Formal testing confirms the weakness of proximal hip girdle muscles noted in the observations already made. The knee jerks are lost relatively early, but the ankle jerks remain active until a late stage, and their preservation is a useful point of distinction from denervating diseases in which they are usually lost early. The plantar responses are generally flexor, though occasional

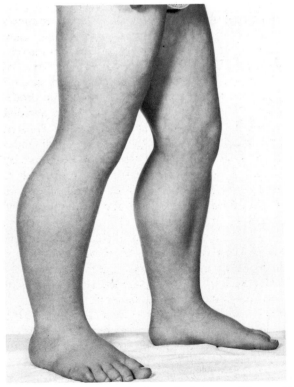
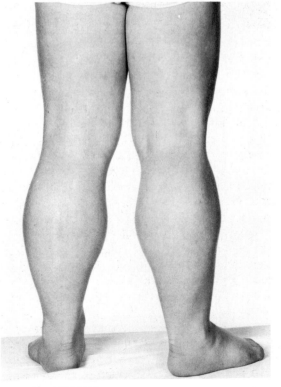

Fig. 3.4 Duchenne muscular dystrophy in boy aged 7 years. Note gross calf enlargement.

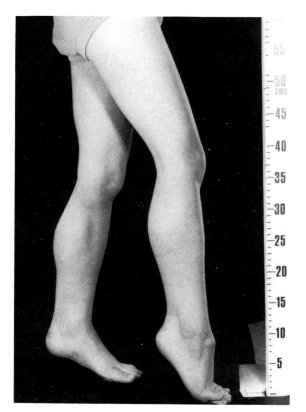

Fig. 3.5 Duchenne dystrophy in 8-year-old boy with calf enlargement and marked equinus deformity.

ligence from an early age, and it may necessitate special educational arrangements at an age when these are not yet necessary on physical grounds. Psychological assessment should be used to define the patient's intellectual status as a guide to suitable school placement.

Cardiac involvement occurs in most, and ultimately probably in all, cases of Duchenne muscular dystrophy. Symptoms and physical signs of this may not be obvious, though a persistent tachycardia is common and some patients die suddenly from myocardial failure. Congestive cardiac failure is rare, in contrast to Friedreich's ataxia. The electrocardiograph shows deep Q-waves in the limb leads and tall R-waves in the right precordial leads.

Severe skeletal deformities result from muscle imbalance and disuse. Rarefaction and narrowing of long bones are seen, with a tendency to fracture with even slight trauma, and severe scoliosis and kyphosis are commonly seen in the later stages.

The course of the disease is relentlessly progressive, even though at an earlier age the acquisition of skills may outstrip the rate of deterioration and give a false impression of improvement. Confinement to bed for medical illnesses, such as common childhood fevers or surgical interventions, may cause a rapid increase in weakness. It is not uncommon for a fracture of a leg to mark the end of independent walking. Surgical intervention should be kept to the minimum, and orthopaedic procedures to the legs in particular should be avoided while the child is still mobile. Affected children have almost always lost the ability to walk independently and become confined to wheel-chairs by the age of twelve years, and often much earlier. Attempts to maintain mobility by means of splints and calipers may succeed for one or two years, but often at a considerable cost.

When the stage of wheel-chair existence is reached, contractures inevitably increase, despite regular physiotherapy, the knees and elbows becoming fixed in flexion, and the spine commonly becomes scoliotic due to increasing weakness of spinal muscles. In time even a wheel-chair life becomes impossible, so severe are the deformities, and the remaining years or months must be spent in bed, with progressive impairment of respiration, speech and swallowing and loss of all voluntary movement except in hands, feet and face, until

extensor responses are seen and in the very late stage of gross weakness the hallux does not move at all. Sensory testing shows no abnormality.

It has been known since the time of Duchenne that intellectual retardation is common in this form of muscular dystrophy and in about one third of patients the intelligence quotient is under 75. The mean IQ has varied in different series. The mental retardation is not progressive, cannot be adequately explained by environmental limitations, and is of unknown cause. The brain showed no significant abnormality in 21 autopsied cases (Dubowitz & Crome 1969), and biochemical investigations have thrown no light on this aspect of the disease. 20 of 30 Japanese cases of Duchenne dystrophy showed slight cerebral atrophy on CT (Yoshioka et al 1980). From a practical point of view the occurrence of intellectual retardation is important, since it can result in delayed recognition of the *physical* disorder when a boy is known to be of dull intel-

death brings relief. This usually occurs by the age of 20, rarely as late as 25, and is due to chest infection with respiratory and sometimes cardiac failure.

Investigations

Since the diagnosis of Duchenne dystrophy is a death-sentence and the genetic implications are so important, there is no room for error. When a boy is seen in whom the diagnosis seems possible or likely, it must be excluded or confirmed by investigation.

The three principal investigations are the measurement of serum CK, electromyography and muscle biopsy. The main differential diagnoses to be considered are the more benign forms of spinal muscular atrophy and polymyositis.

The CK is usually normal in the former. In polymyositis it may be raised but seldom to the very high levels found in Duchenne dystrophy. The level is usually elevated even in the early and presymptomatic stages, but may fall to lower values late in the course of the disease.

The EMG shows myopathic changes in Duchenne dystrophy and often in polymyositis, but changes of denervation in spinal muscular atrophy.

These investigations are not adequate for the diagnosis in the case of a first affected child, and muscle biopsy is essential as the definitive test. The choice of muscle to be biopsied requires some thought. It is wise to avoid a muscle which has been needled for EMG purposes, as inflammatory changes may be found which could wrongly suggest polymyositis. A helpful rule is to allocate one side of the body for EMG and the other for biopsy studies. A grossly wasted muscle is not a good source for a biopsy since it may be largely replaced by fat or connective tissue and give little or no clue to the pathological process. Equally an unaffected muscle should be avoided. At the age, between 5 and 8 years, when most patients with Duchenne dystrophy are first investigated the vastus lateralis or rectus femoris muscles are usually helpful. When these are grossly wasted the biceps may be a better choice. A general anaesthetic is usually employed and is less frightening for the child, but in some circumstances local anaesthesia may be justified.

Whenever muscle biopsies are taken it is essential to use the modern approach (Dubowitz & Brooke 1973, Claireaux & Lake 1978) to examine the tissue. A wide range of special stains is needed to gain as much information as possible from the biopsy, whether it be for a patient with dystrophy, another form of myopathy or a neurogenic lesion.

The appearances in Duchenne dystrophy are not completely specific for this condition. Nonetheless, the biopsy appearances taken in conjunction with the clinical features contribute to the diagnosis. (Fig. 3.6) The degree of change sometimes bears little relation to the severity of the disorder. At a stage of appreciable weakness excessive variation of muscle fibre diameters and proliferation of endomysial connective tissue are the two main features. The numbers of centrally situated nuclei are usually only slightly increased and fibre splitting may be present although usually it is not prominent. Rounded, opaque (strongly eosinophilic) fibres are scattered throughout. Focal lesions include degenerative changes in fibres, with phagocytosis, groups of regenerating fibres and inflammatory reactions due to invasion by histiocytes. Differentiation into fibre types may not be easy using 'ATPase' preparations. Type 1 fibres predominate, as in most myopathies.

Pearson (1962) studied the histopathological features in muscle biopsies from 3 brothers with Duchenne dystrophy of different ages. That from

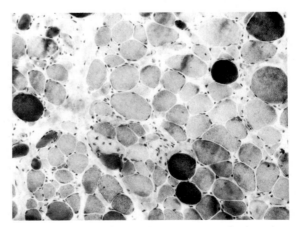

Fig. 3.6 Duchenne muscular dystrophy. Muscle biopsy showing rounded muscle fibres staining darkly (eosinophilic fibres), with a mild increase in endomysial connective tissue and only a few central nuclei. Two fibres undergoing degeneration with invading histiocytes are present.

the youngest, aged 10 months, who had no weakness, showed only moderate variation in muscle fibre diameter and minimal, and in places moderate, increase in interstitial connective tissue. In a boy of 3 years and 4 months with mild weakness present for 6 months the biopsy showed marked changes, with variation in fibre diameter and intensity of staining, fibre regeneration, increase in perimysial and endomysial connective tissue and minimal or no increase in fat. A 5-year-old boy with moderately advanced dystrophy showed typical changes in his biopsy.

Management

The basic biochemical defect in Duchenne and other forms of muscular dystrophy is still unknown, and there is no clear rationale for any basic form of treatment. Various therapeutic measures have been tried and found useless, often after premature claims for their success have raised hopes high only to be dashed when the passage of time has shown them to be unfounded. Recent enthusiastic claims for treatment with allopurinol, for example, (Thomson & Smith 1976) have been unsupported by the findings of other workers (Kulakowski et al 1981).

This lack of a basic effective therapy (a lack which it is hoped will one day be remedied as a result of the continuing interest in and research into Duchenne dystrophy) should not be allowed to induce a laissez-faire attitude towards the sufferers. There are several important points about management which should be borne in mind from the moment of diagnosis.

Obesity should be avoided at all costs, and patterns of healthy eating and exercise should be established from an early age. Mobility is likely to be lost earlier in those who are overweight than those who are spare. This may require strict dietary discipline and sometimes involve the whole family, since fat parents often have fat children.

In some boys with Duchenne dystrophy walking ('ambulation') can be prolonged and the wheelchair stage postponed for a few years by a combination of tenotomies and full-length calipers. The usefulness of the latter has been increased by the introduction of new light-weight materials. Opinion on the value of these methods in general is divided however, and only relatively few clinics use them. Gardner-Medwin (1979b) has reviewed the arguments for and against the aggressive approach to prolonging walking and believes that provision of a well-chosen wheelchair, electrically-powered if necessary, may give a boy much more practical independent mobility than does 'bracing for ambulation' and allow him to concentrate on other objectives — educational, hobbies and travel — in which he can continue to succeed at a less high cost. Nonetheless the question should be seriously considered and discussed with parents, and patient, in advance of ceasing independent walking. The basis of surgery for this purpose is Achilles and ilio-tibial tenotomy to correct, and prevent, contractures. It must be done quickly and with the simplest techniques to minimize the dangerous period of post-operative immobilization. Expert anaesthesia is needed in view of the risks of cardiac dysrhythmia and post-operative respiratory failure. The calipers must extend from the boots to the buttocks, and the boy should actually sit on top of them while walking.

The prevention of deformities, particularly of the spine, is of major importance and should be carefully planned for in advance. Helpful guidance is given by Bossingham et al (1977). Once a deformity has developed it is difficult or impossible to correct it, and prevention is clearly preferable whenever feasible. Boys with Duchenne dystrophy may spend half or more of their life-span in the wheel-chair phase, which follows loss of independent walking at or around the end of the first decade. Their wheel-chair existence should be as comfortable as it can be made and they should remain independent of outside help for as long as possible.

Hip flexion contractures can be delayed by regular movement of the hip joints by physiotherapist and parents while the patient is still walking, but usually become progressively worse after confinement to a wheel-chair.

The problems of the spinal deformity were investigated by Gibson & Wilkins (1975) who analysed the pattern of deformity in 62 patients. They noted five patterns of the spine ranging from the early stage of a straight spine to two alternative final stages. One of these was of gross deformity with a severe lateral curve often with axial rotation of the pelvis and spine. These grotesque deformities render nursing and all activities very difficult. The other end-stage was of a straight or hyper-extended spine with little pelvic obliquity or lateral curve. This posture is vastly preferable to the alternative severe deformity, and is compatible with a better quality of life and relative well-being. Surgical stabilization of the spine by fusion has generally given disappointing results, and Gibson and Wilkins believe that spinal bracing to maintain the spine in hyperextension with the patient seated gives the best hope of achieving the preferred pattern. Kyphosis must be avoided, since in this position the posterior facet joints of the spine open up and facilitate lateral bending and rotation. For unknown reasons some patients assume the hyper-extended spinal position early on in their wheel-chair existence and so protect themselves from the worst deformities. The authors advocate early bracing, when total confinement to a wheel-chair is imminent. The brace is moulded around the iliac crests and extended to the greater trochanters to stabilize the pelvis, and a pad over the thoraco-lumbar area forces the spine into extension, so that pelvis and spine act as a single unit.

Kyphosis may be encouraged if parents, at an early stage of wheel-chair existence, remove the arm supports in order to facilitate propulsion of the chair by the child, since the support given to the spine by the humeri and shoulder girdles is also thereby removed. Further temptation to remove the arm supports is given by the fact that they limit the mobility of the forearms and hands. An adjustable swivel support for the arms can be used so as to combine support and mobility. It is important to centre all the patient's activities to the front of his chair to prevent tilting to either side.

An excellent guide to the problems of 'living with muscular dystrophy' written and illustrated by Welch has been published by the Muscular Dystrophy Group of Great Britain. All parents of of affected boys and those who advise them can learn from this and be helped to plan ahead for the time when the patient will be weaker and more dependent so that difficulties can be anticipated and crises avoided. The minutiae which can make daily living easier and more comfortable are dealt with admirably, especially in relation to toiletting and dressing. For example, a urinal fitted with a non-spill adaptor is particularly useful at night when the child cannot get out of bed. Simple but effective tricks can be used in dressing; for example, in helping a child to put on his shirt an assistant passes his own hand through the shirt-sleeve to grasp the child's hand and gently pulls it into the sleeve.

The importance of the life of the intellect, spirit and imagination in these boys with progressive bodily crippling is often overlooked. Whatever their intellectual endowment their minds should be stretched and stimulated. Life for those who develop a love of reading and an abiding interest in hobbies and pastimes which do not need physical activity will be richer and fuller than for those without these assets, and the wise doctor will encourage investment in these areas at an early age. Life for these boys will be short, but it need not be brutish. 'The wonder of the world, the beauty and the power, the shapes of things, their colours, lights and shades; these I saw. Look ye also while life lasts'.

STRATEGIES FOR THE PREVENTION OF DUCHENNE MUSCULAR DYSTROPHY

Estimates of the incidence of this most frequent form of muscular dystrophy range from 1 in 3000 to 1 in 8000 male births.

There are two main approaches to the problem of prevention, the early detection of cases and, closely linked to it, the detection of carriers. Accurate genetic counselling depends on the fullest possible data on both these aspects.

The importance of these methods was shown by Gardner-Medwin (1978) in his analysis of a series of 155 cases born in the north of England in the years 1952 to 1975. Fifty-five of these might have been prevented by better carrier tracing (28 cases), better counselling (2 cases), better carrier detection methods (1 case), or by earlier diagnosis of a previously affected member of the family (24 cases). Of the 24 boys in the latter group, 15 were conceived *after* their older affected relative had developed symptoms and 9 before, so that about 15% of cases would be theoretically preventable by neonatal screening, and most of these simply by earlier clinical diagnosis. Since about 100 boys with Duchenne dystrophy are born in the United Kingdom each year, neonatal screening might in theory prevent the births of 10 to 15 cases annually on the assumption that all families identified by screening would decide thereafter not to have further children (an assumption which experience has shown is not always correct).

Detection of cases

Very high levels of CK are found in the serum of affected newborn boys and the development of a micromethod applicable to a drop of capillary blood dried on filter paper obtained for the Guthrie test for phenylketonuria (Zellweger & Antonik 1975) has made it possible to screen large populations of newborn babies at little cost. CK levels in normal newborns may be markedly raised on the first day of life but have usually fallen to lower levels by the fourth day, so that the PKU sample, if taken after the third day, is suitable for Duchenne screening (Drummond 1979). Gardner-Medwin (1979) in a discussion of neonatal screening has reviewed the results of four screening projects, from Iowa, West Germany, France and New Zealand, in which the overall incidence of 16 cases in about 56 000 males, or 1 in 3500, approximated to that in previous studies. For genetic counselling to be effective the parents of the newborn child must be told the whole truth about his prognosis, and the effects of this on the bonding process and emotional health and stability of the family may be devastating. For these and allied reasons, many authors believe that screening of total newborn populations should not be implemented until an effective treatment is found for the disease.

Effective alternative approaches to case detection at a later age are the screening by CK estimation of all boys unable to walk at 18 months of age, which might identify 50% of cases (Gardner-Medwin et al 1978) from some 15 000 annual tests, and of all boys with unexplained psychomotor delay or gait disorder in the first 5 years.

Detection of carriers

One third of all cases of Duchenne dystrophy arise as spontaneous new mutations. In these cases the mother does not carry the gene and so will not pass the disease on to further sons or the carrier state to daughters. To distinguish these cases from the commoner cases of classical X-linked recessive inheritance is clearly important. The probability that a case has arisen as a new mutation and that the mother is not at risk of passing the disease on to further children is often the only source of comfort in an otherwise unrelievedly tragic situation.

Sometimes the family history gives clear indications of X-linked inheritance when a brother or maternal uncle of a patient are affected. (See Ch. 21). A negative family history, however, cannot be taken to support or exclude the X-linked pattern or the theory of a new mutation.

Carrier status in females can be detected with a fairly high degree of accuracy. Detection depends on the occurrence of a mild degree of myopathy in most carriers, occasionally associated with muscle hypertrophy or actual weakness, but more often without clinical features. CK levels have been found to be raised in a high proportion of carriers. EMG studies and muscle biopsy seem to be less useful for carrier detection.

Very great benefits for prevention could accrue from more vigorous tracing and counselling of potential carriers of the disease. Screening of large populations of girls such as school-leavers is theoretically possible but should perhaps await the development of more reliable methods of carrier detection. At present it seems more appropriate to focus efforts on screening for carriers in families at risk with a known case of the disease. The largest group (28 patients) in the 55 theoretically preventable cases analysed by Gardner-Medwin (1978) was of cases which might have been prevented by better carrier tracing.

The problem of possible Duchenne muscular dystrophy in girls

It has been suggested that Duchenne dystrophy may occur in girls and an autosomal recessive form has been postulated. This problem has been well assessed and reviewed by Penn et al (1970) who saw 76 typical cases of Duchenne dystrophy in the decade 1957–67. Over the same period they saw 5 girls who might have been considered to have the same disease, but who all differed in some essential respect, such as late age of onset, too slow rate of progression, atypical serum enzyme pattern or conflicting EMG and histological evidence. These authors also analyzed all previous reports of Duchenne dystrophy in girls. Eighty-five cases differed from the disease in boys in important clinical characteristics and there were only 19 in whom the clinical features conformed. In none of these, however, were there adequate laboratory tests to exclude other possible diagnoses such as spinal muscular atrophy, polymyositis or chromosomal abnormality. No case was on record in which an affected girl with adequately documented Duchenne dystrophy had typically affected brothers. On the other hand Japanese workers (Hazama et al 1979) in a review of 6 young girls with muscular dystrophy concluded that in one case the clinical features of the propositus and the family history, with two affected maternal uncles and two affected nephews, supported the diagnosis of Duchenne dystrophy. It seems fair to say that such cases must be very rare, however.

THE BECKER (BENIGN X-LINKED RECESSIVE) FORM OF MUSCULAR DYSTROPHY

In about 10% of all cases of X-linked recessive muscular dystrophy the clinical condition is much milder and the prognosis better than in Duchenne dystrophy. The majority of these milder cases fit into the group described by Becker & Keiner (1955). The onset of this disorder is usually between the ages of 4 and 25 years, the progression of weakness and wasting of pelvic and later pectoral muscles gradual, and the ability to walk is not lost until 25 years or more from onset. Contractures and deformities are uncommon, and cardiac involvement is unusual. The condition is compatible with a normal life span, though some patients have died at an earlier age. Subnormal intelligence probably occurs more often than expected in the general population but not as often as in Duchenne dystrophy. The fact that most patients with the disease, unlike most of those with Duchenne dystrophy, are able to marry and have children, means that they pass on the carrier state to half their daughters and the disease to their grandsons (half

of the sons born to these carrier daughters). A history of affected but ambulant maternal uncles may point towards the diagnosis.

The enlargement of calf muscles common to both may make it difficult at an early stage to distinguish the Becker from the Duchenne type of muscular dystrophy. Often, however, the mildness of the weakness in the former results in the affected boys being regarded as merely clumsy or lazy, being the butt of their schoolfellows on the playing field and being lashed by the tongue of the gamesmaster when they are unlucky enough to attend a school where sport is a major determinant of the pecking order. It is common for the diagnosis to be delayed until the age of 10 or more when neurological referral eventually occurs and examination shows mild but unmistakable signs. Often formal testing shows little weakness, but the pattern of walking, running and stair-climbing shows evidence of mild proximal pelvic girdle weakness. This may be very mild indeed, but enough to constitute a handicap in athletics. In some cases cramp-like pains in the calf muscles on exercise are the main complaint. The course of the illness is so different from that in Duchenne dystrophy, in which walking is grossly laboured by the age of 10, if indeed it is still possible, that there is usually no difficulty in distinguishing the two diseases in older boys.

Laboratory investigations seldom help to distinguish between the two disorders, since the CK usually shows the same high levels and the EMG the same myopathic changes as are found in Duchenne dystrophy.

Similar dystrophic changes are seen in muscle biopsies in both conditions which cannot be distinguished on pathological grounds alone. However, it is said that 'the better the fibre type differentiation in the routine 'ATPase' preparations — the better the prognosis'. In addition to this some patients whose clinical features suggest Becker dystrophy have readily identifiable type 2B fibres which are hypertrophic in contast to the type 1 fibres which are of approximately normal size.

Other varieties of benign X-linked muscular dystrophy have been reported in families in which cardiac involvement, contractures and varying degrees of clinical severity were seen.

EMERY-DREIFUSS MUSCULAR DYSTROPHY

This form of relatively benign X-linked muscular dystrophy, described by Dreifuss & Hogan (1961) and by Emery & Dreifuss (1966), has been well reviewed more recently by Rowland et al (1979) The essential features are (1) inheritance consistent with X-linked recessive, (2) contractures at elbows and neck appearing early in childhood, (3) distribution of weakness with biceps and triceps affected more than scapular muscles and distal muscles in the legs affected earlier than proximal muscles, (4) very slow progression of the myopathy, and (5) cardiac conduction abnormalities appearing in all cases, leading ultimately to atrial arrest. Rowland et al believe that these clinical characteristics define a unique syndrome, although in previous cases myopathic, neurogenic or mixed patterns have been found on muscle biopsy and EMG.

The condition is distinguished from Duchenne and Becker dystrophies by the early contractures and cardiac involvement and the lack of muscle hypertrophy. It can be differentiated from the mitochondrial myopathies by the distribution of weakness, lack of ptosis, ophthalmoplegia, pigmentary retinopathy and other neurological features and by the absence of the characteristic changes on muscle biopsy.

FACIOSCAPULOHUMERAL MUSCULAR DYSTROPHY (LANDOUZY-DÉJÈRINE)

The facial involvement which is an essential feature makes this form of muscular dystrophy easy to recognise: several patterns of inheritance are seen. Most text-book descriptions refer to cases with autosomal dominant inheritance, onset after the age of 7 years, and slow progression compatible with normal longevity.

Our experience at the Hospital for Sick Children, Great Ormond Street, has been largely with sporadic cases of patients without affected siblings or parents, and with an early age of onset. The presenting feature has always been facial weakness, dating from infancy in some patients. Many children had always resented and resisted having their faces washed since, being unable to close their eyes, they could not prevent the soap from getting in. Some were noted to sleep with their eyes slightly open. Most have been unable to whistle. The facial weakness antedated any evidence of limb weakness and in one case had led to a wrong diagnosis of Moebius syndrome being made at the age of 4 years, until the onset of weakness in arms and legs two years later made it clear that the disorder was more widespread. Weakness of orbicularis ori and oculi muscles is seen, with inability fully to close the eyes or to purse the lips, a pouting expression and a transverse smile. The face may be expressionless and the immobility of the upper lip while speaking may put one in mind of the appearance of a ventriloquist's dummy and may make speech indistinct. The facial weakness, like that of the limbs, may be asymmetrical (Fig. 3.7A).

Shoulder girdle weakness usually appears before lower limb involvement. Winging and elevation of the scapulae are seen, (Fig. 3.7B) due to early involvement of serratus anterior and trapezius muscles. The scapulae ride high, especially when abduction of the arms is attempted, and they may be visible from in front of the patient. When held under the axillae the child tends to slide through the examiner's hands.

The sternal heads of the pectoralis major muscles are singled out for atrophy, often asymmetrical, producing an abnormal reversed slope to the anterior axillary folds, which point upwards towards the manubrium sterni instead of downwards towards the xiphoid process. Biceps and triceps are often more weak and wasted than the deltoid muscles. Reduction in muscle bulk in the upper arms in the later stages, contrasting with more normal bulk in the forearms, may give an appearance like that of 'Popeye, the Sailor'. Among forearm muscles brachioradialis is often selectively involved. Truncal weakness with an exaggerated lumbar lordosis may be seen. In the legs weakness of the anterior tibial group may occur early causing footdrop and a flapping gait with tightness of the heel cords and inability to get the heels to the ground. Weakness of pelvic and thigh muscles may be a later feature. The tendon reflexes are usually preserved until the stage of severe weakness. Enlargement of muscles and cardiomyopathy are rare, and

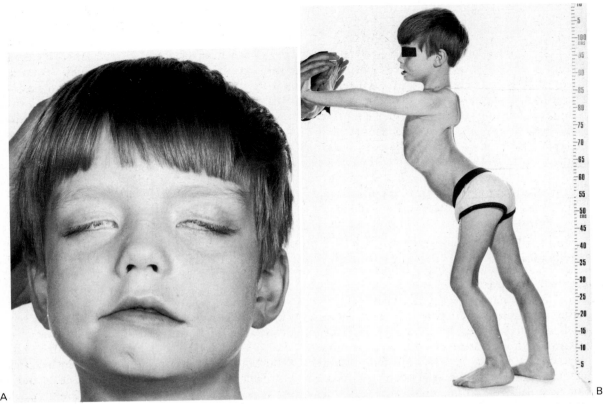

Fig. 3.7 A. Facioscapulohumeral muscular dystrophy in 6 year old boy. Note weakness of eye closure and asymmetrical facial weakness.
B. same patient showing winging of scapulae.

the range of intelligence is normal.

In the sporadic cases described with early onset the rate of progression of weakness is rapid with severe spinal deformity in some cases and a poor prognosis. In cases with onset in the second decade or later the condition is often benign, the patients remaining mobile and active for many years. Episodes of remission with no increase in weakness for periods of up to several years may occur. When two or more siblings are affected, the rate of progression tends to be similar, but some variation may be seen.

The same considerations about maintaining activity, avoiding obesity and preventing deformity apply to this form of muscular dystrophy as to the Duchenne variety.

The CK is often raised, but not usually to the high levels found in Duchenne dystrophy. Myopathic changes are seen on EMG, and muscle biopsies show changes of varying severity.

The changes in the biopsies from younger children with facioscapulohumeral dystrophy are often severe with very marked endomysial fibrosis, surrounding atrophic and grossly hypertrophic fibres. Inflammatory reactions are common (Fig. 3.8). The general appearance, with apparent group atrophy, is reminiscent of the changes found in denervation but the degree of fibrosis is against this. The older patients show much milder pathology with general fibre hypertrophy, foci of inflammatory cells and scattered small angular fibres.

LIMB-GIRDLE MUSCULAR DYSTROPHY

This is an unsatisfactory and heterogeneous group, since this condition has probably been over-diagnosed in the past. Many patients previously so

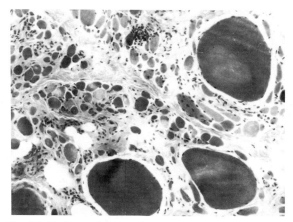

Fig. 3.8 Facioscapulohumeral muscular dystrophy. Muscle biopsy showing marked variation in fibre diameter, increased connective tissue and collections of inflammatory cells. HE × 83

diagnosed have been shown on review to suffer from denervating diseases, particularly the more benign forms of chronic spinal muscular atrophy. Some patients with polymyositis have also been wrongly placed in this diagnostic group.

Genuine cases of limb-girdle dystrophy may be classified as to whether the pelvic or pectoral girdle is predominantly affected. In the former case one sees the pelvi-femoral (or classical Leyden-Moebius) type of dystrophy. The clinical picture closely resembles that of the Kugelberg-Welander syndrome, of some cases of Becker type muscular dystrophy and some cases of congenital myopathy. The scapulo-humeral form, with involvement mainly of pectoral girdle muscles, is less common and may also be difficult to distinguish from denervating diseases.

Recessive, sporadic or dominant forms of inheritance are reported. The age of onset is very variable, and is said to be usually in the second decade. In our experience at the Hospital for Sick Children, Great Ormond Street, the onset has been in the first decade and often in the first five years. The distribution of weakness, whether mainly in pelvic or pectoral girdles, determines the presenting symptoms and clinical picture. Symptoms may resemble those of the Duchenne and Becker dystrophies and be intermediate between them is severity. There may be hypertrophy of calf muscles and vastus lateralis and less often of the deltoids. In the scapulo-humeral form, the muscles affected

early are serratus anterior, trapezii, rhomboids, latissimus dorsi and the sternal heads of pectoralis major. Asymmetry in weakness and wasting are common. Facial weakness is not seen. Tendon reflexes may be lost early, but the ankle jerks are usually retained until a late stage. Cardiac involvement and mental retardation are rare.

Careful thought and investigation are needed before the diagnosis of limb-girdle muscular dystrophy is accepted in a child, since it has so often proved to be wrong in the past.

The CK may not be very helpful since it may not be markedly raised. EMG and nerve conduction studies should allow denervating disorders to be distinguished. Muscle biopsy shows fibre hypertrophy with splitting and increased endomysial connective tissue. Occasional foci of degeneration and regeneration may be seen.

SCAPULOPERONEAL MUSCULAR DYSTROPHY

A syndrome of scapuloperoneal dystrophy has been described by Davidenkow (1939) and more recently by Meadows & Marsden (1969) which appears to be a variant of Charcot-Marie-Tooth disease. A similar clinical picture has been reported by Kaeser (1965) as a form of spinal muscular atrophy. Less often the same features may occur as the result of a progressive muscular dystrophy with no evidence of denervation.

This was the situation in the case of a 9-year-old Arab boy, product of a consanguineous marriage, who developed weakness of the hands. He showed no facial weakness, but had marked weakness of neck flexion, gross wasting of shoulder girdle muscles and upper arms, and marked proximal weakness in both arms. In the legs there was great reduction in muscle bulk below the knees, and gross weakness in the same distribution, especially in dorsiflexion. Proximal muscle bulk and power were more normal. Tendon reflexes were reduced in the arms and at the knees. The CK was raised. The EMG showed myopathic changes in rectus femoris and tibialis anterior with no signs of denervation. Nerve conduction studies were normal. A muscle biopsy from the left quadriceps muscle showed the changes of a muscular dystrophy. It seems reasonable to regard such cases as distinct from facioscapulohumeral muscular dystrophy.

'Ocular muscular dystrophies'

Cases with ocular myopathy or progressive external ophthalmoplegia sometimes associated with more widespread weakness and with other neurological features were regarded in the past as due to a form of muscular dystrophy. Their nosological position has recently been called in question by the demonstration of mitochondrial and other abnormalities in muscle biopsies and their classification and clinical features are discussed later.

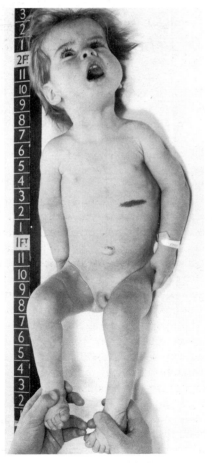

Fig. 3.9 Dystrophia myotonica, 17-month-old boy (the naevus is unrelated.)

MYOTONIC DISORDERS

Myotonia implies the continued active contraction of a muscle persisting after cessation of voluntary effort or stimulation. Clinically the phenomenon is detected by slowness in relaxation of the grip or, as percussion myotonia, by persistent dimpling of a muscle belly such as the thenar eminence or tongue after it has been tapped sharply. The degree of severity determines whether it is complained of as a symptom or merely noted as a sign. In some patients (such as the mildly affected mothers with dystrophia myotonica whose children have the congenital form of the disease) it may be so mild as to be unnoticed, whereas in others it may constitute a disabling symptom in its own right. Orbicularis oculi is often affected, and after closing the eyes the patient has great difficulty in opening them again. The upper eyelids may rise very slowly and the child may extend his neck in an attempt to see more clearly. Ptosis and blepharophimosis may be wrongly diagnosed.

Four hereditary syndromes with myotonia are recognized in children. One of these, dystrophia myotonica, is usually classified as a form of muscular dystrophy. The others, myotonia congenita, paramyotonia congenita and the Schwartz-Jampel syndrome, are myopathies in which deterioration is often absent.

DYSTROPHIA MYOTONICA (STEINERT'S SYNDROME)

Until quite recently this form of muscular dystrophy was regarded as a disease of adolescence or adult life, with the well-known clinical features of myotonia and progressive weakness particularly affecting the face, jaw, neck and distal muscles.

In 1960 Thérèse Vanier from the Hospital for Sick Children, Great Ormond Street, reported six children with dystrophia myotonica whose symptoms dated from early infancy. Since then many series of congenital dystrophia myotonica have been reported from many parts of the world (Dodge et al 1965, Pruzanski 1966, Watters & Williams 1967, Harper & Dyken 1972, Aicardi et al 1974, Harper 1975a).

The clinical picture of the congenital form is

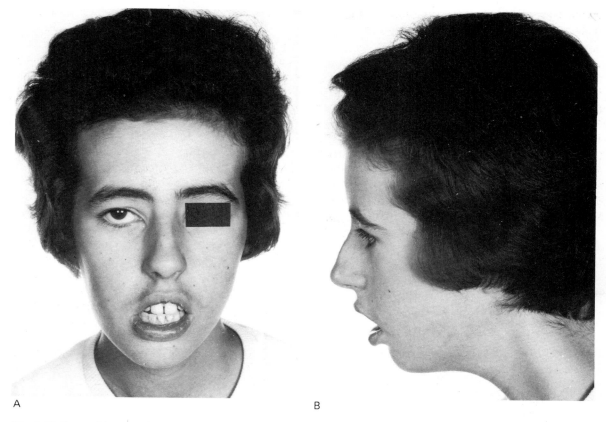

A

B

Fig. 3.10 Dystrophia myotonica, 13-year-old girl;   A. note characteristic face   B. characteristic profile.

striking and quite distinct from the acquired variety. Hypotonia is one of the major features and the disease often presents as the 'limp and floppy baby syndrome'. Myotonia is not detectable at birth and usually not until some years later. Facial diplegia is common and probably invariable, the children having a flat, immobile face, with an open, triangular mouth. (Figs. 3.9 and 3.10) Talipes, congenital dislocation of the hips and other joint deformities are common.

Respiratory problems are frequent. Often there is delay in establishing adequate respiration after birth. In some cases apnoeic or cyanotic attacks occur. Feeding difficulties are common. Death may occur in the newborn period, and there is often a history of neonatal deaths in siblings, suggesting that these infants too may have been affected. The diaphragm may be abnormally high, suggesting eventration.

The presence of congenital talipes and other joint deformities implies onset in utero. This is supported by two other factors commonly noted, the observation by the mother of reduced fetal movements and the occurrence of hydramnios, perhaps explained by a neuromuscular failure in swallowing by the fetus in utero, evidence for which was found by Dunn & Dierker (1973) by intra-amniotic injection of contrast medium.

The severity of the motor deficit in congenital dystrophia myotonica varies and within a sibship one child may be severely and another only mildly affected. Hypotonia, weakness and poor muscle bulk are present in varying degrees. The tendon reflexes may be normal or reduced. Although myotonia may sometimes be seen in infancy in orbicularis oculi when the child blinks or closes his eyes in response to a bright light, myotonia of grasp and on percussion of muscle bellies can rarely be shown in younger patients, and seldom causes symptoms until an older age. In a series of 11 children seen recently at the Hospital for Sick Children, Great Ormond Street, symptomatic myotonia was present in only one patient under the age of 9 years, a girl who had had difficulty in releasing grip from the age of 2 years with severe myotonia from the age of 5, when her mother had to help her to alight from a bus, as she was unable to let go of the rail. Clinically the facial weakness is the most striking feature in younger children: the expressionless face and triangular mouth with tented upper and droopy lower lip, give all affected children a resemblance to one another far greater than to their normal siblings. (The tented upper lip has been shown to persist unchanged over many years of follow-up.)

Although the facial appearance suggests mental retardation this is by no means invariable. The mean IQ of 21 patients collected by Harper (1975a) was 61.1, but 7 of 11 patients in a personal series had intelligence in the normal range, 3 of them with IQs over 100. Psychological assessment is essential in order to avoid the false imputation of mental subnormality.

When the disease is suspected in a child confirmation must be sought from the family history, and the parents must be examined. In the great majority of cases the mother is the affected parent and shows clear evidence of involvement, even though she is often unaware of symptoms or aware only of slight difficulty in releasing her grip in cold weather. (Fig. 3.11) Clinical and electrical myotonia can be shown. With the EMG myotonia is usually readily detected in the extensor muscles of the forearm. There is weakness of eye and mouth closure and sometimes distal limb weakness and wasting. Dyken & Harper (1973) have drawn attention to the pursed appearance of the lips in the affected mothers. The reason why the affected parent is almost always the mother and not the father is debated; one theory is that a maternal intra-uterine effect causes the early development of symptoms in offspring who inherit the disease; another is that affected men are less likely to beget children than are affected women to become mothers. The condition in the affected mothers is usually mild with intelligence in the normal range and it conforms to

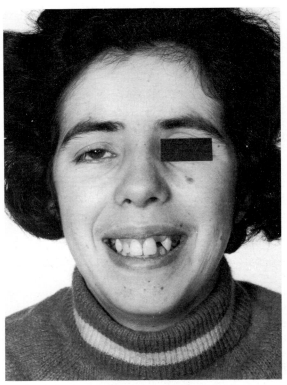

Fig. 3.11 Dystrophia myotonica, mother of patient in Figure 3.9.

the adult pattern of the disease. Often, the affected mother has mildly affected sisters who also have congenitally affected children. A study of the family photograph album can be most rewarding. In the preceding generation the affected grandparent may be either mother or father, and the same is true in earlier generations. There is an impression that in previous generations the disorder may show only minimal expression, often with pre-senile cataract as the only obvious stigma, although a history of diabetes mellitus and hypothyroidism is common. The progressive increase in severity in the three generations is striking.

Differential diagnosis

This includes the many disorders which can underlie the floppy baby syndrome. The facial appearance, the presence of talipes and other joint deformities and recognition of dystrophia myotonica in the mother distinguish the condition from others. In the newborn period apnoeic attacks and feeding difficulties may lead to an incorrect diagnosis of severe congenital heart disease or tracheo-oesophageal fistula, with referral to surgical units. When the diagnosis in the mother is known there should be no difficulty in detecting the disease in the infant. It is advisable for women known to have the disease to have their babies in hospital with full facilities for dealing with respiratory problems.

When there is obvious clinical myotonia other disorders in which this features must be considered. These include myotonia congenita and the Schwartz-Jampel syndrome which differ sufficiently from dystrophia myotonia to be easily distinguished.

In older children a variety of disorders may be wrongly diagnosed. The mean age at diagnosis in 11 children first diagnosed at the Hospital for Sick Children, Great Ormond Street, was 7 years, and other diagnoses previously made had included cerebral palsy (3 cases), Moebius' syndrome (3), Charcot-Marie-Tooth disease (1) and facioscapulohumeral muscular dystrophy (1). In another case school difficulties had caused referral to a Child Guidance Clinic without a physical ailment being recognised.

Investigation

In younger children the most fruitful investigation is electromyography of the affected mother to confirm myotonia. The CK in the mother is usually moderately raised.

The CK in affected children varies: It was within normal limits in most patients in a personal series and moderately raised in two.

Electromyography may show myotonia in affected children even when it is absent clinically, but the absence of electrical myotonia does not exclude the diagnosis in younger children.

Immunoglobulin studies have shown increased catabolism of IgG, and abnormalities of insulin secretion have also been reported.

X-rays of the skull may show hyperostosis of the vault, especially in the frontal bones, and a small sella. X-rays of the limbs may show the distal bones to be slender and muscle bulk reduced. Chest X-rays sometimes show that one dome of the diaphragm is raised.

Muscle biopsy

Congenital myotonic dystrophy is characterised by the presence of small type 1 fibres (hypotrophy) and type 2 fibres which may be hypertrophic. At the young age at which the diagnosis is required the muscle fibres are generally small and slight differences may not be readily apparent. Biopsy of the biceps is said to show the hypotrophy of type 1 fibres to the best advantage. Karpati et al (1973) have shown excessive acid phosphatase activity within muscle fibres from such patients and this apparently specific feature may be helpful in distinguishing this condition from congenital fibre type disproportion or atypical forms of lower motor neuron disorders.

The older patients show markedly increased numbers of central nuclei, not only in the small type 1 fibres but also in the other fibres. Ring fibres, once thought to be a diagnostic feature of myotonic dystrophy, are usually common but are found in many other chronic myopathic disorders.

Prognosis

This depends on the degree of physical and intellectual handicap, which is very variable. As in cerebral palsy, good intelligence may largely compensate for physical difficulties and severe mental retardation may grossly limit the potential of a child with a mild motor deficit.

Although the textbook account of the prognosis in patients with adult onset is one of steady deterioration, it is not yet possible to generalize with regard to the outlook in the congenital form of dystrophia myotonica. In the 70 cases studied by Harper (1975a) only 4 deaths were known to have occurred, of which 3 were in the first year of life. No patient in his study had failed to walk or was in a wheelchair, and most parents of older children reported a steady improvement in their first decade, but later a gradual increase in weakness and wasting, with the appearance of myotonia. Most children have needed special education, usually in schools for the physically-handicapped, or educationally subnormal (moderate). More severely retarded children have needed schools appropriate for their intellectual level. A few with normal intelligence and mild physical defect have coped in ordinary schools.

Treatment

Symptomatic relief for myotonia, when it becomes troublesome, can often be obtained by the use of drugs such as procaine amide and diphenylhydantoin. These have no effect on the weakness. Physiotherapy and judicious orthopaedic surgery can be helpful. Careful assessment of intellectual and physical status is needed in planning for appropriate school placement.

OTHER SYNDROMES WITH MYOTONIA

MYOTONIA CONGENITA (THOMSEN'S DISEASE)

There can be no disputing the eponym for this disorder which was first described by the Danish physician, Julius Thomsen (1876) who himself suffered from it as did members of four generations of his family. Myotonia is the major feature, both as symptom and sign, and the weakness, intellectual and endocrine abnormalities seen in dystrophia myotonica do not occur.

Symptoms often date from infancy when difficulty in opening the eyes after closure on crying or sneezing may be noticed and there may be feeding difficulties and a 'strangled' cry. They may, however, be delayed until later in the first or second decade, with difficulty in releasing grip and in initiating sudden movements. The child may find difficulty in starting to run or walk briskly and his movements remind the observer of a slow-motion film. Usually the myotonia decreases with continued activity, so that he can increase his rate of running to normal and gradually 'work off' the slowness in relaxing his grip. Attempting sudden movements may induce 'intention myotonia' which can cause the child to fall. The myotonia, as in other myotonic disorders, is usually made worse by cold, Myotonia causes delay in eye-opening after strong closure (Fig. 3.12A).

Myotonic lid-lag is sometimes present. When the patient is asked to look upwards at an object held by the examiner and then to follow it downwards, the upper lids are seen to lag behind the movements of the eyeballs instead of accompanying them smoothly on their downward journey (Fig. 3.12B).

Diffuse hypertrophy of muscles is often found which persists throughout life, though the myotonia often shows a gradual diminution. Weakness of the muscles is sometimes found.

The disorder is classically inherited as an autosomal dominant trait, but autosomal recessive inheritance has been reported by Becker (1961) in Germany and by Harper & Johnston (1972) in Britain and may be commoner than is recognised. The parents of affected children should be carefully examined for myotonia as well as questioned since they may be unaware of the symptom or its significance. In the recessive form of the disease the onset of myotonia is often later and it may be more widespread and severe and more often associated with weakness than in the dominant type. In the latter aggravation of myotonia by cold is commoner than in the recessive cases.

The diagnosis is a clinical one, based on a careful history and examination. (One should pay attention to what mothers say; they are often right and have often been wrongly reassured or even ridiculed for reporting what they have observed). The EMG is used as a confirmatory investigation on the patient and the affected parent (who may be either father or mother) to demonstrate electrical myotonia. The CK is often normal.

Muscle biopsy shows only minor non-specific changes with occasional central nuclei and some scattered atrophic fibres. Crews et al (1976) suggested that type 2B fibres are absent, but further studies showed that the abnormal 2B population which they reported was a normal phenomenon in the muscle sampled.

Malignant hyperpyrexia has been reported in one patient with dominantly inherited myotonia congenita.

PARAMYOTONIA CONGENITA

This dominantly inherited disorder, whose nosological status has been much debated since its first description by Eulenberg (1886), combines myotonia with episodes of flaccid paralysis and absence of dystrophic features.

The myotonia is usually present from childhood,

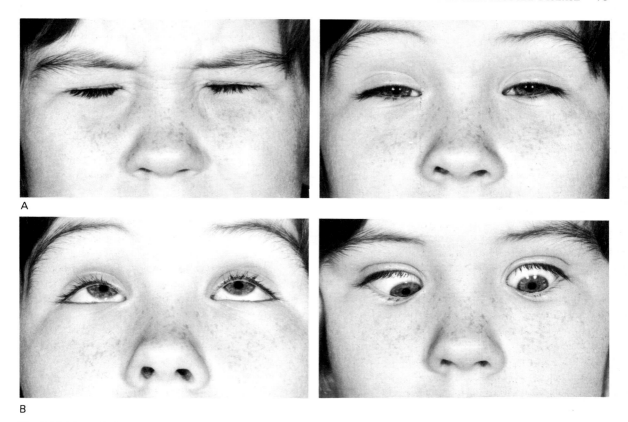

Fig. 3.12 Myotonica congenita, 7-year-old boy. A. (2) showing myotonia of eyelid closure. B (2) showing myotonic lid-lag.

is increased by cold and is described as paradoxical, in that it tends to increase with exercise rather than the reverse. Muscle hypertrophy is present in many patients, some of whom despite this show persistent weakness. A relationship to hyperkalaemic periodic paralysis has been suggested but not proved.

Muscle biopsies from 6 patients in one kindred (Thrush et al 1972) showed marked variation in fibre diameters, and partial or complete loss of differentiation into fibre types.

PERIODIC PARALYSIS

In these rare disorders episodes of periodic, transient paralysis occur with loss of tendon reflexes and of electrical excitability. Three genetic categories have been defined according to the levels of serum potassium found in the attacks, hypoka-laemic, hyperkalaemic and normokalaemic (Pearson 1964). The condition is usually transmitted as an autosomal dominant.

In hypokalaemic periodic paralysis the attacks are often provoked by a large carbohydrate meal and by rest after vigorous exercise. In Europe and the United States the disorder is commoner in males than in females. In Japan the same sex difference is seen in adults but among children the sexes are equally affected.

Treatment of the acute attack with oral or, if necessary, intravenous potassium is usually successful. Prevention involves a diet high in potassium and low in sodium and carbohydrate with potassium salts at night.

Hyperkalaemic periodic paralysis, or adynamia episodica hereditaria, also shows dominant inheritance with brief episodes of weakness starting in the first decade and associated with a rise in serum potassium. Gamstorp (1956) reviewed 68 cases of this disorder and found the attacks lasted about one hour and occurred about once a week. Mytonia can sometimes be found and a relationship to paramytonia has been suggested.

In the normokalaemic variety the attacks of weakness may last several days and are not associated with any change in the level of serum potassium.

THE SCHWARTZ-JAMPEL SYNDROME (CHONDRODYSTROPHIC MYOTONIA)

Though the first report was probably that of Catel (1951), this rare recessively inherited syndrome is usually known by the names of Schwartz and Jampel who described it in 1962. It includes a characteristic facial appearance, a generalized myopathy with marked myotonia and skeletal features. Short stature, joint contractures amounting to arthrogryposis, kyphoscoliosis and pectus carinatum are common in reported cases. Intelligence is normal. The face has a pinched appearance giving an impression of sadness, but shows no actual weakness. Eyelid myotonia is present, so that the eyes are often almost shut, and a false impression of blepharophimosis or blepharospasm is given. Myotonia of the orbicularis oris is responsible for the pinched appearance of the mouth. Myotonia of handgrip and on thenar muscle percussion are present. Mild to moderate weakness of limb muscles and some reduction in tendon reflexes have been reported among the 15 cases reported in the literature.

EMG studies confirm myotonia, which has been found as early as seven months of age. The CK is usually normal. Muscle biopsies have shown only slight, variable and non-specific changes histologically. Biopsies from two children reported by Fowler et al (1974) showed hypertrophy of type II fibres and occasional mild focal atrophy of type I fibres, with changes in succinate dehydrogenase and acetylcholinesterase activity. This may present a retarded, embryonic stage of muscle development, associated with increased sensitivity to acetylcholine, which might lead to continuous muscle fibre activity. The EMG findings in these two patients appeared to differ from classical myotonia in that high frequency discharges were seen on muscle

sampling, which did not wax and wane, and electrical silence of the muscles was never obtained, even under general anaesthesia. Clinically the myotonia behaves as it does in other myotonic disorders, although the degree of facial involvement is unusually severe and it is this which produces the striking facial appearance.

Management of the condition includes orthopaedic connection of talipes and other joint deformities and symptomatic treatment of myotonia with procaine amide or diphenylhydantoin when it is severe.

The differential diagnosis includes other diseases with myotonia and the Morquio-Brailsford form of mucopolysaccharidosis. The facial appearance bears a slight resemblance to that of the whistling face (Sheldon-Freeman) syndrome, but the two conditions can be readily distinguished.

CONGENITAL DISORDER RESEMBLING THE STIFF-MAN SYNDROME (HEREDITARY STIFF BABY SYNDROME)

The stiff-man syndrome is a bizarre, sporadic disorder affecting adults, but a similar rare condition with an hereditary basis has been reported in children. Klein et al (1972) and Sander et al (1979) have described 36 patients in four families.

The main clinical features are similar to those of the sporadic stiff-man syndrome, with attacks of stiffness precipitated by surprise or minor physical contact and with difficulty in making sudden movements as in running. The EMG shows the same features also with continuous electrical activity at rest and normal action potentials. This disappears when diazepam is given. The condition differs from the adult disorder in that the clinical manifestations are milder and are present at or soon after birth. Several children have been born by Caesarean section because stiffness prevented vaginal delivery. Others only became stiff some hours after birth. The initial extreme rigidity decreases in the first day of life but resistance to passive movement of the limbs persists, gradually disappearing over the first few years. Difficulty in swallowing and choking episodes may occur in the first year. Sudden spasms of stiffness occur when the patients are startled and with sudden contact or movement, often causing them to fall down. All the affected children are awkward and clumsy in their movements. Some are made worse by cold.

By 3 years of age muscle tone has become almost normal, but in some cases mild stiffness reappears in adolescence or adult life and spasms may again be provoked by startle.

The condition must be distinguished from other causes of neonatal hypertonia, such as tetany, tetanus, the Schwartz-Jampel syndrome, phenothiazine toxicity, and severe perinatal asphyxia. The clinical and EMG features, together with the relief of both given by diazepam, allow the diagnosis to be made.

The pattern of inheritance seems to be autosomal or X-linked dominant. Very few cases of non-familial stiff-man syndrome have been reported in children (Sander et al 1979).

CONGENITAL MYOPATHIES WITH SPECIFIC HISTOLOGICAL AND HISTOCHEMICAL FEATURES

A variety of congenital myopathies, previously undreamed of, have been recognised by the use of careful histological and histochemical examination of muscle biopsies from patients previously undiagnosed or included within the histological ragbag of 'benign congenital hypotonia' or its ancestor, 'amyotonia congenita'.

In general these disorders are present at birth (and indeed prenatally) even though they may not develop their pathological hallmark until later life and their diagnosis may therefore be delayed. Most are relatively benign and non-progressive, though there are exceptions among them. Joint contractures and arthrogrypotic features may occur, as in any neuromuscular disease of early onset. Evidence of denervation is generally absent. The inheritance usually shows an autosomal dominant pattern, though sporadic cases are seen. The affected parent may deny symptoms and show only mild signs, so that careful examination may be needed to detect abnormality. Affected siblings usually show a similar degree of abnormality, but exceptions are seen in some families.

The clinical features of these disorders are similar, with variations on the theme of weakness,

muscle wasting, hypotonia, delayed motor development and joint contractures. There are no pathognomonic clinical features, so that although the diagnosis may be suspected clinically it must be confirmed by muscle biopsy. In some cases the muscle enzymes and EMG are normal.

The diseases are named from the appearances of the muscle biopsy. This pathological nomenclature of clinical disorders is necessary in view of the lack of other distinctive features.

CENTRAL CORE DISEASE

This condition was recognised in 1956 by Shy & Magee as a 'new congenital non-progressive myopathy'. Five patients in three generations of one family were affected, showing hypotonia, delayed motor development and mild non-progressive weakness. (Fig. 3.13)

The disorder is inherited as an autosomal dominant and the affected parent may be unaware of weakness or have accepted a mild degree of weakness as 'just one of those things'. It is therefore important to examine both parents carefully. The condition may present as 'the limp and floppy baby syndrome' and congenital talipes, kyphoscoliosis and hip dislocation may occur, as in other congenital myopathies. The severity of involvement may vary from one affected sibling to another. This was well shown by one family with all four children affected in which the first born, a girl, (Fig. 3.14) had severe scoliosis, chest deformity and a vital capacity of only 250 ml at the age of 11 years, whereas the three younger children (Fig. 3.15) were only mildly affected (Brett et al 1974).Their father showed mild weakness of facial and shoulder girdle muscles but was able to work as a gardener.

Routinely stained sections from muscle biopsies show very little apart from a hint of amorphous-looking areas in some fibres. These areas are only visible to the keen eye and are best demonstrated with methods to show mitochondrial enzyme activity or phophorylase activity. (Fig. 3.16) These 'central cores' show loss of mitochondria and hence the mitochondrial enzyme methods show these areas as devoid of activity. The cores are not necessarily central but may be peripheral, single or multiple. Some confusion can be caused with 'tar-

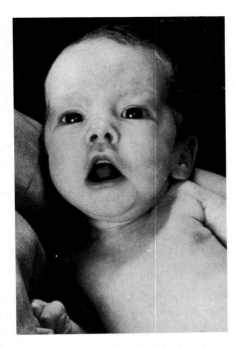

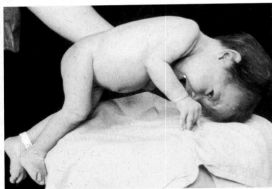

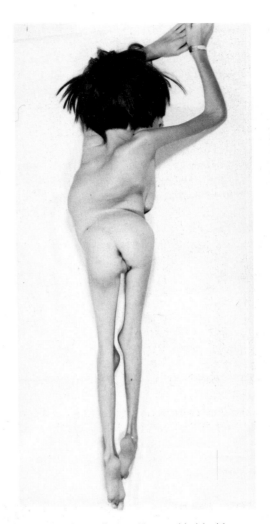

Fig. 3.14 Central core disease. 10-year-old girl with severe kyphoscoliosis, contractures and gross muscle wasting.

Fig. 3.13 Central core disease. 10-week-old girl.
A. Face. Note myopathic appearance.
B. Ventral suspension.

get fibres' found in denervation and some authors prefer the term 'core-targetoid fibre' to underline the difficulty in distinguishing these two features. Most cases show type 1 fibre predominance.

The number of cores does not correlate with the clinical severity of the condition; this is well illustrated by the family mentioned above (Figs. 3.14 and 3.15). The diagnostic central cores were abundant in the father's muscle biopsy but were absent in biopsies from two of his affected children and present in only about 12% of the muscle fibres in

the girl, who later died from respiratory insufficiency.

MYOPATHY WITH MINICORES (MULTICORE DISEASE)

Two children with a non-progressive myopathy with lesions resembling those of central core disease, but smaller and more abundant, were reported by Engel and his colleagues (1971) under the title *Multicore Disease*. The term 'minicore' was preferred by Currie et al (1974). It prevents confusion with central core disease in which multiple cores are often found, and emphasises the fact that the changes on electron microscopy, with distortion and irregularity of Z-lines, are shorter in extent than in the latter condition.

The clinical picture is a rather non-specific one with moderate non-progressive weakness, more marked proximally, hypotonia and hyporeflexia. Facial weakness is present in about half the reported cases (Lake et al 1977). Intelligence is usually normal. The CK is generally normal and EMG abnormalities are minimal.

NEMALINE OR ROD-BODY MYOPATHY

Thread-like bodies in the muscle biopsy of a 4-year-old girl with a congenital myopathy, who had graduated from being a floppy infant to a moderately weak child, led Shy and his colleagues (1963) to dub it nemaline myopathy, from the Greek word for a thread. Later reports have shown that some patients are more severely affected than others. Reported cases have shown dominant inheritance or sporadic occurrence. Reduction in muscle bulk is often a striking feature.

Many patients show 'dysmorphic' skeletal features, such as pigeon-chest, kyphoscoliosis, pes cavus, high arched palate and a long face with prognathic jaw, which are rather reminiscent of Marfan's syndrome. (Fig. 3.17) Such features may suggest the diagnosis, which can only be established, however, by muscle biopsy.

The pathological hallmark of this disorder is the presence of red-staining rod-like structures within the muscle fibres when the Gomori trichrome method is applied. (Plate 1) These rods may be numerous, apparently filling the whole fibre, or may be scattered. Two main histological patterns may be seen; one in which there is type 1 fibre predominance and uniformity of fibre size; and one in which there are two distinct populations of fibre sizes appearing not unlike fibre type disproportion. Patients presenting in the early months of life with hypotonia and respiratory problems usually die with fulminating pneumonia before the first birthday.

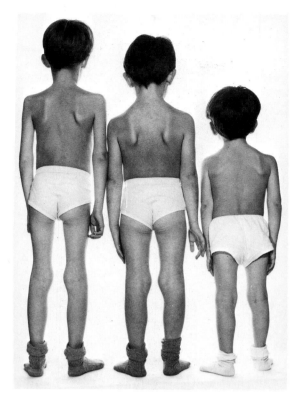

Fig. 3.15 Central core disease. 3 brothers of the above patient, aged 8, 6 and 4 years, with milder degree of disease.

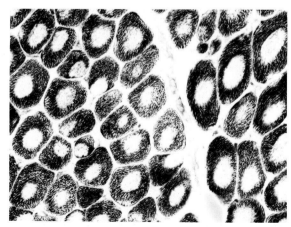

Fig. 3.16 Central core disease. A muscle biopsy stained for NADH tetrazolium reductase activity shows central (and peripheral) areas devoid of activity. These areas are cores and show disorganized ultrastructure with depletion of mitochondria. NADH tetrazolium reductase × 224

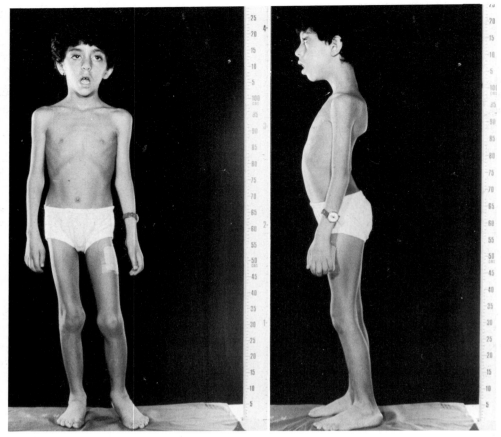

Fig. 3.17 Nemaline myopathy in 10-year-old boy. Note markedly myopathic face.

MYOTUBULAR OR CENTRONUCLEAR MYOPATHY

Spiro et al (1966), who first described this disorder in a 12-year-old boy, were impressed by the resemblance of his muscle biopsy to the myotubes of fetal muscle, and therefore suggested the name myotubular myopathy. The clinical picture in reported patients is of varying degrees of limb weakness often with ptosis and external ophthalmoplegia. The onset is most often in infancy but occasionally in later childhood, and the disorder is usually nonprogressive. There is some uncertainty as to the mode of inheritance, which may well be autosomal dominant.

By contrast in the Netherlands cases of myotubular myopathy with X-linked recessive inheritance have been recognized (Van Wijngaarden et al 1969, Barth et al 1975). In the pedigree reported by Barth et al, 13 boys died in the neonatal period from asphyxia. Poor fetal movements and hydramnios were noted in many cases, attesting the presence of the disorder prenatally. It appears that insufficient expansion of the chest in the affected infants caused their death by suffocation. Clinically the mothers of the children were normal, but myotubes, centronuclear fibres and type 1 fibre atrophy were found in the patients and in some of the female carriers. There was no evidence of anterior horn cell involvement.

CONGENITAL FIBRE TYPE DISPROPORTION

The size of type 1 and type 2 fibres in the muscles

of most normal children is roughly similar. Variations are seen in several conditions, and a histological picture with type 1 fibres smaller than type 2 seems to be associated with a specific non-progressive congenital myopathy (Brooke 1973). The presentation is with hypotonia in infancy, often with contractures and congenital dislocation of one or both hips. Weakness is variable, but has not been seen to increase after two years of age. Most reported patients have had short stature: kyphoscoliosis and foot deformities are common. Children with more severe degrees of weakness may be misdiagnosed as cases of Werdnig-Hoffmann disease and an unnecessarily gloomy prognosis may be given.

Muscle biopsy shows two populations of fibre sizes. (Fig. 3.18) The larger fibres, often longer than normal for age, have type 2 (A and B) characteristics and the smaller fibres, with normal or slightly reduced diameters, have type 1 fibre characteristics. The mean diameter of type 1 fibres is at least 12% smaller than the mean diameter of either or both of the type 2 fibres. The distribution of fibre types is normal and there are no other features in the biopsy, although moth-eaten fibres have been described. The changes are not present in every muscle and the prognosis, although usually favourable, may not be so, particularly if there

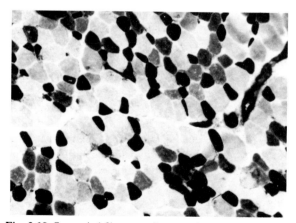

Fig. 3.18 Congenital fibre type disproportion, muscle biopsy. The only abnormality present in this histological diagnosis is the disproportion in size of the fibre types. Type 1 fibres, stained darkly, are small, while Type 2A (stained lightly) and most type 2B fibres (intermediate) are larger. There does not seem to be much correlation between the histological appearance and the clinical presentation and prognosis. Reversed ATPase × 134

is severe respiratory difficulty (Spiro et al 1977, Cavanagh et al 1979).

The differentiation of congenital fibre type disproportion from infantile myotonic dystrophy may be impossible unless the acid phosphatase activity in the latter is increased. Another difficulty which may be encountered is the very small difference in fibre diameters needed to establish the diagnosis in very young infants. A difference of as little as 2 μm in the mean diameter at 2 months of age is enough for the histological diagnosis of congenital fibre type disproportion. The spectrum of this disorder is enlarging and time will eventually allow us to decide whether, as is now suspected (Cavanagh et al 1979), it is merely a histological appearance with a variable prognosis.

THE METABOLIC MYOPATHIES

The metabolic defects which probably underlie the muscular dystrophies and the congenital myopathies described in the previous section have not yet been defined. By contrast with these, there is a small group of metabolic myopathies in which defects in glycogen or lipid metabolism or mitochondrial abnormalities have been shown.

THE GLYCOGENOSES

Muscle involvement is common in the various disorders with abnormalities of glycogen metabolism due to specific enzyme deficiencies.

In *type II glycogenosis* due to acid maltase deficiency there is widespread involvement of many tissues: skeletal muscle, heart, liver, CNS and kidneys. The clinical picture in infancy (Pompe's disease) is of severe paralysis and hypotonia, or of cardiac and respiratory symptoms. Muscle weakness is due to primary involvement of muscle and to anterior horn cell affection causing muscle weakness through denervation. When weakness is severe, the clinical picture resembles that of Werdnig-Hoffmann disease and the prognosis for survival is as poor. In some juvenile cases the myopathy is much milder and may simulate a limb girdle muscular dystrophy, with or without cardiac involvement.

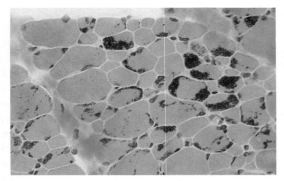

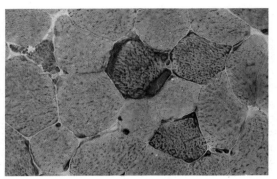

Plate 1 Muscle biopsy; nemaline myopathy. Cryostat section stained with the modified Gomori trichrome method showing numerous red/purple granular rods present in many fibres. Variation in fibre diameters is also evident

Plate2 Muscle biopsy; mitochondrial cytopathy. Cryostat section stained with the modified Gomori trichrome method showing subsarcolemmal accumulations of red-staining material which correspond to collections of abnormally structured mitochondria

A more benign disorder, *type III glycogenosis*, is associated with deficiency of the 'debranching' enzyme, amylo-1, 6-glucosidase. Muscle involvement may be absent or mild, causing some hypotonia and weakness, but hepatic problems predominate with hepatomegaly and mild hypoglycaemia. Rossignol et al (1979) have reported on three patients who had severe muscle weakness, one of whom died from cardiac involvement at $4\frac{1}{2}$ years of age.

Type V glycogenosis, due to deficiency of myophosphorylase, is eponymously named McArdle's disease and its effects are limited to skeletal muscle. McArdle in 1951 showed that blood lactic acid failed to rise in the normal way after ischaemic exercise in a man who complained of muscle cramps on exercise. Deficiency of myophosphorylase was later demonstrated. The symptoms in this condition can be classified into three groups: easy fatiguability in childhood and adolescence, cramps and weakness on exertion and transient myoglobinuria from the age of 20, and weakness and wasting of proximal muscles at a later stage. It is unusual for the diagnosis to be made until adult life, partly because the disorder is not considered and partly because muscle cramps are not common in childhood but develop later. The youngest reported patient was a 12-week-old girl, who died, described by Di Mauro & Hartlage (1978). Sengers et al (1980) have recently described the case of a 12-year-old boy who from the age of 6 had the classical features of fatiguing and muscle pain on exercise with a 'second wind phenomenon'

so that after slowing down he was able to resume walking without any difficulty. His symptoms were for a time regarded as psychogenic in origin, as with so many unusual disorders. McArdle's disease should be considered in the differential diagnosis of exercise intolerance in childhood. Some familial cases have been reported, suggesting an autosomal recessive pattern of inheritance, but a dominant and X-linked mode have also been considered. No specific treatment is yet available and it is advisable for patients to limit their activities to the degree tolerated and learn to live with the disorder.

Rather similar clinical features and failure of blood lactate to rise with ischaemic exercise are seen in *type VII glycogenosis*, associated with deficiency of the enzyme phosphofructokinase (Tarui et al 1965).

Muscle structure in Pompe's disease is severely distorted and shows massive glycogen deposition and strong acid phosphatase activity related to the lysosomal storage. (Fig. 3.19) Biopsy should not be necessary since ECG changes are considered to be fairly specific and the deposition of glycogen in lymphocytes in a peripheral blood film is almost pathognomonic (Fig. 3.20) Assay of acid maltase in cultured fibroblasts is the investigation of choice.

The milder forms of *type II glycogenosis* show less severe muscle involvement with a lesser degree of patchy glycogen deposition. Acid phosphatase activity is associated with the glycogen deposits as in the severe form.

Glycogen deposition in McArdle's disease may

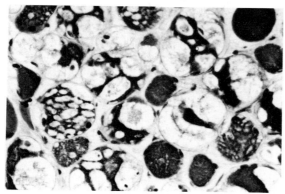

Fig. 3.19 Glycogenosis type II: juvenile. Marked vacuolar changes are present in a muscle biopsy from a 7-year-old boy presenting with 'a muscular dystrophy'. The vacuoles are filled with glycogen.
HE × 208

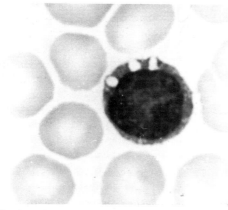

Fig. 3.20 Pompe's disease (GSD II). Peripheral lymphocytes show small discrete cytoplasmic vacuoles which can be shown to contain glycogen.
MGG × 1920

not be marked and only the total lack of skeletal muscle phosphorylase in histochemical preparations is diagnostic. Smooth muscle phosphorylase (in blood vessel walls) is preserved.

MYOPATHIES WITH MITOCHONDRIAL AND LIPID ABNORMALITIES

Mitochondrial cytopathy

Various myopathies have recently been recognized in which muscle biopsy has shown striking abnormalities of mitochondria and lipid, alone or in combination.

The most dramatic of these conditions is a clinicopathological syndrome first described by Kearns & Sayre (1958) and variously known as oculocraniosomatic neuromuscular disease with 'ragged-red fibres' (Olson et al 1972), Kearns & Sayre's ophthalmoplegia, and 'ophthalmoplegia plus'. Many cases previously regarded as 'ocular muscular dystrophy' were probably examples of this or related conditions. Most examples were thought to be sporadic but two affected brothers have been reported (Schnitzler & Robinson 1979). Progressive external ophthalmoplegia, which can occur in other diseases, is seen as the cardinal feature of this disorder in association with short stature, ptosis and with a wide variety of other neurological abnormalities. These include retinitis pigmentosa, ataxia, sensorineural deafness, mental retardation and muscle weakness in the limbs. Defects of cardiac conduction, sometimes necessitating an artificial pacemaker, impaired growth and raised CSF protein are often present. In most reported cases the onset has been in childhood as early as 6 years of age, but in some cases in the third or fourth decades. The earliest symptoms to be noticed apart from short stature are usually ocular; either gradually progressive ptosis (Fig. 3.21) and external ocular palsy or visual loss due to pigmentary retinopathy may be the presenting defects. Limb weakness and reduction of tendon reflexes may be mild.

Biopsy of skeletal muscle in such cases shows the characteristic 'ragged red' fibres in the trichrome preparations which indicate mitochondrial disturbances (Plate 2). These fibres show strong mitochondrial enzyme activity (succinate dehydrogenase) and with the electron microscope abnormal intramitochondrial inclusions can be found, Lipid and glycogen may also be prominent in these fibres. The presence of these distinctive features is not pathognomonic for 'ophthalmoplegia plus', as it is sometimes called, since they have been described in several other myopathic conditions. They are sometimes referred to as 'myopathies with abnormal mitochondria'. Although the term 'ocular dystrophy' has been used, there is rarely any dystrophic process and 'myopathy' is the preferred term.

The more widespread nature of the condition has recently been emphasised by Egger et al (1981) who

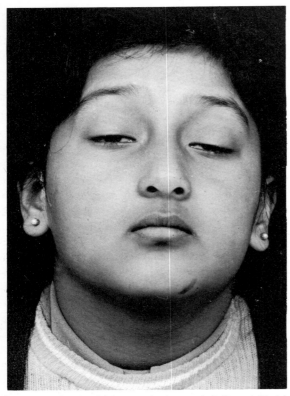

Fig. 3.21 Mitochondrial cytopathy (myopathy). 9-year-old girl with ptosis.

have described it as a multisystem disorder with 'ragged red fibres' on muscle biopsy and have suggested the term 'mitochondrial cytopathy'. These authors have stressed the varied clinical picture in their 13 patients, with short stature as the usual presenting feature and with a wide variety of neurological features, as well as involvement of the heart, gastro-intestinal tract, endocrine organs and kidneys, occurring in different combinations. The clinical spectrum in affected relatives of the 13 children varied from isolated symptoms to the complete syndrome with 'ragged red fibres' and seems to be consistent with an autosomal dominant mode of inheritance with variable expressivity. Some cases of Leigh's disease (subacute necrotizing encephalomyelopathy) (Ch. 8) may be examples of mitochondrial cytopathy (Egger et al 1981).

The radiological changes in the brain with CT have been reviewed by Egger & Kendall (1981) in 11 proven cases of mitochondrial cytopathy. Focal low density lesions were seen in the basal ganglia and white matter with cerebral atrophy which varied from slight to severe. On serial examination the changes were seen to increase. Calcification in the basal ganglia has been reported previously in this form of leucoencephalopathy, but was not seen in this series.

An apparently different condition combining abnormalities of mitochondria, lipid and glycogen was described by Jerusalem et al (1973). At the age of 7 weeks the patient was profoundly weak in all but her ocular muscles, and had hypotonia, hyporeflexia, hepatomegaly and macroglossia. A muscle biopsy at that age showed marked excess of lipid with glycogen deposits and mitochondrial abnormalities. Thereafter her motor development was delayed, but intellect was normal and her macroglossia disappeared. At 22 months of age muscle biopsy was repeated and the abnormalities were much less striking. We have seen two similar cases both with dramatic elevations of serum lactic acid. These levels gradually subsided over several weeks and the patients have progressed from extreme hypotonia and requiring tube-feeding as neonates to near normality at 2 years of age.

Muscle biopsy in these two cases showed changes identical to those in Jerusalem's case. There was marked vacuolation of muscle fibres and accumulation of deposits of fat and glycogen in the vacuoles. Many fibres also showed red staining in trichrome preparations associated with mitochondrial excesses. There was no increase in acid phosphatase activity so this disorder can be easily differentiated from Pompe's disease. Electron microscopy showed deposits of glycogen and fat among severely damaged mitochondria whose outer membranes were not intact and there was proliferation of the cristae. Virus-like particles were seen in one biopsy.

It is important to recognize this disorder since in spite of the dramatic changes in the biopsy, the patients improve and the prognosis appears good.

MYOPATHY WITH CARNITINE DEFICIENCY

A lipid storage myopathy responsive to prednisone treatment was reported by Engel & Siekert (1972) in a 19-year-old girl with progressive weakness.

Her muscle was later shown to have a very low level of carnitine, a substance intimately associated with the transport of fatty acids across the mitochondrial membrane where they undergo β-oxidation. Carnitine deficiency thus leads to a lipid storage and increased ω-oxidation causing raised excretion of dicarboxylic acids.

Since the original description, several other cases have been recorded and at least two types have been recognized: (a) systemic carnitine deficiency with low or absent liver-, serum-, and muscle-carnitine and (b) muscle-carnitine deficiency. Each type presents with muscle weakness and easy fatiguability. The recent report by Scholte et al (1979), however, casts doubt on the validity of such a distinction. The disease may also present in the newborn period with hepatomegaly and hypotonia. Such cases have a poor prognosis.

Although prednisone produced a good response in the original cases, treatment with large doses of oral carnitine has been much more encouraging.

Muscle biopsy, essential for diagnosis, shows numerous lipid droplets in type 1 fibres without other features (Fig. 3.22). Assay of the carnitine levels is important since there are other causes of lipid myopathy which have the same histological appearance.

In an allied condition the activity of one or other of the carnitine-palmityl transferases may be deficient. This condition does not cause any problems unless the patient takes strenuous exercise when muscle pain, cramps and myoglobinuria may occur. A biopsy may then show some lipid accumulation but at other times it will appear normal on microscopy.

POLYMYOSITIS AND DERMATOMYOSITIS

Dealing as they do with so many crippling neurological illnesses which they are powerless to alleviate, the paediatric neurologist and paediatrician must always be on the alert for treatable conditions. When a disorder, adequately treated, carries a better prognosis in childhood than in adult life there is strong motivation not to miss a case.

Polymyositis, on both these grounds, should be kept in mind in all cases of muscle weakness in childhood. The term covers a trinity of disorders with muscle weakness as their cardinal feature. The commonest of these is an uncomplicated polymyositis, the second a form in which polymyositis or dermatomyositis are associated with connective-tissue disorders, and the third a variety with polymyositis and malignant disease. The last is apparently not seen in childhood, and the second type is not common. The aetiology in the common simple form is uncertain, but the frequent occurrence of viral infections of various kinds shortly before the onset suggests an immunological mechanism with delayed hypersensitivity.

In most cases of polymyositis the onset of symptoms is in adult life, but in 17% of cases in several collected series the onset was under the age of 15 years. Very rarely it is congenital causing hypotonia and weakness in the newborn period (Walton 1956). An excess of girls over boys is present in most reported series.

The presentation is usually subacute in childhood, but may be acute or chronic and insidious. Weakness often starts in the proximal leg muscles and may be acute or subacute in onset. It may also involve shoulder girdle muscles. Its distribution is often asymmetrical, but when symmetrical may simulate a limb-girdle form of muscular dystrophy. (Fig. 3.23) Distal muscles may also be involved and a common presentation is with calf muscle involvement causing contractures and toe-walking. (Fig. 3.24) Pain and tenderness in the muscles may be prominent in the early stages.

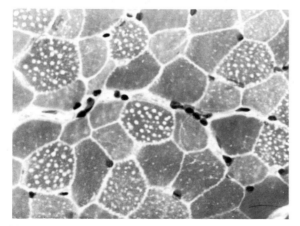

Fig. 3.22 Carnitine deficiency. Muscle biopsy showing vacuolation of some muscle fibres (Type 1 fibres) containing fat droplets. Type 2 fibres are less severely affected. HE × 301

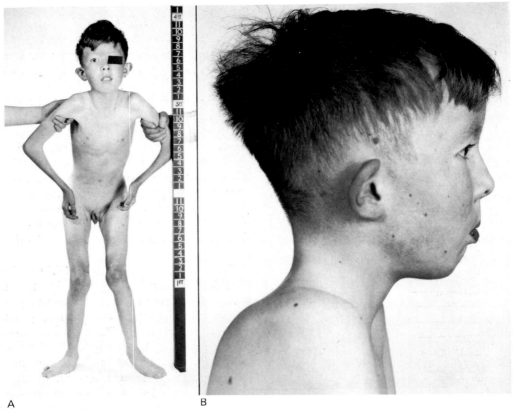

A   B

Fig. 3.23 A. Polymyositis with severe contractures and wasting in 11-year-old boy. B. Polymyositis showing fixed facial expression in same patient.

Joint pain may also be complained of, but in some cases it is difficult to decide whether pain is in muscles or joints. Fever is not uncommon. The child may appear generally unwell with anorexia and weight loss, even when afebrile, and is often very miserable indeed, so much so that his misery and apathy may prevent recognition of his weakness for a time. It may be difficult to decide whether the failure of a child to walk is a case of 'can't' or 'won't'. Co-operation in formal testing of power is unlikely, but observation of the pattern of walking, of Gowers' manoeuvre on rising from the floor, of rising from a low chair and of attempts to reach up for a proferred sweet will indicate the degree of weakness. The anterior neck muscles are often affected, causing weakness of neck flexion, which together with asymmetry of weakness when present helps to distinguish the disease from muscular dystrophy. The muscles supplied by the cra-

nial nerves are not usually affected, apart from the sternomastoids and trapezii. Tendon reflexes may be normal, but are reduced in many cases, and pyramidal and sensory signs are absent.

Lesions of the skin or subcutaneous tissue are common in various sites and the term 'dermatomyositis' is applied to these cases. Such changes were seen in 11 of the 16 patients reported by Rose (1974). There is often a dusky, erythematous, lilac-coloured rash in the butterfly area of the face, and the eyelids and periorbital skin are generally affected (Fig. 3.23). Sclerodermatous changes may be seen in the hands and arms. Calcification is sometimes seen in the skin and subcutaneous tissue in more chronic cases and may occur in extensive sheets. This calcinosis was noted in 50% of Rose's patients, both treated and untreated and in 5 of the 8 children reported by Goel & Shanks (1976), in one of whom it was decreased by treat-

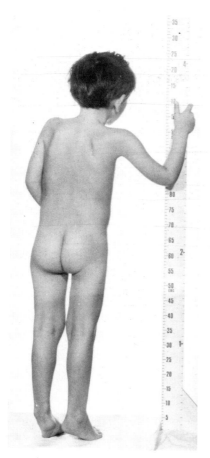

Fig. 3.24 Polymyositis. Milder case with heel cord contractures in 7-year-old boy.

ment with ethanehydroxydisphosphonate. Severe ulceration of the skin is sometimes seen in areas without calcinosis.

Dysphagia is common in adults, occurring in 29% of the mainly adult patients reported by Vignos et al (1964), but seems to be rarer in children. It was present in only two of the 16 children in Rose's series (1974).

Fluctuation in the illness may occur in untreated cases with relapses and remissions.

Investigations

The ESR may be raised to very high levels but may sometimes be normal. Muscle enzymes, particularly CK, are often but not invariably raised; their

levels are usually lower than those seen in Duchenne muscular dystrophy.

The EMG often shows a characteristic pattern of abnormality, combining myopathic features (polyphasic, short duration potentials on voluntary contraction) with spontaneous fibrillation potentials similar to those found in denervating disorders.

Confirmation of the diagnosis depends, in the opinion of most experts, on the finding of typical changes in muscle biopsy material. As always, the choice of muscle to biopsy is important. Muscles which are unaffected clinically and those with chronic fibrotic changes should be avoided. It is particularly important to avoid biopsying a muscle at the site of previous EMG needling where inflammatory changes can persist and mislead the pathologist.

Dermatomyositis presents a fairly easily recognizable pathological picture in the muscle. (Fig. 3.25) Collections of inflammatory cells are found in the muscle septa, not usually infiltrating between muscle fibres. Perifascicular atrophy may be present due to loss of capillaries at the periphery of muscle bundles. Some muscle fibres show irregular loss of enzyme staining ('moth-eaten fibres') and electron microscopy may show undulating tubular elements present in vessel endothelia. These tubular elements bear some resemblance to the paramyxovirus nucleocapsids. Inflammatory

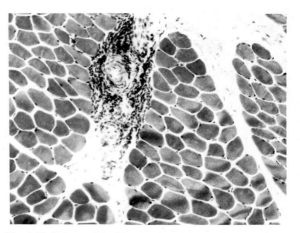

Fig. 3.25 Polymyositis. Muscle biopsy showing marked perivascular collections of inflammatory cells in the perimysium.
HE × 96

cells are present in the skin around its appendages. Unfortunately the collections of inflammatory cells and perifascicular atrophy are not always found.

Polymyositis often presents a picture of marked degenerative and regenerative changes with inflammatory changes not confined to the septa. Undulating tubules are said not to occur, but in one of our cases they were present in the endothelial cells of capillaries.

Treatment

The natural history of polymyositis has been greatly altered by corticosteroid treatment. The prognosis generally is better in younger than older patients: in Rose & Walton's series (1966) no deaths occurred in those with onset under the age of 30, whereas the mortality rose progressively in each decade thereafter. Disability in untreated children is usually greater than in those who are treated, and early treatment gives better results than delayed. In his study of 16 children with polymyositis or dermatomyositis followed up for 6 to 16 years, Rose (1974) found that most of the 10 patients treated initially with steroids in high dosage for an average of 2.5 years had only a short period of severe disability and made an excellent recovery. Three children whose treatment was delayed for 17 to 36 months after onset made a less complete, but functionally satisfactory recovery. Six patients who were never treated with steroids had a much longer period of severe disability but nonetheless made a good recovery eventually. Not all untreated patients do as well as this, however, and occasional children are seen with 'burnt-out' polymyositis who are severely crippled by joint contractures, weakness and wasting.

These good therapeutic results were probably related to the high initial doses of prednisone given, usually 60 to 80 mg per day, maintained until there was a response, or for a minimum period of 6 weeks. The response was judged clinically and by following the CK level. After clinical improvement, which often followed a fall in CK and occurred within 2 to 6 weeks, the dose of steroid was gradually reduced over two or three months to a maintenance level. This was the minimum dose which just prevented recurrence of clinical symptoms, and was usually 5 to 10 mg per day. This dose was continued for at least two years. Vigorous physiotherapy and early mobilization to prevent contractures are an important part of treatment. The natural history of the disease usually shows an active phase of two or three years duration, and the aim of treatment is to maintain mobility and independence by suppressing the severer symptoms and preventing relapses during this time. Steroid treatment has nothing to offer in patients with burnt-out disease unless they show signs of renewed activity of the disease clinically or by a rise of CK.

Long-term maintenance treatment with low doses of steroids after remission is obtained by initial high doses as described above has been the usual policy, but Dubowitz (1976) has recently suggested that there are advantages to a schedule of short-term treatment with moderate doses, gradually tapering the dose as soon as there is clinical improvement without waiting for full remission, and trying to stop the steroids when possible within 6 months. In a personal series of 8 children so treated he found this policy to be generally effective, and no cases of calcinosis were seen. He believes that prolonged steroid treatment may have been a factor in the chronicity of the disease and failure of adequate response in many reported cases. Dubowitz favours the use of other drugs such as azothioprine, cyclophosphamide or methotrexate in patients showing no response to prednisone after 4 to 6 weeks. Such immunosuppressant drugs have been advocated by other workers such as Currie & Walton (1971) when steroids are ineffective or are contra-indicated for any reason.

TRANSIENT ACUTE MYOSITIS IN CHILDHOOD

Myalgia and muscle weakness of short duration occur from time to time in children with viral upper respiratory tract infections. Complete recovery is the rule in these cases which can be easily distinguished from polymyositis. Lundberg (1957), under the title 'myalgia cruris epidemica', described 74 children with acute pain and weakness in the calf muscles and Middleton et al (1970) reported severe myositis in 26 children, many of whom had raised CK levels and evidence of infection with influenza A or B virus.

McKinlay & Mitchell (1976) reported eight cases of transient acute polymyalgia with weakness in childhood. The symptoms were symmetrical and the calf muscles were affected in all but one child. The affected muscles were tender and the children were reluctant to use them for this reason rather than because of actual weakness, which was usually assessed as MRC grade 4. Serum CK levels were raised in all cases, sometimes to very high levels, but all fell quickly to normal with clinical recovery which took place within 72 hours. Four of the children had a transient neutropenia and six had thrombocytopenia, but serological studies gave no evidence of specific virus infection. Four similar cases of benign acute childhood myositis were reported by Antony et al (1979).

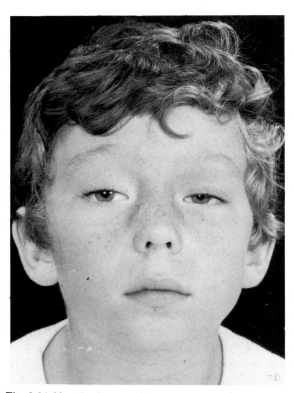

Fig. 3.26 Myasthenia gravis. 5-year-old boy with ptosis and facial weakness.

MYASTHENIA GRAVIS AND MYASTHENIC SYNDROMES

Myasthenia gravis has a prevalence of about 2 to 4 per 100 000 (Hokkanen 1969), but is much rarer than this in childhood. Only 51 of the 447 patients (11%) attending the myasthenia gravis clinic of the Massachusetts General Hospital between 1935 and 1959 developed symptoms under the age of 17 years (Millichap & Dodge 1960). Those with age of onset under 10 years make up about 4.3% of all cases.

There have been striking advances in this field in recent years. The variety of myasthenic syndromes seen in infancy and childhood is much wider than that seen in adult life. Fenichel (1978) in an excellent review has described no less than ten clinical syndromes of defective neuromuscular transmission in the paediatric age group. It is important to distinguish between myasthenia proper and the rarer myasthenic syndromes associated with other disorders. Many of the former are congenital, but the classical juvenile form will be described first.

JUVENILE OR LATE-ONSET MYASTHENIA

This is the commonest form of myasthenia in childhood and closely resembles the adult disease. The clinical picture is as variable, and can be as confusing, as in older patients. 35 of the patients in the series of Millichap & Dodge (1960) had their onset after 2 years of age, most often in the second decade of life. 53 of Bundey's (1972) patients developed symptoms after the age of two. Involvement of eye muscles and ptosis occurred in all but two of these. (Fig. 3.26) Ptosis, with or without ophthalmoplegia, was a common mode of presentation, occurring in 20 cases, but in only 3 patients, all with onset under the age of 8, did weakness remain confined to the eyes. In 18 children weakness of limbs was a presenting complaint. A slowly progressive course was usual in the early stages before treatment was started, with relapses and remissions lasting up to several months. 8 children showed an initially rapid and severe course. The onset of weakness may be insidious, but is often sudden, and sometimes seems to be precipitated by an infection or an emotional disturbance.

Recognition of the diagnosis may be delayed. All too often it has not been thought of, because it is considered a rarity in childhood. Confusion with other diseases is easy. A variable ptosis may be attributed to ophthalmoplegic migraine; if there is a history of a recent virus infection a mild encephalitis may be postulated. The very variability of the weakness and fatiguability of muscles, which are diagnostic features of the disease, may be misinterpreted as due to conversion hysteria or other psychological disorder especially if symptoms begin soon after an emotional upset. An expressionless face in a myasthenic patient may be attributed to depression. When weakness comes on soon after an infection, as commonly happens, polyneuritis or even poliomyelitis may be suspected. External ophthalmoplegia in such cases may suggest the Miller-Fisher syndrome.

A few cases of late-onset myasthenia with a limb-girdle distribution of weakness in adolescence have been reported (Fenichel 1978) as perhaps representing a specific variety with probable autosomal recessive inheritance.

CONGENITAL FORMS OF MYASTHENIA

Four syndromes of congenital myasthenia are now recognized, two of which are much rarer than the others.

1. Transient neonatal myasthenia

This rare category is of practical concern mainly to the neonatologist but is of great interest. It was probably first recognized by Stickroot et al (1942) who reported the case of a myasthenic mother whose newborn infant developed generalized weakness on the third day of life and died on the seventh day from respiratory failure. The condition has since been reported many times and affects about one in seven of the live-born children of myasthenic mothers. Surviving children recover completely within a few weeks and do not relapse, the disorder being a transient one, possibly due to an immune reaction between the infant's muscles and a placentally transmitted maternal antibody. The severity of the infant's symptoms shows no correlation with the severity or duration of his mother's myasthenia. Previous thymectomy in the mother does not prevent the condition from developing in her newborn baby. In the severest cases the infant is so weak and hypotonic that he cannot feed and respiration and survival are in jeopardy. Treatment is needed urgently with neostigmine or pyridostigmine to overcome these problems. Tube-feeding may be necessary and assisted respiration is occasionally needed. In the two cases reported by Stern et al (1964) treatment was required for 47 and 40 days, after which the babies were normal. It is important for women with myasthenia to be delivered in hospital with facilities for the supportive care and specific treatment of their affected infants, who are in a similar vulnerable position to that of the babies of women with dystrophia myotonica.

2. Congenital persistent myasthenia

In contrast to the transient cases of neonatal myasthenia in the offspring of myasthenic mothers are children of normal mothers who show mild but persisting weakness from the newborn period. There were 6 such cases among the 51 in the series of Millichap & Dodge (1960). The main presenting features are ptosis, a weak cry and generalized weakness. The ptosis persists and the children are often found later to have an external ophthalmoplegia which has probably been present in the newborn period but overlooked. Limb weakness does not usually persist, and weakness of bulbar and respiratory muscles is not common or severe in contrast to the later onset form of childhood myasthenia. The diagnosis in such cases may be long delayed and the fact that the ptosis and ophthalmoplegia tend to be unresponsive to treatment with cholinergic drugs often leads to a mistaken diagnosis of congenital ptosis or ocular myopathy. The mildness of the condition in some patients makes the suffix 'gravis' seem inappropriate, and one feels tempted to speak of 'myasthenia mitis'.

In milder cases abnormality may escape detection in the newborn period and the condition may be congenital in some patients in whom it is only recognized after some months or even years. Bundey (1972), in a genetic study of infantile and juvenile myasthenia gravis based on four London hospitals, distinguished between an early-onset form (5 patients) with symptoms starting under two years of age, in which the illness was milder but more persistent and often associated with myasthenia in siblings, and a late onset group (53 patients) with onset between 2 and 20 years of age which clinically resembles adult myasthenia and is associated with auto-immunity and an increased incidence of thyroid disorders. In the early onset myasthenic syndrome there is no detectable antibody to acetylcholine receptors in contrast to the acquired form (Newsom-Davis et al 1978), and immunological methods of treatment and plasma exchange are of no avail.

3. Familial infantile myasthenia

This term has been applied to a small number of cases of congenital myasthenia which seem to show autosomal recessive inheritance. The mothers of these children are normal but their siblings may be affected. The onset is with severe respiratory and feeding difficulties at birth, and episodes of hypotonia and apnoea, sometimes provoked by intercurrent infections, may be a major problem, sometimes requiring respiratory assistance. In this regard and also in the absence of involvement of the extra-ocular muscles this syndrome differs from the milder congenital persistent form of myasthenia described above. There is also a tendency to spontaneous remission. The patient reported by Robertson and his colleagues (1980) had no further apnoeic attacks after 23 months of age and later remained well apart from easy fatiguability and generalized weakness, most marked proximally, after exercise. A case of congenital myasthenia with decreased fetal movements and arthrogryposis multiplex congenita (Smit & Barth 1980) may have been an example of this condition.

The severe respiratory problems make diagnosis and treatment of these cases very important. The condition may account for some cases of the 'sudden infant death syndrome' and perhaps also for some cases of unexplained respiratory distress.

4. Acetylcholinesterase deficiency

Engel and his colleagues (1977) have reported one case of this myasthenic syndrome with end-plate acetylcholinesterase deficiency, small nerve terminals and reduced acetylcholine release. A 5-day-old boy was noted to have ptosis which improved after sleeping. Acetylcholinesterase treatment was ineffective.

MYASTHENIC SYNDROMES

The Eaton-Lambert syndrome, a defect in neuromuscular transmission in association with malignant tumours, particularly bronchial carcinoma, is well recognized in adults. There is only one documented report in a child (Shapira et al 1974). This concerned a 10-year-old boy who developed a myasthenic syndrome and was later found to have leukaemia.

Myasthenic syndromes have also been reported in a girl who later developed a rapidly progressive form of systemic lupus erythematosus (Hackett et al 1974) and in another girl with juvenile rheumatoid arthritis (Aarli et al 1975).

A myasthenic syndrome has also been noted in previously well patients receiving antibiotics (as distinct from exacerbation of pre-existing myasthenia by antibiotics). In the review by McQuillen et al (1968) of 23 cases of antibiotic-induced myasthenia from the literature 8 of these had their onset under 10 years of age, and 2 were aged one and two days. In 7 cases neomycin was the antibiotic involved and in one case streptomycin. The onset of weakness was usually immediately after surgery, performed for a variety of indications.

Infantile botulism (Ch. 22), which is associated with severe weakness and hypotonia, is caused by in vitro production of botulinus toxin which interferes with neuromuscular transmission.

Diagnosis

Once the diagnosis of myasthenia has been considered it is usually easily confirmed. The most helpful investigation is generally a therapeutic test with cholinergic drugs to confirm that the weakness is of myasthenic type. Edrophonium chloride (Tensilon) is best used for this, a small dose being given preferably intravenously. A dose of 0.1 ml (1 mg) may be used in an infant and a larger dose in older children up to the adult dose of 1 ml (10 mg). Unfortunately the results can sometimes be difficult to interpret in some young and unco-operative children. If ptosis or external ophthalmoplegia is the main feature the response can be difficult to judge in a crying child. It may be necessary to set up an intravenous infusion with saline, wait until the child has settled down and then inject the dose into the set. Sometimes an intramuscular injection of neostigmine may be more helpful with a more delayed but prolonged result than with the intravenous route which usually produces improvement in half to one minute. The Tensilon test is also useful in treated patients in distinguishing between myasthenic weakness from undertreatment and cholinergic weakness from over-treatment. It is possible for some muscles to be 'overdosed' and others 'underdosed'. Thus in severely affected patients it is important to test respiratory and bulbar muscles carefully, lest these be 'overdosed' and dangerously weakened, rather than the less important ocular muscles.

Since thymomas are common in older myasthenic patients, though rare under the age of 30 (Schultz & Schwab 1971) it is advisable to arrange for tomographic radiographs of the chest in children to avoid missing an occasional tumour.

Neurophysiological investigations may show a decrement in the amplitude of muscle action potentials in response to repeated nerve stimulation which disappears after a dose of Tensilon. In young children this rather painful procedure may be poorly tolerated, and their cooperation cannot be counted on for the recording of action potentials from individual muscle fibres within a single motor unit to show the presence of neuromuscular block at individual junctions. (See Ch. 24).

Treatment

Medical treatment is aimed at overcoming the defect in neuromuscular transmission which underlies the weakness and fatiguability of myasthenia. Anticholinesterase drugs are used to increase the effectiveness of acetycholine by inhibiting the enzyme cholinesterase which normally destroys it rapidly at the neuromuscular junction.

Neostigmine bromide or Progstigmine is used for its relatively short-term effect, lasting about 3 hours. The drug, supplied in 15 mg tablets, has a fairly rapid action but its effect may also wear off rapidly, so that the longer acting Pyridostigmine bromide or Mestinon, which also has a smoother absorption from the gut, is often preferred. The 60 mg tablets are equivalent to the 15 mg tablets of Neostigmine. The dose and timing required must be assessed by careful observation. When bulbar weakness and dysphagia are a problem a dose should be taken half an hour before meal times. In severe cases differential weakness of various muscles makes management difficult, since some muscles may be overtreated and others undertreated. A careful watch must be kept for weakness of respiratory and bulbar muscles which can be dangerous.

Neuromuscular transmission may be impaired by several antibiotic drugs, including streptomycin, gentamicin, kanamycin, viomycin, polymyxin and colistin. These should be avoided or used with great caution. Care should also be taken for the same reason with curare, quinine, quinidine, and procainamide. Barbiturates, morphine and chloropramine in large doses may also be dangerous.

A possible immunological basis for myasthenia has been suggested by its association with other immune disorders (mainly in adults) and by the finding of similar changes in the thymus glands of patients to those seen in the thyroid gland in Hashimoto's disease. Antibodies to skeletal muscle are found in many patients with myasthenia, and in the vast majority of those with thymomas. Such considerations have led to attempts at treatment with immunosuppressive drugs, which have been disappointing (Rowland 1971), and with ACTH and cortical steroids. Short courses of ACTH in high doses are often followed by a remission, but severe deterioration often occurs during the course and may necessitate assisted respiration. Improvement is usually short-lived, so that repeated courses have been needed, but in some adult patients remission has been maintained by a single weekly injection of 100 units after an intensive course. Encouraging results have also been obtained with oral prednisone in high doses given on alternate days in order to decrease side-effects.

Thymectomy has been used in the treatment of myasthenia for many years. Most reported cases have been in adults. In patients without thymomas remission can be expected in about 50%. In one large series (Papatestas et al 1971) the time of onset of remission was directly related to the activity of the germinal centres in the removed thymus glands. The percentage of patients in remission increased with each post-operative year, and 90% followed up for five years or more were in remission or had shown improvement. Sex, age and duration of symptoms did not markedly affect this trend. There were only 4 patients under the age of 10 years in the 111 non-thymomatous cases. Few childhood cases have been reported. Among these is a series of 14 patients treated by thymectomy under the age of 20 (Fonkalsrud et al 1970). Their average age at operation was 13.3 years and average duration of symptoms $2\frac{1}{2}$ years. Only 2 patients, both aged 19, were found to have thymomas. Significant objective improvement was seen in all but one case. There was only one death in the series, occurring two years after operation. Cavanagh (1980) has reviewed the role of thymectomy in childhood myasthenia, analysing 8 series which have included children. He found 38 patients who were under 15 years of age at the time of operation. The age of onset of myasthenia ranged from 2 to 15 years, and its duration from 6 months to 10 years. No thymomas were reported. Cavanagh found that it was difficult to draw any firm conclusions about the role of thymectomy in view of the inadequacy of the details given in many cases as to pre- and postoperative status, and recommended much more precise documentation. It might be suspected that the mild early onset cases would respond less well to surgery than the later onset cases, but this is not clear.

The indications for operation in myasthenia are usually taken to be an increasing need for anticholinesterase drugs and a poor response to medication. Early surgery has been said by some to give better results than delayed operation, but prolonged duration of symptoms need not be considered a contraindication (Papatestas et al 1971).

Recent evidence points to a post-synaptic defect in myasthenia gravis. Studies have shown marked simplification of the post-synaptic folds and a reduced number of funtioning acetylcholine receptors. Raised titres of antibodies to these receptors have been found in patients with acquired myasthenia, but not in the congenital (persistent) form.

In adults with myasthenia gravis plasma exchange allows the antibody titres to be lowered and an inverse relation can be shown between these titres and clinical indices of muscle strength, with a minimum time lag of two days for the clinical response. (Newsom-Davis et al 1978). So far there is little experience of plasma exchange in children with myasthenia.

DENERVATING DISEASES
THE SPINAL MUSCULAR ATROPHIES

In this group of disorders, usually but not invariably inherited as autosomal recessive characters, the basic lesion lies in the anterior horn cells of the spinal cord. It is probably related to a metabolic defect, but, as with most of the genetically determined myopathies and neuropathies, the nature of this defect is still unknown and, by the same token, no effective treatment is available. The clinical features of the spinal muscular atrophies are compounded of paralysis, hypotonia, and reduced or absent tendon reflexes, sometimes with bulbar involvement and skeletal deformities related to weakness. As with the other paralytic disorders of childhood, the picture is modified by age of onset, rate of progression, and presence and degree of respiratory and bulbar problems. At one end of the scale the presentation is as the floppy infant syndrome, and at the other as a disease which may be slowly progressive or even become arrested. In the past, examples of the more benign varieties have often masqueraded under the labels 'amyotonia congenita' and 'benign congenital hypotonia', and others have been misdiagnosed as various forms of muscular dystrophy, particularly the limb-girdle type.

The classification of the spinal muscular atrophies has been much discussed in recent years, and there is still disagreement about the position of certain cases.

SPINAL MUSCULAR ATROPHY TYPE I.
ACUTE SPINAL MUSCULAR ATROPHY:
WERDNIG-HOFFMANN DISEASE

Werdnig (1891, 1894) and Hoffmann (1893) are

usually credited with the first description of the disease which traditionally bears their names. (Gardner-Medwin (1977) has pointed out that the cases which they described were not of this type, but that the misnomer is now indelible.) Werdnig-Hoffmann disease conventionally refers to the acute, infantile variety of spinal muscular atrophy with onset in the first 6 months of life and often in prenatal life. Most cases are recessively inherited, and the incidence in the United Kingdom is one per 20 000 births (Pearn et al 1973). In a consecutive series of 76 cases of acute Werdnig-Hoffmann disease seen at the Hospital for Sick Children, Great Ormond Street (Pearn & Wilson 1973) the onset was prenatal in at least one third of cases. This was based on a history of reduced fetal movements in pregnancy or the presence of orthopaedic deformities at birth. These included deformities of wrists or feet, which were unilateral in some cases, and are attributable to imbalance between synergist and antagonist muscle groups. The infants were often hypotonic and weak at birth, and had failed to cry strongly after delivery and shown prolonged cyanosis. Feeding difficulties were sometimes prominent in the newborn period and always became severe at a later stage. Signs of the disease were present by 4 months of age in 95% of cases and delay in motor milestones was evident by 5 months of age in all. Only one of the 76 children was ever able to sit unsupported and only 20 could ever lift their heads from the bed, even momentarily. Most affected children were unable to kick off the bedclothes as normal infants do, and were seen to move their legs very little. Parents are often aware of the relative immobility of the legs compared with the arms at a stage before the arms show obvious weakness.

The clinical picture is dominated by profound hypotonia and weakness with resultant delay in motor milestones, and the presence of abnormal postures similarly determined. The infant usually lies in a characteristic frog-like position when supine with limbs abducted and flexed, and the flexed legs externally rotated so that the outer sides of the knees lie on the bed. (Fig. 3.27) When placed in a sitting position he falls forward on to his face with his spine curved, and when the examiner attempts to hold him up horizontally supported under his trunk he dangles limply like an

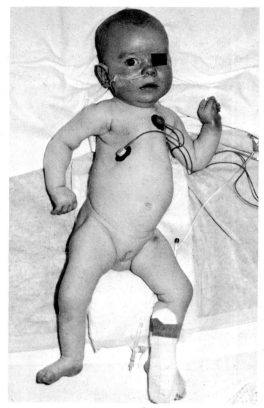

Fig. 3.27 Werdnig-Hoffmann disease. 3-month-old girl with pneumonia (note bell-shaped chest).

inverted U. When held under the axillae he tends to slide through the examiner's hands. The face is often lacking in expression with an open mouth due to facial weakness, despite an obviously normal degree of alertness and social responsiveness with a ready, if feeble, smile. The cry is often very weak. Tendon reflexes are normally absent at an early stage.

The features so far described do not distinguish Werdnig-Hoffmann disease from certain other severe paralytic disorders, including myopathies, but further examination will often show fasciculation and signs of intercostal muscle paralysis, which are almost pathognomonic. Fasciculation is usually seen best in the tongue, which is often wasted in the later stages. It should be examined with a good light, preferably when the infant is not crying, and is often made easier by the fact that the mouth is kept open spontaneously. When a spatula or tongue-depressor is inserted into the mouth it is often impossible to decide whether fasciculation is present or not. Fasciculation is usually difficult to detect in the limb muscles of young children, due to overlying fat, but may sometimes be seen in the muscles of the thenar eminence. Sometimes small-range, irregular, jerky movements of the fingers may be seen, related probably to fasciculation in the interossei. Occasionally on auscultation over the hands with a stethoscope intermittent, fine crackling noises can be heard.

Weakness of intercostal muscles is shown at first by intercostal recession as the baby cries, but later there is severe breathing difficulty, with paradoxical respiration, the abdomen bulging outwards and the ribs and intercostal spaces indrawing on inspiration due to strong action of the diaphragm. Infants with the intrauterine onset of the disease have been shown to have significantly smaller lung volumes than those with later onset (Cunningham & Stocks 1978), in keeping with the view that fetal breathing movements may be one of the main requirements for normal development of the fetal lung.

The weakness progresses inexorably until the child becomes almost immobile, though remaining watchful and alert. The progressive nature of the weakness distinguishes Werdnig-Hoffmann disease from the cases of early onset spinal muscular atrophy with a more benign course. Feeding becomes more and more difficult, and choking may occur during the course of a feed, which may take an hour or more. Tube-feeding is needed to prolong life and is usually justified, though it buys only a limited amount of time, and death from pneumonia is inevitable from a combination of respiratory inefficiency and inhalation of food. In Pearn and Wilson's series 95% of patients were dead by 18 months of age and all by 27 months, the mean life expectancy from birth being 5.9 months. The clinical course and prognosis are very similar in affected siblings, so that the history of a previously affected child provides a fairly reliable guide to his sibling's prognosis, in contrast to the more chronic forms of spinal muscular atrophy, in which differences between siblings may be much greater.

The differential diagnosis includes the more chronic and benign forms of spinal muscular atrophy, from which the 'test of time' allows distinction, and all the varied conditions which can give

rise of the floppy infant syndrome. It is particularly important to recognise the few treatable disorders such as myasthenia gravis, polymyositis and some cases of polyneuritis. The presence of fasciculation and intercostal muscle weakness are important clinical pointers. Some cases of acid maltase deficiency (Type II glycogenosis) with involvement of anterior horn cells as well as of muscle may closely simulate Werdnig-Hoffmann disease, but are much rarer.

The most helpful investigations are usually neurophysiological. Motor nerve conduction velocity is generally normal. The EMG may show a poor interference pattern. Fibrillation potentials are frequent, but not invariable. Regularly discharging motor units at 5 to 15 second intervals may often be seen at rest or with sedation (Buchthal & Olsen 1970). The CK level is usually normal. There is no cardiac involvement and the ECG shows no intrinsic abnormality, but it may nonetheless be diagnostic in cases of spinal muscular atrophy showing, as an artefact, a tremor of the baseline probably due to fasciculation in skeletal muscles (Dubowitz 1978).

Muscle biopsy should not be lightly undertaken in this disease, since general anaesthesia carries some risk for the infant and deaths have occurred following it earlier than would otherwise have been anticipated. Local anaesthesia is safer in the child with poor respiratory reserve.

At autopsy the main findings in the CNS are severe loss of large neurons from the anterior horns of the spinal cord with atrophy of anterior roots and motor nerves and severe loss of large myelinated nerve fibres.

INTERMEDIATE SPINAL MUSCULAR ATROPHY (TYPE 2)

The existence of cases of childhood spinal muscular atrophy with a more chronic and benign course and a later age of onset has been recognized for many years. Survival to later childhood or beyond, even into the second or third decades, has been reported in many series of patients (Byers & Banker 1961, Dubowitz 1964, Gamstorp 1967, Gardner-Medwin et al 1967, Munsat et al 1969, Fried & Emery 1971, Pearn et al 1973, Pearn & Wilson 1973). Fried & Emery (1971) have arbitrarily defined as the intermediate (type 2) form of spinal muscular atrophy those cases with proximal muscular weakness with onset of symptoms usually between 3 and 15 months of age, and survival beyond 4 years, often into adolescence or later. These cases certainly differ markedly from those of acute Werdnig-Hoffmann disease, defined by Pearn & Wilson (1973) as having their onset by 5 months of age and with death by 27 months, but there is still debate (Gardner-Medwin 1977) as to whether they are genetically distinct from cases with later onset sometimes associated with the names of Kugelberg & Welander (1956).

The age of onset in the more chronic forms of spinal muscular atrophy varies greatly and may differ in affected siblings, in contrast with the situation in the acute form. The onset may be very early and even prenatal, with feeble fetal movements, talipes and other skeletal deformities, and fasciculation of the tongue. Among a total of 166 cases of spinal muscular atrophy reviewed by Pearn & Wilson (1973) at the Hospital for Sick Children, Great Ormond Street, there were 18 children with chronic generalized spinal muscular atrophy, or 'arrested Werdnig-Hoffmann disease'. The median age of onset in these patients was 6 months, and their weakness was so severe that none had even achieved the ability to crawl. The life-span varied from 2 years to the third decade, and severe deformities of the spine and joints developed. In addition to 76 cases of acute fatal Werdnig-Hoffmann disease, the authors' series included 70 children with chronic spinal muscular atrophy with relatively severe proximal involvement. The age of onset and severity in this group vary, cases with earlier onset often showing more severe weakness. With onset under two years of age normal walking is seldom possible but walking may be achieved with the help of calipers. Hypotonia, weakness more proximal than distal, areflexia, and sometimes fasciculation are found in varying degrees. (Fig. 3.28) Skeletal deformities are prominent, and progressive kyphoscoliosis is a major problem (Fig. 3.29) but can often be prevented by spinal bracing. The children are vulnerable to respiratory infections which may result in death earlier than would otherwise occur. In some cases there is clearly progressive increase in weakness and disability, and in others the condition worsens more

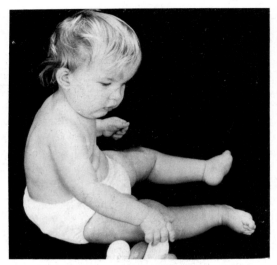

Fig. 3.28 Intermediate type spinal muscular atrophy, 17-month-old boy.

slowly so that, as with Duchenne dystrophy at an earlier stage, it may be difficult to be certain of deterioration. The affected children are of normal intelligence and may learn trick movements and methods of circumventing their weakness. They are sometimes extremely demanding and tyrannize over their parents like little potentates.

Examples of the most benign form of chronic spinal muscular atrophy are often labelled Wohlfart-Kugelberg-Welander disease, or type 3 spinal muscular atrophy. These patients develop, between the age of 2 years and adult life, slowly progressive limb weakness starting in the legs and usually with a proximal emphasis. A waddling gait is often the first symptom and Gowers' manoeuvre may be used to rise from the floor. In these and other ways the disorder may mimic muscular dystrophy, so that it has been called 'pseudomyopathic'. The condition is most often misdiagnosed as a limb-girdle muscular dystrophy. Asymmetry of muscle involvement is common. The face is rarely affected. Fasciculation can often be seen in the tongue and other muscles, but is not invariable.

The variability in the ages of onset and severity of weakness in siblings with the more chronic forms of spinal muscular atrophy make decisions based on these factors of doubtful value. Genetically also the situation is less clear-cut than with acute Werdnig-Hoffmann disease. Bundey and

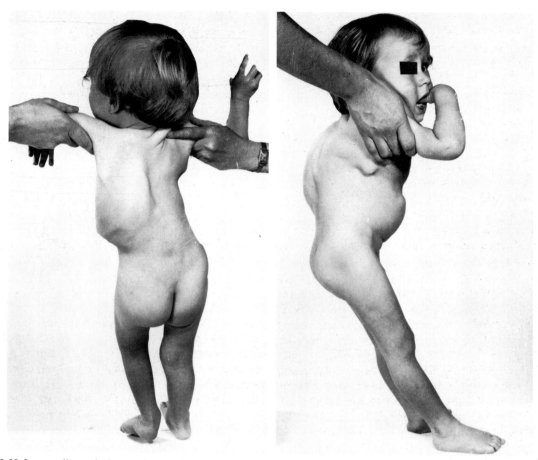

Fig. 3.29 Intermediate spinal muscular atrophy, 22-month-old boy with severe spinal deformity.

Lovelace (1975) in a study of 33 patients with onset in infancy or childhood found that the siblings of those with onset before 2 years showed an incidence of disease of 1 in 5, due to most patients having an autosomal recessive disorder. By contrast, among the families of patients with onset *after* 2 years, the incidence in sibs was only 1 in 15, and among their children it was 1 in 8. Thus both autosomal recessive and autosomal dominant forms occurred in this age group, but it seemed likely that nearly half of those with onset after 2 had non-genetic disease.

Investigations in the more chronic forms of spinal muscular atrophy give similar results to those in the acute form, but slowing of motor nerve conduction velocity is sometimes found, and the EMG may show myopathic features in long-standing cases. The CK is usually normal but may be raised when there are secondary myopathic changes.

Pathology

Disease affecting the anterior spinal nerve roots, anterior horn cells and perhaps also motor areas of the brain stem will produce the changes associated with Werdnig-Hoffman disease, but will not necessarily be specific for this disorder. Similar changes are seen in poliomyelitis, some cases of arthrogryposis and in the syndrome of anterior horn cell disease with retardation and pontocerebellar hypoplasia described recently by Goutières et al (1977).

Selective loss of nerve fibres or anterior horn cells will produce selective atrophy of the muscle fibres they innervate. Thus the first change noted

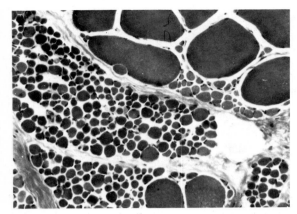

Fig. 3.30 Chronic spinal muscular atrophy. Muscle biopsy showing grouping of large and small fibres without increase in connective tissue.
HE × 122

is atrophy of some muscle fibres (usually of both fibre types). The remaining, initially normal fibres become hypertrophied, perhaps as a compensatory effect, and the picture is complicated by collateral sprouting of intact nerve fibres reinnervating some of the atrophied fibres. A biopsy from such patients shows groups of large fibres (often with type 1 characteristics) interspersed with groups of small atrophic fibres (usually with type 2 characteristics). (Fig. 3.30) The groups of muscle fibres may be separated by wide bands of perimysial connective tissue.

The appearances in the less severe cases may be almost normal with routine staining methods, but type grouping (groups of normal sized type 1 fibres and groups of normal sized type 2 fibres) will be found with the appropriate ATPase method.

Secondary myopathic changes, with degenerative changes, centrally situated nuclei and increased endomysial connective tissue may be the predominant feature in biopsies from patients with chronic spinal muscular atrophy. These changes may be almost indistinguisable from those of limb-girdle dystrophy.

Treatment in the more chronic forms of spinal muscular atrophy

In the more benign forms with uncertain or good expectation of life, careful management is needed to ensure that the quality of life is as good as pos-sible. The child should be kept mobile for as long as possible by all reasonable means. Many children can be helped to walk or enabled to continue to do so with light calipers. The prevention of spinal deformity is a major concern, and well-fitting braces are essential, as with Duchenne dystrophy. Guidance is given by Bossingham et al (1977).

Wheel-chairs and seats at home and at school must be tailor-made for the individual child, and re-tailored to cope with growth. Special attention must be paid to support for the feet to prevent equinus and equinovarus deformity. Contractures should be prevented as far as possible by physio-therapy, and exercise against resistance within the limits set by fatigue may be of value in maintaining, or perhaps even increasing, the strength of mus-cles. Exercise brings other rewards also in a sense of well-being and achievement, and a reduction of the risk of becoming obese, especially when com-bined with sensible dietary habits (shared and encouraged by the child's whole family).

Careful thought must be given to education. A school for physically handicapped children is usu-ally most appropriate, providing physiotherapy and suitable education, although the children are often more intelligent than most of their fellow-pupils. Occasionally, with some concessions, education in a normal school is possible, but problems of phys-ical management may necessitate a special atten-dant to take the child to the toilet, for example, and move him from one classroom to another. The bet-ter the education the child can receive, the better his chances of becoming self-supporting on leaving school despite his physical limitations.

RARER VARIATIONS ON THE THEME OF SPINAL MUSCULAR ATROPHY IN CHILDHOOD

Fazio-Londe's disease (progressive bulbar palsy)

Although atrophic changes in neurons of lower cra-nial nerve nuclei have been found in many cases of spinal muscular atrophy in childhood (Brandt 1950, Thieffry et al 1955, Byers & Banker 1961) the clinical effects of these lesions are oversha-dowed in most cases by the profound weakness of limb muscles. By contrast rare cases of progressive bulbar palsy are seen in children between the ages of 1 and 12 years in which spinal muscular atrophy occurs as a later and less striking feature. The cranial nerve palsies are dramatic with inspiratory stridor, dysphagia, palatal palsy, tongue involvement, facial diplegia and external ophthalmoplegia. (Fig. 3.31) These features may suggest the diagnosis of a brain-stem neoplasm, but the expected pyramidal signs do not appear in the limbs, in which instead evidence of denervation develops with flaccid weakness, loss of tendon reflexes and fasciculation. The condition is sometimes known as Fazio-Londe's disease from the authors of early reports of cases which were not examined pathologically. In the case of Gomez (1962), a girl who developed bulbar features at 33 months of age and died 17 months later, depletion of nerve cells was found in the 3rd, 4th, 6th, 7th, 10th and 12th motor cranial nerve muscles, with degeneration of

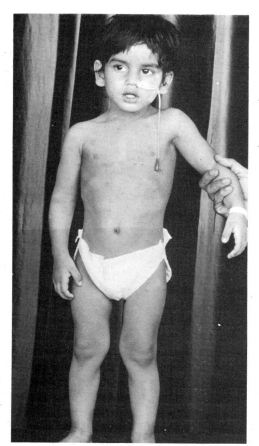

Fig. 3.31 Fazio-Londe disease. 2-year-old boy

neurons in the anterior horns in the cervical and upper dorsal regions of the spinal cord. The pyramidal tracts were not involved.

The condition, which is rare in relation to other forms of spinal muscular atrophy, may affect siblings and in these cases seems to be recessively inherited. No effective treatment is available and the disease is usually fatal.

Juvenile amyotrophic lateral sclerosis

Rarely children are seen with a progressive disorder showing both upper and lower motor neuron weakness and resembling adult amyotrophic lateral sclerosis (ALS), but with recessive inheritance and sometimes a more rapidly progressive course. Two sisters, aged 13 and 15 years, reported by Gordon Holmes (1905) seem to have conformed to this pattern, but survived at the time of the report. Nelson & Prensky (1972) reported the clinical and pathological findings in a case of sporadic juvenile amyotrophic lateral sclerosis and reviewed the four other autopsied cases. The patient developed a rapidly progressive flaccid weakness of all four limbs at 12 years of age with later pyramidal signs and died one year from onset. In this and in the other autopsied cases there was degeneration and loss of anterior horn cells, with involvement of brain stem motor nuclei, bilateral corticospinal tract degeneration and loss of myelin and axons in the white matter of the spinal cord and medulla. Many of these juvenile cases of ALS showed neuronal inclusions which are not seen in sporadic adult cases of the disease.

Hereditary distal spinal muscular atrophy

This distal form of anterior horn cell disease accounted for about one in 8 of the 262 cases of 'peroneal muscular atrophy' (using the term in a purely descriptive sense) reviewed by Thomas & Harding (1980c).

The subject is reviewed by Marsden (1975) and Harding & Thomas (1980). The latter analysed a series of 34 patients with hereditary distal spinal muscular atrophy. They comment that the condition resembles Hereditary motor and sensory neuropathy (HMSN) types I and II, but differs from them in showing less weakness in the upper limbs, relative preservation of tendon reflexes and an entirely normal clinical sensory examination. Neurophysiologically motor nerve conduction velocity and sensory nerve action potentials are normal with EMG evidence of denervation. Almost all the patients developed symptoms under the age of 20 years and most in the first decade. All had weakness in the legs and one quarter also had weakness in the arms. Pes cavus was seen in over three-quarters and was severe in more than half of these. Scoliosis was present in three cases. The ankle jerks were preserved in two thirds of cases and in 80% the knee jerks and upper limb reflexes were normal, an important point of distinction from HMSN (peroneal muscular atrophy of the Charcot-Marie-Tooth type).

In this series there were 14 patients with autosomal dominant and two with autosomal recessive inheritance. The disorder seems to be sporadic in many cases.

Marsden's (1975) review showed the age of onset varying from infancy to middle life, with the rate of progression slow in all cases. The prognosis seemed to be particularly good in those with childhood onset, who remained only mildly or moderately disabled in their 50s and 70s. The arms became affected later in about half the patients.

Anterior horn cell disease associated with pontocerebellar hypoplasia in infants

Goutières et al (1977) described three siblings who presented with an identical clinical picture of severe mental retardation, cortical blindness and extensive peripheral paralysis of lower motor neuron type, and died before one year of age. In one necropsied case spinal cord lesions indistinguishable from those of Werdnig-Hoffmann disease were associated with extreme hypoplasia and atrophy of the cerebellum and with atrophy of the ventral part of the pons. Despite grossly reduced motor and sensory nerve conduction velocities in two infants no prominent abnormalities were found in the nerves studied pathologically. Somewhat similar cases have been reported by previous authors and the condition may be less rare than it seems. It should be suspected when the clinical features of Werdnig-Hoffmann disease are associated with severe mental retardation. The inheritance is as an autosomal recessive trait and the prognosis is clearly very poor.

Anterior horn cell disease with agenesis of the corpus callosum

A rare recessively inherited syndrome in which anterior horn cell disease is associated with absence of the corpus callosum, and dysmorphic features has been reported from Canada (Andermann et al 1976). The patients present with psychomotor retardation and progressive flaccid tetraplegia and show absence of sensory action potentials as well as evidence of denervation on neurophysiological investigation. The high incidence of the condition makes it a major health problem in Charlevoix County, where it was first recognized.

Dominantly inherited spinal muscular atrophy

A small number of cases of spinal muscular atrophy have been noted to show an autosomal dominant mode of inheritance in addition to those with the distal form mentioned above. Zellweger et al (1972) have reported a family with 21 affected individuals in 6 generations. All showed proximal weakness, more marked in the legs than the arms. The severity of the weakness varied from one patient to another and males were generally worse than females. The rate of deterioration in muscle strength was very slow. Muscle biopsies showed the changes of neurogenic atrophy with some superimposed myopathic changes, the latter perhaps accounting for the raised CK levels found in some cases.

Hereditary distal spinal muscular atrophy with vocal cord paralysis

A large kindred of 9 patients in two generations has recently been reported (Young & Harper 1980) with an unusual form of spinal muscular atrophy most often presenting in the teens with wasting of the small hand muscles, involving particularly median nerve innervated muscles. Vocal cord paralysis is a characteristic and potentially hazardous feature. Distal weakness and wasting developed later in the lower limbs.

POLIOMYELITIS-LIKE ILLNESS ASSOCIATED WITH ACUTE ASTHMA IN CHILDHOOD (ASTHMATIC AMYOTROPHY, HOPKINS' SYNDROME)

An acute illness with flaccid paralysis in 10 children aged under 10 years was reported from Melbourne by Hopkins (1974). In each case an acute asthmatic illness had preceded the onset of paralysis by between 4 and 7 days. All the children had previously been immunised against poliomyelitis and viral studies showed no evidence of polio or other viruses. The clinical features and CSF findings (moderate elevation of protein level and a pleocytosis of between 8 and 497 cells per cubic mm) resembled those of the paralytic phase of poliomyelitis, suggesting that the anterior horn cell is the site of the lesion. Neurophysiological studies in some of these cases and in the patient reported by Danta (1975) supported this and gave no evidence for a peripheral neuropathy. Residual weakness in the paralysed muscle groups has usually been severe, though some recovery occurred in less severely affected muscles.

In three children with this syndrome Manson & Thong (1980) found evidence of non-specific immune deficiency including raised serum IgM and IgE levels. Evidence of viral invasion was inconclusive. These authors suggest that a combination of immune deficiency with the stress of the acute asthma attack may have rendered their patients susceptible to invasion of the anterior horn cells by a viral agent, which may have been of external origin or have existed in a latent form within the host.

THE PRADER-WILLI SYNDROME

This syndrome is mentioned here because of the profound hypotonia which is a prominent feature and which results in the affected children presenting as examples of the floppy infant syndrome. Dubowitz (1969) considered that many of those labelled earlier as cases of 'benign congenital hypotonia' were examples of the Prader-Willi syndrome.

Described by Prader and his colleagues (Prader et al 1956, Prader & Willi 1963), and well reviewed by Stephenson (1980) the syndrome pre-

sents with gross hypotonia at birth usually with feeding difficulty often needing tube-feeding. Fetal movements may have been feeble and delivery is often by the breech. The birth weight is often low and the eyes are almond-shaped often with up-slanting palpebral fissures. The mouth may be triangular and open. The hypotonia usually improves and the motor milestones are achieved late, with walking usually after the age of two. Micropenis and cryptorchidism (Fig. 3.32) allow the condition to be more easily recognized in the male. Hypoplastic labia are a valuable clue in girls in the newborn period. Gross obesity is another cardinal feature and usually develops after the child has learned to walk. The stature is short with the hands and feet being particularly small by mid-childhood. Mental retardation is usual with the IQ

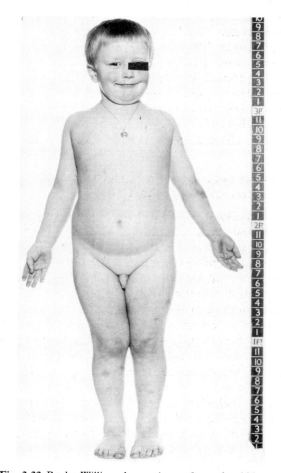

Fig. 3.32 Prader-Willi syndrome. 4 years 9 months-old boy.

generally less than 80, and commonly between 40 and 60.

The condition is sometimes rather jocularly entitled the HHHO or H₃O syndrome from the initial letters of its main features (hypotonia-hypomentia-hypogonadism-obesity) (Zellweger & Schneider 1968).

The disorder is usually sporadic. Detailed investigations (CK, neurophysiological tests and muscle biopsy) give normal results.

The natural history shows decrease in hypotonia, so that mental retardation and obesity constitute the major problems in the older child. Obesity can often be avoided by early and strict dietary control. The importance of this is shown by the very poor prognosis in the grossly obese patients. In a recent series of 24 patients with the Prader-Willi syndrome after the age of 15 years (Laurance et al 1981) obesity was the main handicap, associated with an insatiable appetite. Three patients developed diabetes mellitus. Scoliosis was present in 15 and required operative correction in two. Somnolence was an almost universal symptom, especially in the grossly obese patients, who slept excessively and would often fall asleep and become cyanosed within a few minutes of sitting down (the 'Pickwickian syndrome'). The prognosis is very poor in such patients who will die from cor pulmonale unless weight loss can be achieved, and these children can be said to 'dig their own graves with their teeth'. Nine other patients with the syndrome had died between the ages of 3 and 23 years, the cause of death being cor pulmonale in most cases.

The differential diagnosis is from various congenital neuromuscular disorders producing the floppy infant syndrome, particularly from dystrophia myotonica and from some of the congenital myopathies carrying a good prognosis.

MALIGNANT HYPERPYREXIA AND MYOPATHY

Certain individuals react abnormally to agents used in general anaesthesia, especially halothane and suxamethonium, with a rapid and progressive rise in body temperature and generalized muscular rigidity. The subject has been reviewed by Lenard and Ketler (1975), among others. The incidence of the condition is about one in 10 000 anaesthetics and the mortality rate is high, about 65%. There is often a family history of similar episodes, suggesting a genetic component, and in some patients clinical or laboratory evidence of neuromuscular disease may be found.

Anaesthetists are now well aware of the problem but it is also important to the paediatrician and paediatric neurologist since almost 40% of patients have been under 14 years of age.

The clinical features in the affected individuals and their relatives have varied greatly in the reported cases of malignant hyperpyrexia. In some affected families there is evidence of a subclinical myopathy with raised CK levels. Often this shows an autosomal dominant mode of inheritance, as in the family with 5 generations reported by Isaacs & Barlow (1970) in which 3 members died from hyperpyrexia. About half of the family members had raised CK levels. In a series of cases of malignant hyperpyrexia from Australia and New Zealand (King & Denborough 1973) all 18 propositi were males aged 4 to 54 years, 12 of them being under 20. There were 7 survivors of 18 episodes and the 6 tested all showed raised CK levels. There were 9 cases with raised CK levels in other family members and 9 with normal levels. In all 9 families with raised levels in relatives the results suggested autosomal dominant inheritance. In one family raised levels were found in the propositus and in 23 relatives. Many of these showed overt evidence of a myopathy which varied in its clinical severity and increased with advancing age. The survey also showed 5 young males, of whom only one survived, with similar physical abnormalities, including short stature, cryptorchidism, low-set ears, small chin and eyes with an antimongoloid slant. These patients did not have relatives affected by either similar physical features or malignant hyperpyrexia. Pre-existing physical abnormalities have also been reported in other patients who developed hyperpyrexia (Britt & Kalow 1970). These include kyphoscoliosis, squint and hernias, defects which have led to surgery and to the development of this serious reaction.

A few affected patients have shown evidence of a more specific myopathy, e.g. myotonia congenita with dominant inheritance (King & Denborough 1973) and central core disease (Denborough et al 1973).

The concept of a 'malignant hyperpyrexia myopathy' has been proposed by Harriman et al (1974), but it seems more likely that a *variety* of mild, mainly subclinical myopathies may underlie the liability to this disorder. The subject is not yet fully understood, but awareness of the potential problem should prompt close co-operation between paediatricians and their anaesthetist colleagues whenever the family or past history is suspicious. A history of anaesthetic deaths or mishaps in close relatives should suggest the possibility, and a raised CK level will increase suspicion. Unfortunately the CK is not reliable as a screening method for this purpose. Abnormal results have been found with in vitro testing of biopsied muscle from patients and relatives, the muscle showing an abnormal fall in ATP concentration (Harrison 1971) and an abnormal contraction response (Ellis et al 1971).

In suspected cases it would seem wise to avoid halothane and suxamethonium for anaesthesia. Prevention is clearly preferable to treatment since the management of malignant hyperpyrexia when it develops is difficult and the mortality high. Vigorous cooling of the patient is important. Harrison (1971) has suggested a method of treatment based on experiments with susceptible Landrace pigs. Intravenous procaine was used to treat the established syndrome in 5 pigs, 2 of which survived. Previous trials of treatment with active cooling, correction of acidosis and tubocurarine had proved ineffective. In addition to intravenous procaine Harrison suggests immediate cessation of the anaesthetic, rapid correction of acidosis and hypokalaemia, and isoprenaline to support the circulation. ECG monitoring is essential.

CONGENITAL ABSENCE OF MUSCLES

Congenital absence of one or more muscles is not uncommon in childhood as an isolated anomaly. The pectoral muscles, major and minor, the former in its sternal portion, are those most often affected. The condition may be unilateral or bilateral. Other muscles often affected are trapezius, sternomastoid, serratus anterior and quadriceps femoris. In some cases the condition is familial with autosomal recessive or dominant inheritance. Figures 3.33A, 3.33B show a 7-year-old boy with bilateral absence of pectoralis major, sternomastoids, serratus anterior and other muscles, including the abdominal muscles in their lower parts. His 5-year-old sister was similarly affected but their parents were normal so that autosomal recessive inheritance was the presumed pattern of inheritance. Patients with marked deficiency of abdominal wall musculature may also have congenital anomalies of the renal tract and hydronephrosis (prune belly syndrome). Abnormalities of the arm, breast or thorax on the same side are often found with absence of the pectoral muscles. The commonest association is with syndactyly (Poland's Syndrome) and this 'anomalad' is usually sporadic and shows a male to female ratio of about 3:1. It is well reviewed by Mace et al (1972).

TRANSVERSE MYELITIS OR MYELOPATHY

Myelitis often occurs as part of a post-infectious encephalomyelitic illness (Miller et al 1956) and in such cases the spinal cord problems are often overshadowed by the encephalitic features, at least initially.

A syndrome of transverse myelitis or myelopathy is also seen in children with the sudden onset of rapidly increasing weakness of the limbs, sensory loss and impairment of sphincter control. Many cases have a history of a preceding respiratory infection of probable, or proven, viral aetiology, and the interval between this and the onset of weakness is similar to that in the Guillain-Barré syndrome (from which the disorder must be distinguished), measuring from a few days to 4 weeks. Some cases are related to *mycoplasma* infection.

The subject was well reviewed by Paine & Byers (1953). In their series of 25 children aged from 6 months to 15 years, 15 had had a recent acute infectious disease while 10 had no such history. The preceding illnesses included measles, varicella, and smallpox vaccination and the time interval var-

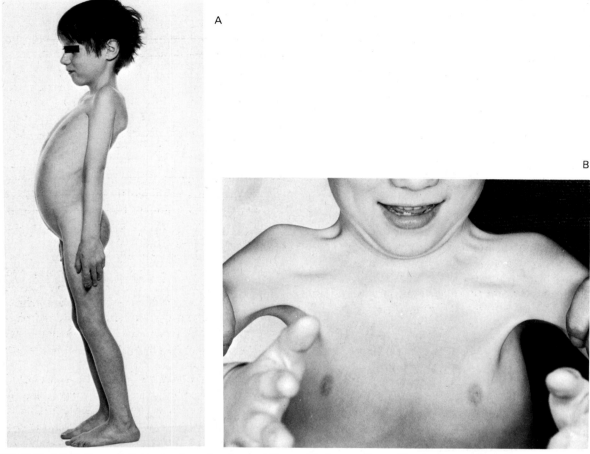

Fig. 3.33 A & B. Congenital absence of muscles. 5-year-old boy, with absence of sternal heads of pectoralis major, sternomastoids, serratus anterior and partial absence of abdominal wall muscles. Note winging of scapulae and bulging abdominal wall.

ied from one to 21 days. Pain in the limbs and/or back was a common presenting symptom and was soon followed by the onset of weakness. This most often began in the legs and in some cases extended no further, but more often spread rapidly upwards to involve the arms. Similar findings were noted in a series of 20 children aged between 6 months and 13 years with transverse myelitis at the Hospital for Sick Children, Great Ormond Street (Eggerding, personal communication 1981) 16 of whom had a history of recent infection, usually of the upper respiratory tract.

A clinical picture of 'Landry's ascending paralysis' is often seen and respiratory problems may ensue when the intercostal muscles are paralysed. The paralysis is initially flaccid but pyramidal signs may appear after a short interval with exaggerated deep tendon reflexes and extensor plantar responses. When the cervical region is affected a motor level can often be found with weakness of the triceps and loss of its tendon reflex, while the biceps is strong with a preserved reflex. Bladder and bowel involvement are common. Sensation is impaired below the level of the lesion. In older children a clear sensory level can often be detected; this was found in 9 of Eggerding's 20 patients. It is often possible to show a dissociated sensory loss with pain and temperature sensation affected while joint position and vibration sense are preserved. Light touch may or may not be impaired. A zone of hyperaesthesia can often be found just above the sensory level. The motor and sensory defects are usually fairly symmetrical on the two sides of the body. Localised spinal tenderness may be found at the level of the lesion and neck stiffness is sometimes present.

Paine and Byers found that the sensory level in their 10 'idiopathic' cases was in the upper or mid-thoracic region, as reported by several previous authors, while in the post-infectious cases it was often in the lumbar region. They argued plausibly for a vascular origin in many cases of transverse myelitis, since the clinical features are those of the 'anterior spinal artery syndrome' with sparing of posterior column sensation.

Investigations

The CSF may be normal, but commonly shows an increase in protein level and sometimes in cell count. In 6 of Eggerding's 20 patients the fluid was normal. In the others protein levels of up to 100 mg per 100 ml and white cell counts of between 11 and 110 per cu mm (mainly lymphocytes) were found.

The role of radiology is to exclude a spinal cord tumour or a lesion compressing the cord. Myelography should be preformed whenever there is doubt about the diagnosis. 12 of Eggerding's patients underwent this investigation. The results were normal in all but one case in which there was abnormal expansion of the cord in the lower thoracic region which was examined after laminectomy and showed no sign of a tumour.

Nerve conduction studies may be helpful when it is difficult clinically to distinguish between transverse myelitis and the Guillain-Barré syndrome (occasionally the two disorders occur simultaneously). However, normal conduction velocity does not exclude polyneuritis.

An encephalitic component to the illness may be suggested by drowsiness, irritability and an abnormal EEG. These features were present in 5 of Eggerding's patients.

Prognosis

The prognosis is often remarkably good with many severely paralysed children recovering dramatically in a matter of days or weeks. Recovery in 15 of the 25 patients in Paine and Byers' series was classed as 'good' or better and only 4 failed to achieve some useful return of function. In Eggerding's series 8 patients became normal, 7 had mild residual deficits and 5 were more severely handicapped. The interval between the nadir of weakness to the first sign of recovery may be very short and in one case was as little as 4 hours. There is no good evidence that the prognosis is altered by the use of ACTH or corticosteroids, though these are sometimes used in the hope of reducing any oedema of the spinal cord that may be present.

In patients with respiratory insufficiency intubation and respiratory support are needed, and their management is similar to that of severe cases of the Guillain-Barré syndrome or of poliomyelitis. The bladder may need to be catheterised, and physiotherapy to chest and limbs and meticulous care of the skin at pressure points to prevent ulceration are also important.

The differential diagnosis includes spinal cord tumour, vascular malformation, or compression by epidural abscess or haematoma, poliomyelitis and the Guillain-Barré syndrome. The striking sensory and motor levels make the last two conditions unlikely. Spinal cord compression may cause confusion but can be distinguished by myelography. Infantile botulism may need to be considered, but this usually affects younger children than does transverse myelitis. Finally the possibility that an episode of 'transverse myelitis' may be the first event in the development of disseminated sclerosis in a child should be considered, but this appears to be very rare indeed, optic or retrobulbar neuritis being probably the commonest presentation (Ch. 8).

REFERENCES

Aarli J A, Milde E–J, Thunold S 1975 Arthritis in myasthenia gravis. Journal of Neurology, Neurosurgery and Psychiatry 38: 1048–1055

Aicardi, J, Conti D. Goutières F 1974 Les formes néo-natales de la dystrophie myotonique de Steinert. Journal of the Neurological Sciences 22: 149

Andermann, E, Andermann F, Carpenter S, Karpati G, Eisen A, Melancon D, Bergeron J 1976 Familial agenesis of the corpus callosum with sensorimotor neuropathy: a new autosomal recessive syndrome originating in Charlevoix County. Journal Canadien des Sciences Neurologiques. Scientific Programme of the 11th Canadian Congress

Antony J H, Procopis P G, Ouvrier R A 1979 Benigh acute childhood myositis. Neurology 29: 1068–1071

Banker B Q, Victor M, Adams R D 1957 Arthrogryposis multiplex due to congenital muscular dystrophy. Brain 80: 319

Barth P G, Van Wijngaarden G K, Bethlem M D 1975 X-link myotubular myopathy with fatal neonatal asphyxia. Neurology 25: 531–536

Becker P E 1961 Heterogeneity of myotonia. In: Excerpta Medica International Congress Series No 32, E 79–80, Amsterdam

Becker P E, Keiner F 1955 Eine Neue X-chromosomale muskeldystrophie. Archiv für Psychiatrie und Nervenkrankheiten 193: 427

Bossingham D H, Williams E, Nichols P J R 1977 Severe childhood neuromuscular disease. The management of Duchenne muscular dystrophy and spinal muscular atrophy. Muscular Dystrophy Group of Great Britain

Brandt S 1950 Werdnig-Hoffmann's infantile progressive muscular atrophy: clinical aspects, pathology, heredity and relation to Oppenheim's Amyotonia Congenita and other morbid conditions with laxity of joints or muscles in infants. Ejnar Munksgaard Forlag, Copenhagen.

Brett E M, Morgan-Hughes J A, Lake B D 1974 Heterogeneity in two families with central core disease. Transactions of the American Neurological Association 99: 132–134

Britt B A, Kalow W 1970 Malignant hyperthermia: A statistical review. Canadian Anaesthetists' Society Journal 17: 293

Brooke M H 1973 A neuromuscular disease characterized by fibre types disproportion. In: Kakulas B A (ed) Proceedings of 2nd International Congress on Muscle Diseases, Perth, Australia, Nov 1971, ICS No 282, Excerpta Medica, Amsterdam

Buchthal F, Olson P Z 1970 Electromyography and muscle biopsy in infantile spinal muscular atrophy. Brain 93: 65

Bundey S 1972 A genetic study of infantile and juvenile myasthenia gravis. Journal of Neurology, Neurosurgery and Psychiatry 35: 41–51

Bundey S, Lovelace R E 1975 A clinical and genetic study of chronic proximal spinal muscular atrophy. Brain 98: 455

Byers R K, Banker B Q 1961 Infantile muscular atrophy. Archives of Neurology 5: 140–164

Catel W 1951 Differential Diagnostische Symptomatologie von Krankheiten des Kindesalters, 2nd edn. Georg Thieme Verlag, Stuttgart

Cavanagh N P C, Lake B D, McMeniman P 1979 Congenital fibre type disproportion myopathy: a histological diagnosis with an uncertain clinical outlook. Archives of Disease in Childhood 54: 735–743

Cavanagh N P C 1980 The role of thymectomy in childhood myasthenia. Developmental Medicine and Child Neurology 22: 668–670

Collier, J, Wilson S A K 1908 Amyotonia congenita. Brain 31: 1

Crews J, Kaiser K K, Brooke M H 1976 Muscle pathology of myotonia congenita. Journal of the Neurological Sciences 28: 449–457

Cunningham M, Stocks J 1978 Werdnig-Hoffmann disease: the effects of intrauterine onset on lung growth. Archives of Disease in Childhood 53: 921

Currie S, Walton J N 1971 Immunosuppressive therapy in polymyositis. Journal of Neurology, Neurosurgery and Psychiatry 34: 447

Currie S, Noronha M, Harriman D 1974 'Minicore disease'. Excerpta Medica, International Congress Series 334: 12

Danta G 1975 Electrophysiological study of amyotrophy associated with acute asthma (asthmatic amyotrophy). Journal of Neurology, Neurosurgery and Psychiatry 38: 1016–1021

Davidenkow S 1939 Scapulo-peroneal amyotrophy. Archives of Neurology and Psychiatry (Chicago) 41: 694

Denborough M A, Dennett X, Anderson R M 1973 Central core disease and malignant hyperpyrexia. British Medical Journal 1: 272

Di Mauro S, Hartlage P L 1978 Fatal infantile form of muscle phosporylase deficiency. Neurology 28: 1124–1129

Dodge P R, Gamstorp I, Byers B K, Russell P 1965 Myotonic dystrophy in infancy and childhood. Pediatrics 35: 3

Donner M, Rapola J, Somer H 1975 Congenital muscular dystrophy: a clinico-pathological and follow-up study of 15 patients. Neuropädiatrie 6: 239–258

Dreifuss F E, Hogan G R 1961 Survival in X-chromosomal muscular dystrophy. Neurology 11: 734–737

Dubowitz V 1964 Infantile muscular atrophy. A prospective study with particular reference to a slowly progressive variety. Brain 87: 707–718

Dubowitz V 1969 The floppy infant. Clinics in Development Neurology No. 31 Spastics International Medical Publications and William Heinemann Medical Books, London

Dubowitz V 1976 Treatment of dermatomyositis in childhood. Archives of Disease in Childhood 51: 494–500

Dubowitz V 1978 Muscle disorders in childhood. Major problems in clinical paediatrics. W B Saunders, London

Dubowitz V 1980 The floppy infant. Clinics in Development Medicine No 76, 2nd edn. Spastics International Medical Publications and William Heinemann Medical Books, London

Dubowitz V, Brooke M H 1973 Muscle biopsy: a modern approach. W B Saunders, London.

Dubowitz V, Crome L 1969 The central nervous system in Duchenne muscular dystrophy. Brain 92: 805–808

Duchenne de Boulogne G B A 1868 Récherches sur la paralysie musculaire pseudohypertrophisme, ou paralysie myo-sclérosique. Archives Générales de Médecine (6 sér) 11: 5, 179, 305, 421, 552

Dunn L J, Kierker L J 1973 Recurrent hydramnios in association with myotonia dystrophica. Obstetrics and Gynaecology 42: 104

Dyken P R, Harper P S 1973 Congenital dystrophia myotonica. Neurology (Minneapolis) 23: 465–473

Egger J, Lake B D, Wilson J 1981 Mitochondrial cytopathy. A multisystem disorder with ragged red fibres on muscle biopsy. Archives of Disease in Childhood 56: 741–752

Egger J, Kendall B E 1981 Computed tomography in mitochondrial cytopathy. Neuroradiology 22: 73–78.

Egger J, Kendall B E, Erdohazi M, Lake B D, Wilson J, Brett E M 1983. Involvement of the central nervous system in congenital muscular dystrophies. Developmental Medicine and Child Neurology 25: 32–41

Ellis F R, Harriman D G F, Keaney N P, Kyei-Mensah K, Tyrell J H 1971 Halothane-induced muscle contracture as a cause of hyperpyrexia. British Journal of Anaesthetics 43: 721

Emery A E H, Dreifuss F E 1966 Unusual type of X-linked muscular dystrophy. Journal of Neurology, Neurosurgery and Psychiatry 29: 358–362

Engel A G, Roelofs R, Olson W H 1971 Multicore disease: a

recently recognised congenital myopathy associated with multifocal degeneration of muscle fibres. Mayo Clinic Proceedings 46: 666–681

Engel A G, Siekert R G 1972 Lipid storage myopathy responsive to prednisone. Archives of Neurology 27: 174

Engel A G, Lambert E H, Gomez M R 1977 A new myasthenic syndrome with end-plate acetylcholinesterase deficiency, small nerve terminals and reduced acetylcholine release. Annals of Neurology 1: 315–330

Eulenberg A Von 1886 Ueber eine familiäre, durch 6-generationen verfolgbare form congenitaler paramyotonie. Neurologisches Zentralblatt 5: 265–272

Fenichel G M 1978 Clinical syndromes of myasthenia in infancy and childhood. A review. Archives of Neurology 35: 97–103

Fonkalsrud E W, Herrmann C, Mulder D G 1970 Thymectomy for myasthenia gravis in children. Journal of Pediatric Surgery 5: 157–165

Fowler W M, Layzer R B, Taylor R G, Eberle E B, Sims G E, Munsat T L, Philippart M, Wilson B W 1974 The Schwartz-Jampel syndrome. Its clinical physiological and histological expression. Journal of the Neurological Sciences 22: 127

Fried K, Emery A E H 1971 Spinal muscular atrophy Type II. A separate genetic and clinical entity from Type I (Werdnig-Hoffman disease) and Type III (Kugelberg-Welander disease). Clinical Genetics 2: 203–209

Fukuyama Y, Haruna H Karazura M 1960 A peculiar form of congenital progressive muscular dystrophy. Report of 15 cases. Pediatria Universitatis Tokyo 4: 5–8

Gamstorp I 1956 Adynamia episodica hereditaria. Acta paediatrica scandinavica (Uppsala) supplement 108

Gamstorp I 1967 Progressive spinal muscular atrophy with onset in infancy or early childhood. Acta paediatrica scandinavica 56: 408–423

Gamstorp I 1974 Encephalo-myelo-radiculoneuropathy. Involvement of the CNS in children with Guillain-Barré-Strohl syndrome. Developmental Medicine and Child Neurology 16: 654–658

Gardner-Medwin D 1976 Duchenne muscular dystrophy: early diagnosis and screening. Archives of Disease in Childhood 51: 982 (letter)

Gardner-Medwin D 1977 Children with genetic muscular disorders. British Journal of Hospital Medicine 17: 314–340

Gardner-Medwin D 1978 Strategie per la prevenzione della distrofia muscolare di Duchenne. In: Distrofia Muscolare: Alla Ricerca Di Nuove Frontiere, Mario Negri Institute for Pharmacological Research and the Carol Besta Neurological Institute, Milan, p 4–9

Gardner-Medwin D 1979a Controversies about Duchenne muscular dystrophy. I. Neonatal screening. Developmental Medicine and Child Neurology 21: 390–393

Gardner-Medwin D 1979b Controversies about Duchenne muscular dystrophy. 2. Bracing for ambulation. Developmental Medicine and Child Neurology 21: 659–662

Gardner-Medwin D, Bundey S, Green S 1978 Early diagnosis of Duchenne muscular dystrophy. Lancet 1: 1102

Gardner-Medwin D, Hudgson P, Walton J N 1967 Benign spinal muscular atrophy arising in childhood and adolescence. Journal of the Neurological Sciences 5: 121–158

Gibson D A, Wilkins K E 1975 The Management of spinal deformities in Duchenne muscular dystrophy. A new concept of spinal bracing. Clinical Orthopaedics and Related Research 108: 41–51

Gilboa N, Swanson J R 1976 Serum creatine phosphokinase in normal newborns. Archives of Disease in Childhood 51: 283–285

Goel K M, Shanks R A 1976 Dermatomyositis in childhood: review of eight cases. Archives of Disease in Childhood 51: 501–506

Gomez M R, Clermont V, Bernstein J 1962 Progressive bulbar paralysis in childhood (Fazio-Londe's disease). Report of a case with pathologic evidence of nuclear atrophy. Archives of Neurology 6: 317

Goutières F, Aicardi J, Farkas E 1977 Anterior horn cell disease associated with pontocerebellar hypoplasia in infants. Journal of Neurology, Neurosurgery and Psychiatry 40: 370

Gowers W R 1879 Pseudo-hypertrophic muscular paralysis. A clinical lecture. Churchill, London

Hackett E R, Martinez R D, Larson P K, Paddison R M 1974 Optic neuritis in systemic lupus erythematosus. Archives of Neurology 31: 9–11

Harper P 1975a Congenital myotonic dystrophy in Britain I. Clinical aspects. Archives of Disease in Childhood 50: 505–513

Harper P 1975b Congenital myotonic dystrophy in Britain. II. Genetic aspects. Archives of Disease in Childhood 50: 514–521

Harper P S, Dyken P R 1972 Early-onset dystrophia myotonica. Evidence supporting a maternal environmental factor. Lancet 2: 53

Harper P S, Johnston D M 1972 Recessively inherited myotonia dystrophica. Journal of Medical Genetics 9: 213–215

Harriman D G F, Ellis F R, Currie S, Sumner D W 1974 Malignant hyperpyrexia myopathy. 3rd International Congress on Muscle Disease, Newcastle. Excerpta Medica, International Congress Series No 334: 52

Harrison G G 1971 Anaesthetic-induced malignant hyperpyrexia: A suggested method of treatment. British Medical Journal 3: 454–456

Hazama R, Tsujihata M, Masataka M, Mori K 1979 Muscular dystrophy in six young girls. Neurology 29: 1486–1491

Hoffman J 1893 Ueber chronische spinale muskelatrophie im kindesalter auf familiärer basis. Deutsche Zeitschrift für Nervenheilkunde 3: 427–470

Hokkanen E 1969 Epidemiology of myasthenia gravis in Finland. Journal of the Neurological Sciences 9: 463–478

Holmes G 1905 Familial spastic paralysis associated with amyotrophy. Review of Neurology and Psychiatry 3: 256–263

Hopkins I J 1974 A new syndrome: poliomyelitis-like illness associated with a acute asthma in childhood. Australian Paediatric Journal 10: 273–276

Hosking G P, Bhat U S, Dubowitz V, Edwards R H T 1976 Measurements of muscle strength and performance in children with normal and diseased muscle. Archives of Disease in Childhood 51: 957–963

Isaacs H, Barlow M B 1970 Malignant hyperpyrexia during anaesthesia: possible association with subclinical myopathy. British Medical Journal 1: 275

Jerusalem F, Angelini C, Engel A G, Groover R V 1973 Mitochondrial-lipid-glycogen (MLG) disease of muscle. Archives of Neurology 29: 162–169

Kaeser H E 1965 Scapuloperoneal muscular atrophy. Brain 88: 407–418

Karpati G, Carpenter S, Watters G V, Eisen A A, Andermann F 1973 Infantile myotonic dystrophy. Neurology 23: 1066–1077

Kearns T P, Sayre G P 1958 Retinitis pigmentosa, external ophthalmoplegia and complete heart block. Archives of Ophthalmology (Chicago) 60: 280

King J O, Denborough M A, Zapf P W 1972 Inheritance of malignant hyperpyrexia. Lancet 1: 365–370

King J O, Denborough M A 1973 Malignant hyperpyrexia in Australia and New Zealand. Medical Journal of Australia 1: 525–528

Klein R, Haddow J E, De Luca C 1972 Familial congenital disorder resembling stiff-man syndrome. American Journal of Diseases of Children 124: 730–731

Krijgsman J B, Barth P G, Stam F C, Slooff J F, Jaspar H H J 1980 Congenital muscular dystrophy and cerebral dysgenesis in a Dutch family. Neuropädiatrie 11: 108–120

Kugelberg E, Welander L 1956 Heredofamilial juvenile muscular atrophy simulating muscular dystrophy. Archives of Neurology and Psychiatry (Chicago) 75: 500–509

Kulakowski S, Renoirte P, De Bruyn C H H M 1981 Dynamometric and biochemical observations in Duchenne patients receiving allopurinol. Neuropediatrics 81: 92–94

Lake B D, Cavanagh N, Wilson, J 1977 Myopathy with minicores in siblings. Neuropathology and Applied Neurobiology 3: 159–167

Laurance B M, Brito A, Wilkinson J 1981 Prader-Willi syndrome after age 15 years. Archives of Disease in Childhood 56: 181–186

Lebenthal E, Scochet S R, Adam A, Seelenfreund M, Fried A, Najenson T et al 1970 Arthrogryposis multiplex congenita — 23 cases in an Arab kindred. Pediatrics 46: 891–899

Lenard H G, Ketler 1975 Malignant hyperpyrexia and myopathy. Neuropädiatrie 6: 7–12

Lunberg A 1957 Myalgia cruris edidemica. Acta paediatrica 46: 18–31

McArdle B 1951 Myopathy due to a defect in muscle glycogen breakdown. Clinical Science 10: 13

Mace J W, Kaplan J M, Schanberger J E, Gotlin R W 1972 Poland's syndrome. Report of seven cases and review of the literature. Clinical Pediatrics 11: 98–102

McKinlay I A, Mitchell I 1976 Transient acute myositis in childhood. Archives of Disease in Childhood 51: 135–137

McQuillen M P, Cantor H E, O'Rourke J R 1968 Myasthenic syndromes associated with antibiotics. Archives of Neurology 18: 402–415

Manson J I, Thong Y H 1980 Immunological abnormalities in the syndrome of poliomyelitis-like illness associated with acute bronchial asthma (Hopkins' syndrome). Archives of Disease in Childhood 55: 26–32

Marsden C D 1975 Inherited Neuronal Atrophy and Degenerations Predominantly of Lower Motor Neurons. In: Dyck P J, Thomas P K, Lambert E H (eds) Peripheral neuropathy W B Saunders, Philadelphia, Vol 2

Meadows J C, Marsden C D 1969 A distal form of chronic spinal muscular atrophy. Neurology (Minneapolis) 19: 53

Mendell J R, Wiechers L 1979 Lack of benefit of allopurinol in Duchenne dystrophy. Muscle and Nerve 2: 53

Middleton P J, Alexander R M, Szymanski M T 1970 Severe myositis during recovery from influenza. Lancet 2: 533

Miller H G, Stanton J B, Gibbons J L 1956 Para-infectious encephalomyelitis and related syndromes. Quarterly Journal of Medicine 25: 427

Millichap J C, Dodge P R 1960 Diagnosis and treatment of myasthenia gravis in infancy, childhood and adolescence. Neurology (Minneapolis) 10: 1007–1014

Munsat T L, Woods, R, Fowler W, Pearson C M 1969 Neurogenic muscular atrophy of infancy with prolonged survival. Brain 92: 9–24

Nelson J S, Prensky A L 1972 Sporadic juvenile amyotrophic lateral sclerosis. A clinicopathological study of a case with neuronal cytoplasmic inclusions containing RNA. Archives of Neurology 27: 300–306

Newsom-Davis J, Pinching A J, Vincent A, Wilson S G 1978 Function of circulating antibody to acetylcholine receptor in myasthenia gravis: investigation by plasma exchange. Neurology 28: 266–272

Nichols P J R, Wilshere E R 1980 Equipment for the Disabled Child 4th edn, Portslade, Sussex. Equipment for the Disabled, 2 Foredown Drive

Olson W, Engel W K, Walsh G O, Einaugler R 1972 Oculocraniosomatic neuromuscular disease with 'ragged-red' fibres. Archives of Neurology 26: 193–211

Oppenheim H 1900 Ueber allgemeine und localisierte atonie der muskulatur (myatonie) im frühen kindesalter. Montaschrift für Psychiatrie und Neurologie 8: 232

Paine R S, Byers R K 1953 Transverse myelopathy in childhood. American Journal of Diseases of Children 85: 151–163

Papatestas A E, Alpert L I, Osserman K E, Osserman R S, Kark A E 1971 Studies in myasthenia gravis: effects of thymectomy. Results on 185 patients with nonthymomatous and thymomatous myasthenia gravis 1941–1969. American Journal of Medicine 50: 465

Pearn J H, Carter C O, Wilson J 1973 The genetic identity of acute infantile spinal muscular atrophy. Brain 96: 463–470

Pearn J H, Wilson J 1973 Chronic generalised spinal muscular atrophy of infancy and childhood: arrested Werdnig-Hoffman disease. Archives of Disease in Childhood 48: 768

Pearson C M 1962 Histopathological features of muscle in the preclinical stages of muscular dystrophy. Brain 85: 109–120

Pearson C M 1964 The periodic paralyses: differential features and pathological observations in permanent myopathic weakness. Brain 87: 341

Penn A S, Lisak R P, Rowland L P 1970 Muscular dystrophy in young girls. Neurology (Minneapolis) 20: 147

Prader A, Labhart A, Willi H 1956 Ein Syndrom von Adipositas, Kleinwuchs, Kryptorchismus und Oliogophrenie nach Myotonieartigem Zustand im Neugeborenalter. Schweizerische Medizinische Wochenschrift 86: 1260

Prader A, Willi H 1963 Das Syndrom von Imbezillitat, Adipositas, Muskelhypotonie, Hypogonadismus and Diabetes Mellitus mit 'Myotonie'-Anamnese. Verhand 2nd International Kongress der Psychiatrie und Entwicklungsstorungen die Kindesalter, Vienna 1961. Karger, Basel and New York, part 1

Pruzanski W 1965 Congenital malformations in myotonic dystrophy. Acta neurologica scandinavica 41: 34

Robertson W C, Chun R W M, Kornguth S E 1980 Familial infantile myasthenia. Archives of Neurology 37: 117–119

Rose A L 1974 Childhood polymyositis. A follow-up study with special reference to treatment with corticosteroids. American Journal of Diseases of Children 127: 518–522

Rose A L, Walton J N 1966 Polymyositis: a survey of 89 cases with particular reference to treatment and prognosis. Brain 89: 747

Rossignol A-M, Meyer M, Rossignol B, Palcoux M-P, Raynaud E-J, Bost M 1979 La myocardiopathie de la glycogenose type III. Archives françaises de Pédiatrie 36 (3): 303–309

Rowland L P, Fetell M, Olarte M, Hays A, Singh N, Wanat F E 1979 Emery-Dreifuss muscular dystrophy. Annals of Neurology 5: 111–117

Sander J E, Layzer R B, Goldsobel A B 1979 Congenital stiff-man syndrome. Annals of Neurology 8: 195–197

Santavuori P, Leisti J, Kruss S 1977 Muscle, eye and brain disease: a new syndrome. Neuropädiatrie suppl 8, 533

Schnitzler E R, Robertson W C 1979 Familial Kearns-Sayre syndrome. Neurology 29: 1172–1174

Schultz M D, Schwab R S 1971 Results of thymic (mediastinal) irradiation in patients with myasthenia gravis. Annals of the New York Academy of Science 183: 303–307

Schwartz O, Jampel R S 1962 Congenital blepharophimosis associated with a unique generalized myopathy. Archives of Ophthalmology 68: 52

Sengers R C A, Stadhouders A M, Jasper H H J, Lamers K J B, Trijbels J M F, Notermans S L H 1980 Muscle phosporylase deficiency in childhood. European Journal of Pediatrics 134: 161–165

Shapira Y, Cividalli G, Szabo G, Rosin R, Russell A 1974 A myasthenic syndrome in childhood leukaemia. Developmental Medicine and Child Neurology 16: 668–671

Shy G, Magee K R 1956 A new congenital non-progressive myopathy. Brain 79: 610

Shy G M, Engel W K, Somers J E, Wanko T 1963 Nemaline myopathy. A new congenital myopathy. Brain 86: 793

Smit L M E, Barth P G 1980 Arthrogryposis multiplex congenita due to congenital myasthenia. Developmental Medicine and Child Neurology 22: 371–374

Smith D 1976 Recognizable patterns of human malformation. Major problems in clinical pediatrics. W B Saunders Company, Philadelphia, vol 7

Spiro A J, Shy G M, Gonatas N K 1966 Myotubular myopathy. Archives of Neurology 14: 1–14

Stephenson J B P 1980 Prader-Willi syndrome: neonatal presentation and later development. Developmental Medicine and Child Neurology 22: 792–795

Stern G M, Hall J M, Robinson D S 1964 Neonatal myasthenia gravis. British Medical Journal 2: 284

Stickroot F L, Schaeffer R L, Bergo H L 1942 Myasthenia gravis occurring in an infant of a myasthenic mother. Journal of the American Medical Association 120: 1207

Tarui S, Okuno J, Ikura Y, Tanaka T, Suda M, Nishikawa M 1965 Phosphofructokinase deficiency in skeletal muscle. A new type of glycogenosis. Biochemical and Biophysical Research Communications 19: 517–523

Thieffry S, Arthuis M, Bargeton E 1955 40 cas de maladie Werdnig-Hoffmann avec 11 examens anatomiques. Revue neurologique 93: 261

Thomsen J 1876 Tonische krämpfe in willkürlich beweglichen muskeln in fulge von erester psychischer disposition (ataxia muscularis). Archiv für Psychiatrie und Nervenkrankheiten 6: 706–718

Thomson W H S, Smith I 1976 X-linked recessive (Duchenne) muscular dystrophy (DMD) and purine metabolism. Lancet 2: 805

Thrush D C, Morris C J, Salmon M V 1972 Paramyotonia congenita: a clinical, histochemical and pathological study. Brain 95: 537–552

Vanier T M 1960 Dystrophia myotonica in childhood. British Medical Journal 2: 1284

Van Wijngaarden G K, Fleury P, Bethlem J, Meijer A E F H 1969 Familial 'myotubular' myopathy. Neurology (Minneapolis) 19: 901–908

Vignos P J, Bowling G F, Watkins M P 1964 Polymyositis: effect of corticosteroids on final results. Archives of Internal Medicine 114: 263

Walton J N 1956 'Amyotonia congenita'; a follow-up study. Lancet 1: 1023–1027

Watters G V, Williams T W 1967 Early onset myotonic dystrophy. Archives of Neurology 17: 137

Welch D C 19   Living with muscular dystrophy. The Muscular Dystrophy Group of Great Britain. Nattrass House, 35 Macaulay Road, Clapham SW4 0QP

Werdnig G 1891 Swei frühinfantile hereditäre falle von progressiver muskeldystrophie unter dem bilde der dystrophie, aber auf neurotische grundlage. Archiv für Psychiatrie Und Nervenkrankheiten 22: 437–480

Werdnig G 1894 Die Frühinfantile progressive spinale amytrophie. Archiv für Psychiatrie Und Nervenkrankheiten 26: 706–744

Wharton B A 1965 An unusual variety of muscular dystrophy. Lancet 1: 248–249

Yoshioka M, Okuna T, Honda Y, Nakano Y 1980 Central nervous system involvement in progressive muscular dystrophy. Archives of Disease in Childhood 55: 589–594

Young I D, Harper P S 1980 Hereditary distal spinal muscular atrophy with vocal cord paralysis. Journal of Neurology, Neurosurgery and Psychiatry 43: 413–418

Zellweger H, Afifi A, McCormick W F, Mergner W 1969a Benign congenital muscular dystrophy. A special form of congenital hypotonia. Clinical Pediatrics 6: 655

Zellweger H, Afifi A, McCormick W F, Mergner W 1967b Severe congenital muscular dystrophy. American Journal of Diseases of Children 114: 591–602

Zellweger H, Schneider H J 1968 Syndrome of hypotonia-hypomentia-hypogonadism-obesity (HHHO) or Prader-Willi syndrome. American Journal of Diseases of Children 115: 588–598

Zellweger H, Simpson J, McCormick W F, Ionasescu V 1972 Spinal muscular atrophy with dominant inheritance: report of a new kindred. Neurology 22: 957–963

Zellweger H. Antonik A 1975 Newborn screening for Duchenne muscular dystrophy. Pediatrics 55: 30–34

4

Neuromuscular disorders: II. Peripheral neuropathy

E. M. Brett

Peripheral neuropathy affecting many nerves (polyneuritis or polyneuropathy) may occur alone or with other neurological deficits. The field has been reviewed by Thomas (1975). Many of the disorders reviewed are rare in childhood, e.g. the neuropathies associated with toxic substances, diabetes mellitus, uraemia, liver disease, hypothyroidism, carcinoma and amyloidosis. Others are common in childhood or limited to this age group. Many of the latter are described elsewhere in this book.

Various conditions in which a neuropathy is associated with progressive disease affecting myelin in the central and peripheral nervous systems have been described in Chapter 5. In these diseases the involvement of the CNS with progressive dementia and ataxia is the most striking feature. In Friedreich's ataxia and ataxia-telangiectasia (Ch. 8) the effects of the peripheral neuropathy are overshadowed by the more dramatic ataxia and other features. In Fabry's disease (Ch. 5) pain is the main feature of the neuropathy.

In certain other diseases the effects of the peripheral neuropathy itself upon motor and sensory function make a more important contribution to the clinical picture. In some of these a metabolic defect is known and in others suspected. These disorders will be considered here together with the Guillain-Barré syndrome which, though sporadic, acquired and usually self-limited, produces profound effects on motor function.

PERONEAL MUSCULAR ATROPHY: CHARCOT-MARIE-TOOTH DISEASE

Hereditary motor and sensory neuropathy (Types I and II)

In 1886, the French neurologists Charcot and Marie, and the Englishman Tooth, in his thesis for the degree of MD, Cambridge, separately described a form of progressive muscular atrophy starting in the feet and legs and later affecting the arms. The initial involvement of the peroneal muscles caused Tooth to name the disease the peroneal type of progressive muscular atrophy. In France the eponym *maladie de Charcot-Marie* is now usual, and in the English-speaking world it is known as peroneal muscular atrophy or Charcot-Marie-Tooth disease. (In justice neither of these eponymous titles should be used since the condition was reported by several physicians in earlier publications.) Peroneal muscular atrophy is one of the commonest inherited neurological disorders, with an estimated prevalence in the Newcastle region of northern England of 4.7 per 100 000 (Davis et al 1978) which may well be an underestimate.

The inheritance of the disease may be autosomal dominant or recessive, and it is particularly important not only to enquire carefully for a family history, but also to *examine* parents and siblings for minor evidence of involvement such as degress of pes cavus, and to arrange nerve conduction studies when suspicious signs are found.

The disease can be one of the mildest of the heredodegenerative disorders of the nervous system and compatible with a full life span. This was well demonstrated by an interesting report by Alajouanine and his colleagues (1967) on a patient who had been examined by Charcot in 1891 at the age of 13 having first shown signs of the disease at the age of 7. Until the age of 75 she led an active life and could walk with the aid of calipers and sew and write without serious difficulty. She was frequently examined by many neurologists and showed the characteristic distal atrophy, pes cavus and sensory impairment in the legs, later developing bilateral optic atrophy which caused severe blindness. She died at the age of 80.

If the term is used in a purely descriptive sense progressive peroneal muscular atrophy can theoretically result from disease of the anterior horn cell, the peripheral nerve or of muscle. In the 1950s it was shown (Gilliatt & Thomas 1957) that some patients with peroneal muscular atrophy had severely reduced motor nerve conduction velocity while others did not. The work of Dyck and Lambert (1968a, b) has shown that there are two distinct disorders with neurogenic peroneal muscular atrophy. One type affects predominantly the peripheral nerve and the other the anterior horn cell and dorsal root ganglion cell neurons, although some overlap exists between these two categories.

1. Dominantly inherited form of peroneal muscular atrophy with peripheral neuropathy of hypertrophic type (Hereditary motor and sensory neuropathy type I)

This group includes kinships similar to those reported by Charcot & Marie (1886) and Tooth (1886) and is the type most often seen in paediatric practice. The earliest sign is usually a foot deformity with high arched feet, pes cavus or hammer toes. Parents often complain of difficulty in finding shoes to fit their children's feet. Affected parents, who themselves have pes cavus, can often detect it at an early age in their affected children. In other cases the foot deformity is only recognised in retrospect, after gait disorder has led to medical consultation and enquiry. Abnormality in walking or running usually develops in the second half of the first decade or in the second decade. Walking is clumsy and awkward. Weakness of ankle dorsiflexion causes foot drop which necessitates a compensatory exaggerated lifting of the knees in walking. The gait is 'slapping' since, instead of the heel hitting the ground first followed by the normal rocking heel-toe action, the forefoot is the first to touch the floor. This slapping gait is as easily heard as seen, and can be recognised when the patient is still out of sight. When at a later stage weakness of ankle plantar flexion is prominent as well as of dorsiflexion, there is difficulty in fixing the ankles sufficiently to stand still and maintain balance.

Some children will then shift their feet continuously in fidgety fashion and others will stand with their knees bent in an attempt to achieve stability.

Difficulty in manipulation and weakness of the hands are not usually complained of until the second decade of life, although mild wasting and weakness of the small muscles of the hand may be found on examination before any disability is admitted to. In the later stages there may be severe weakness and wasting of the hands with a claw hand deformity and thinning of the distal forearm muscles, but more often the involvement is mild.

Examination of the legs shows a foot deformity which tends to increase with age and a slapping gait with inability to stand on the heels and evidence of peroneal muscle weakness on more formal testing 'on the bed'. Muscle wasting is seen below the knee and may slowly increase, spreading later to involve the lower thirds of the thighs, although weakness is not usually marked in the quadriceps muscles. Severe degrees of wasting have been graphically described as like ostrich or stork legs or the appearance of an inverted champagne bottle. This gross degree of below knee wasting is uncommon in children, and according to Dyck & Lambert (1968) is not seen in this group. Fasciculation may rarely be seen in the weak muscles.

Tendon reflexes are successively lost in the order of ankle jerks, knee jerks and arm reflexes. Signs of pyramidal dysfunction are not seen. The plantar responses remain flexor until abolished altogether by gross weakness of the muscles of the feet.

Sensory testing, especially in the later stages, may show impairment first in the toes and later in the fingers and hands. Sensory loss tends to affect joint position and vibration sense and two-point discrimination. It is not often found in younger children.

Peripheral nerves in the feet, neck and elbow may be palpably thickened and these nerves should always be carefully felt.

Spinal deformity, cardiac abnormality and diabetes are not common, in contrast to the situation in Friedreich's ataxia.

Investigation of the family will often show an affected parent and siblings. The clinical features in some of the affected relatives may be so mild, limited perhaps to high arched feet, that recognition of the disease may be difficult. In some cases the affected parent is unaware of any abnormality in himself, or may admit to having trouble with his feet, but attribute it to other causes such as poliomyelitis, trauma or a 'slipped disc'. (One affected father attributed his pes cavus to prolonged immersion in the sea when torpedoed in the Pacific: many such specious explanations could probably be quoted by other neurologists.) Peroneal muscular atrophy was found in one third of a series of 77 patients investigated for 'idiopathic' pes cavus by Brewerton and his colleagues (1963) and was the commonest single cause of this. It is essential therefore to arrange for nerve conduction studies which will usually show unequivocal evidence of peripheral neuropathy.

Conduction velocity studies are the most important form of investigation. Dyck & Lambert (1968a) regard low conduction velocities in peripheral nerves as the hallmark of this disorder. They found that the velocities of the ulnar, median and lateral popliteal nerves of those affected were on average less than half the values in unaffected subjects. The mean amplitude of the muscle action potential was also decreased by more than half, and the distal latencies were more than three times greater. Sensory nerve action potentials are also reduced or absent.

Nerve biopsy in this condition shows evidence of extensive segmental demyelination and remyelination with 'onion bulb' formations due to concentric Schwann cell proliferation. These changes were found by Thomas and his colleagues (1974) in nerve biopsies regardless of whether the nerves were palpably thickened or not.

2. Dominantly inherited form of peroneal muscular atrophy of neuronal type (Hereditary motor and sensory neuropathy type II)

This disorder differs from the hypertrophic variety in that clinical enlargement of peripheral nerves, hypertrophic neuropathy, segmental demyelination and diffuse slowing of motor nerve conduction velocity are not seen. The age of onset is also usually later than in the commoner hypertrophic condition; the commonest presentation is with difficulty in walking, which began in the fifth decade or later except in one kinship reported by Dyck and Lambert (1968b) in which it began in the first or second decades. Weakness of the small hand muscles is less severe but that of the plantar flexor muscles of the ankles is more severe with more marked atrophy than in the hypertrophic form of the disorder. Pes cavus was present in four of the eight patients reported by Dyck and Lambert. The mean conduction velocity of peripheral nerves was much higher than that of patients with hypertrophic neuropathy, but was slightly lower than that of unaffected relatives and other controls.

Thomas and his colleagues (Thomas et al 1974; Harding & Thomas 1980a, b) have confirmed these two strikingly different varieties of peroneal muscular atrophy, which have come to be known as hereditary motor and sensory neuropathy (HMSN) Types I and II. Harding and Thomas in a detailed review of 228 patients with HMSN, comprising 120 index cases and 108 affected relatives, separated these into two genetically distinct categories, Types I and II, on neurophysiological criteria, depending on whether motor nerve conduction velocity in the median nerve was below or above 38 metres per second. (The median nerve was chosen rather than the peroneal nerve since the abductor pollicis brevis muscle is less often totally denervated than the extensor digitorum brevis). Type I cases were more numerous (173). Most showed autosomal dominant inheritance (139 cases in 39 families), 8 cases in 4 families were probably recessive and 26 sporadic. The patients with probable recessive inheritance showed significantly slower motor conduction velocity. The peak age of onset in the Type I cases was in the first decade of life. When compared with the later onset Type II cases they tended to show greater weakness of the hands, tremor and ataxia in the upper limbs, generalised areflexia and more extensive distal sensory loss, sometimes with acrodystrophic changes. Deformities of the feet and spine were more frequent. Thickening of peripheral nerves was confined to Type I cases.

The peak age of onset in the 55 Type II cases was in the second decade with many developing symptoms much later, sometimes as late as the seventh decade. 37 patients showed dominant and 3 recessive inheritance, while 15 cases were sporadic.

Among 262 patients with the clinical syndrome of 'peroneal muscular atrophy' Harding and Thomas (1980c) have found 34 cases of hereditary distal spinal muscular strophy. It resembles HMSN Types I and II in some ways, but differs from them in showing less weakness in the arms, relative preservation of tendon reflexes and entirely normal sensory findings. Motor and sensory nerve function is normal on electrophysiological testing. 24 of the patients were male and 10 female. Inheritance was autosomal dominant in 14 patients and recessive in 2, the other cases being sporadic. Almost all the patients developed symptoms under the age of 20 and most in the first decade. All had weakness of the legs and a quarter had arm weakness. The ankle jerks were lost in about one third, but in over 80% the knee jerks and arm reflexes were normal. Pes cavus was present in over 75% and was severe in half of these, but scoliosis was present in only 3 patients. The changes of denervation were found on EMG but peripheral nerve function was normal on neurophysiological investigation.

Autosomal recessive forms of hereditary motor and sensory neuropathy

Under this title Harding & Thomas (1980) have described six families with probable autosomal recessive inheritance of the disorders. Four of these were classified as HMSN type I and two as type II. There was a high consanguinity rate suggesting that the recessive genes involved are rare.

Compared with the classical dominantly inherited forms of these disorders the mean age of onset was significantly earlier for the type II cases (12 years compared with 24.5 years), but did not differ for the type I patients. The motor nerve conduction velocity was significantly lower for the recessive type I but not for the type II cases compared with the dominant form. The severity of the clinical features tended to be greater for the recessive type I cases compared with the dominant form, and their distinction from cases of Friedreich's ataxia is important.

Variant forms of hereditary motor and sensory neuropathy

Previously two eponymous forms of genetic polyneuropathy have been considered as clinical entities distinct from all others. These are hereditary hypertrophic polyneuritis (Déjèrine-Sottas disease) and the Roussy-Lévy syndrome, in which a static tremor of the arms and ataxic gait are associated with features of peroneal muscular atrophy. Thomas and his colleagues (1974) believe that these are not distinct genetic entities although they may describe individual cases. Patients with these particular features are better regarded as variations on the theme of hereditary motor and sensory neuropathy of autosomal dominant inheritance. Hypertrophic polyneuropathy is not peculiar to any one condition but is found in many inherited and acquired neuropathies and seems to be a non-specific result of repeated segmental degeneration and regeneration.

TREATMENT IN PERONEAL MUSCULAR ATROPHY

The slow rate of deterioration in many patients with this disorder should encourage attempts to improve the gait by orthopaedic measures. In some patients the foot-drop may be helped by a toe-spring. In many cases surgery has much to offer and discussion with an experienced orthopaedic surgeon soon after the diagnosis is made is advisable so that plans can be made. The topic is reviewed by Levitt and his colleagues (1973) who obtained excellent or good results in 9 of 12 patients treated surgically. All but one of those with satisfactory results had triple arthrodesis. Many had previous soft-tissue procedures, but operations designed to correct only one part of the deformity without stabilizing the hind-part and the mid-part of the foot, that is without concomitant triple arthrodesis, were less successful.

Sadly surgery has nothing comparable to offer in the upper limbs and the severe weakness, wasting and deformity of the hands seen in some patients is a grave handicap. Mechanical aids, such as electric typewriters, tape-recorders and the POSSUM machine as used in severe cerebral palsy (Ch. 11) may help partially to compensate for this.

ABETALIPOPROTEINAEMIA

(*Bassen-Kornzweig disease*) (Bassen & Kornzweig 1950)

The biochemical defect in patients with abetalipoproteinaemia is an inability to synthesize an apolipoprotein for the formation of very low-density and low-density lipoprotein, and chylomicrons. As a result triglycerides accumulate within small intestinal cells, fat-soluble vitamins are not absorbed and there is deficiency of vitamins A and E with low levels of cholesterol in plasma. Increased cholesterol in red cell membranes contributes to the formation of acanthocytes, red cells with thorn-like projections.

This rare disorder is inherited as an autosomal recessive with gastro-intestinal symptoms predominating in infancy but subsiding later, and with neurological and retinal degenerative features developing in childhood or adolescence, worsening for some years and then slowing down or becoming stationary.

Coeliac-like symptoms occur in infancy with frequent, bulky, offensive stools which float and sometimes with abdominal distension and growth retardation. A gluten-free diet gives no relief but restricted fat intake may reduce the diarrhoea. Biopsy of the small intestine shows a normal villous pattern but mucosal cells, especially at the tips of the villi, are filled with liposomes containing triglycerides. Acanthocytes are seen in wet preparations of fresh blood from all patients. These thorny, normocytic and normochromic red cells do not form rouleaux and hence the erythrocyte sedimentation rate is low.

Neurological features may include early delay in motor milestones or mental retardation, but grosser signs of central and peripheral nerve disorder develop later in childhood or in adolescence, giving a clinical picture similar to that of Friedreich's ataxia. This includes ataxia of gait and manipulation with intention tremor, dysarthria, hyporeflexia, weakness and reduced posterior column sensation (joint position and vibration). Scoliosis and equinovarus deformity of the feet are common.

Clinical features of a peripheral neuropathy occur in about a third of patients with reduced appreciation of pain and temperature in a 'glove and stocking' distribution. Nerve conduction studies have shown a mild slowing of motor nerve conduction velocity and the few biopsy and autopsy studies of peripheral nerves have shown demyelination in several cases with associated axonal loss in one.

Retinal abnormalities seem to be invariable. They may be found in early childhood but usually present in adolescence with night blindness, followed later by scotomas and finally by reduced visual acuity. Ophthalmoscopy shows small punctate granules in the peripheral retina and sometimes at the macula, and later clumps of pigment appear but without the 'bone corpuscle' appearance seen in some other conditions with retinal pigmentary degeneration. The electroretinogram (ERG) is progressively reduced. Pallor of the optic discs and attenuation of retinal arteries may develop later.

Myocardial fibrosis with arrhythmias and heart failure has been reported in several adults but is rare in childhood.

Acanthocytosis is not unique to Bassen-Kornzweig disease. It has been seen in hepatic failure, pyruvate kinase deficiency and Wolman's disease. Several families with inherited neurological disorders and acanthocytosis, but with normal plasma lipoproteins, have been reported. In one family the disease presented in adult life showing autosomal dominant inheritance (Critchley et al 1968).

TANGIER DISEASE (FAMILIAL α-LIPOPROTEIN DEFICIENCY)

This rare disorder was discovered (Frederickson et al 1961) in a 5-year-old from an isolated fishing community in Tangier island in Chesapeake Bay after his tonsils, removed surgically, were found to be bright yellow-orange with large amounts of cholesterol esters and free cholesterol in foam cells. Similar cells are also found throughout the reticuloendothelial system, in the liver, spleen, lymph nodes, bone marrow, skin and rectal mucosa and lamina propria. Hepatosplenomegaly is common and may cause abdominal discomfort and hypersplenism with thrombocytopenia, anaemia and reticulocytosis. Corneal infiltration and cardiac involvement were reported in several adult patients. Cholesterol levels are very low in the plasma and α-lipoproteins are absent.

The condition is inherited as an autosomal recessive and has a variable clinical spectrum. Neurological features, in the form of a severe motor and sensory peripheral neuropathy, occur in many patients. A neuropathy was present in 7 of the 14 patients with Tangier disease reported up to 1975 (Pleasure 1975). Their clinical features were very varied, symptoms starting between early childhood and middle age, with severity ranging from a single transient episode of weakness to a progressive neuropathy causing generalized weakness, wasting, fasciculation and almost complete sensory loss. Some patients had features suggesting a mononeuritis or 'mononeuritis multiplex', particularly involving the third, sixth and seventh cranial nerves, but often with loss of function only in muscles innervated by terminal twigs, so that an isolated ptosis or weakness of eye closure resulted.

REFSUM'S SYNDROME (HEREDOPATHIA ATACTICA POLYNEURITIFORMIS)

This rare disorder was first reported in 1945 by Refsum and more fully described by him in 1946. Its clinical features are those of a chronic polyneuropathy combined with pigmentary retinal degeneration, ataxia and other cerebellar signs and an increase in the protein level in the CSF with a normal cell count. Neurogenic hearing loss and cardiomyopathy are also present in most cases. Less common signs are icthyosiform skin changes, pupil abnormalities, lens opacities, anosmia and skeletal abnormalities. Accumulation of phytanic acid has been shown, and Steinberg (1978) has termed this inborn error of metabolism 'phytanic acid storage disease'. This biochemical defect, due to reduced capacity to oxidize phytanic acid, is the only pathognomonic feature of the disease, since the clinical manifestations may occur in other syndromes.

The condition is inherited as an autosomal recessive with males and females equally affected and a high proportion of consanguineous marriages in the parents, who are clinically normal. It was first described in Norway and most reported cases have come from Norway, Sweden, the British Isles, Germany and France. The age of onset has varied from early childhood to the third decade. The onset may be difficult to determine precisely. In four children presenting between 4 and 7 years of age (Refsum et al 1949) the onset was insidious with loss of appetite, unsteady gait, dry, scaly skin and progressive deafness. Sometimes symptoms seem to be precipitated by infections. Dramatic exacerbations and remissions of symptoms may occur spontaneously.

Ophthalmological disturbances

Pigmentary retinal degeneration or night blindness (hemeralopia) are present in all cases and Refsum believes they are essential for the diagnosis. Night blindness is often the earliest symptom and may be present for years before the diagnosis is made. Gradual concentric constriction of the visual fields develops until finally only tubular vision is left. For many years central vision may remain only slightly impaired or even normal. Rarely, optic atrophy, cataracts and vitreous opacities occur and contribute to the visual impairment. Ophthalmoscopically fine granular or 'pepper and salt' pigmentation is seen, usually peripherally but occasionally at the macula. The ERG is absent or reduced. The pupils are normal in children, though in many adults they show poor reactions to light, convergence and accommodation. Nystagmus has been noted in some cases.

Neurological features

A chronic, progressive peripheral neuropathy, which is usually symmetrical and initially distal causing muscular atrophy and weakness, is the second cardinal manifestation of the disease. It may develop some years after visual and auditory impairment. The distal weakness and wasting with progressive reduction of tendon reflexes starting with the ankle jerks may simulate peroneal muscular atrophy of the Charcot-Marie-Tooth type. Motor and sensory nerve conduction velocity are greatly reduced, motor velocities of under 10 m per second being common. EMG studies show evidence of denervation. Deep sensation is often impaired with loss of joint position sense distally. Cutaneous hypaesthesia with a 'glove and stocking' distribution may be found, and some patients complain of painful paraesthesiae. There may be palpable thickening of peripheral nerves (ulnar, peroneal and greater auricular).

Progressive hearing loss of cochlear type may start early and become almost complete. Anosmia and hyposmia may also occur. Ataxia and nystagmus of cerebellar type are present in many cases. In others unsteadiness of gait and manipulation are due mainly to weakness and sensory loss.

Cardiomyopathy is present in most cases as shown by cardiac enlargement, tachycardia, conduction disturbances and ECG changes, and has probably been the cause of sudden death in some patients.

Skin changes are more marked in children than in adults. Their severity varies from a dry, scaly skin to an icthyosis-like condition and may decrease during remissions (spontaneous or diet-induced) of the neurological symptoms.

Skeletal manifestations include abnormalities of the metatarsal bones, which may be short or elongated, pes cavus, hammer toes and epiphyseal dysplasia of the shoulders, elbows and knees.

Pathology

Changes are always seen in the peripheral nerves but their severity varies. They show irregular hypertrophy with myelinated nerve fibres reduced in number and Schwann cell processes giving rise to typical 'onion bulb' formations. In the CNS axonal reaction in the anterior horn cells and posterior column degeneration are seen secondary to the peripheral lesions. Further lesions include tract degenerations in the medial lemniscus and in cerebellar connexions, particularly the olivocerebellar fibres.

Investigations

The CSF protein is increased in almost all cases to between 100 and 700 mg per 100 ml or even higher. The cell count is normal so that the albuminocytological dissociation seen in the Guillain-Barré syndrome and in some other forms of polyneuritis is present.

The diagnostic test is the demonstration of phytanic acid (3, 7, 11, 15-tetramethylhexadecanoic acid) in the serum. This compound is not normally present in humans but accounted for 5 to 30% of the total fatty acids of the serum lipids in 9 patients investigated by Kahlke (1964). It is thought to be of exogenous dietary origin, its accumulation in Refsum's syndrome being due to failure of its α-hydroxylation to α-hydroxyphytanic acid. The mode of action of phytanic acid in producing neurological dysfunction is not clear, but the peripheral neuropathy could perhaps result from its incorporation into myelin making the structure of the latter less stable than normal.

Treatment

Two therapeutic approaches have been tried in Refsum's syndrome. Two patients with very high levels of phytanic acid were treated as an emergency by plasmapheresis once a week for several months in combination with dietary treatment.

The dietary approach aims at excluding from the diet phytanic acid, which is found in many animal fats, and phytol, its precursor, which is found in plant lipids in green vegetables. Most of the calories are supplied as carbohydrates. (Stokke & Eldjarn 1975 give details of the revised diet.) Three adult Norwegian patients were so treated (Eldjarn et al 1966). The results in two were excellent with normal serum levels of phytanic acid and no clinical relapses. One of these two patients died from an apparently unrelated intrapontine haemorrhage and showed no histological features of Refsum's disease and no accumulation of phytanic acid in his organs. The surviving patient showed improvement in nerve conduction velocity and a fall in CSF protein. Similar improvement with diet has been found by other workers.

HEREDITARY SENSORY NEUROPATHY

Sensory loss with insensitivity to pain is a feature of some rare congenital syndromes of hereditary sensory neuropathy (HSN) seen in childhood and also of hereditary sensory radicular neuropathy (HSN Type I) (Denny-Brown 1951) which presents in adult life with dominant inheritance. The term 'congenital indifference to pain' is sometimes applied to these syndromes but is inapt as it suggests a cerebral lesion for which evidence is lacking. The various forms of HSN have been classified by Thomas (1975).

The childhood syndromes are:

a. Congenital sensory neuropathy; (HSN Type II in Thomas' classification)
b. Congenital sensory neuropathy with anhidrosis; (HSN Type IV)
c. Congenital insensitivity to pain, and
d. Familial dysautonomia (the Riley-Day syndrome) (HSN Type III)

They are reviewed by Vassella et al (1968), Barry et al (1974), Thomas (1975), and Dyck & Ohta (1975).

More recently a syndrome of hereditary spastic paraplegia with sensory neuropathy has been reported, with analgesia leading to severe problems of injury and infection (Cavanagh et al 1979).

The differential diagnosis of these syndromes includes the Lesch-Nyhan syndrome (Ch. 8) in which self-mutilation is common, and conditions with mental retardation in which it may occur (Ch. 13).

a. Congenital sensory neuropathy (Thévenard 1942, Johnson & Spalding 1964, Barry et al 1974) (HSN Type II)

This is a rare autosomal recessive disorder with onset in infancy or childhood, in which there is gross impairment of appreciation of all modalities of cutaneous and sometimes kinaesthetic sensation, hypotonia and absence of tendon reflexes. The sensory loss is distal in distribution and may lead to a mutilating neuropathic arthropathy with paronychia, ulcers of the fingers and feet and often unrecognized fractures of the limbs. Intelligence is usually normal and there is no impairment of autonomic function with normal production of tears but some loss of sweating. Two unrelated infants with this condition were reported by Barry et al (1974). They showed delayed motor development and were unresponsive to pain, one child damaging his fingers by chewing them. Touch sensation and corneal reflexes were absent. In one case light and electron microscopy studies of skin from peripheral sites showed no free nerve endings though normal nerves were seen in more proximal skin. Unmyelinated fibres with only an occasional

small myelinated fibre were present in the sural nerve in one case, while no sural nerve tissue was found in the other. The prognosis in this disorder seems to be reasonably good, though the children are at risk of severe painless injuries, ulceration and infection of the extremities. Amputation of chronically infected digits may be needed.

b. Congenital sensory neuropathy with anhidrosis (Swanson et al 1965, Vassella et al 1968) (HSN Type IV)

This condition with autosomal recessive inheritance shares some features with the preceding one, but differs from it in its preservation of light touch sensation and association with inability to sweat and with mental subnormality. There is wide spread congenital absence of pain and temperature appreciation with self-mutilation by biting of the fingers and tongue, with normal appreciation of light touch and preserved corneal reflexes. The children are mentally retarded, the IQs of seven reported patients being between 40 and 80 (Vassella et al 1968). This factor makes the prevention of severe injury very difficult. All patients have shown unpredictable rises of temperature probably related to their inability to sweat normally. Histological examination of the skin showed normal free nerve endings, nerve receptors and sweat glands in the case of Vassella et al, but another case at necropsy (Swanson et al 1965) showed absence of the small primary sensory neurons in the posterior root ganglia, posterior roots and Lissauer's tract.

c. Congenital insensitivity to pain

This term has been applied to a rare clinical entity with absence of normal appreciation of and reaction to pain but no other neurological deficits. The condition is typified by the four siblings reported by Thrush (1973) lacking pain sensation from birth but with normal appreciation of other sensory modalities, normal tendon reflexes and normal sweating. These features distinguish this from the two previously described syndromes. The children had sustained many severe, painless injuries causing disfigurement, fractures and Charcot joints. Self-mutilation by biting, head-banging and scratching were common. Three patients had intelligence levels in the dull normal range, as did two unaffected siblings, and one had an IQ of 57. They were overactive, mischievous children who would often injure themselves through bravado by jumping from heights. Fortunately their behaviour improved with age and they seemed to learn to use other clues to help avoid injury, though remaining unaware of pain.

Motor and sensory nerve conduction studies gave normal results. A sural nerve biopsy showed a reduction in numbers of large myelinated fibres.

d. Familial dysautonomia (the Riley-Day syndrome)

As the name implies the neuropathy in this disorder involves autonomic as well as peripheral nerves, both of which show absence of unmyelinated nerve fibres. The condition is almost restricted to those of Ashkenazi Jewish descent from Eastern Europe and shows autosomal recessive inheritance though a few a typical cases in Gentiles have been reported. An early feature is severe feeding difficulty with failure to thrive. Developmental retardation becomes evident as time passes and it also becomes clear that the affected children do not feel pain, do not cry tears and sweat excessively. Hypotonia and reduced or absent tendon reflexes are other features of the neuropathy with absent corneal reflexes and postural hypotension. The normal fungiform papillae of the tongue are absent. Excessive sweating, defective temperature control, frequent chest infections and recurrent vomiting create great problems of management. Many patients die in infancy or childhood from aspiration pneumonia. Sepsis and cor pulmonale may be terminal complications at a later age. Inadequate management of dehydration and extreme hyperpyrexia with infections and vomiting crises may also prove lethal.

The diagnosis can be strongly suspected in older children but may be difficult to distinguish in infancy from other causes of feeding problems and failure to thrive. Absence or great reduction in overflow tears is invariable and should strongly suggest the disease. A smooth, pale tip to the tongue due to absence of fungiform papillae makes it even more likely.

Confirmation of the diagnosis is obtained by two tests.

1. Histamine test

The intradermal injection of 0.03 to 0.05 ml of 1 in 1000 solution of histamine normally causes pain and erythema followed quickly by a central wheal surrounded by a flare. In dysautonomia the pain is much less and there is no axon flare. The test is reliable with no false negative results. False positive results (with absent flare in non-dysautonomic patients) are seen in congenital sensory neuropathy which may be excluded clinically and by

2. The methacholine (mecholyl) test

2.5% methacholine when instilled into the conjunctival sac has no effect on the normal pupil but in most patients with dysautonomia causes miosis.

Treatment

The problems of management are severe especially in infancy, when feeding difficulties and dysphagia predominate and aspiration pneumonia is a threat. Tube-feeding may be needed. Vomiting crises occur after the age of three years and may cause dehydration, aspiration of vomit and haematemesis. Respiratory infections, spinal deformity and anaesthesia are important hazards. Seizures occur in about 40% of patients, often associated with the hyperpyrexia to which they are liable. Intelligence is below normal in many patients and academic under-achievement is common due to immaturity, emotional lability and frequent absence from school through illness. The eyes are vulnerable to trauma, being unprotected by tears and lacking the normal corneal sensitivity as a warning of irritants such as foreign bodies. Keratitis, blepharitis, corneal ulcers and scars are the result in many patients.

A vigilant and comprehensive approach to management is needed in view of the hazards of the disease. These problems are well reviewed by Axelrod et al (1974) who consider that a more aggressive and informed approach to treatment is extending the life span with patients now surviving to the third and fourth decades.

Hereditary spastic paraplegia with sensory neuropathy

Cavanagh et al (1979) have reported five patients

with spastic paraplegia present from early childhood and a progressive ulcerating distal sensory neuropathy affecting arms and legs (Fig. 4.1A, 4.1B). In 3 cases the paraplegia and neuropathy were clinically evident at an early age. This condition differs from the previously recognized categories of sensory neuropathy (Thomas 1975) in the progressive sensory impairment and gradual loss of tendon reflexes with the greater involvement of pain and temperature sensation. The inheritance may have been by an autosomal recessive mechanism, although in a pair of half-brothers born to

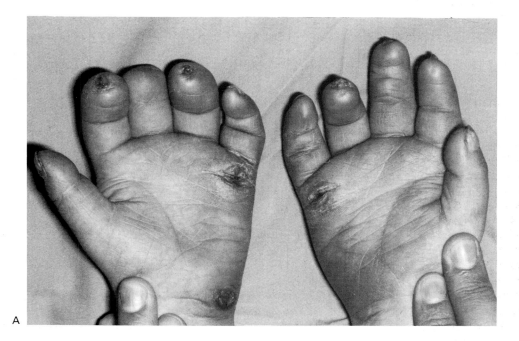

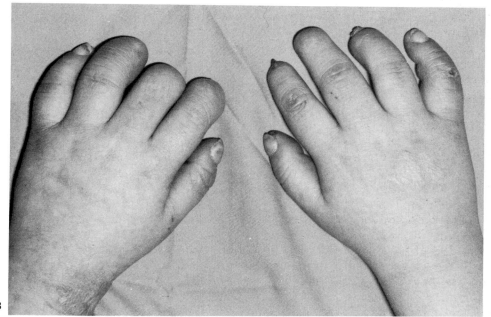

Fig 4.1A & B Hereditary spastic paraplegia with sensory neuropathy in 7-year-old boy, showing severe deformities of hands.

the same mother but of uncertain paternity an X-linked dominant mode is possible.

The prognosis in this condition is poor. One patient died aged 29 of renal failure due to a nephrotic syndrome associated with amyloidosis, and the outlook in those presenting at a younger age appears even worse with osteomyelitis a severe problem.

Hereditary neuropathy with liability to pressure palsies

There are many reports of families suffering from an inherited disorder of peripheral nerves which show an increased susceptibility to pressure and traction. Isolated nerve palsies occur with the sudden or gradual onset of weakness, often with pain. Gradual recovery is usual but there may be residual weakness. The CSF has been normal when examined. The degree of trauma involved is often very slight and a pre-existing abnormality of peripheral nerves seems likely, since widespread electrophysiological abnormalities have been found in many patients in nerves which seemed clinically unaffected (Earl et al 1964). In some families autosomal dominant inheritance is shown by involvement of many generations. The nerves affected include most peripheral nerves but the brachial plexus has been very commonly involved. The age of onset of symptoms varies but has been as early as $2\frac{1}{2}$ years in the family reported by Jacob et al (1961).

In this family and in that reported by Guillozet & Mercer (1973) the patients had asymmetrical faces with close-set eyes. This disorder is distinct from a form of epidemic brachial neuritis occurring in adults and described by Wyburn-Mason (1941) and Spillane (1943).

Painful brachial plexus neuropathy

A disorder with the rapid onset of pain followed by muscle weakness usually affecting one arm has been recognized for many years. It may occur at any age from a few months onwards but is much commoner in adults than children. In some cases the symptoms have started soon after vaccination or injection of serum. Most cases seem not to be familial, though Taylor (1960) reported a family with 119 individuals in five generations with a strong tendency towards recurrent attacks of neuritis. He described it as heredofamilial mononeuritis multiplex with brachial predilection. Though brachial plexus involvement was commonest, the cranial nerves and multiple peripheral nerves were also affected in this family. Excruciating pain was followed by the onset of muscle weakness, atrophy and sensory loss, with functional recovery after many months though residual deficits were seen. In half of the affected females the attacks were associated with pregnancy. The onset was as early as 4 years of age, and the inheritance was clearly as an autosomal dominant.

Most reported cases have not been familial, however, and in the series of 99 patients reported by Tsairis et al (1972) with brachial plexus neuropathy, a family history seemed likely in only one case. Seven of these patients had the onset of symptoms under 20 years of age, the youngest being 3 months old. Fourteen patients gave a history of recent vaccination or foreign serum injection, but the clinical features in these seemed no different from the rest. In most cases weakness began within two weeks of the onset of pain. Sensory loss most often affected the territory of the circumflex nerve or the radial surface of the forearm. The brachial plexus could be affected in the upper or lower parts or in its entirety and often bilaterally. Recurrences occurred in four patients. Most patients had recovered within three years. In a series of five children with acute brachial neuritis, with a sixth suffering from 'neuralgic amyotrophy' of one leg, four were left with some residual weakness and a previously undescribed shortening of the affected limb (Day, personal communication 1982).

THE GUILLAIN-BARRÉ SYNDROME (ACUTE INFECTIOUS POLYNEURITIS: ACUTE IDIOPATHIC POLYNEURITIS)

In 1916, Guillain, Barré and Strohl described a syndrome of 'radiculoneuritis' with acute flaccid paralysis and with an increase in protein in the CSF but without a cellular reaction. (Cases of ascending paralysis described by Landry in 1859 may have been examples of the same condition.)

The Guillain-Barré syndrome is not rare in childhood and is the commonest form of peripheral neuropathy affecting children. Wiederholt et al (1964) in their series of 97 cases from the Mayo clinic found that it occurred at all ages with peaks in the first and fifth decades. Many series have shown a male to female ratio of between 2 to 1 and 3 to 2.

Clinical features

Flaccid weakness of the limbs develops, often following a prodromal upper respiratory or gastro-intestinal illness of probable or proven viral origin. The interval between the preceding illness and the onset of polyneuritis is between one and 28 days, usually between 10 and 14. This illness is most often a common cold, but pharyngitis, tonsillitis and gastro-intestinal disorder are also frequent precursors. Occasionally a more specific virus infection such as mumps, chicken-pox, infectious mononucleosis, herpes simplex, zoster or cytomegalovirus, is implicated by clinical features, virus isolation or rising antibody titres, but the syndrome in general cannot be regarded as related to one virus infection more often than any other. It is unusual for more than one member of a family to develop the condition, even though all may be stricken by the preceding infectious illness. The aetiology of the syndrome and its relationship to the previous illness is obscure. An allergic or auto-immune mechanism has been suggested and is given some support by the cases with identical clinical features in which paralysis has closely followed an immunizing procedure. The most recent example of this is the dramatic increase in cases of Guillain-Barré syndrome in individuals who had received swine influenza vaccine in the United States (Grouse 1980; Marks & Halpin 1980). Evidence from other species also lends some support to this idea: experimental allergic neuritis (EAN) in animals was shown by Waksman & Adams (1955) to resemble the Guillain-Barré syndrome in man clinically and pathologically and to be associated with the presence of circulating antibodies. In the acute phase of the human illness circulating demyelinating factors were shown by Cook et al (1971) and this may have implications for therapy in a disease for which no treatment is of proven value (Brettle et al 1978).

Weakness of the limbs is usually acute in onset, bilateral, and often symmetrical. Often generalized, it commonly starts in the legs, spreading upwards to involve the arms, giving the picture of so-called 'Landry's ascending paralysis'. Weakness is more likely to affect the legs alone than the arms alone. It may be equal in proximal and distal muscles and, if unequal, is more often greater distally than proximally. The muscles of respiration and those supplied by the cranial nerves may be affected, as in poliomyelitis, producing a more serious threat than that caused by limb weakness alone.

The onset of paralysis is sometimes subacute, and in some children it is difficult to be certain when it began since they may have been confined to bed as a result of the preceding infectious illness and are only noticed to be weak when they have recovered from this and are expected to get up and about again.

Sensory symptoms are usually less striking than paralysis, but in some cases paraesthesiae of the hands and feet, often painful, are complained of before the onset of weakness, or may accompany this. In younger children, less able to describe their symptoms, a history of sensory disorder is less likely than in older children or adults, but it should be enquired for. Occasionally back pain or severe pain in the limbs with muscle tenderness are prominent features.

Involvement of cranial nerves is common, and often more than one nerve is affected. The facial nerve is the most frequently involved, often bilaterally. Other cranial nerve feature include dysphagia, a nasal voice, ptosis, diplopia, and disorders of external eye movements. Occasionally papilloedema is present, particularly in cases with very high levels of protein in the CSF.

Mental clarity is usually fully preserved, although the children are often understandably frightened by their symptoms. An encephalitic or myelitic component occurs in some cases, and is suggested by drowsiness, headache, irritability, opisthotonos or neck stiffness. Gamstorp (1974) found evidence of CNS involvement, as judged by such features and EEG changes, in ten children with the Guillain-Barré syndrome. Striking changes in mood and behaviour were present early and persisted long after the motor symptoms had disappeared. In order to stress the common involvement of the CNS, at least in childhood,

Gamstorp suggested the term 'encephalo-myelo-radiculoneuropathy', but brevity and euphony will probably continue to recommend the eponyms to most clinicians.

On examination in the early stages the major finding is flaccid, often symmetrical, paralysis of variable distribution. Wasting of the muscles is not usual, but they are often tender on palpation. The tendon reflexes are usually absent and, when present, almost always reduced. The plantar responses are generally flexor, unless weakness has abolished them. Occasionally a transiently extensor plantar response is seen. Sensory testing may show anaesthesia with a distal, often 'glove and stocking' distribution in older and co-operative children. Impairment of postural sensation in small or even larger joints can sometimes be shown on testing and is often an important factor contributing to the difficulty in walking or causing inco-ordination in the upper limbs. When loss of postural and superficial sensation is severe the resultant unsteadiness and impairment of co-ordination may mimic cerebellar ataxia. Guillain himself (1936) referred to ataxia in several adult patients and commented that some patients might present a pseudotabetic appearance like that associated with diphtheritic neuritis.

The course of the illness is usually a progressive increase in weakness to a peak, often followed by a plateau with no further deterioration, and finally improvement, usually with complete recovery. The time relations of these phases can vary. The interval from onset of the illness to maximum weakness was about 10.5 days in the series of Eberle et al (1975). Recovery usually starts within one or two weeks from the attainment of greatest weakness, but may be delayed, and the rate at which it occurs is also variable. Relapses and remissions are quite common.

Biopsies of peripheral nerves, which are rarely justified in children with acute polyneuritis, usually show segmental demyelination and sometimes foci of inflammatory cells. Similar changes are found in the rare cases which come to autopsy.

Differential diagnosis

This is from other causes of acute paralysis. Poliomyelitis, (which has become rarer in the United Kingdom than the Guillain-Barré syndrome) may be difficult to distinguish, but usually produces a less symmetrical distribution of weakness, and is not associated with paraesthesiae, though muscle tenderness may occur. Previous immunization against poliomyelitis makes the disease less likely but does not exclude it. Tendon reflexes are absent or reduced in severe paralysis due to poliomyelitis, but are more likely to be preserved in unaffected muscles than is the case in polyneuritis. There may be particular diagnostic difficulty in the rare cases in which the Guillain-Barré syndrome comes on soon after oral polio vaccine has been given. The typical CSF changes of polyneuritis and the common finding of slowing of motor nerve conduction velocity help to distinguish the two disorders in most cases. Transverse myelitis must also be considered in the differential diagnosis; a clear motor and sensory level is often found.

Acute flaccid paralysis in infancy may be due to infantile botulism (Ch. 22) a condition reported recently in the United States and only once so far recognized in Britain. It is unusual for the Guillain-Barré syndrome to affect children as young as this. The neuropathy of acute intermittent porphyria is rare in childhood but can produce a symmetrical flaccid paralysis.

Polymyositis may need to be considered, but points of distinction include the asymmetry commonly seen in the weakness, the frequent preservation of tendon reflexes, the relative rarity of weakness of bulbar muscles and the commonly associated skin lesions. A raised CK level also favours polymyositis, and the neurophysiological investigations give different results in the two disorders (Ch. 24).

The combination of weakness, hypotonia and inco-ordination caused by loss of postural sensation may produce a clinical picture very suggestive of cerebellar disorder, and young children with polyneuritis are often admitted to hospital with the referring diagnosis of a cerebellar tumour. If a lumbar puncture has been performed (highly inadvisable with such a suspicion), the finding of a raised CSF protein may seem to strengthen this possibility. The occasional occurrence of papilloedema may be even more misleading.

Severe pain in the back with back or neck stiffness and paralysis of the limbs may suggest a neo-plasm or other pathology affecting the spinal cord. The finding of a raised CSF protein in this situation may lend spurious support to this idea, and some unfortunate children with the Guillain-Barré syndrome have been subjected to myelography on this acccount. When pain in the limbs is severe, rheumatic fever or other forms of arthropathy may be strongly suspected.

Prognosis

Although severe respiratory and cranial nerve involvement may be life-threatening, these problems can usually be dealt with in the acute stage of the illness and the patient tided over until improvement begins, either spontaneously or in association with treatment.

Most children who survive the acute stage can be expected to make a complete recovery. In a few cases the outlook is less benign, since recovery may be delayed and incomplete, and relapses and recurrences can occur.

Factors related to incomplete recovery have been examined by Eberle et al (1975) who found the most useful predictor of eventual incomplete recovery to be the time taken for improvement to begin after weakness had become maximum. If 16 days elapsed without improvement after reaching the nadir of weakness, there was a 96% probability that full recovery would not occur, and if more than 18 days passed without improvement incomplete recovery was almost certain. The interval from the onset of weakness to maximum weakness or to the start of improvement did not seem to correlate well with eventual recovery. Incomplete recovery was also associated with a higher incidence of absent deep tendon reflexes and of severe weakness in distal muscles.

Investigations

The CSF changes generally conform to the classical 'albuminocytological' dissociation, with a rise in protein level to between 100 and 300 mg per 100 ml and often higher, yet without the pleocytosis which accompanies most inflammatory diseases. The cells usually number 5 or less per cubic mm, the cell type being lymphocytic. The diag-nostic value of these changes is lessened by the fact that they may not occur at an early stage of the illness, so that the CSF may be normal when first obtained, and changes may only be detected by serial examination. The maximum elevation of protein in the series of 26 children with the Guillain-Barré syndrome studied by Peterman et al (1959) occurred from 10 to 25 days after onset. In Marshall's (1963) mainly adult cases the peak was between the fourth and eighteenth days. A natural desire to avoid repeating lumbar puncture in children may result in the raised protein being undetected. The return to normal levels is often slow, lagging behind clinical improvement.

Neurophysiological studies of motor and sensory nerve conduction are helpful in establishing the diagnosis (see Ch. 24) and in following improvement.

Relapses, with worsening of the condition before it has fully recovered, and recurrences, implying further episodes after complete recovery from the original illness, can occur in polyneuritis. In children they probably occur in fewer than 10% of cases. Like the primary episode of polyneuritis, they tend to follow upper respiratory or gastro-intestinal infections. Recurrent and chronic relapsing Guillain-Barré polyneuritis was reviewed by Thomas et al (1969) who reported five cases, including three children. Occasionally relapses may occur at intervals over a period of a year or more.

That different immunopathogenic mechanisms may operate in acute idiopathic and in chronic relapsing polyneuropathy is suggested by the finding in 14 of 15 patients with the latter of a 'monoclonal' (single) IgG band in the CSF which was unchanged on repeated examination and unaffected by corticosteroid treatment (Dalakas et al 1980). By contrast, in acute idiopathic polyneuropathy, transient oligoclonal IgG bands were found in 19 of 47 patients and these disappeared when the neurological signs subsided. The authors suggest that the stable IgG band in the chronic relapsing condition may reflect the response to a persisting antigenic stimulation and may in time prove to be of prognostic value early in the course of the illness and perhaps help in therapeutic decisions.

Treatment

Treatment is basically symptomatic and supportive, aimed at relieving symptoms and maintaining respiration and nutrition, when these are threatened by respiratory and bulbar paralysis, until improvement begins.

Death, when it occurs, is usually due to respiratory failure, so respiratory function must be regularly monitored and vigorous efforts made to maintain adequate ventilation with tracheostomy and assisted respiration. The situation is similar to that in severe cases of paralytic poliomyelitis, except that the prognosis is better, and skilled medical and nursing care are essential. Urinary retention may occur and requires the use of catheters.

Analgesia may be needed for painful paraesthesiae. Physiotherapy should be directed towards passive movement of paralysed limbs and the prevention of contractures and deformity as well as assisting postural drainage of the chest.

The use of steroid treatment has been controversial. It is difficult to assess its effect in a condition which usually improves spontaneously. Several authors have found steroids to be without benefit (Plum 1953, Marshall 1963, Ravn 1967), but Graveson (1961) and Swiek & McQuillen (1976) reported more encouraging results. The numbers of patients in these series were small, and larger numbers are needed for a controlled trial and statistical analysis in order to try to resolve this question. The results of the recently published London multicentre controlled trial of prednisolone (Hughes et al 1978) indicated that steroid treatment was not helpful and could be detrimental, with three relapses in the prednisolone group but none among the controls. For the doctor faced with the individual child patient with the Guillain-Barré syndrome it seems logical to reserve steroids for patients who are deteriorating rather than to use them in milder cases. The mode of action of steroids in polyneuritis, if they are effective in some cases, is still unknown as in other neurological diseases in which they are used. The dose required is usually high and may give rise to the features of Cushing's syndrome and other side-effects. These can sometimes be limited by giving very high doses on alternate days.

One adult patient with severe and progressive paralysis was recently treated by plasma exchange and showed a dramatic and abrupt improvement (Brettle et al 1978). Though this cannot be proved to be due to the treatment it is consistent with the removal of a humoral factor such as a myelinotoxic antibody.

THE MILLER-FISHER SYNDROME

Ophthalmoplegia is rare in the Guillain-Barré syndrome, but occurs in a syndrome regarded as an unusual variant, (Fisher 1956). The clinical features of the Miller-Fisher syndrome are external ophthalmoplegia, areflexia and ataxia without gross weakness of limbs or trunk. Facial and other cranial nerve palsies may be present. The CSF usually shows the same changes as in the classical Guillain-Barré syndrome. The condition is benign, usually with complete recovery, though relapses and remissions can occur. There is often a history of a preceding upper respiratory infection but, as with the Guillain-Barré syndrome proper, there is no constant relationship with a particular virus.

The defect of external eye movements is severe. There may be total lack of eye movements, both voluntary and reflex. By contrast ptosis is often slight and the pupil reactions may be relatively spared. Parallelism of the eyes is often preserved. Sometimes there may be greater impairment of either horizontal or vertical conjugate movements and the recovery of one or other of these movements may occur before the other. The site of the lesion causing the ophthalmoplegia is uncertain, but there may be both a peripheral and central involvement of the oculomotor system (Tripp 1975).

Differential diagnosis

Despite its rarity, it is important to recognize the syndrome in view of its benign prognosis in contrast to that of many diseases causing ophthalmoplegia. The condition must be distinguished from myasthenia gravis, in which ptosis is usually more marked, tendon reflexes are usually present, the CSF normal and the tensilon test positive. A pontine glioma may have to be considered when sixth and seventh cranial nerve palsies are present, but these are rarely as symmetrical in the early stages as they are in the Miller-Fisher syndrome, and are often associated with signs of pyramidal tract dysfunction.

Peripheral neuropathy in acute intermittent porphyria

The commonest form of porphyria in north-western Europe is the acute intermittent variety, and neuropathy is its most dangerous complication and the commonest cause of death (Ridley 1969). Death is usually due to respiratory failure from paralysis of the muscles of respiration. The abdominal crises of porphyria, though distressing and diagnostically puzzling, are less of a threat to life. Though rare in childhood, the diagonosis should be considered in older children with acute neuropathy.

In Ridley' series the youngest patient with neuropathy was aged 18 years but about half the patients had experienced one or more attacks with abdominal symptoms before the first episode in which neuropathy occurred. Muscle weakness, usually symmetrical, was the commonest presentation in the neuropathic attacks, often preceded by aching, cramp-like pain or stiffness in the affected muscles. A few attacks began with sensory symptoms with paraesthesiae or numbness, and urinary hesitation or retention occurred in several cases. The cranial nerves were affected in many attacks, especially the seventh and tenth nerves. Loss or reduction of tendon reflexes was almost invariable. Mental disturbances were common and could precede or coincide with the onset of neuropathy. They often occurred in patients who had recently received barbiturates. Fits occurred in six attacks.

Pathological changes in the nervous system in acute porphyria were reviewed by Hierons (1957). His five cases included two in which symptoms, in the form of abdominal pain, began at the ages of 9 and 13 years. In the former case neurological symptoms were delayed until 24 years later, but in the latter convulsions, paralysis, papilloedema and hypertension developed acutely within 18 months and death occurred two months later.

The neuropathy of the Chediak-Higashi syndrome

In this rare disease haematological features (anaemia, leucopenia and thrombocytopenia) are associated with defective hair pigmentation, a liability to infection and lymphoreticular malignancy and neurological problems. The latter include mental retardation, seizures and muscular weakness.

Lockman et al (1967) have described a peripheral neuropathy in which giant lysosomal bodies are present in Schwann cells. The patient was an 11 year old girl who had developed weakness two years previously in muscles supplied by the right ulnar and both peroneal nerves.

FACIAL PARALYSIS

Paralysis of the facial muscles, like that of other voluntary muscles, may be due to lesions of the upper or lower motor neuron at various levels.

Upper motor neuron facial weakness is common in cerebral palsy. It is common in both congenital and acquired hemiplegia and also in bilateral hemiplegia or tetraplegia, but rare in spastic and spastic-ataxic diplegia. It may also occur in cerebral hemisphere tumours, usually accompanied by some weakness in the ipsilateral upper limb. Facial palsy of upper motor neuron origin can usually be readily distinguished from lower motor neuron weakness, since the upper part of the face is spared in the former, whereas the whole of the face on one side is affected with peripheral facial paralysis.

Facial weakness may be due to lesions of many kinds at the various levels of the lower motor neuron from the nucleus of the facial nerve to the muscle fibre.

Nuclear lesions include congenital absence or hypoplasia of the nuclei as in Moebius' syndrome (often associated with bilateral sixth nerve palsies), brain stem tumours, infections such as poliomyelitis, degenerative disorders such as progressive bulbar palsy of Fazio-Londe type and rare cases of syringobulbia and hydrobulbia.

Muscle disorders causing facial weakness, discussed in Chapter 3, include dystrophia myotonica, facioscapulo-humeral muscular dystrophy, various congenital myopathies, mitochondrial myopathies and myasthenic syndromes. The weakness is invariably bilateral in these cases. Lower motor neuron facial weakness, usually bilateral, is common in the Guillain-Barré syndrome.

Lower motor neuron facial paralysis (Bell's palsy)

Unilateral facial weakness of acute onset without dysfunction of other cranial nerves or tracts is usually due to involvement of the facial nerve at some point between the pons and the facial muscles. The nerve has a long course, much of which runs within the petrous bone, with a close relationship to the middle ear.

The term 'Bell's palsy' refers to lower motor neuron facial paralysis of undetermined cause. In most cases of acute facial palsy no cause is found, but it often presents soon after or during the course of a mild upper respiratory infection. Sometimes there is a more obvious and severe illness such as mumps parotitis, otitis media, herpes zoster or meningitis. The onset is often associated with pain in the face or ear. This is followed shortly by weakness of the face so that the mouth is drawn to the opposite side and the eyelid cannot be closed nor the forehead wrinkled on the affected side. In severe cause the lower lid falls away from the eyeball so that tears cannot drain into the lacrimal punctum and run down on to the cheek.

Involvement of the branches of the facial nerve may lead to other symptoms. Thus when the petrosal nerve is affected lacrimation is impaired in the ipsilateral eye. With involvement of the chorda tympani nerve salivation and taste over the anterior two thirds of the tongue are impaired. When the nerve to the stapedius muscle is affected the patient may complain that noises appear unduly loud and painful on the affected side, and tests of acoustic impedance give abnormal results.

Treatment of Bell's palsy with corticosteroids is often recommended within the first 48–72 hours from onset when its beneficial effect may be due to the reduction of oedema and hence of compression of the nerve in the facial canal. Treatment is given for 1–2 weeks. Spontaneous improvement tends to begin within a few weeks of onset and is usually complete within a few months, so that the effects of therapy are difficult to assess. An eye patch may be needed to protect the cornea from damage.

In many series of acute facial weakness in children hypertension has been found to be the cause, and the blood pressure should be checked in all cases (Ch. 19). The weakness is unilateral, tends to improve with control of hypertension and may recur when the blood pressure rises again. It may be due to haemorrhage or oedema in the facial canal

with pressure on the facial nerve. Birth trauma during a difficult delivery with or without forceps, or skull fractures may cause facial paralysis. Local tumours affecting bone, such as various sarcomas and metastases may also present with facial weakness.

Unilateral or bilateral facial palsy with a tendency to spontaneous remission and recurrence is seen in Melkersson's syndrome in association with chronic facial oedema.

SCIATIC NERVE INJURY

Sciatic nerve injury is a hazard of intramuscular injections into the buttocks. This can occur at any age if the injection site is incorrect, but newborn and especially premature infants are most vulnerable. In dissections of the gluteal region in two stillborn infants Gilles & French (1961) found that the maximal depth of tissue covering the sciatic nerve was less than 1 cm. Penicillin, streptomycin, vitamin K and many other drugs may be involved. Damage may be due to the injection of material into the nerve, to the needle or to ischaemia. Weakness appears after one or more days from the injection, but its precise onset may be difficult to date in a sick infant under treatment for an infection. In the neonate injections of drugs into the umbilical artery may cause sciatic paralysis (San Agustin et al 1962).

The site of injury to the sciatic nerve or its branches may be surmised from the pattern of weakness of muscles and confirmed by electromyography which may give evidence of denervation in these muscles. Damage to the sciatic nerve before it divides into the common peroneal nerve and the nerve to the hamstrings may pick out the peroneal portion with sparing of the hamstrings and gastrocnemius. Foot-drop is the commonest motor feature, due to weakness of the ankle dorsiflexors, and the foot is held in plantar flexion and inversion. 20 of the 21 patients with post-injection sciatic palsies reported by Gilles and French (1961) had obvious foot-drop, while the other had hamstring weakness as the sole deficit. Sensory features may be prominent in older children, with pain and dysaesthesiae in the foot and with loss of sensation.

The differential diagnosis includes infections

causing paralysis (poliomyelitis, herpes zoster or diphtheria). Spinal cord tumour should also be considered, but is less likely with unilateral weakness, a non-progressive course and absence of pyramidal tract involvement.

In severe cases the prognosis for recovery is poor. Complete recovery occurs in about one third of cases, and footdrop often fails to improve. Arrest of growth in the affected foot is common; it occurred in 9 of the 21 cases of Gilles and French, all the children being under $3\frac{1}{2}$ years of age at the time of the injury. A granuloma palpable in the buttock at the site of injection indicates a poor prognosis for recovery and surgical exploration should be considered, when no improvement in weakness is seen, with a view to attempting to remove the granuloma and deal with any adhesions around the nerve.

Prevention of sciatic nerve injury is best achieved by attention to the placing of intramuscular injections. The buttock is better avoided in favour of the lateral aspect of the thigh at the junction of the middle and lower thirds, where there is a relatively large muscle mass with no important underlying nerves or blood vessels. If the buttock is used, its outer and upper segment is the safest site.

The carpal tunnel syndrome

This syndrome, with compression of the median nerve at the wrist by the flexor retinaculum and related structures, is rare in children. It may occur in certain of the mucopolysaccharidoses, especially types II and IV.

TOXIC NEUROPATHIES

These may be divided into the *iatrogenic* neuropathies and those related to *industrial and environmental hazards*. They are reviewed by Thomas (1975). Many drugs capable of causing neuropathy are not used in children. Those which may be used include *Isoniazid* for the treatment of tuberculosis, which can cause a distal mixed sensory and motor neuropathy by interfering with the activity of pyridoxine. Isoniazid neuropathy has become rare since lower doses and pyridoxine supplements have been employed. A neuropathy due to *Nitrofurantoin* may

develop in children treated with this drug for urinary tract infections especially in the presence of renal failure. Paraesthesiae and distal sensory loss are early features. *Vincristine*, used in the treatment of leukaemia and malignant reticuloses, quite commonly causes a peripheral neuropathy. This starts distally in the limbs with loss of tendon reflexes and paraesthesiae followed by sensory loss and weakness, usually affecting the hands first and later the feet.

Metallic poisoning of various kinds may induce neuropathy. *Lead* has been mentioned elsewhere in this connexion; it is very rare as a cause of childhood neuropathy in Britain. *Arsenical* neuropathy is also rare in Britain, but common in the United States due to chronic exposure to arsenical compounds used for agricultural or medicinal purposes. A distal sensorimotor neuropathy develops, the sensory symptoms usually predominating with painful paraesthesiae and often with the acute onset of paralysis, so that the Guillain-Barré syndrome may be closely simulated. Gastro-intestinal symptoms, skin pigmentation and hyperkeratosis of the palms and soles point to the diagnosis. Accidental or even intended suicidal ingestion of *Thallium* by children may cause a polyneuropathy with mainly sensory symptoms. Gastro-intestinal symptoms and renal failure may occur in the acute phase. Hypertension and tachycardia are common. Delayed alopecia, two to four weeks after ingestion, is typical and provides a useful clue to the cause of the illness.

Paraneoplastic polyneuropathy

Though well recognised in adults as a non-metastatic complication of malignant disease, polyneuropathy of this aetiology is rare in childhood. Kurczynski et al (1980) reported a 13-year-old boy with Hodgkin's disease who developed acute polyneuropathy and auto-immune haemolytic disease and who showed significant axonal degeneration in peripheral nerves and in the dorsal funiculus. Their review of the literature showed only one similar case in childhood.

Giant axonal neuropathy

The case of a 6-year-old girl with progressive weakness over 3 years was reported by Asbury et al (1972) and Berg et al (1972). She showed muscle wasting without fasciculation, weakness, areflexia and impairment of touch, postural and vibration sense. She had remarkably kinky hair and splaying out of her lower legs. The CSF was normal. Neurophysiological studies gave results consistent with peripheral neuropathy but with normal conduction velocities in surviving fibres.

Biopsy of a sural nerve showed argentophil masses representing gross segmental enlargement of axons. Ultrastructurally these axons were distended by masses of tightly woven microfilaments. Similar findings were present in a three year old boy reported by Carpenter et al (1974) whose hair, when examined chemically, showed a decrease in disulphide bonds and an increase in thiol groups.

The condition is a rare progressive mixed polyneuropathy, which can only be diagnosed by biopsy, though it can be suspected from the unusual frizzy or kinky appearance of the hair and the stance and gait with adducted knees and splayed out lower legs. (It is quite distinct from Menkes' disease, and affects both sexes.)

The first British case has now been recognized (Ackroyd, personal communication 1982). Autosomal recessive inheritance is indicated in the Japanese family with two sisters affected by giant axonal neuropathy born to consanguineous parents (Takebe et al 1981). One of these girls suffered from mental retardation and epilepsy and the other from precocious puberty.

REFERENCES

Alajouanine T, Castaigne P, Cambier J, Escourolle R 1967 Maladie de Charcot-Marie. Etude anatomo-clinique d'une observation suivie pendant 65 ans. Presse médicale 75: 2745

Asbury A K, Gale M K, Cox S C, Baringer J R, Berg B O 1972 Giant axonal neuropathy — a unique case with segmental neurofilamentous masses. Acta neuropathologica (Berlin) 20: 237–247

Axelrod F B, Nachtigal R, Dancis J 1974 Familial dysautonomia: diagnosis, pathogenesis and management. In: Schulman I (ed) Advances in pediatrics.

Barry J E, Hopkins I J, Neal B W 1974 Congenital sensory neuropathy. Archives of Disease in Childhood 49: 128–132

Berg B O, Rosenberg S H, Asbury A K 1972 Giant axonal neuropathy. Pediatrics 49: 894–899

Brewerton D A, Sandifer P H, Sweetnam D R 1963 'Idiopathic' pes cavus. An investigation into its aetiology. British Medical Journal 2: 659–661

Carpenter S, Karpati G, Andermann F, Gold R 1974 Giant axonal neuropathy. A clinically and monphologically distinct neurological disease. Archives of Neurology 31: 312–316

Cavanagh N P C, Eames R A, Galvin R J, Brett E M, Kelly R E 1979 Hereditary sensory neuropathy with spastic paraplegia. Brain 102: 79–94

Charcot J M, Marie P 1886 Sur une forme particulière d'atrophie musculaire progressive, souvent familiale, débutant par les pieds et les jambes et atteignant plus tard les mains. Revue de Médecine, Paris 6: 97–138

Dalakas M C, Houff S A, Engel W K, Kadden D L, Sever J L 1980 CSF 'monoclonal' bands in chronic relapsing polyneuropathy. Neurology 30: 864–867

Davis C J F, Bradley W G, Madrid R 1978 The peroneal muscular atrophy syndrome. (Clinical, genetic, electrophysiological and nerve biopsy studies). Journal de Génétique Humaine 26: 311–349

Dyck P J, Lambert E H 1978a Lower motor and primary sensory neuron disease with peroneal muscular atrophy. 1. Neurologic, genetic and electrophysiological findings in hereditary polyneuropathy. Archives of Neurology, Chicago 18: 603–618

Dyck P J, Lambert E H 1978b Lower motor and primary sensory neuron disease with peroneal muscular atrophy. 11. Neurologic, genetic and electrophysiological findings in various neuronal degenerations. Archives of Neurology, Chicago 18: 619–625

Dyck P J, Ohta M 1975 Neuronal atrophy and degeneration predominantly affecting peripheral sensory neurons. In: Dyck P J, Thomas P K, Lambert E H (eds) Peripheral neuropathy. W B Saunders, Philadelphia

Earl C J, Fullerton P M, Wakefield G S, Schutta H S 1964 Hereditary neuropathy with liability to pressure palsies (a clinical and electrophysiological study of four families). Quarterly Journal of Medicine 33: 481

Fisher M 1956 An unusual variant of acute idiopathic polyneuritis (syndrome of ophthalmoplegia, ataxia and areflexia). New England Journal of Medicine 255: 57–65

Gilles F H, French J H 1961 Postinjection sciatic nerve palsies in infants and children. Journal of Pediatrics 58: 193–204

Gilliatt R W, Thomas P K 1957 Extreme slowing of nerve conduction in peroneal muscular atrophy. Annals of Physical Medicine 4: 104–106

Grouse L D 1980 Swine flu sequelae. Journal of the American Medical Association 243: 2489

Harding A E, Thomas P K 1980a Genetic aspects of hereditary motor and sensory neuropathy (Types I and II). Journal of Medical Genetics 17: 329–336

Harding A E, Thomas P K 1980b Autosomal recessive forms of hereditary motor and sensory neuropathy. Journal of Neurology, Neurosurgery and Psychiatry 43: 669–678

Harding A E, Thomas P K 1980c Hereditary distal spinal muscular atrophy. Journal of the Neurological Sciences 45: 337–348

Harding A E, Thomas P K 1980d The clinical features of hereditary motor and sensory neuropathy Types I and II. Brain 103: 259–380

Johnson R H, Spalding J M K 1964 Progressive sensory neuropathy in children. Journal of Neurology, Neurosurgery and Psychiatry 27: 125

Hierons R 1957 Changes in the nervous system in acute porphyria. Brain 80: 176–192

Kurczynski T W, Choudhury A A, Horwitz S J, Roessmann U, Gross S 1980 Remote effects of malignancy on the nervous system in children. Developmental Medicine and Child Neurology 22: 205–222

Lockman J A, Kennedy W R, White J G 1967 The Chediak-Higashi syndrome: electrophysiological and electron microscopic observations on the peripheral neuropathy. Journal of Pediatrics 70: 942–951

Marks J S, Halpin T J 1980 Guillain-Barré syndrome in recipients of a New Jersey influenza vaccine. Journal of the American Medical Association 243: 2490–2494

Pleasure D E 1975 Abetalipoproteinemia and Tangier disease. In: Dyck P J, Thomas P K, Lambert E H (eds) Peripheral neuropathy. W B Saunders, Philadelphia

Qaqundah B Y, Taylor W F 1970 Miller Fisher syndrome in a 22-month-old child. Journal of Pediatrics 77: 868–870

Ridley A 1975 Porphyric neuropathy In: Dyck P J, Thomas P K, Lambert E H (eds) Peripheral neuropathy W B Saunders, Philadelphia, London, Toronto, ch 46

San Agustin M, Nitowsky H M, Borden J N 1972 Neonatal sciatic palsy after umbilical vessel injection. Journal of Pediatrics 60: 413

Stokke O, Eldjarn L 1975 Biochemical and dietary aspects of Refsum's disease. In: Dyck P J, Thomas P K, Lambert E H (eds) Peripheral neuropathy W B Saunders, Philadelphia

Swanson A G, Buchan G C, Alvord E C 1965 Anatomic changes in congenital insensitivity to pain: absence of small primary sensory neurons in ganglia, roots and Lissauer's tract. Archives of Neurology 12: 12

Swick H M, McQuillen M P 1976 The use of steroids in the treatment of idiopathic polyneuritis. Neurology 26: 205–212

Takebe Y, Koide N, Takahashi G 1981 Giant axonal neuropathy: report of two siblings with endocrin logical and histological studies. Neuropediatrics 12: 392–404

Taylor R A 1960 Heredofamilial mononeuritis multiplex with brachial predilection. Brain 83: 113–137

Thévenard A 1942 L'acropathie ulcéro-mutilante familiale. Revue neurologique 74: 193

Thomas P K 1975 Peripheral neuropathy. In: Matthews W B (ed) Recent advances in clinical neurology. Churchill Livingstone, Edinburgh

Thomas P K, Calne D B 1974 Motor nerve conduction velocity in peroneal muscular atrophy, evidence for genetic heterogeneity. Journal of Neurology, Neurosurgery and Psychiatry 37: 68–75

Thomas P K, Calne D B, Stewart G 1974 Hereditary motor and sensory polyneuropathy (peroneal muscular atrophy). Annals of Human Genetics 38: 111–153

Thrush D C 1973 Congenital insensitivity to pain — a clinical, genetic and neurophysiological study of four children from the same family. Brain 96: 369–386

Tooth H H 1886 The peroneal type of progressive muscular atrophy. H K Lewis, London

Tripp J H 1975 Miller-Fisher polyneuritis. Proceedings of the Royal Society of Medicine 68: 301–302

Tsairis P, Dyck P J, Mulder D W 1972 Natural history of brachial plexus neuropathy: report on 99 patients. Archives of Neurology 27: 109–117

Van Allen M W, Macqueen J C 1964 Ophthalmoplegia, ataxia and the Syndrome of Landry-Guillain-Barré. A report of four cases with comments on the ophthalmoplegia. Transactions of the American Neurological Association 89: 98–103

Vassella F, Emrich H M, Kraus-Ruppert R, Aufdermaur T, Tönz O 1968 Congenital sensory neuropathy with anhidrosis. Archives of Disease in Childhood 43: 124–130

5

Progressive neurometabolic brain diseases

E. M. Brett and B. D. Lake

The neurometabolic disorders include a number of rare but important progressive degenerative diseases of the nervous system. Most are inherited in an autosomal recessive fashion and show involvement of different parts of the central and sometimes peripheral nervous system with a variety of progressive deficits, especially dementia, epilepsy, blindness, ataxia and disorders of tone and reflexes. Their classification is complex, and is confused by a welter of eponyms and also by a terminology based sometimes on outmoded concepts. Advances in neuropathology, biochemistry and enzymology now require that a full classification should be based on criteria from all these fields, but in some of these conditions our knowledge of the basic defect is still incomplete, and in such cases classification cannot be regarded as final. In the following account, a composite classification is used which is partly clinical, but refers also to pathological and chemical findings.

From the neuropathological standpoint, two main groups of these diseases can be distinguished. In the first, the neuronal storage diseases (neurolipidoses) the grey matter of the brain is principally affected, and in the second, the leucodystrophies or disorders of white matter, demyelination is the main feature, although there is some overlapping of these categories. In both groups metabolic defects are known or suspected, due to inherited deficiencies of specific enzymes, so that these diseases are regarded as inborn errors of metabolism and thus analogous to phenylketonuria and other amino-acidurias. No effective basic treatment is yet possible in these conditions which are uniformly fatal. Diagnostic accuracy is essential so that parents may be advised of the grim prognosis and also of the genetic implications with the high risk of recurrence in later pregnancies. Accurate diagnosis is also necessary for monitoring of future pregnancies. Prenatal diagnosis is possible in all those with known enzyme defects.

THE NEURONAL STORAGE DISEASES

In these diseases an abnormality of complex lipid metabolism due to deficiency of a lysosomal enzyme results in the accumulation of various metabolites within neurons. The word 'storage' applied to this accumulation is not ideal, but is traditionally used for want of a better term. Similar storage of metabolites may also occur in the cells of other organs. In one form of Niemann-Pick disease, for example, the reticulo-endothelial system, liver, spleen and other viscera are involved, in addition to neurons, but in another form the neurons are not affected. In Gaucher's disease also liver and spleen are always affected, and the nervous system additionally in some cases.

Analysis of biopsy material from the nervous system and other affected organs by means of histochemistry, chemical analysis and thin-layer chromatography will in many cases allow the stored material to be defined. Electron microscopy allows the ultrastructure of this material to be examined.

The gangliosidoses are a group of related neuronal storage disorders in which neurons contain abnormal amounts of the complex lipids known as gangliosides, and ultimately die. Advances in the understanding of these diseases have been more complete than in some other neurometabolic conditions; a biochemically-based terminology seems logical today, and preferable to the vague and inaccurate terms 'amaurotic family idiocy' and 'cerebromacular degeneration' formerly used for them (and for other unrelated conditions) which have outlived their usefulness. Eponyms also have obvious disadvantages, but in some cases are so hallowed by tradition as to be assured of longer survival.

The biochemical relationships of these diseases are well reviewed by Brady (1976) Dawson and Tsay (1976) and Stanbury et al (1978). An excellent introduction to the inborn errors of metabolism has been given recently by Ellis (1980)

THE G_{M2}-GANGLIOSIDOSES

TAY-SACHS DISEASE: INFANTILE G_{M2}-GANGLIOSIDOSIS

Clinical features

Clinically this condition is the most distinct entity and was the first of the neurometabolic diseases to be recognized, although its aetiopathogenesis was unsuspected when it was first described in 1881 by the London ophthalmologist Waren Tay and soon afterwards by the New York neurologist, Bernard Sachs, (1887) who later coined the name 'amaurotic family idiocy'. It is now known to be caused by an accumulation of G_{M2}-ganglioside (using Svennerholm's classification (1964)) in neurons resulting from deficiencies of the lysosomal enzyme, hexosaminidase (Table 5.1). The ganglioside occurs in the brain in concentrations from 100 to 300 times the normal.

It is inherited as an autosomal recessive trait and affected families show an increased incidence of parental consanguinity. Though it is common in Ashkenazi Jews of Eastern European origin, in Britain most of the affected families are non-Jewish, while in New York most are Jewish. In the United States the gene frequency is 1 in 30 among Ashkenazi Jews and only 1 in 380 among other groups.

The disease begins in the first year of life. Our experience of 32 cases shows that the onset was very early in 28 of these. Twenty-four children never learned to sit alone. In the other 4, who had achieved independent sitting, deterioration with loss of skills began at about 7 months of age. Blindness and spasticity develop and seizures are com-

Table 5.1 Showing relationships between enzymes and stored products in brain and kidney of patients with G_{M2}-gangliosidosis, G_{M1}-gangliosidosis and Fabry's disease. cer = ceramide; glu = glucose; gal = galactose

	G_{M1}-ganglioside	
G_{M1}-gangliosidosis	↓ β-galactosidase	
	G_{M2}-ganglioside	*Brain*
G_{M2}-gangliosidosis	↓ Hexosaminidase A	
	G_{M3}-ganglioside	
	cer-glu-gal-gal-N-acetylgalactosamine	
Sandhoff's disease	↓ Hexosaminidase B	
	cer-glu-gal-gal	*Kidney*
Fabry's disease	↓ α-galactosidase	
	cer-glu-gal	
	cer-glu-gal-N-acetylgalactosamine-gal	*Brain*
G_{M1}-gangliosidosis	↓ β-galactosidase	
	cer-glu-gal-N-acetylgalactosamine-gal	
G_{M2}-gangliosidosis	↓ Hexosaminidase A (& ?B)	
	cer-glu-gal	

mon. An exaggerated startle response (Schneck et al 1964) is often the earliest symptom, though frequently only recognised in retrospect; it is provoked by sudden noise and consists of extension, abduction and elevation of the arms. Episodes of laughter (gelastic attacks) are often noted, sometimes in relation to seizures and sometimes independently. On ophthalmoscopy optic atrophy is commonly found and in about 90% of cases a cherry-red spot is seen at one or both maculae

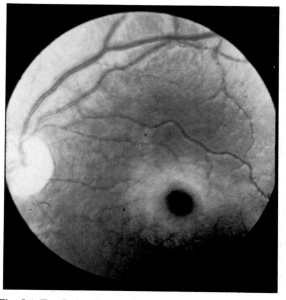

Fig. 5.1 Tay-Sachs disease: cherry red spot at macula

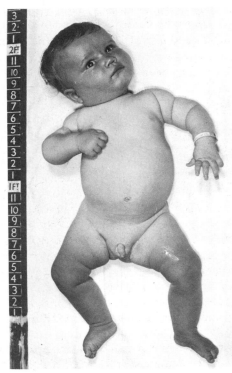

Fig. 5.2 Tay-Sachs disease: 12-month-old boy

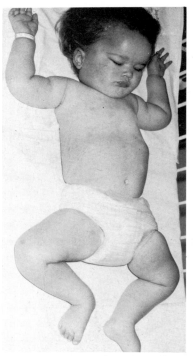

Fig. 5.3 Tay-Sachs disease: same patient aged 2½ years showing enlarged head

(Fig. 5.1). Similar lesions may be seen in some other diseases, but in the setting described the sign is almost pathognomonic of Tay-Sachs disease. Tendon reflexes are increased, but tone is often reduced at first and later increased with a decerebrate picture. The brain and head may be markedly enlarged due to the neuronal storage, particularly in the later stages (Figs 5.2 and 5.3). Survival after the age of 4 years is rare. The average age at death in our series was 2 years and 5 months.

The diagnosis can now be made by the assay of hexosaminidase in the blood. The enzyme exists as two components, A and B, and three patterns of deficiency are recognised, of which the commonest is a marked deficiency of component A with high levels of B (type 1 G_{M2}-gangliosodosis). In Sandhoff's disease (type 2) components A and B are both grossly reduced. The third type is exceedingly rare and hexosaminidase A and B are both normal (Conzelmann & Sandhoff, 1979). Clinical differences between these three types are minimal. Levels of the enzyme in both parents, who are carriers, are reduced to heterozygote levels (i.e. about 50%

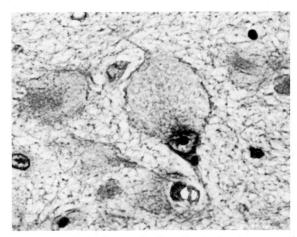

Fig. 5.4 Tay-Sachs disease. Section of brain showing neuronal cytoplasm grossly distended by storage of ganglioside. HE × 198

of normal). In each type marked accumulation of G_{M2}-ganglioside is found in the brain and in other tissues including intestinal neurons (Figs 5.4 and 5.5). When reliable enzyme assay is available, however, biopsy is unnecessary and unjustified. The

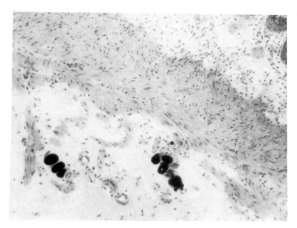

Fig. 5.5 Tay-Sachs disease; rectal biopsy. The large and foamy ganglion cells in the submucosa are strongly positive with the periodic acid-Schiff reaction. PAS × 83

EEG changes in 20 cases of Tay-Sachs disease have been reviewed (Pampiglione et al 1974). Abnormalities in the first year of life were relatively mild but there was rapid deterioration thereafter until death. The electroretinogram remained unaffected.

A very unusual case of Sandhoff's disease has been reported (Johnson et al 1977) with the onset of slowly progressive ataxia in a 2½-year-old boy who was found to have cherry red macular lesions but did not develop dementia, seizures or other deficits over the next 2 years.

Treatment

No effective treatment is at present available to halt the inexorable deterioration or improve function. Attempts at enzyme replacement have been made by the intravenous route and also by intraventricular and intrathecal injection of hexosaminidase preparations (Von Specht et al 1979), but have been unsuccessful. Symptomatic treatment involves attempted control of seizures with anticonvulsant drugs.

Prenatal diagnosis

Prenatal diagnosis is possible at about 12 to 16 weeks of pregnancy by measuring the enzyme content of cultured amniotic fluid cells. However, since 82% of cases of Tay-Sachs disease are first-affected children in the family, only 18% can be detected prenatally if the indication for prenatal screening is the birth of a child with the disease. Mass screening in at-risk Ashkenazi Jewish populations with a carrier rate of 1 in 30 will detect many heterozygotes and, in theory at least, offers much better hope of prevention through genetic counselling. The experience of mass screening programmes in large Jewish populations in North American cities is under assessment for its effectiveness, co-operation of those concerned, and psychological effects. The cost-effectiveness of such programmes when compared with the cost of caring for a child with Tay-Sachs disease from birth to death is high. In communities such as London, where the disease is commoner in non-Jewish people than in Jews, screening programmes are much less efficient.

LATE ONSET G_{M2}-GANGLIOSIDOSIS

An identical accumulation of G_{M2}-ganglioside has been found in neurons in occasional children with a genetically distinct disease with progressive dementia and epilepsy starting after 18 months of age (i.e. beyond the age-range of Tay-Sachs disease). In one series of late onset cases (Brett et al 1973) 4 patients presented before the age of 2 years and 4 between 3½ and 10 years. Gait disturbance, dementia and fits were prominent symptoms. An exaggerated startle reaction to sound developed at 14 months in one patient who also showed an unusual type of cherry red spot at the maculae. Hexosaminidase assays showed a partial deficiency of component A in 2 cases and a profound deficiency in 4, with no correlation between the age of onset and degree of enzyme deficiency. Pathological changes are similar to those in Tay-Sachs disease, and it is not clear why the onset of neurological symptoms should be delayed in these cases.

Chronic G_{M2}-gangliosidosis simulating Friedreich's ataxia

An unusual form of G_{M2}-gangliosidosis in 11 Ashkenazi Jewish patients has been reported recently from the United States (Willner et al 1981). The patients developed cerebellar ataxia at an early age and later features of upper and lower motor neuron disorder. In three older patients dementia or recurrent psychotic episodes occurred.

Membrane-bound lamellar cytoplasmic inclusions, consistent with lysosomal ganglioside accumulation, were seen in rectal ganglia. The activity of β-hexosaminidase-A was markedly reduced in the patients and moderately reduced in their parents in keeping with autosomal recessive inheritance. The disorder has not yet been described in other communities, but further reports are to be expected.

THE G_{M1}-GANGLIOSIDOSES

INFANTILE G_{M1}-GANGLIOSIDOSIS (GENERALISED GANGLIOSIDOSIS: LANDING'S DISEASE: PSEUDO-HURLER'S DISEASE)

A less common biochemical aberration occurs when deficiency of the enzyme β-galactosidase, transmitted as an autosomal recessive character, causes accumulation within neurons of the ganglioside G_{M1} and within the viscera of compounds containing a terminal β-galactose residue (Table 5.1). The condition is inherited as an autosomal recessive trait and shows no obvious ethnic predilection. Children are usually affected at birth or in early infancy with failure to thrive, hepatosplenomegaly, coarse facial features and often kyphosis, (Fig. 5.6) giving a superficial resemblance to Hurler's syndrome, whence the synonym 'pseudo-Hurler's disease'. Retarded development is present from the beginning and in our experience these children usually have poor head control and never learn to sit alone or to grasp. Regression with loss of their few abilities soon follows. Fits occur in some patients. A cherry-red spot may be seen as in Tay-Sachs disease (and the misleading synonym 'Tay-Sachs disease with visceral involvement' has been used), but there should be no difficulty in distinguishing the two conditions. Peripheral oedema may be present. Death usually occurs by the age of 2 years. Low levels of β-galactosidase are found in leucocytes and skin fibroblasts in patients

and heterozygote levels in their carrier parents. Neurons in brain and intestine contain increased amounts of ganglioside G_{M1}, the staining reactions of which are identical with those of G_{M2}-ganglioside. The liver, spleen and reticulo-endothelial system, including bone-marrow (Fig. 5.7), contain foamy histiocytes which have recently been shown to contain a complex carbohydrate with a terminal galactose (formerly thought to be a mucopolysaccharide). Neural biopsy may be avoided by enzyme assay of white blood cells, and marrow biopsy is helpful, although a precise diagnosis cannot be based on the latter alone.

Lateral X-rays of the spine may show anterior 'beaking' in lumbar vertebrae as in the mucopolysaccharidoses.

LATE INFANTILE AND JUVENILE G_{M1}-GANGLIOSIDOSIS

Analogous to the later onset form of G_{M2}-gangliosidosis are cases in which low levels of β-galactosidase are associated with neuronal accumulation of G_{M1}-ganglioside in children whose illness begins between one and 5 years of age. Progressive mental and motor deterioration occur and fits are common. Spastic tetraplegia develops and cerebellar and extra-pyramidal features may be seen. Decerebrate rigidity occurs finally and death usually follows between 3 and 9 years of age. Coarse facial features, hepatosplenomegaly and macular lesions are absent, but minor X-ray changes may be found in the lumbar vertebrae with 'beaking' as seen in Hurler's syndrome. This may be a useful clue, in an otherwise rather non-specific clinical picture, to the diagnosis which is confirmed by low levels of leucocyte β-galactosidase.

In addition to radiological changes and enzyme assay, examination of blood films and bone marrow may be helpful in the G_{M1}-gangliosidoses. Lymphocytes in peripheral blood are markedly vacuolated in the infantile but not in the late infantile form of the disease.

In the infantile form May-Grünwald-Giemsa preparations of marrow films contain many large vacuolated storage cells which resemble Niemann-Pick cells and show strong acid phosphatase activity. In the late infantile condition storage cells in

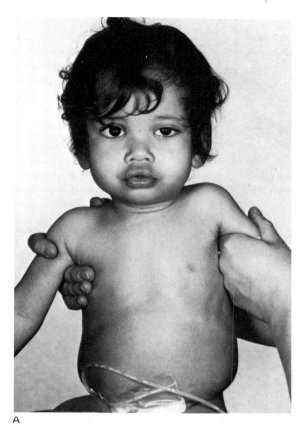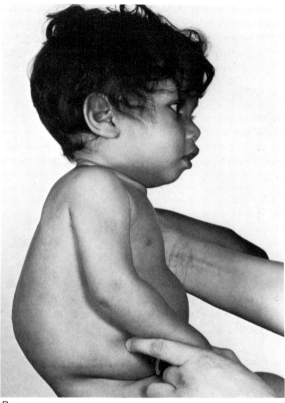

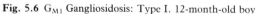

Fig. 5.6 G$_{M1}$ Gangliosidosis: Type I. 12-month-old boy   A. Front view   B. Lateral: note kyphos

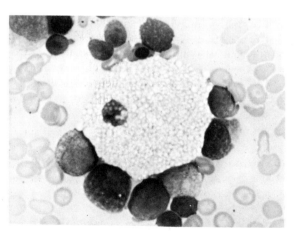

Fig. 5.7 G$_{M1}$-Gangliosidosis: Type I. Large foamy storage cell present in a film from a marrow aspirate. The appearances are similar to those of Niemann-Pick (type A) disease but, unlike the latter, they do not stain with Sudan Black.
May-Grunwald-Giemsa × 576

marrow are fewer in number and different in appearance. They have some resemblance to Gaucher cells, staining a distinctive sky-blue colour with a fibrillary wrinkled appearance to their cytoplasm suggestive of wrinkled tissue-paper.

Neurons in brain and intestine show similar changes in both forms of the disease.

Prenatal diagnosis is possible by enzyme assay of cultured amniotic fluid cells obtained at amniocentesis.

BATTEN'S DISEASE ('NEURONAL CEROID LIPOFUSCINOSIS')

Historical background

In the earlier stages of development of knowledge of the 'neuronal storage diseases' starting in the late 19th century confusion was rife. Zeman in an admirable contribution (1972) on the historical development of the nosological concept of 'amaurotic family idiocy' has charted the way through this confusion. When the approach to these disorders was necessarily clinical and histological it was natural that various conditions to which ballooning of neurons with contained material was common should be lumped together as cases of 'amaurotic family idiocy'. This was the term coined by Sachs for the disorder which later came to bear the eponym Tay-Sachs disease. Sachs' designation 'amaurotic family idiocy' unfortunately persisted and soon came to be used in a far wider sense than was first intended, being applied to cases, regardless of their clinical features, in which the brain showed neuronal ballooning similar to that seen in Tay-Sachs disease.

It was against this background that clinical descriptions of a condition very different from Tay-Sachs disease began to appear, first from what may be called 'the London school', principally F. E. Batten and M. S. Mayou, and later, in 1905, from the German neurologist Vogt and psychiatrist Spielmeyer.

In 1903 Frederick Batten published a detailed report of two sisters with similar macular changes combined with a cerebral degeneration beginning at the ages of 4 and 6 years. The London ophthalmologist, Mayou, in 1904 described a similar condition starting at the age of 6 with visual failure and mental deterioration in 3 of 7 children born to consanguineous parents. F. E. Batten later saw 5 more patients in 2 sibships with the same condition and made histopathological studies of 2 brains and, together, with Mayou, of the retinae.

In 1914 F. E. Batten described the clinical picture of 'family cerebral degeneration with macular change', suggesting that his own cases, with those of Mayou and of several European workers, formed a definite entity which was clinically and anatomically distinct from Tay-Sachs' disease. In the same report Batten also described 3 siblings whose illness differed from that of his other patients since it began between 3 and 4 years of age with convulsions, death occurring at 4, 7 and 8 years; one of these children showed macular changes. He emphasised the non-Jewish origin of these patients and the variable age of onset and rate of deterioration in contrast to Tay-Sachs disease. Pathologi-

cally he described uniform atrophy of the brain, neuronal distension with granular lipid inclusions, and atrophy of the retinal neuro-epithelium, contrasting with its preservation in Tay-Sachs disease. Most unfortunately, by subtitling his paper 'so-called juvenile form of family amaurotic idiocy' he weakened his argument for the separation of these cases from Tay-Sachs disease and strengthened the hand of the 'Unitarian school' or 'lumpers'.

The contribution of Vogt in 1905 is the basis on which the Unitarian concept of 'amaurotic family idiocy' came to be founded, so that this term came in time to embrace — for some at least — such diverse conditions as Tay-Sachs disease, Batten's disease in its various forms, Hurler's syndrome, Niemann-Pick and even Gaucher's disease. Vogt in 1905 described 8 patients from 3 families with a progressive neurological illness with blindness, dementia and paralysis starting between 2 and 8 years and a course lasting from one to 10 or more years. These he regarded as examples of the juvenile form of 'familial amaurotic idiocy' in contrast to Tay-Sachs disease. In the same year 4 siblings with a similar clinical picture were reported by Spielmeyer. (1905) Arguments from ophthalmological evidence for separating Spielmeyer's cases from Tay-Sachs disease were put forward by Stock (1908) who commented on the degeneration of the neuro-epithelium with preservation of the remaining nervous elements including the optic nerves, and shrewdly recognised their similarity to the 3 earlier cases of Mayou (1904). The observations of Jansky (1908) and Bielschowsky (1913) further expanded the widening concept of 'amaurotic familial idiocy'. These concerned 7 children in two families with a progressive neurological illness starting at about 3 years of age with convulsions as an early feature followed by mental deterioration and blindness and death within 3 or 4 years of onset. Pigmentary retinal changes were not see. Thus the eponym Bielschowky-Jansky disease came to be applied to a late infantile form of 'amaurotic familial idiocy' with an earlier age of onset than in the cases of Spielmeyer or most of those of Vogt. The age of onset was now being used as an alternative to the long list of eponyms which is reminiscent of a roll-call of the French Foreign Legion, in which the names of their own compatriots understandably, but confusingly, find favour with later workers. A late or adult form of 'amaurotic familial idiocy' was described by Kufs in 1925, affecting two siblings in their late twenties with dementia but without blindness, so that the descriptive term, now hallowed by long misuse, was clearly a misnomer. The list was further enlarged in 1931 by Sjögren who reported 115 patients from 50 Swedish families with 'juvenile amaurotic idiocy', most developing blindness at 5 to 8 years. In some circles the name of Sjögren is customarily added to those of Spielmeyer and Vogt for the so-called juvenile form of amaurotic familial idiocy, while in others Stock completes the trio.

The nature of the material accumulating within nerve cells in some of the neuronal storage diseases was speculative until the advent of sophisticated chemical methods and electron microscopy. A major advance was the demonstration by Klenk in 1939 of a marked increase in a complex lipid substance, later identified by Svennerholm (1962) as ganglioside G_{M2}, in the brains of two patients with Tay-Sachs disease; by contrast the brains of 5 patients with juvenile amaurotic idiocy, 4 of them from Sjögren's (1931) material, did not show any increase in ganglioside. These advances led to the concept of the gangliosidoses, which were further clarified when the enzyme defect was defined. The unitarian concept of amaurotic familial idiocy, however, lingered on for some years but received a further blow when advances in electron-microscopy allowed Terry and Korey (1960) to show the ultrastructure of the intraneuronal ganglioside accumulation in Tay-Sachs disease in the form of a previously unknown lamellated structure, the membranous cytoplasmic body (MCB). The lipid granules in several cases of late infantile and juvenile amaurotic idiocy were examined by Zeman & Alpert (1963), who showed that they were strongly auto-fluorescent and had the staining characteristics of ceroid or lipofuscin (the 'wear and tear pigment' found in neurons from normal people of advancing age), so that the name neuronal ceroid-lipofuscinosis (NCL) was proposed as a suitable biochemical term for these disorders. In the same year Zeman and Donahue showed that the ultrastructure of these lipid organelles differed from the MCB of Tay-Sachs disease; a wide range of patterns has been seen which can be correlated with the clinical subgroups.

The origin and nature of the lipopigment are still in some doubt. It has been suggested that it may derive from an intermediate product of the oxidation of polyunsaturated fatty acids, so that there may be a defect of peroxidation. Deficiency of peroxidase has been shown in peripheral leucocytes by Armstrong et al (1974) and this provided the basis for a form of anti-oxidant treatment suggested by Zeman (1974). More recently, however, doubt has been cast on the role of peroxidase deficiency by the finding that the iso-enzyme components were similar in patients with the late infantile, juvenile and adult forms of Batten's disease and in controls (Pilz et al 1976). Also many workers have shown that the peroxidase assay is not consistent and that most patients show no such deficiency. Even more recently, Wolfe and his colleagues in Montreal (1977) showed that retinoic acid is a component of the stored material in late infantile Batten's disease and have suggested that a diet low in vitamin A might be helpful.

The term NCL has gained widespread currency in recent years and has the merit of implying a clear separation from the gangliosidoses, sphinogomyelinoses, mucopolysaccharidoses and other inborn metabolic errors. However, the precise nature of the stored material is still unproven and in the absence of an assured biochemical nomenclature the use of eponyms still has some justification. In the clinical account which follows, the term Batten's disease will be used, although Bielschowsky-Jansky and Spielmeyer-Vogt may be preferred by some physicians.

Clinical features of the various forms of Batten's disease

In childhood three major clinically and genetically distinct patterns are seen, all inherited in autosomal recessive fashion. These will be described separately.

Late infantile form

In this condition, often associated with the names of Bielschowsky and Jansky, development of the affected children is normal in the first and usually for most of the second year of age. The first symptom is an abnormality in developmental progress, usually taking the form of a slowing down in the rate of progress or a plateau in development, followed by loss of skills and profound dementia. Among 41 patients at the Hospital for Sick Children, Great Ormond Street, the mean age of onset was 22 months. Seizures occur as a later feature; their mean age of onset was 36 months in the same series and in 89% of cases they began after the age of 30 months. The attacks take various forms; major convulsions, myoclonic attacks and 'drop attacks' are seen. At times continuous myoclonic jerking of the limbs may occur. Drug treatment of the seizures tends to give disappointing results, especially in the later stages. Cerebellar ataxia is common, but it may only be clearly recognizable at an earlier stage since it is often later obscured by myoclonic jerking and eventually overshadowed by increasing spasticity. Other pyramidal signs are seen with exaggerated tendon reflexes and extensor plantar responses.

Pigmentary changes in the maculae and retinae are commonly seen and optic atrophy develops, but cherry red spots are not seen. The assessment of vision is made difficult by the dementia but visual failure is not an early feature in these patients.

Treatment can only be symptomatic with anticonvulsants, and death usually occurs by the age of 6 or 7 years, after the child has become increasingly helpless, unable to feed, and very vulnerable to chest infections.

Skull X-rays commonly show thickening of the bones of the vault, suggestive of cerebral atrophy which is often confirmed if air-encephalograms or CT scans are carried out.

More specific diagnostic help is given by neurophysiological investigations, since combined recordings of the electroretinogram (ERG) and the cortical visual evoked response from the occipital are (VER) with the EEG have shown absence of the ERG, in keeping with a gross loss of function of retinal receptor elements, together with a grossly enlarged VER, up to 20 times higher in amplitude than in controls, in response to photic stimulation at low rates of flash (one per second) (Harden et al 1973). These electrical findings in our experience are pathognomonic for the late infantile form of Batten's disease.

Cerebral biopsy, usually taken from the right frontal lobe, as a full neurosurgical procedure, allows neurons to be examined. These contain a PAS-positive, sudanophilic and autofluorescent material which resists extraction in embedding procedures. This is in contrast with the ganglioside deposition disorders in which the gangliosides are removed by processing and so cannot be demonstrated in 'paraffin' sections. Electron microscopy of the brain biopsies shows a variety of inclusions with a predominance of those described as curvilinear. Intestinal biopsy, of rectum (full thickness) or appendix, gives neural tissue in the myenteric plexuses in which similar diagnostic neuronal changes can be shown. In addition, deposits with similar staining characteristics are present in vascular endothelium and in the smooth muscle cells. The ultrastructure of the deposited substance in the rectal biopsies is constant from case to case and is always of curvilinear type. The intestinal approach to biopsy is preferable, in terms of lower morbidity and mortality, to the more drastic brain biopsy, but considerations of surgical and pathological expertise are involved in the choice.

Recent work has shown that even less traumatic procedures may be used to confirm the clinical diagnosis. Skin biopsies examined by electron microscopy show the characteristic curvilinear bodies in the sweat gland epithelium, vessel endothelium and in smooth muscle cells. Fibroblasts do not appear to be involved. Lymphocytes, while showing no changes on light microscopy, contain curvilinear deposits and thus the diagnosis can be confirmed by EM examination of the buffy coat from 2 ml of blood. Suction rectal biopsies, taken without anaesthetic and without apparent discomfort, can also be used provided that sufficient care is exercised in using all the stains necessary. Examination of autofluorescence in unfixed sections is probably the most sensitive index.

Diagnostic difficulty is common in the earlier stages of the illness before gross deterioration has suggested the possibility of a progressive brain disease. Even then, the occurrence of severe, intractable seizures may suggest that the problem is basically one of epilepsy of non-progressive aetiology and the diagnosis is thus often delayed. When a sibling is known to have the disease, the diagnosis is usually made early, and parents are often aware of developmental slowing at an earlier age in a second affected child than a first. The mean age of diagnosis among 41 patients at the Hospital for Sick Children, Great Ormond Street, was 50 months.

Juvenile form

This condition, often called Spielmeyer-Vogt disease, has a very characteristic clinical picture and is one of the most easily recognized of the degenerative brain disorders. The presentation is almost invariably with progressive visual failure at the age of 5 to 7 years, occasionally as late as 8 years, associated with a pigmentary retinopathy which becomes more obvious with time, and later with optic atrophy. The electroretinogram is reduced or absent, and may be abnormal before retinopathy is clinically detectable. In a series of 17 patients seen at the Hospital for Sick Children, Great Ormond Street, the mean age of onset was 6.2 years.

Fits are common, but are not seen as a presenting symptom, the interval from onset of visual failure usually being at least one year with mean age of onset 9.7 years in the same series. Major convulsions and myoclonic attacks occur and tend to worsen, often becoming intractable in the later stages.

Dementia also occurs at a late stage and its recognition may be long delayed because learning difficulties and behaviour problems are often attributed to the blindness and its psychological effects. Many children have been regarded as hysterical because no cause has initially been found for their visual failure. Others, though known to have visual loss and a pigmentary retinopathy, are not recognized as suffering from progressive brain disease until fits and dementia develop. Many patients have been causing concern to the teachers in their schools for the blind or partially-sighted for some years before the diagnosis is finally made and referral for investigation has often been made at the insistence of the teachers. The mean age at diagnosis in the series of 17 patients referred to was 10.6 years, varying between 7 and 15 years.

Pyramidal, extrapyramidal and cerebellar signs may all develop in the course of time but are often long delayed, the patients remaining mobile for many years (Fig. 5.8).

The diagnosis may be readily suspected from the clinical features and confirmed by neurophysiol-

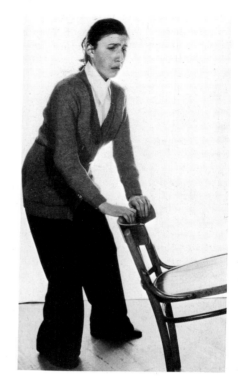

Fig. 5.8 Juvenile Batten's disease: 15-year-old girl.

ogical and biopsy studies. The finding of an absent or reduced response on the electroretinogram with an abnormal EEG is strongly suggestive. Neural biopsy, from brain or intestine shows neurons with characteristic staining properties.

Rectal or appendix biopsy are fully adequate for diagnosis in skilled hands and it should seldom be necessary to resort to cerebral biopsy. The neuronal changes in the rectal biopsy consist of the deposition of a PAS positive, sudanophilic, autofluorescent granular substance (Fig. 5.9 and Plate 3) which shows a fingerprint-like structure when examined by electron microscopy. Smooth muscle cells are similarly affected. The diagnosis can be made using the suction rectal biopsy method — with the same caveat as in the diagnosis of late infantile Batten's disease. Skin biopsy does not seem to be sufficiently reliable to be depended on as a diagnostic method in Juvenile Batten's disease. The fingerprint deposits may be present, often resembling curvilinear deposits, but may be absent.

A helpful finding in this form of Batten's disease

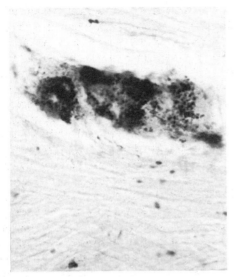

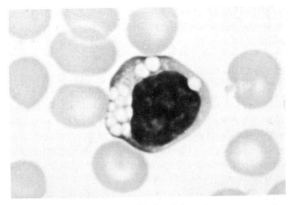

Fig. 5.10 Juvenile Batten's disease. A lymphocyte present in the tail of a blood film shows prominent bold vacuoles. Similar lymphocytes are seen in G_{M1}-gangliosidosis type 1. MGG × 1472

Fig. 5.9 Juvenile Batten's disease, rectal biopsy. The neurons contain a granular sudanophilic substance which is also present in some smooth muscle cells. Sudan black × 538

is vacuolation in lymphocytes of peripheral blood, which may be present in some 25% of cells (Fig. 5.10).

Electron microscopy shows that the fingerprint bodies characteristic of juvenile Batten's disease in the rectal biopsy may be present in a small proportion of the vacuoles in lymphocytes but are not constantly found.

The course of the disease is progressive deterioration, at a rate which may vary from one case to another, so that death may occur as early as 13 years or be deferred occasionally until 20 years or more. Survival in a demented, blind and paralysed state for many years makes this one of the most tragic diseases encountered in the whole field of child neurology.

Treatment until recently has been symptomatic in this and other forms of Batten's disease. In recent years treatment with vitamins E and C, and butylated-hydroxytoluene (Zeman 1974) has been tried in the hope of reducing the formation of lipid peroxides and thus inhibiting the build-up of lipopigment. Our experience so far in a small series of patients has been disappointing, as has that of a trial of diet low in vitamin A, suggested more recently by the finding of retinoic acid deposition (Wolfe et al 1977).

Infantile form

Recently in Scandinavia (Santavuori et al 1973, Haltia et al 1973, Hagberg et al 1974) cases have been reconnized of a neurological illness starting between 8 and 18 months of age with progressive mental deterioration, ataxia, visual failure and myoclonic jerks, the rate of progression being very rapid. The early onset of this condition distinguishes it from the late infantile (Bielschowsky-Jansky) form of Batten's disease, with which in the past it was often confused. The disorder appears to be particularly common in Finland, where it is the commonest progressive encephalopathy in children under two years of age, although cases are being reported increasingly from other countries. Ten cases have now been recognised at the Hospital for Sick Children, many of them in retrospect, since they had previously been classified as examples of the late infantile disease.

Slowing in developmental progress is usually first noticed at about 12 months of age, but sometimes slightly earlier. Later the child loses the skills of walking and manipulation and such speech as he has acquired and becomes progressively less responsive socially. Hypotonia and ataxia develop, the latter sometimes being very severe. The head shows marked slowing in its rate of growth, so that microcephaly is a prominent feature. Visual failure develops early and causes the children to bump into things from 12 months of age. Optic atrophy and brownish discolouration of the maculae may be seen on ophthalmoscopy, but pigmentation of the peripheral retina is not increased. Myoclonic jerks start at about 2 years of age and may be very striking, at times amounting to myoclonic status. Sometimes movements with a bizarre character which have been aptly compared to the movements of knitting are seen. These tend to disappear after a few months. Generalized convulsions may also occur.

The rapid progression of the disease leads to a 'burnt-out' stage in the third year of life. By this age the affected children are completely unresponsive socially and show no willed activities. Myoclonic attacks tend to decrease in the later stages. Tone in the limbs is at first decreased, but later the children become hypertonic with flexion contractures. Signs of pyramidal dysfunction are seen with hyperreflexia and extensor plantar responses.

Patients may survive in a totally deteriorated condition for many years, and death has been delayed in some cases until the age of 8 or 9 years, a later age paradoxically than is seen in the *late* infantile form of Batten's disease.

Neurophysiological investigations are helpful and show a pattern different from that in other forms of Batten's disease, or indeed in any other

disorder. The EEG is invariably abnormal with slowing of rhythmic activity, often with generalized irregular bursts of sharp and slow waves and of spike-wave discharges. Later, usually after some months, there is progressive diminution in amplitude so that the records become largely or completely isoelectric after the age of three. The electroretinogram is reduced and eventually extinguished in all cases. The visual evoked responses from the occipital region are also reduced, indicating involvement of the visual pathways from the retina, and/or the visual cortex. The abnormal photic responses to slow rates of flicker seen in the late infantile form are not seen in this variety.

Brain biopsies have shown a marked gliosis with neuronal and astrocytic deposition of a PAS-positive, sudanophilic, autofluorescent substance. A similar substance is found in neurons of the appendix and rectum and in the smooth muscle cells. Ultrastructural studies show rather amorphous deposits known as granular osmiophilic deposits or, more colloquially, as 'Finnish snowballs'.

Skin biopsies show these deposits particularly in the vascular endothelium, but also in smooth muscle cells. Electron microscopy of buffy coat preparations from 2–3 ml of blood shows granular osmiophilic inclusions which are membrane-bound in the cytoplasm of lymphocytes although under

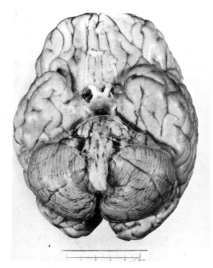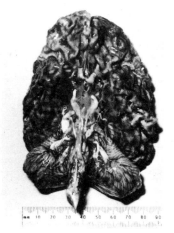

Fig. 5.11 Infantile Batten's disease.
Ventral view of the brain of a 9-year-old patient showing extreme shrinkage of the cerebral hemispheres, cerebellum and brain stem. Compare with normal control on the left

the light microscope no abnormality may be seen.

In the autopsied cases the brain is very small with weights between 325 and 420 g in 8 Finnish cases with the mean age at death 7.6 years (normal weight 1270 g at 7.5 years) (Fig. 5.11). This is in keeping with the progressive slowing in growth of head size leading to severe microcephaly. Diffuse cerebral gyral atrophy is seen and the cerebellum is also affected, but the brain stem and spinal cord are relatively less affected. The cerebral and cerebellar cortex show gross depletion of neurons, the thin remaining cortical rim being made up mainly of a network of fibrillary astroglia with scattered macrophages and blood vessels.

'Early juvenile' subgroup

Detailed analysis of clinical, electrophysiological and rectal biopsy appearances in about 120 cases of Batten's disease at the Hospital for Sick Children, Great Ormond Street, has shown in most cases a good correlation between the age of onset, clinical course, electrical and biopsy features. In a few cases this correlation is imperfect, and among these exceptional cases are 5 with similar features constituting a small subgroup which is best described as 'early juvenile' (Lake & Cavanagh 1978). In their clinical and electrical features and in the absence of vacuolated lymphocytes these patients resemble the late infantile form, showing ataxia as the presenting symptom followed soon by grand mal fits or drop attacks, and a rapidly deteriorating course. In this, and in the fact that visual failure is a later feature, they differ from the juvenile cases whereas the biopsy findings are identical to those of the juvenile form. The authors have suggested that the genes of the late infantile and juvenile forms of Batten's disease are allelic and that the 'early juvenile' subgroup is a genetic compound presenting as an intermediate phenotype.

A most unusual family has been reported by Proops & Green (1981), in which three and possibly four children in a sibship of seven had the late infantile form of neuronal ceroid lipofuscinosis and also suffered from an arthropathy. The electron-microscopic findings showed some overlap between those characteristic of the late infantile and of the juvenile form of the disease. Skin biopsies were studied in four children, being abnormal in three.

In one of these a synovial biopsy showed similar abnormalities to those in skin, with inclusions of both curvilinear and fingerprint type. This family may represent a further sub-group of the disorder.

NIEMANN-PICK DISEASE AND RELATED DISORDERS

A radical re-appraisal of the condition known as Niemann-Pick disease has taken place since it was first described by Niemann (1914).

Crocker & Farber (1958) in their review of 18 patients so diagnosed recognised that the condition had a broader range of biological behaviour than was then usually stated. Three years later Crocker (1961) divided the disease into four sub-groups based on combined clinical and chemical criteria. The lipid accumulating in the nervous tissues of patients with Niemann-Pick disease is sphingomyelin, and there is a deficiency of the enzyme sphingomyelinase. Cerebral (neurovisceral) and visceral forms (without CNS involvement) occur. All are inherited in autosomal recessive fashion.

The commonest group, and that which the paediatrician is most likely to see, is Crocker's group A which makes up about 85% of all cases. This is the 'classical', infantile form of the disease. It is common in people of Ashkenazi Jewish origin, like Tay-Sachs and Canavan's disease, but also affects Gentiles. The disorder starts very early and a prenatal onset is suggested by the fact that the children are often born light for dates. Early jaundice is common and hepatosplenomegaly is present from an early age. Failure to thrive is a severe and early feature so that coeliac disease, lactose intolerance or Hirschsprung's disease are sometimes wrongly suspected. Development is slow from the start and most patients do not achieve independent sitting. Head retraction and squint are common and seizures may occur. A cherry-red spot is sometimes present at the macula. Deterioration with loss of abilities and increasing spasticity lead to death between 7 months and 3 years of age with an average age of 2 years. Pulmonary infiltration is seen on chest X-rays and in some cases osteoporosis with expansion of long bones, modelling defects and widening of the metacarpals.

In Crocker's group B, the visceral or chronic

form of Niemann-Pick disease, the central nervous system is not involved but there is massive visceral enlargement with sphingomyelin storage in viscera only and deficiency of sphingomyelinase less severe than in type A. The onset is from two years of age to adult life. Patients may have a muddy-brown complexion and be subject to recurrent bronchitis, their chest X-rays showing more obvious pulmonary infiltration than occurs in type A. Radiological changes in bones also tend to be more severe than in the infantile form of the disease. Haematological problems are common and often related to abnormalities of platelets.

Pathology

The characteristic Niemann-Pick cell is morphologically similar to those found in many of the visceral storage diseases with the result that 'Niemann-Pick cells' are found in a variety of disorders including histiocytosis X, mucopolysaccharidosis, Wolman's disease and G_{M1}-gangliosidosis. The large cell, with a foamy-looking cytoplasm, is readily found in bone marrow aspirates and this may be one of the simplest investigations necessary for the diagnosis (Fig. 5.12). Although similar-appearing cells occur in other disorders, various staining procedures make a confident diagnosis possible. The Niemann-Pick cells often stain weakly with Sudan black and show a red birefringence in polarised light after staining. They react variably with the PAS stain and contain cholesterol. Niemann-Pick cells occur throughout the reticuloendothelial system (spleen, liver, lymph nodes) and deposits of sphingomyelin are also found in hepatocytes, smooth muscle cells and lymphocytes. The neurons in the brain and rectum appear similar to those in Tay-Sachs' disease and there is marked demyelination in the brain. Suction rectal biopsies may be used for diagnosis and excessive sphingomyelin deposition may be demonstrated by thin layer chromatography of solvent extracts of these biopsies.

In Type B Niemann-Pick disease presenting in childhood it may be possible to show the characteristic cell in the bone marrow but in those patients presenting later with haematological problems the marrow contains numerous 'sea-blue histocytes' (Long et al 1977). Lymphocytes, which

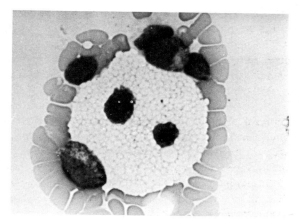

Fig. 5.12 Niemann-Pick disease type A. A bone marrow film shows large foamy Niemann-Pick cells which will stain weakly with Sudan Black.
MGG × 576

show discrete vacuolation in Type A, do not show any abnormality in Type B. Sphingomyelinase assay of white cells or cultured fibroblasts can be used for diagnosis. Liver, spleen and smooth muscle are affected as in Type A but neuronal involvement is not seen.

NEUROVISCERAL STORAGE DISEASE WITH VERTICAL SUPRANUCLEAR OPHTHALMOPLEGIA ('OPHTHALMOPLEGIC LIPIDOSIS')

The classification of Crocker's groups C and D previously classed with Niemann-Pick disease is still unsatisfactory but an important advance has been the recognition (Neville et al 1973) of a progressive neurological disease with ataxia, dementia and seizures later in the disease. A vertical supranuclear ophthalmoplegia is found in many of the patients but this is not apparent in the early stages and may not occur until late in the course of the disease. There is neuronal and reticuloendothelial storage of an as yet unidentified substance which shows characteristic ultrastructure different from other storage conditions. Sphingomyelinase activity is always normal.

The bone marrow contains cells which bear a superficial resemblance to Niemann-Pick cells but the vacuoles are not uniform in size and their contents do not stain with Sudan dyes. An occasional, rare sea-blue histiocyte may be found. Peripheral blood lymphocytes show no vacuolation.

The clinical features are distinctive. Early jaundice and failure to thrive were seen in several patients in the series of Neville et al. Splenomegaly was common, and hepatomegaly rather less so. The age of onset of neurological symptoms varied between one and eight years. Seizures were frequent, being mainly grand mal in type. Myoclonic attacks were not seen in contrast to the situation in the various forms of Batten's disease in which they are often common.

A striking defect of voluntary eye movement was seen in seven patients. Horizontal movements were normal, but vertical eye movements were grossly limited on attempted following of visual lures, particularly in a downward direction. 'Head thrusting' and blinking was sometimes used by the patients in an attempt to obtain vertical eye movements. Difficulty in walking downstairs and in seeing objects in low-lying situations was mentioned as a complaint in the histories of some patients, and others had episodes in which the eyes became 'stuck' in elevation. By contrast a full range of elevation and depression of the eyes was usually seen with the doll's head manoeuvre (when the patient was asked to fix his gaze on a point and the neck passively extended and flexed). Although supranuclear defects of ocular movements may occur in certain other diseases (ataxia-telangiectasia, Huntington's chorea, Parkinson's disease, juvenile Gaucher's disease, kernicterus and 'the Sylvian aqueduct syndrome'), a purely vertical supranuclear ophthalmoplegia in the setting of progressive neurological deterioration appears to be pathognomonic of this rare disease. Bone marrow and rectal biopsy allow the diagnosis to be confirmed.

Some authors (Karpati et al 1977) prefer to use the term 'juvenile dystonic lipidosis' for this condition but since dystonia is not a readily identifiable sign we feel it is inappropriate. Indeed, the first patient considered to have this disorder (Elfenbein 1968) showed no clear evidence of dystonia.

Fredrickson has suggested that the term type D Niemann-Pick disease should be restricted to those patients originating from Nova Scotia, but it is more logical at present to include both Crocker's types C and D in the group with ophthalmoplegic lipidosis until an enzyme defect is discovered.

GAUCHER'S DISEASE

Since the first description by Gaucher in 1882 of the disease which bears his name its nosological position has changed greatly. Several forms of the condition are now recognized, having in common the presence of numerous large 'Gaucher' cells in the bone-marrow and reticulo-endothelial system. As with Niemann-Pick disease, some forms show neuronal involvement and in others visceral involvement is seen without neurological features.

In all forms of Gaucher's disease there is a defect of cleavage of glucose from glucosyl ceramide due to a deficiency of the enzyme glucocerebrosidase, and as a result glucocerebrosides accumulate in the reticulo-endothelial cells.

Type I Gaucher's disease, the commonest form, sometimes called the adult or non-neuronopathic type, is a slowly progressive disorder with marked enlargement of liver and spleen, often with haematological problems due to hypersplenism, and with pain and fractures due to bony involvement. This non-neuronopathic form may rarely be present at birth or in early childhood.

It contrasts with Type II, the acute infantile variety, which presents in infancy with early feeding difficulties. Development is retarded from the start. The children are often described as placid and slow, as in non-progressive mental retardation, and they do not learn to sit unsupported. Fits may occur. Head retraction and spasticity develop with bulbar signs. Cherry-red spots are seen at the maculae in occasional patients.

The liver and spleen are enlarged at an early age, the spleen usually more than the liver. Anaemia and thrombocytopenia are common and the serum acid phosphatase level is raised.

Death usually occurs by one year of age.

The demonstration of Gaucher cells in biopsies of bone-marrow, spleen or liver, or (where available) enzyme assay of white blood cells or cultured fibroblasts, allows the condition to be distinguished from the infantile form of Niemann-Pick disease and other neurovisceral disorders.

A subacute neuronopathic juvenile form of Gaucher's disease, known as Type III, is also recognized, most patients in this group coming from the province of Norrbotten in northern Sweden (Herrlin & Hillborg 1962, Dreborg et al 1980). The clinical severity in this Norrbottnian type of Gaucher's disease (Dreborg et al 1980) may vary greatly not only between families but also within an affected sibship with malignant forms in children who die early, adults only slightly or moderately affected, and transitional forms. Until 1965 splenectomy was performed at or soon after diagnosis but since that time the operation has been deferred or avoided. Deterioration seems to have been more rapid after early splenectomy with regard to skeletal complications and, later, to intellectual impairment and ataxia.

The age of onset in the 22 patients was between birth and 14 years, with a median of 12 months. A large abdomen due to splenomegaly was the main feature. Unexplained fever and increased sweating and appetite were other early symptoms. The diagnosis was made at a median age of $2\frac{1}{2}$ years.

Growth in height was normal in the first 6 months but was often progressively retarded over the next 18 months or so. Skeletal abnormalities were noted in all cases and included thinning of the cortex especially of the distal femur with an Erlenmeyer flask deformity and thoracic kyphosis without vertebral collapse. Necrosis of the femoral heads and necks was common with fractures at various sites. Splenic enlargement was progressive and often massive with less striking hepatomegaly. Anaemia, thrombocytopenia, leucopenia and a bleeding tendency were common.

Psychomotor development appeared normal in most patients in the first year of life, but deterioration was noted later in some. Seizures occurred in 6 patients. Oculomotor apraxia was found in 10 children. 8 patients died, at ages between 2.9 and 25.2 years.

An unusual variant of juvenile neuronopathic Gaucher's disease has recently been described in a African family (Tripp et al 1977). Three of eight siblings were affected by a rapidly progressive neurological illness with myoclonus, splenomegaly, Gaucher cells in bone-marrow and spleen and raised acid phosphatase levels. The onset was at the age of 8 years with death by 14. A striking defect of voluntary eye movements in the horizontal plane was seen due to a supranuclear ophthalmoplegia, contrasting with normal eye movements on the doll's head monoeuvre. (This defect seems more severe than the oculomotor apraxia described in some of the Swedish cases mentioned above.) This unusual form of Gaucher's disease can be recognized in the later stages by careful examination of eye movements, just as the syndrome described by Neville et al (1973) can be detected by the *vertical* supranuclear ophthalmoplegia.

No effective treatment for Gaucher's disease is yet available and the prognosis of the progressive neurological variants is inevitably one of continuing deterioration to death. Anticonvulsant therapy is of limited benefit. Splenectomy has been performed in some patients for symptomatic relief, as the massive spleen is a handicap to the patients and hypersplenism also causes problems. Splenic transplantation has been tried (Groth et al 1971) in one adult patient in the hope that the high activity of glucocerebrosidase in the spleen might replace the deficient enzyme. Some encouraging metabolic changes were noted, but the graft was later rejected and death ensued. A more promising therapeutic approach at least for the non-neuronopathic varieties of Gaucher's disease is by attempted replacement of glucocerebrosidase (Brady et al 1974, 1975). When exogenous enzyme was given to two patients with Gaucher's disease there was a 26% reduction in the glucocerebroside level of their livers (Brady et al 1974). The raised blood level of glucocerebroside fell to normal figures and remained there for some months after the enzyme had been given. The authors have calculated that in these two patients four and thirteen years accumulation of glucocerebroside were catabolized (Brady et al 1975). This approach is unlikely to be useful, however, in the infantile, neuronopathic form of the disease, unless it proves possible to deliver the enzyme to the brain and reverse the changes that must have occurred in utero.

The characteristic Gaucher cells found abundantly in bone marrow aspirates are readily distinguishable from those of Niemann-Pick disease on the morphological appearance alone. The cytoplasm of the cells has a wrinkled, striped appear-

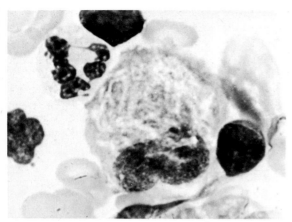

Fig. 5.13 Gaucher's disease. A large binucleate Gaucher cell in a film prepared from a marrow aspirate. The cytoplasm of the cell has a striated appearance.
May-Grunwald-Giemsa × 1216

ance which stains a blue-grey colour in the routine May-Grünwald-Giemsa procedure (Fig. 5.13). Marrow films should always be examined in preference to sections because morphology is easier to assess and the staining reactions are more easily applied to the cells which retain their contents in air-dried films. Gaucher cells, and all other storage cells, show a strong acid phosphatase reaction and this method readily identifies their presence even at low power examination. Gaucher cells stain positively with PAS but only weakly with Sudan black. They are distributed widely in the liver as enlarged Kupffer cells, throughout the spleen and in lymph nodes. Liver cells and neurons of the frontal cortex and gastrointestinal tract are not involved in the storage of glucocerebroside. The distribution of cells does not appear to differ in the different forms although in the infantile form the numbers of cells in the portal areas is much greater than in the juvenile and adult forms where Gaucher cells are much more scattered throughout the liver.

FABRY'S DISEASE: (ANGIOKERATOMA CORPORIS DIFFUSUM)

Since it is a disorder of sphingolipid metabolism this very rare disorder is included in this section, although its clinical features make it an uneasy bedfellow for the diseases previously described.

Excessive amounts of ceramide trihexoside (cer-amide-glucose-galactose-galactose), usually found only in small amounts in plasma and kidneys, are present in affected tissues, as a result of deficiency of the enzyme ceramide-trihexosidase which normally cleaves the terminal α-galactose from the chain.

The condition is inherited as an X-linked trait. It presents as a systemic disease, the affected boys usually developing a punctate-rash as the dermatological name implies. This is most marked in the 'bathing-trunk' area. Episodic pain in the feet and hands may be a prominent feature and is at times disabling; patients may be unable to bear weight on their feet during these episodes. Fever and weight loss may occur. Renal involvement in older patients due to vascular changes may cause hypertension, cerebrovascular accidents and renal failure leading to death, but survival to the forties or later is common.

Peripheral nerve involvement in a 46-year-old man with Fabry's disease has been shown by study of a sural nerve biopsy (Kocen & Thomas 1970). The patient had a long history of attacks of pain in the limbs but showed no evidence of peripheral neuropathy on clinical examination and had normal results on nerve conduction studies. The nerve showed a moderate depletion of myelinated nerve fibres, particularly affecting the smaller fibres. There was no evidence of segmental demyelination.

Treatment until recently has been purely symptomatic with analgesics for relief of pain. Sometimes phenytoin (dilantin or diphenylhydantoin) is helpful. A more basic approach is now possible by attempted replacement of the deficient enzyme. When the enzyme, isolated from human placental tissue, was infused into two patients with Fabry's disease, there was a fall in the raised blood level of ceramidetrihexoside (Brady et al 1973), and there is some evidence that the enzyme continued to exert a beneficial effect after it had been cleared from the circulation, possibly by activating an inactive protein, since more enzyme activity was found in the liver after infusion than had actually been administered (Brady et al 1975).

CEREBROTENDINOUS XANTHOMATOSIS

This curious and very rare familial disease, first

described by van Bogaert and his colleagues in 1937, combines dementia and slowly progressive cerebellar ataxia with the finding of massive xanthomas of tendons and lungs, and of cataracts. The onset is usually in later childhood and deterioration may be very slow. Large amounts of free and esterified cholestanol are stored within the nervous system. This sterol is also increased in the tendinous xanthomas, but in these cholesterol predominates. The basic enzyme defect is still unknown. Evidence of peripheral neuropathy has recently been found in 4 patients (Kuritzky et al 1979).

ALPERS' DISEASE

The status of certain neurological diseases is often called in question on re-assessment of pathological material. The term 'Alpers' disease', or 'poliodystrophia cerebri progressiva', is sometimes applied, following reports by Alpers (1931, 1960) of diffuse progressive degeneration of the cerebral grey matter, to a syndrome starting in early life with convulsions and leading to neurological deterioration with spasticity and dementia. While it is possible that some of the reported cases represent a specific clinico-pathological entity, it seems that the eponym has also been used for a motley collection of other conditions, including cases of birth injury, post-epileptic atrophy and post-encephalitic sequelae (Blackwood & Corsellis 1976). Certainly the symptoms of dementia and severe seizures are found in so many specific degenerative diseases of the brain, most of which can be suspected on clinical grounds and confirmed by appropriate investigations, that the diagnosis of Alpers' disease should be viewed with strong suspicion.

Nonetheless a good case for a specific recessively inherited clinico-pathological syndrome with features of Alpers' disease has been made by Huttenlocher and his colleagues (1976). They reported 4 children with progressive degeneration of the cerebral cortex and hepatic cirrhosis and considered that these, and 4 previously described cases, (Blackwood et al 1963, Wefring & Lamvik 1967) represented a distinct form of hepatocerebral degeneration with its onset between 1 and 3 years

of ages. Mild developmental delay was sometimes present, but most characteristic was the explosive onset of intractable convulsions, leaving the child in a stuporous and demented state. Clinical features of hepatic disease occurred late if at all. The children died within 10 months of the onset of convulsions. In 3 cases the pathological features were indistinguishable from those of Alpers' disease. The liver showed cirrhosis or subacute hepatitis with fatty infiltration of hepatocytes.

PROGRESSIVE MYOCLONIC EPILEPSY: FAMILIAL MYOCLONUS EPILEPSY: LAFORA BODY DISEASE

Myoclonic seizures, which are sudden, shock-like, involuntary contractions of one or more muscles or parts of muscles, are common in childhood and occur in different settings. Often their cause is unknown, particularly when they affect otherwise normal children. Sometimes they occur in children with other evidence of neurological dysfunction, such as cerebral palsy, retardation and other forms of seizure, and in these cases it is reasonable to attribute them to the brain pathology responsible for these other deficits such as brain damage due to perinatal problems, intrauterine infections or postnatal encephalopathy. Anoxic brain damage is sometimes followed by the development of myoclonus. Infantile spasms (Ch. 12) are a particular and striking type of myoclonic seizure of varied aetiology, sometimes described, especially in North America, as 'massive myoclonic seizures'. Myoclonic fits are seen in several of the progressive degenerative disorders described above, such as Gaucher's disease and the various forms of Batten's disease.

In addition myoclonic seizures are seen as an early and prominent symptom of another familial disorder, first described by Unverricht in 1891, in association with progressive intellectual deterioration. This specific form of progressive myoclonus epilepsy is distinguished from the infantile and late infantile varieties of Batten's disease by its age of onset, which is between 7 and 10 years, and from the juvenile type by the absence of pigmentary retinopathy and altered ERG. The disease presents with major convulsions and myoclonic fits which are often induced and increased by attempted manipulation so that these attempts are thwarted by shock-like jerkings of the hands and arms which may mimic cerebellar ataxia. These often vary under the influence of emotional factors, being worse under conditions of stress and better when the patient is calm. Photic stimulation may also aggravate the attacks. Intellectual deterioration is insidious at first, becoming more profound as time passes and after some years the patient reaches a pre-terminal stage with dementia, spasticity and almost continuous myoclonic jerking.

Lafora bodies, particularly common in the perikarya of neurons in the cerebral cortex, thalamus, globus pallidus and sustantia nigra, are strongly PAS-positive polyglucosan bodies. Smaller but much more numerous bodies are present throughout the neuropil. These bodies (larger and smaller) have much in common with corpora amylaceae (Robitaille et al 1980). Lafora bodies are not found in all cases with the clinical features of progressive myoclonic epilepsy, and clinically there seems little to distinguish cases in which they are not present.

The EEG is usually abnormal, often with bilateral spikes and sharp waves. Halliday (1967) and Halliday & Halliday (1970) have demonstrated that most patients with this disorder show abnormally large somato-sensory evoked responses recorded from the parietal 'hand' area when the contralateral median nerve is stimulated electrically. The amplitude of these responses is many times larger than those of normal controls or sufferers from benign familial essential myoclonus. It is thought that the jerks in the latter condition may arise at lower levels in the brain-stem, while those in progressive myoclonic epilepsy also involve the cerebral cortex and pyramidal system.

No effective treatment is available for this disease which leads to death within 10 or 15 years. Treatment is symptomatic with anticonvulsants in an attempt to suppress the severe and distressing jerks. Nitrazepam, clonazepam and sodium valproate are among the drugs which have proved most helpful, but in the later stages little or no relief is obtained from any medication and the terminal stage is of total helplessness and jerking amounting at times to status myoclonicus.

DENTATORUBRAL ATROPHY (RAMSAY HUNT SYNDROME)

An even rarer familial disorder in which myoclonus is prominent, but associated with true cerebellar ataxia, was described by Ramsay Hunt (1921) under the title 'dyssynergia cerebellaris myoclonica — primary atrophy of the dentate system'. His four patients developed myoclonus and other seizures in late childhood or adolescence followed later by cerebellar ataxia. Dementia was not a prominent feature. This condition is so rare that its precise status is hard to define, but it may not be a homogeneous disease, since myoclonus is often associated with cerebellar dysfunction in other progressive diseases, and can at times mimic cerebellar ataxia. The pathological basis of the disease, however, was thought to be specific, as autopsy showed involvement of the dentate nucleus, dentato-rubral and spinocerebellar tracts, and superior cerebellar peduncle.

THE LEUCODYSTROPHIES

Introduction

In this large group of distinctive disorders the pathological hallmark is widespread, often symmetrical demyelination, often with striking sparing of the arcuate fibres, or failure of normal formation of myelin in the central white matter of the brain. This may be softened and cavitated or hard and gliotic. In some members of the group peripheral nerves are affected and show segmental demyelination. Clinically these diseases of white matter tend to present with motor symptoms such as ataxia and paralysis, in contrast to the 'grey matter diseases' or neuronal storage disorders already considered in which dementia and seizures are common early features. The distinction between these two groups of disorders is helpful, but cannot be pushed too far, since demyelination may occur in the grey matter diseases and two of the leucodystrophies (metachromatic and Krabbe's) are known to be due to inherited defects of enzymes with resultant metabolic error and are associated with storage of lipid material, so that they could logically be classed as sphingolipidoses.

The classification of the leucodystrophies is difficult and unsatisfactory. Figures and lingering attitudes from the past contribute to the confusion. The contribution of Paul Schilder must be considered in order to set this classification in an historical context, since the term 'Schilder's disease' was, and sometimes still is, used as a generic term for these diseases.

Poser & van Bogaert (1956) have provided a helpful review of the 'Natural history and evolution of the concept of Schilder's diffuse sclerosis'. The term 'diffuse sclerosis' had been in neuropathological use for some decades when Schilder published his report in 1912 of a 14-year-old girl who died after an illness of four and a half months' duration with mental deterioration and raised intracranial pressure. The histological findings were of extensive bilateral demyelination with almost complete sparing of axons and subcortical U-fibres. Schilder concluded that this represented a new pathological entity, a diffuse disease of the white matter in childhood. He coined the name 'encephalitis periaxialis diffusa' in view of the relative axonal sparing.

In 1913 Schilder published a study of the brain of a case previously studied by others and included it in his new category. In 1924 he published his third case in which the pathology showed marked inflammatory changes and perivascular lymphocytic infiltrates.

Unfortunately many later writers applied the name 'Schilder's disease' or 'diffuse sclerosis' to a host of unrelated and heterogeneous conditions which have since been recognized as belonging to quite different categories. British and American authors particularly have tended to retain all these superficially similar disorders under the name 'Schilder's disease'. Poser and van Bogaert have used Schilder's original three cases as prototypes for the classification of disorders of white matter,

Table 5.2 Summary of the clinical features of the different forms of metachromatic leucodystrophy

Group	Age at which symptoms started	Symptoms	Age at diagnosis	Motor signs at diagnosis	Fits	Death
1. Late infantile (n = 24)	6*–25 months (mean 17)	Gait disorder, followed within months by a general loss of abilities	15–60 months (mean 34)	Mainly pyramidal and cerebellar. Ankle reflexes absent in 11 in presence of extensor plantars in 7 of the 11	Later in 5	5 months to 8 years after onset
2. Intermediate or early juvenile (n = 7)	4–6 years (mean 5)	Gait disorder with simultaneous educational and behavioural problems in 4	$5\frac{1}{2}$–12 years (mean $8\frac{1}{4}$)	Mainly extrapyramidal but also cerebellar and pyramidal. Ankle reflexes absent in one	Early in 1, later in 5	$3\frac{1}{2}$ to over 17 years from onset
3. Juvenile (n = 6)	6–10 years (mean 8)	Educational and behavioural problems, followed 6 months to 4 years later by gait disorder	$8\frac{1}{2}$–14 years (mean 11)	Predominantly extra-pyramidal and some pyramidal. Ankle reflexes absent in one	Later in 4	5 to over 11 years from onset
4. Atypical (n = 1)	13 years	Mild gait disorder followed 3 years later by intellectual deterioration	16 years	Extrapyramidal	–	Alive 6 years after onset

* Only one patient younger than 12 months

using his first case to represent true diffuse sclerosis, his second case for the degenerative, genetic diseases of myelin, the leucodystrophies, and his third case for the subacute encephalitides typified by van Bogaert's subacute sclerosing leucoencephalitis.

METACHROMATIC LEUCODYSTROPHY (SULPHATIDE LIPIDOSIS)

This interesting condition, of which Schilder's second (1913) case may well have been an example, was one of the first to be separated off from the varied diseases included under his name and under the term diffuse sclerosis. Its separation was brought by the unusual staining properties shown by many tissues due to the presence of excess sulphatides.

Like many other progressive neurometabolic diseases, metachromatic leucodystrophy (MLD) occurs in three forms in childhood, a late infantile variety (the commonest), a rarer juvenile form and an intermediate or early juvenile type (MacFaul et al 1982) (Fig. 5.14 and Table 5.2). There is also a very rare adult form.

Common to all these forms is the finding of excess sulphatides in many tissues, including the central (Fig. 5.15) and peripheral nervous system, demyelination of the white matter of the cerebrum, cerebellum and spinal cord, and segmental demyelination in peripheral nerves. Sulphatide, cerebroside-3-sulphate, a sulphuric acid ester of cerebroside, is present in excess due to impaired hydrolysis of sulphatide to cerebrosides as a result of deficiency of the enzyme cerebroside-sulphatase (aryl-sulphatase A). Progressive neurological deterioration occurs in all subgroups. The age of onset and clinical course are similar within affected families, a fact of some value in recognizing whether a sibling of a known sufferer from the disease is affected or not.

The late infantile form

Sometimes known as Greenfield's disease, this is the most homogeneous group. The 24 children with this variety of MLD in the series of MacFaul et al (1982), presented between the ages of 6 and

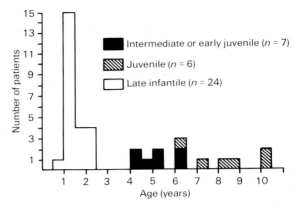

Fig. 5.14 Age at which symptoms started in 37 patients with metachromatic leucodystrophy

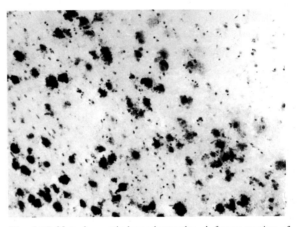

Fig. 5.15 Metachromatic leucodystrophy. A frozen section of brain showing sulphatide accumulation in macrophages in the white matter. The cortex (top right) is unaffected. Sulphatide shows a strong purple-red metachromasia in the brain with toluidine blue.
Toluidine blue × 83

25 months (with a mean of 17 months), with a delay or deterioration in walking, followed by a general loss of ability. Eight children never walked alone. In 7 children an immature, toddler type of gait persisted and in 12 deterioration occurred in walking ability. The gait disorder is due partly to ataxia and partly to spasticity of the legs, but is often attributed to the normal toddler unsteadiness of gait and only when it persists and is followed by slowing down of motor and social progress does suspicion of a pathological condition arise. The mean age of

diagnosis in this series was 34 months — twice the mean age of onset. Later the loss of previously acquired skills confirms this suspicion. As in many progressive degenerative diseases of childhood, it may be difficult to be certain from the history precisely when the symptoms began. Concern has often been present for some months before medical advice is sought. It is common for parents to be reassured that the child is normal and that they should not worry; this is inevitable when signs are subtle and minimal, but it sometimes has the effect of destroying parental confidence in their medical advisers. Parents who have had one or more affected children are much quicker to recognize abnormality in a second child, and in their anxiety may even anticipate the onset of symptoms, sometimes realizing intuitively in some indefinable way that the child is 'different'.

As time passes increasing dementia and spasticity develop. Seizures are not a prominent symptom and occurred in only 6 of the 24 patients of MacFaul et al.

Clinical examination shows a combination of ataxia with spasticity and intellectual deterioration. An important clinical clue is the finding of reduced or absent tendon reflexes as evidence of peripheral neuropathy. This paradoxical finding in the presence of increased tone and extensor plantar responses should suggest the presence of metachromatic or Krabbe's leucodystrophy. Positive toe jerks, a form of stretch reflex obtained by tapping on the dorsum or sole of the foot and sometimes over a wider area of the lower leg, are commonly seen in these two diseases and when combined with areflexia are highly suggestive of the diagnosis. Ophthalmoscopic examination may show optic atrophy in the later stages, and an atypical cherry red spot at the macula has been seen in several cases.

The prognosis is uniformly bad, with death at a mean age of $4\frac{3}{4}$ years and seldom later than the age of 8.

The widespread nature of the disease, with involvement of the renal tract, gall bladder and intestine as well as the central and peripheral nervous system, provides a wide choice of diagnostic investigations. The peripheral neuropathy may be confirmed by neurophysiological methods with study of motor nerve conduction velocity in the ulnar, lateral popliteal or other nerves (Fullerton 1964). Conduction velocity tends to become slower with the passage of time and may be as slow as 10 or 12 metres per second in the later stages. The CT scan often shows areas of low attenuation in the central cerebral white matter (Fig. 5.16).

The EEG is usually abnormal and may be helpful (Fig. 24.6). In the 22 children studied by Mastropaolo et al (1971) the normal rhythmic activity appropriate for the age of the child tended gradually to disappear early in the course of the disease, but spikes or complex wave forms were uncommon, and 3 per second spike and wave complexes were never seen. The responses to photic stimulation are well preserved in the earlier stages but later disappear. The electroretinogram is preserved. The CSF commonly shows a raised level of protein, but this finding is not specific for the disease. In the pre-enzyme era, biopsy of neural tissue was necessary for diagnosis and cerebral biopsy was often performed.

Today neural biopsy in MLD is difficult to justify, since alternative, less traumatic diagnostic methods are available. Deposits of sulphatides are

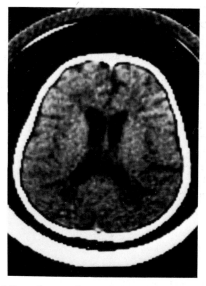

Fig. 5.16 Juvenile metachromatic leucodystrophy. 10-year-old girl with slowly progressive intellectual deterioration and behaviour disorder for 12 months
CT. Note low attenuation adjacent to frontal horns and trigones and diffusely enlarged cortical sulci. The lateral and third ventricles were moderately dilated.

widespread throughout the body and are particularly concentrated in the distal and collecting tubules of the kidneys. These cells are shed into the urine and can be seen in the urinary sediment together with other epithelial cells. The demonstration of intracellular metachromatic material in the urine provides a 'spontaneous biopsy' which has proved a very reliable test in our experience.

A fresh specimen of urine is desirable since the precipitation of phosphates and urates is likely to be minimal. Early morning specimens may contain lysed cells, and very dilute specimens may contain no cells, so both should be avoided. The latter may result in a false negative result and the laboratory report should specify, if no intracellular material is seen, whether or not cells are present in the sediment, so that further specimens can be examined if necessary.

The urine sample is centrifuged and three slides are prepared from the deposit, air-dried, fixed in formaldehyde vapour at 60°C and stained overnight with 0.01% toluidine blue in McKilvaine buffer pH 5.0.

Sulphatides in urinary epithelial cells give a golden-yellow metachromasia with toluidine blue which appears greenish in polarized light (Plate 4). The presence, within cells, of such metachromasia is pathognomonic for metachromatic leucodystrophy (and mucosulphatidosis) and is found in all forms of the disease. *Extracellular* deposits are not pathognomonic but, if they are present, suspicion is heightened and further samples should be examined.

Confirmation of the diagnosis is by enzyme assay for aryl-sulphatase A in white blood cells or cultured fibroblasts. The enzyme may also be measured in the urine. In patients the enzyme level is deficient. Carrier levels are found in the heterozygous parents of affected children.

If a neural biopsy is considered necessary the logical choice is the sural nerve, in which metachromatic deposits can be shown in Schwann cells and macrophages (Plate 5).

The juvenile form

In this group the patients are 'middle-aged' children with the onset between 6 and 10 years of age.

The juvenile form is less common than the late infantile. In two earlier series of children with MLD from the Hospital for Sick Children, Great Ormond Street, there were 26 of the late infantile and 13 of the juvenile condition (Schutta et al 1966, Mastropaolo et al 1971). The 38 cases of MacFaul et al, of which 11 had been reported previously, included 6 juvenile cases.

The onset of the disease tends to be more insidious and the course slower in the juvenile than in the earlier onset cases, and the diagnosis is often long delayed as a result. Whereas motor problems, particularly gait disorder, are the commonest presenting feature in the late infantile cases, in the juvenile form the presentation is often with changes in behaviour, falling off in school work and mental deterioration at about 8 years of age. It is often difficult to be certain of the exact age of onset, and the rather non-specific problems of behaviour and poor school performance may be regarded as of psychological origin, with punitive measures or the kinder but equally unproductive psychiatric referral as a consequence. Outbursts of aggression, antisocial behaviour and general 'naughtiness' persist and increase until in time it becomes clear that a dementing process is present. Motor difficulties appear later due to extrapyramidal features alone or associated with pyramidal and/or cerebellar dysfunction, so that a rather Parkinsonian appearance may be produced. Areflexia is less common in this group than in the late infantile form. Optic atrophy and visual failure occur as late features.

Fits occurred in 4 of the 6 children in this group at between 8 and 14 years of age.

Two patients in this series died, age 11 and 15 years, 5 years from onset of their illness. Three others were still alive between 6½ and 11 years after onset.

Intermediate or early juvenile form

A small subgroup of 7 patients previously classified as 'juvenile' has been recognized by MacFaul et al, at the Hospital for Sick Children, Great Ormond Street, with a rather earlier onset at between 4 and 6 years of age (mean 5 years). Their presentation was with gait disorder alone or associated with dementia. In those presenting with gait disturbance

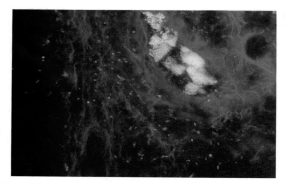

Plate 3 Rectal biopsy; juvenile Batten's disease. Cryostat section unstained, showing marked autofluorescence of the neuronal and smooth muscle deposits. Viewed under dark ground illumination with excitation at 360 nm, barrier at 410 nm

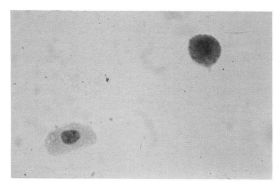

Plate 4 Urinary deposit; metachromatic leucodystrophy. Stained with toluidine blue showing a normal bladder epithelial cell (lower right) and a renal tubular cell containing abundant brown metachromatic sulphatide

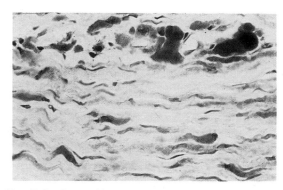

Plate 5 Sural nerve biopsy; metachromatic leucodystrophy. Cryostat section stained with toluidine blue showing brown and red metachromatic deposits of sulphatide in macrophages and Schwann cells

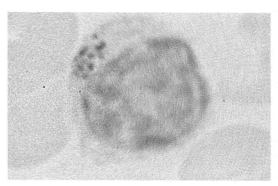

Plate 6 Peripheral blood lymphocyte; MPS II (Hunter). Stained with the toluidine blue method of Muir, Mittwoch and Bitter showing red metachromatic inclusions in the cytoplasm

alone, evidence of intellectual deterioration followed after an interval of between 8 and 26 months. Fits occurred in 3 patients. Extrapyramidal, pyramidal and cerebellar signs were present, but the ankle reflexes were absent in only one patient in this group. The course of the illness varied, two patients dying within 4 and 6 years from onset while others were still surviving between 9 and 17 years after onset.

Diagnostic investigations in the two later onset forms of MLD are similar to those for the late infantile disease, examination of urine for intracellular metachromatic material and assay of arylsulphatase-A in urine and white blood cells giving the simplest and most reliable confirmation of the diagnosis when laboratory facilities are available. The presence of a peripheral neuropathy may be confirmed by the finding of slowed motor nerve conduction velocity. Neural biopsy should not be necessary. The CT scan shows similar changes in the white matter to those in the late infantile variety (Fig. 5.16). Prenatal diagnosis can be made in all forms of the disease by amniocentesis, fetal cells being cultured and their enzyme content measured.

Despite the relatively advanced stage of present knowledge about MLD, no effective treatment is yet available. Although cultured fibroblasts from affected children have been shown to take up the enzyme in vitro (Wiesmann et al 1972), attempts to adminster arylsulphatase-A to a patient were unsuccessful (Greene et al 1969). Another therapeutic appraoch has been with a diet low in vitamin A, which seems to act as a coenzyme in the synthesis of active sulphate. A five-fold reduction in urinary sulphatide was obtained in a child treated for 4 months with a vitamin A-deficient diet, but no clinical benefit was seen (Melchior & Clausen 1968). Progression of the disease seemed to become arrested for 2 years in another child so treated (Moosa & Dubowitz 1971). In the patient treated by Warner (1975) a low vitamin A diet produced neither clinical improvement nor reduction in urinary sulphatide levels. It seems likely that any treatment, to be effective, would need to be applied at a very early age. Studies of affected fetal brain have shown involvement before 20 weeks' gestation.

KRABBE'S GLOBOID BODY LEUCODYSTROPHY

The Danish neurologist Krabbe in 1916 described 'a new familial, infantile form of diffuse brain-sclerosis.' The condition had probably been recognized earlier, but he was the first to comment on the globoid cells in the affected cerebral white matter which are regarded as its pathological hallmark.

The disease has distinct analogies with metachromatic leucodystrophy, though it is rarer. Both can be regarded as diseases of white matter with demyelination in central and peripheral nervous systems, and both are associated with accumulation of complex lipids due to deficiency of lysosomal enzymes. In Krabbe's disease there is an excess of galactocerebrosides due to deficiency of galactocerebroside beta-galactosidase (galactocerebrosidase).

Like metachrometic leucodystrophy, Krabbe's disease occurs in an early and a later onset form.

The commoner infantile form often presents in the early weeks or months of life with vomiting and poor feeding and weight gain. Apathy, irritability and inconsolable crying are prominent from a few weeks of age onwards. There is severe retardation and the children usually fail to sit alone, regressing and losing the few abilities they have gained from about 5 months of age. Variable increase in tone and head retraction are common. Episodes of unexplained fever may occur. An exaggerated startle reaction to noise may be an early symptom and may raise the suspicion of Tay-Sachs disease but a cherry-red spot is not seen, though optic atrophy and blindness usually develop. Seizures are rare.

Clinical evidence of peripheral neuropathy in the form of depressed or absent tendon reflexes is mentioned in many earlier reports, including that of Krabbe, who noted that the knee jerks could not be obtained in any of his five patients and that a flaccid state succeeded spasticity in the terminal stages of the disease. In a series of 7 British and Canadian patients (Dunn et al 1969) a peripheral neuropathy was present with depressed or absent tendon reflexes, grossly reduced motor nerve conduction velocity (between 10 and 15 metres per second) and impaired sensory conduction. Segmental demyelination in peripheral nerves was found on biopsy and later autopsy. Positive toe jerks are often seen in combination with reduced tendon reflexes and extensor plantar responses, as in metachromatic leucodystrophy, and this combination of signs in the setting of progressive neurological deterioration with its onset at 2 to 6 months of age is highly suggestive of Krabbe's disease.

Death usually occurs between 9 and 30 months of age.

Cases of Krabbe's disease have sometimes been mistaken for cases of cerebral palsy but a careful history, with a period of normality before the onset of symptoms should prevent this mistake.

Tay-Sachs disease, which enters into the differential diagnosis in view of the rather similar age of onset and the fact that an exaggerated startle reaction to sound may be seen in both conditions, can be excluded clinically by the signs of peripheral neuropathy, the rarity of fits and the absence of a cherry-red spot at the macula. The infantile (Hagber-Santavuori) form of Batten's disease, and the infantile forms of Niemann-Pick and Gaucher's disease, in which a cherry red spot may be seen, can usually be differentiated also by their lack of peripheral nerve involvement and by other positive features such as hepatic and splenic enlargement.

Suspicion of the diagnosis of infantile Krabbe's disease can be strengthened by nerve conduction studies. The CSF protein is often raised to very high levels and the EEG may be diffusely abnormal. Assay of galactocerebrosidase activity in white blood cells shows very low levels, and heterozygote levels are found in the parents. Biopsy of a peripheral nerve such as the sural shows segmental demyelination. The brain shows profound loss of myelin (Fig. 5.17). Cerebral biopsy, to be of any value, must include adequate white matter, which shows demyelination and large, spherical, multinucleated globoid cells, 20 to 25 μm in diameter, which contain stored galactocerebroside (Fig. 5.18). The CT scan shows low attenuation in the central white matter (Fig. 5.19).

A much rarer form of Krabbe's disease has been recognized in a few children with its onset after two years of age. Progressive neurological deterioration is seen but the clinical picture is less specific than in the infantile form, and peripheral neuropathy may not be present. Neuropathy was absent in the three cases reported by Crome et al (1973), repeated nerve conduction studies giving normal results, and a sural nerve biopsy from one of these patients showing no demyelination. A thorough search for demyelination in autopsy material from this case showed no abnormality. Elevation of the CSF protein level seems to be less common in the

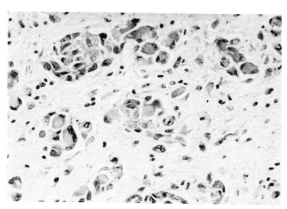

Fig. 5.18 Krabbe's leucodystrophy. Clusters of globoid cells are present in the demyelinated white matter. The globoid cells are PAS positive and may be multinucleate. HE × 198

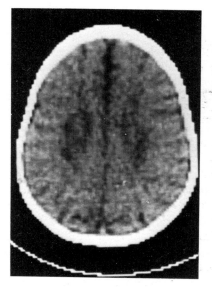

Fig. 5.19 Krabbe's globoid body leucodystrophy. 14 month old girl with history of developmental standstill from age of 6 months and regression from 8 months.
CT. There is low attenuation in the central white matter with moderate dilatation of the third and lateral ventricles.

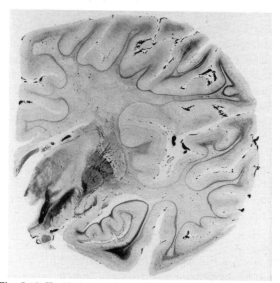

Fig. 5.17 Krabbe's leucodystrophy.
Section of cerebral hemisphere stained for myelin showing profound loss of myelin with relative preservation of the subcortical arcuate fibres and the basal ganglia

late onset form of Krabbe's disease than in the infantile cases. In a recent case described by Dunn et al (1976) no globoid cells were found in the brain of a patient in whom the galactocerebrosidase activity was deficient. There was, however, massive demyelination.

ADRENAL LEUCODYSTROPHY (ADDISON-SCHILDER'S DISEASE: X-LINKED DIFFUSE SCLEROSIS WITH ADRENAL INSUFFICIENCY)

Among the cases previously diagnosed as Schilder's disease it seems clear that some were examples of this leucodystrophy associated with adrenocortical insufficiency and features of Addison's disease. If eponyms are ever justified, the name of Schilder is reasonably perpetuated for this disorder, linked with that of Addison, though the term Addison-Scholz disease is preferred by some.

The older literature contains reports of boys noticed to have 'melanoderma' at an early age who later developed progressive neurological symptoms leading to death with the finding at autopsy of diffuse cerebral sclerosis and adrenal atrophy.

The clinical syndrome is now more clearly defined (Hoefnagel et al 1962, Aguilar et al 1967, Gray 1969, De Long et al 1982). The typical disease occurs only in males and behaves as an X-linked condition with several boys in a sibship often affected and sometimes with a family history of maternal uncles having died of Addison's disease or of a progressive neurological illness which was regarded at the time as Schilder's disease. The age of onset of neurological symptoms is usually between 5 and 9 years. The features of adrenal insufficiency may precede or follow those of the brain disorder. Sometimes the insidious nature of both sets of symptoms makes it difficult to decide when they began. In some cases a definite diagnosis of Addison's disease has been made, because of increased pigmentation, episodes of vomiting and catastrophic reactions to intercurrent infections, before any neurological disorder in evident. In others neurological deterioration may have continued for some years without endocrine symptoms appearing, and sophisticated investigations may be needed to show evidence of adrenocortical dysfunction. There may be great variation in the pattern of presentation and rate of deterioration within an affected family. The relationship between the endocrine and neurological disorders is far from clear; it is certainly not a cause and effect relationship, since many affected patients have now been adequately treated by replacement therapy for their adrenocortical deficiency without the slightest effect on the neurological symptoms which show inexorable progression to death, usually within a few years of their onset. Recent biochemical advances (Moser et al 1981) could conceivably lead in time to some form of effective treatment.

The earliest neurological symptoms are often vague and their onset may be difficult to date with accuracy. As with many of the progressive degenerative brain diseases, parents have often been aware from an early age of a slight, indefinable difference between the behaviour of the affected boys and that of their normal siblings. Often more severe symptoms seem to date from school entry (which in Britain is normally at about the age of five) when the child fails to meet the demands to sit still and conform in the class and may show disruptive behaviour. (In more permissive schools this may not excite comment.) Failure to make progress with learning may be evident at this age or later, and teachers may comment on poor coordination. Worsening behaviour at home and at school is usually regarded as due to naughtiness and regular punishment may result. A childhood psychosis may be suspected and the unhappy child and his parents may be referred to a psychiatrist. Months or years of psychiatric treatment, with drugs, psychotherapy and 'case-work' with parents may follow, until deteriorating school performance and other evidence of dementia, motor disorder, visual failure, sometimes due to cortical blindness, deafness or convulsions force recognition of the organic nature of the disease. Symptoms of adrenal insufficiency may develop at any stage and these may also cause the physician at last to turn his attention from psyche to soma.

Neurological examination is usually normal in the earlier stages but later pyramidal, extrapyramidal, and sometimes cerebellar signs develop, with obvious dementia. Optic atrophy is seen and occasionally papilloedema is present. Signs of peripheral neuropathy are not usually a feature of the disease, but nerve conduction studies and sural nerve biopsy have given evidence of a neuropathy with a disorder of myelination, with additional loss of both myelinated and unmyelinated axons (De Long et al 1982).

Symptoms suggestive of Addison's disease may be obvious with diarrhoea or vomiting, hypotension and pigmentation which may be gross, but in

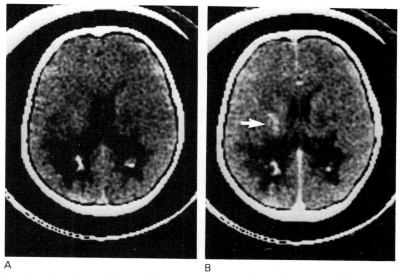

Fig. 5.20 Adrenal leucodystrophy. 7-year-old boy with progressive intellectual deterioration for 16 months.
CT. Note low attenuation in cerebral white matter around trigones and occipital horns and right internal capsule. Enhancement of left internal capsule with contrast (B) (arrowed)

many cases pigmentation may be absent or detected only in the buccal mucous membranes; it is helpful to examine the palmar creases and any scars from operations or trauma since pigmentation may be seen in these, including chicken-pox scars.

The CT scan is extremely helpful in this disease, showing the appearances of a leucodystrophy, often most marked in the occipital regions and often with enhancement of the internal capsules (Fig. 5.20). Other investigations are most usefully directed to the demonstration of adrenocortical dysfunction, since this is pathognomonic of the disease in the context of progressive neurological disorder of boys with the CT appearances described. Urinary excretion of 17-hydroxycorticosteroids and 17-oxosteroids may be reduced or normal, so that the test should not be relied on for a diagnosis. The levels of plasma cortisol before and after injection of tetracosactrin (Synacthen, Ciba) 0.25 mg/70 kg body weight, are measured and a minimal or negative response confirms the adrenal disorder. Unfortunately a normal response may be misleading, since this was found in 2 of 5 boys with adrenal leucodystrophy studied by Rees et al (1975). These authors suggested that estimation of plasma ACTH may be a more reliable and sensitive method for detecting adrenal disease since raised levels were found in all 5 patients and also in the symptom-free

brother of one of these.

Moser and his colleagues (1981) have shown increased plasma levels of saturated very long chain fatty acids (C26 fatty acid) in 16 boys with adrenal leucodystrophy (ALD) (and also in two patients with adrenomyeloneuropathy) as well as in most heterozygotes for ALD. These authors believe that the technique can be used for diagnosis and carrier detection, and also for the assessment of the results of any therapy.

The CSF may show a raised level of protein and sometimes a moderate increase in lymphocytes but these changes are non-specific and not very helpful, so that lumbar puncture is not indicated in most cases.

Neurophysiological investigations are also of limited diagnostic value, the EEG usually showing a severe generalized abnormality in the later stages. The visual evoked responses from the occipital area are often reduced or absent suggesting impairment of the visual pathways and/or visual cortex. This may be found at an early stage when cortical blindness is present. The electroretinogram is not affected. Nerve conduction studies and nerve biopsy have given evidence of peripheral neuropathy in some cases (De Long et al 1982).

Adrenal biopsy has been used for diagnosis by electronmicroscopy, showing the characteristic crys-

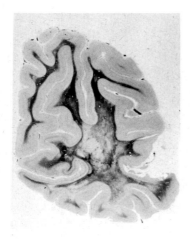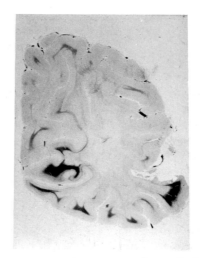

Fig. 5.21 Adrenal leucodystrophy (Addison-Schilder's disease). Adjacent sections of occipital lobe stained for myelin (R) and glial fibrils (L) showing marked demyelination and glial replacement

talline inclusions in the enlarged cortical cells (Powers & Schaumburg 1974). The inclusions are thought to represent long-chain fatty acid esters. Although the peripheral nerves may show similar changes, these are not consistent or specific.

Brain biopsy is difficult to justify in this condition, since the diagnosis can be made more easily by endocrine studies, the necessarily small amount of tissue removed at biopsy may not include sufficient white matter to allow the pathologist to show the characteristic changes, and the procedure may be poorly tolerated.

At autopsy the brain is often shrunken and lighter than normal (Fig. 5.21). The central white matter may be cystic and cavitated on section or alternatively greyish and indurated. Histologically there is widespread demyelination of the white matter with sudanophilic extra- and intracellular debris, probably derived from myelin breakdown. The neurons are usually normal except in more advanced cases in which neuronal loss may be seen. An inflammatory-like appearance with some perivascular cuffing by mononuclear cells is often present.

The adrenal glands show gross atrophy of the cortex, the medulla being normal (Fig. 5.22). The zona reticularis and fasciculata are particularly affected with ballooned cortical cells in which a striated appearance of the cytoplasm may be seen. A lymphocytic infiltration is occasionally seen.

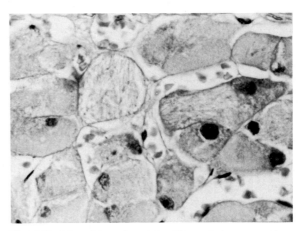

Fig. 5.22 Adrenal leucodystrophy. Fine striations are evident in the enlarged cells of the zone reticularis in an atrophied adrenal gland.
HE × 480

A congenital case of adrenal leucodystrophy has been reported in a male infant dying at 17 months of age with severe neurological features but without clinical signs of adrenal insufficiency. The brain showed gross demyelination and also micropolygyria (Ulrich et al 1978).

The concept of the disease has been further widened by O'Neill et al (1981) under the title 'the adrenoleukomyeloneuropathy complex'. In a kindred of four generations, and both sexes, varying combinations of leucodystrophy, myeloneuropathy

(Ch. 8), peripheral neuropathy and primary Addison's disease were noted.

SPONGY DEGENERATION OF THE BRAIN: SPONGIFORM LEUCODYSTROPHY: CANAVAN'S (VAN BOGAERT-BERTRAND) DISEASE

Spongy change, 'status spongiosus' and spongiform leucodystrophy are terms given to a distinctive appearance of the brain which may be gross enough to be visible to the naked eye or detectable only with the microscope. These changes affect the deeper layers of the cerebral cortex and the underlying white matter and have been seen in a variety of neurological diseases. In older patients they may be associated with Alzheimer's and Jakob-Creutzfeldt disease, arteriosclerosis, hypertension and some post-infectious syndromes (Seitelberger 1967). In childhood similar changes have been described in some neurometabolic disorders, such as homocystinuria, hyperglycinaemia, arginosuccinic acidaemia, phenylketonuria, and maple-syrup urine disease.

Spongiform changes are also seen in children with a rare progressive neurological disease without, as yet, a known metabolic basis. The disorder sometimes known as Canavan's disease was reported in 1931 by Myrtelle Canavan under the title 'Schilder's encephalitis periaxialis diffusa'. Van Bogaert & Bertrand (1949) were responsible for defining the condition clinically and pathologically, and their names are sometimes applied to it in preference to Canavan's. The clinical picture of Canavan's disease appears to be a fairly distinctive one, with the onset in the first year of life of developmental delay and regression, with hypotonia followed by increased muscle tone, optic atrophy, seizures and excessive crying. The condition is inherited as an autosomal recessive and most of the earlier reported patients were of Ashkenazi Jewish origin, their families deriving from the same areas (Lithuania, Eastern Poland and the Ukraine) whence the families of many children with Tay-Sachs disease originate. Non-Jewish children have also been affected. In 15 of 26 cases reported up to 1965 symptoms had started by the age of 3 months, and in all by 6 months (Hogan & Richardson 1969).

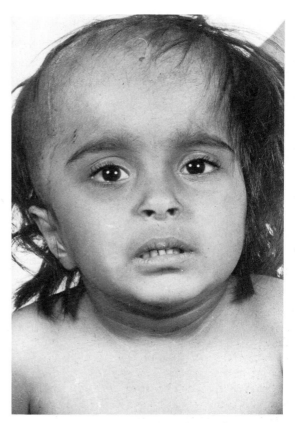

Fig. 5.23 Spongiform leucodystrophy: 4-year-old girl; note large head

Striking enlargement of the head is a common feature which helps to distinguish the condition from some other degenerative diseases with onset in the first year, but which sometimes leads to a wrong suspicion of obstructive hydrocephalus (Fig. 5.23). Progressive deterioration leads to a decorticate condition and to an early death, the average age of which was 19 months in the collected series analysed by Hogan & Richardson (1969).

Spongiform changes of similar type may be seen in children with recessively inherited progressive neurological disease of later onset and rarely in infants with symptoms dating from birth.

Examination of the CSF may show a raised protein level and the EEG is usually abnormal, but these results are non-specific. Nerve conduction studies give normal results. Skull X-rays may show enlargement of the skull vault sometimes with separation of the sutures. Air encephalography may

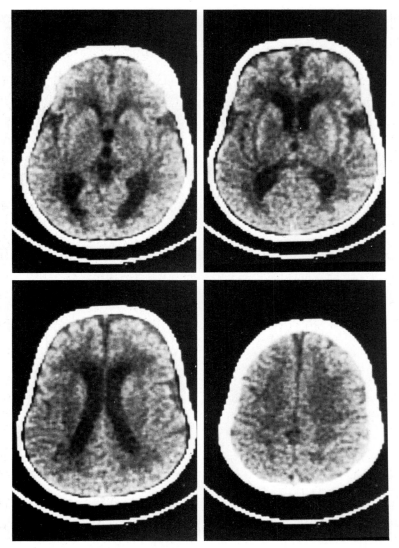

Fig. 5.24 Spongiform leucodystrophy. 14-month-old boy with gross developmental delay, increased reflexes and poor vision. CT. Note widespread low attenuation of the white matter including the external capsules and, to a lesser extent, the internal capsules. Also low attenuation in the thalami. There is cerebral atrophy with a large third and lateral ventricles and wide sylvian fissures and convexity sulci

indicate enlargement of the ventricular system without obstruction, and the CT may show gross changes suggesting involvement of central white matter (Fig. 5.24).

The diagnosis, though it may be strongly suspected on clinical grounds, is basically a pathological one and can only be confirmed in life by brain biopsy and the finding of the characteristic spongy changes. The spongiform leucodystrophies are among the few remaining conditions for which biopsy is still necessary and justified (Boltshauser & Wilson 1976).

The striking histological features are in the white matter and the deeper cortical layers with rarefaction and numerous vacuoles coalescing to form larger cavities giving an appearance like that of a sponge, (Fig. 5.25) which may even be visible to the naked eye. These changes are probably not spe-

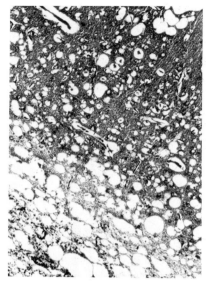

Fig. 5.25 Spongiform leucodystrophy (Canavan). Marked vacuolar changes present in the white matter (lower right/left) and perivascularly in the cortex (upper left/right) are particularly prominent at the junction of cortex and white matter.
Glees × 48

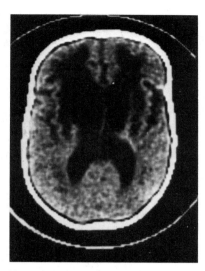

Fig. 5.26 Alexander's leucodystrophy. 6-year-old girl with progressive intellectual deterioration and large head. CT. All the ventricles were dilated with enlargement of the sylvian fissures and cortical sulci. Low attenuation in the white matter most marked in the frontal region

cific to one clinical entity, although an infantile disorder corresponding to the description of Canavan's disease is probably the commonest clinical correlate of this pathological picture.

ALEXANDER'S LEUCODYSTROPHY

There is little specific about the clinical features of this rare condition, first described by Alexander in 1949, which appears to be a clinicopathological entity, occurring sporadically without clear familial incidence. Whereas most of the other diseases of white matter may often be strongly suspected from careful assessment of the clinical evidence, the progressive neurological deterioration in this disorder may start in infancy or later childhood with dementia, seizures and spasticity, and may be so insidious that its progressive nature may not be appreciated for some years. Enlargement of the brain and skull are common, as in spongiform leucodystrophy, and this may be a valuable clue. This megalencephaly may contrast strikingly with emaciation in the later stages and wrongly suggest the diagnosis of a diencephalic syndrome due to a neoplasm. Persistent

hiccup was the presenting feature in a recent case (Wilson et al 1981).

There are no pointers to the biochemical basis of the disorder and laboratory investigations are unhelpful with the exception of the CT scan, which shows ventricular enlargement and low attenuation in the cerebral white matter (Fig. 5.26) and brain biopsy which is diagnostic. Histological examination shows diffuse demyelination and rarefaction of

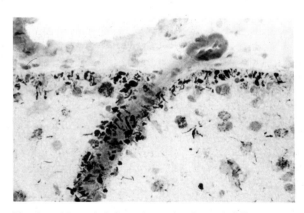

Fig. 5.27 Alexander's leucodystrophy. Rosenthal fibres, present in subpial and perivascular regions, are also found scattered throughout cortex and white matter. They represent accumulations of fibrillary material in astrocytic processes.
Luxol fast blue × 224

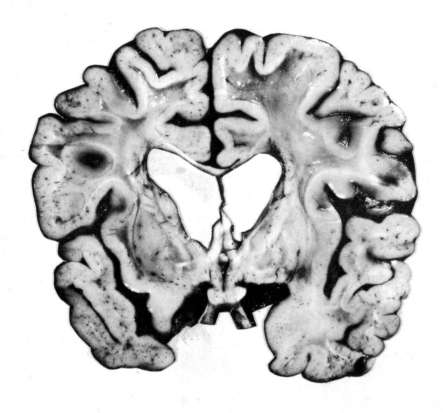

Fig. 5.28 Alexander's leucodystrophy. Coronal slice of brain through basal ganglia showing grey depressed centrum semiovale with frank degeneration in some areas. Note thinned corpus callosum and enlarged ventricles

white matter with little or no sparing of the arcuate fibres. Rosenthal fibres are present particularly in the sub-pial regions and around vessels in the cortex and white matter (Fig. 5.27). These are astrocytic processes containing fibrillary aggregates. Macroscopically the large brain shows indurated cortex contrasting with underlying white matter which is softened, jelly-like and cavitated (Fig. 5.28).

The importance of establishing a definite diagnosis in this disease lies mainly in the prognostic implications with invariable deterioration and death. The genetic implications involved in the other disorders described above are lacking in most cases, but the non-genetic nature of the disease is a factor of great importance in advising the parents of an affected child, and is indeed the only element of consolation in a tragic situation. Alexander's leucodystrophy and spongiform degeneration are among the very few degenerative disorders in which cerebral biopsy is still essential for a diagnosis.

THE MUCOPOLYSACCHARIDOSES (MPS)

In these genetically-determined storage diseases with deficiencies of specific lysosomal enzymes, there is accumulation of acidic polysaccharides in various organs. Certain clinical features occur in varying combinations in the different syndromes and suggest the diagnosis which should be confirmed biochemically. The clinical features commonly seen are mental retardation, corneal clouding, enlargement of spleen and liver, bony deformities, dysmorphic facial appearance, broad hands with short, spade-like fingers, a large protruding tongue, a depressed nasal bridge and dry, coarse skin. These features tend to increase with age so that the diagnosis may not be suspected for some years. Normal intelligence is present in some syndromes.

The term 'gargoylism' was introduced many years ago for patients suffering from the syndromes then recognized, who were often referred to as 'gargoyles' from their grotesque facial features. The term was distressing and insulting and, like the archaic name 'mongolism', is falling into deserved disuse.

As with many other syndromes nosology offers a choice of a chemical terminology or the use of eponyms: the mucopolysaccharidoses (MPS) remains the preferred term for the whole group of syndromes (although logically the newer chemical term 'glycosaminoglycans' should be used with the suffix 'osis', the neologism has little to recommend it). Recent biochemical progress has led to greater understanding of these disorders, the underlying enzyme defect being known in many cases, and this has necessitated a change in terminology.

The main polysaccharide substances accumulating in the MPS are listed below, with the older and the new nomenclature (Table 5.3).

The polysaccharides normally undergo step-wise degradation by hydrolytic cleavage of component molecules by various enzymes. Lack of specific enzymes is responsible for the different MPS syndromes. These have been partially reclassified in recent years on the basis of the enzyme defects.

Table 5.3 Nomenclature of polysaccharides in the mucopolysaccharidoses

Old	New
Chondroitin sulphate B	Dermatan sulphate
Heparitin sulphate	Heparan sulphate
Keratosulphate	Keratan sulphate

Table 5.4 shows their present and previous classifications with the enzyme deficiencies responsible.

The clinical features of the various MPS syndromes will be described. All are inherited in autosomal recessive fashion except for MPS II (Hunter's syndrome) which is X-linked.

MPS IH (Hurler's syndrome) (Hurler 1919)

This disorder is the best known of the MPS group and heads the list of eponyms, though its description by Hurler in 1919 came two years after Hunter's report of the syndrome which bears his name. A more detailed account of this condition will be given since it serves as a useful exemplar of the group.

It is the severest disorder with clinical features evident in infancy and progressive intellectual and physical deterioration usually leading to death by 10 years of age. Early features include a lumbar kyphos, stiff joints, chest deformity and nasal discharge. The child becomes dwarfed after the first year and skeletal X-rays are grossly abnormal. Progressive corneal clouding occurs. Umbilical and inguinal herniae are common. Hepatosplenomegaly develops and increases with age. The coronary arteries and heart valves are also affected. Respiratory infections and cardiac failure are the usual causes of death. In the first year or two intellectual development often seems normal but after this regression and loss of speech, social and motor skills is the usual pattern. Obstructive hydrocephalus may occur from meningeal involvement and may contribute to the intellectual problems.

The head is large with a prominent forehead and is often scaphocephalic with a ridged sagittal suture. The nasal bridge is flat and the nostrils are wide. The lips are large and often parted to disclose the large tongue, hypertrophied gums and alveolar ridges and widely spaced peg-like teeth. The coarse, grotesque features with the obvious mental retardation may suggest cretinism but the two conditions are easily distinguished clinically and radiologically. The neck is short and the chest deformed both by the spinal kyphos and the flaring of the lower thorax due partly to the massive liver and spleen. The hands are broad and the short fingers often show flexion contractures producing a

Table 5.4 The mucopolysaccharidoses — classification, biochemical and enzyme features

New terminology	Syndrome Aslo known as	MPS excreted in urine	Enzyme deficient
MPS I H	Hurler's syndrome	Dermatan sulphate	α-L-Iduronidase
MPS I S	Scheie's syndrome	Heparan sulphate	α-L-Iduronidase
	(Formerly called MPS V)	Dermatan sulphate	α-L-Iduronidase
MPS I H/S	Hurler-Scheie compound	Heparan sulphate	
		Dermatan sulphate	
		Heparan sulphate	
MPS II A	Hunter's syndrome — severe form	Dermatan sulphate	Sulpho-iduronate sulphatase
MPS II B	Hunter's syndrome — mild form	Heparan sulphate	Sulpho-iduronate sulphatase
		Dermatan sulphate	
		Heparan sulphate	
MPS III A	Sanfilippo syndrome A	Heparan sulphate	Heparan-sulphate sulphatase
MPS III B	Sanfilippo syndrome B	Heparan sulphate	N-acetyl-α-D-glucosaminidase
MPS III C	Sanfilippo syndrome C	Heparan sulphate	Acetyl CoA-α-glucosaminide-N-acetyl transferase
MPS IV	Morquio's syndrome	Keratan sulphate	Chondroitin-sulphate-N-acetyl-hexosamine-sulphate-6-sulphatase
MPS VI A	Maroteaux-Lamy syndrome — severe form	Dermatan sulphate	Chondroitin sulphate-N-acetylgalactosamine-sulphate-4-sulphatase (aryl sulphatase B)
MPS VI B	Maroteaux-Lamy syndrome — mild form	Dermatan sulphate	
MPS VII	β-glucuronidase deficiency	Dermatan sulphate	β-Glucuronidase

claw-hand deformity. Larger joints are also involved, with flexion deformities of the knees and elbows caused by thickening of peri-articular ligaments and tendons.

Ocular features

Corneal clouding is invariable in MPS IH. It increases with age, being mild in the earlier stages and needing slit-lamp examination for confirmation. Buphthalmos, megalocornea and retinal changes have also been described so that many factors may contribute to the progressive visual impairment. Optic atrophy from compression of the optic nerves or chiasm by arachnoid cysts may also play a part.

Ear, nose and throat aspects

Deafness may occur, but is less severe than in MPS II. It may be due to bony compression of the auditory nerve, to deformity of the ossicles, to the increased liability to middle ear infections or to a combination of these factors. Nasal congestion and frequent upper respiratory infections are very com-

mon: some patients have had their tonsils and adenoids removed before the diagnosis is made.

Cardiac features

Cardiac murmurs are common and appear to be due to deformation rather than primary malformation of heart valves, with resultant stenosis or regurgitation. Nodular thickening of the aortic and mitral valves is almost invariably found at autopsy. In some cases the tricuspid and pulmonary valves are involved, in some all four valves and in others the coronary arteries, aorta and pulmonary artery.

Radiological findings

Striking abnormalities are seen on X-rays of various bones in MPS 1H and other members of the group. *Skull*: the sella turcica is unusually long and deep with an anterior pocket. Its shape is variously described as like that of a shoe, a fish-hook, the letter 'J' or the Greek letter 'Ω'. (Fig. 5.29) Arachnoid cysts are sometimes found in this and other MPS disorders: these may cause visual loss by compressing or distorting the optic chiasm and may

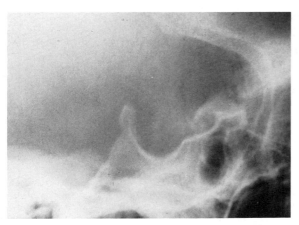

Fig. 5.29 MPS IS. Skull X-ray. 13-year-old girl. The pituitary fossa is enlarged. There is depression of the pre-sellar sphenoid creating the shape that was formerly described as fish-hook (this is often associated with a suprasellar arachnoid cyst).

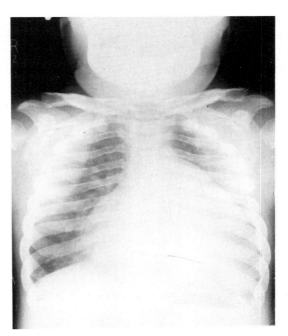

Fig. 5.31 AP Chest radiograph of a 12-year-old boy with Type II MPS. The heart is enlarged. The ribs and clavicles are broad and heavy and there is a symmetrical varus deformity of the proximal humeri

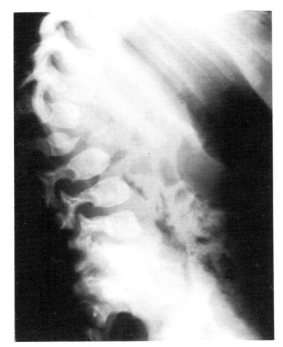

Fig. 5.30 Lateral dorso-lumbar spine of a 3-year-old boy with Type IH MPS. There is a dorso-lumbar gibbus associated with inferior 'hooks' anteriorly on the bodies of L1 and L2. The vertebral bodies elsewhere have an immature oval configuration.

cause erosion of the anterior clinoid processes and body of the sphenoid bone. The vault is large and may show premature synostosis of the sagittal and later of other sutures. *Spine*: the first and second lumber vertebrae at the apex of the gibbus are wedge-shaped and 'beaked' with an anterior projection from the lower parts of their bodies (Fig. 5.30). The *ribs* are oar-shaped, being very broad anteriorly but narrow posteriorly (Fig. 5.31). The *long bones* show changes mainly in the upper limbs and diaphyses (Fig. 5.32). Their shafts are enlarged from expansion of the medullary cavity and the cortex may be thinned. *Hands*: the metacarpals are broad, malformed and pointed at their proximal ends (Fig. 5.33). The hips may show flaring of the wings of the ilia and hypoplasia of their bases with abnormal capital femoral epiphyses (Fig. 5.34).

MPS IS (Scheie's syndrome) (Scheie et al 1962)

Although the same enzyme, α-L-iduronidase, is deficient in this syndrome as in MPS IH, the clinical features are very different. The two disorders have in common corneal clouding, hand deformity and aortic valve involvement, but in MPS IS in-

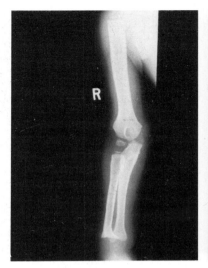
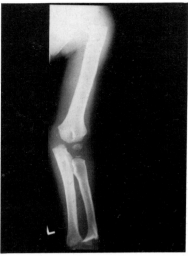

Fig. 5.32 AP radiograph of the upper limbs of a 10-year-old boy with Type VI MPS. There is a varus deformity of the proximal humerus. The diaphyses are wide. There is irregularity and splaying of the distal radial metaphysis and the bone age is delayed

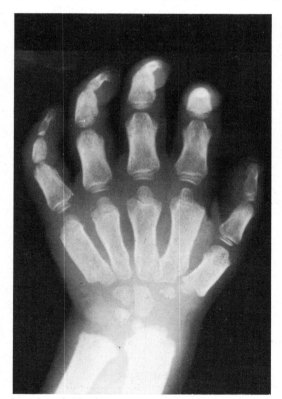

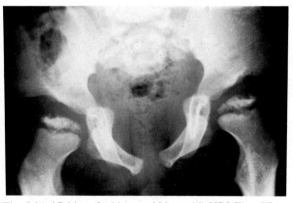

Fig. 5.34 AP hips of a 10-year-old boy with MPS Type VI. The iliac wings flare laterally and there is hypoplasia of the bases of the ilia. There is coxa valga. The capital femoral epiphyses are flattened, fragmented and sclerotic.

telligence and stature are usually normal, the face does not show the grotesque features of 'gargoylism' and joint deformities and radiological abnormalities are milder. The progressive corneal clouding is the major or only problem for many patients and unfortunately cannot be relieved surgically since corneal grafts become opacified. Pigmentary retinopathy may also develop. Some patients survive into their fifties.

A 'Hurler-Scheie compound' of MPS IH and IS has been postulated (McKusick et al 1972) in which the Hurler gene is on one chromosome and the Scheie gene on the other.

Fig. 5.33 PA radiograph of the left hand of a 12-year-old boy with MPS Type II. There is a 'claw' deformity due to inability to straighten the fingers. The phalanges are short and broad. There is proximal pointing of the second to fifth metacarpals. The carpal centres are small and irregular and the bone age is retarded

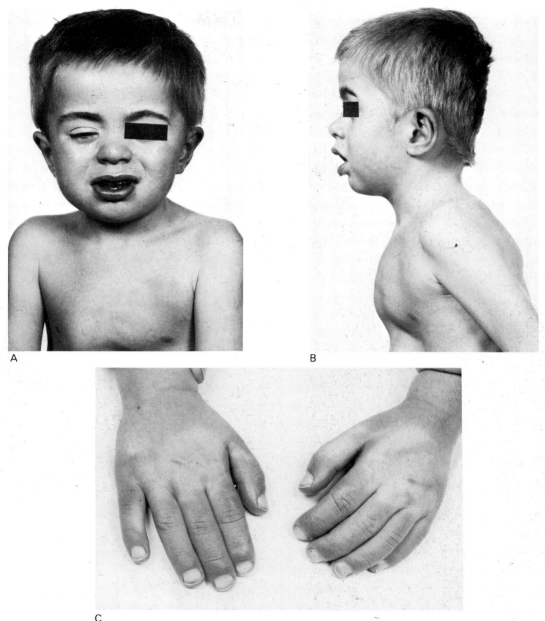

Fig. 5.35 Hunter's syndrome (MPS II) in 4 years and 9 months old boy, (A) front view, (B) lateral, (C) hands

MPS II (Hunter's syndrome) (Hunter 1917)

The main clinical differences of this syndrome from MPS IH (Hurler's syndrome) are the absence of corneal clouding, the greater frequency of deafness, the longer survival in most cases and inheritance as an X-linked recessive. Mental deterioration is slower and a lumbar gibbus is usually absent. Stiffness of joints, dwarfing, hepatosplenomegaly, heart disease and grotesque facies are common to MPS IH and MPS II (Fig. 5.35). Retinal changes occur in MPS II with reduction in the ERG: these changes are easier to detect than in the syndromes with corneal clouding. Median nerve compression in the carpal tunnel may give rise to the carpal tunnel syndrome with sensory symptoms and weakness and wasting of the muscles of the thenar eminence (this is also seen in MPS IV and VI).

A milder (type B) and a severer (type A) form of MPS II are recognized based on length of survival and severity of neurological problems (McKusick 1972), patients with the severe form dying before the age of 15 years.

MPS III (Sanfilippo syndrome) (Sanfilippo et al 1963)

Three clinically identical forms of this syndrome occur with different enzyme deficiencies. The basic clinical features are a combination of severe and progressive mental retardation with relatively mild somatic features and without corneal clouding. Hepatosplenomegaly, stiffness of joints, dwarfing

and skeletal changes are mild or moderate. The facial features resemble those of MPS IH, II and VI but are much milder and the diagnosis is therefore more likely to be missed (Fig. 5.36). Cardiac defects are absent. Some patients may survive to the third or fourth decade and the combination of severe mental defect with aggressive behaviour and normal strength can create major problems in management.

MPS IV (Morquio's or Morquio-Brailsford syndrome; chondro-osteodystrophy) (Morquio 1929)

Described independently in Uruguay and England in 1929, this syndrome, though chemically a MPS disorder, is of greater importance orthopaedically than neurologically, apart from the secondary effects of spinal cord compression.

The face is normal but dwarfing is severe. Pro-

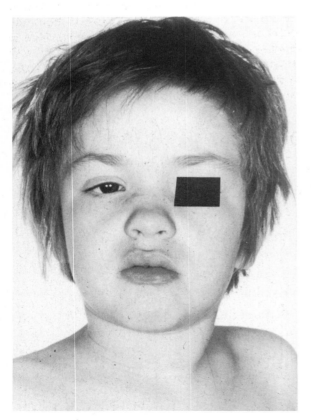

Fig. 5.36 Sanfilippo's syndrome (MPS III) 5 and a half-year-old girl

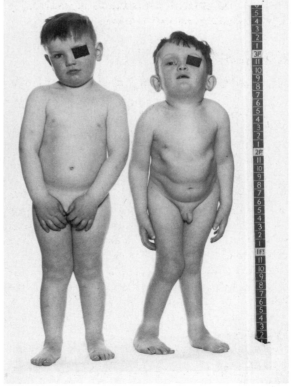

Fig. 5.37 Morquio's syndrome (MPS IV) 5 and a half-year-old boy with control of same age

gressive skeletal abnormalities develop after the first year of life, with dorsal kyphosis, flared thorax, bulging sternum, prominent joints and knock knees (Fig. 5.37). The stance is semi-crouching and the gait awkward. Intelligence is normal and there are no abnormal neurological signs in the earlier stages. Corneal clouding starts later and progresses more slowly than in other MPS disorders, not being easily detected until after the age of 10. Progressive sensorineural deafness begins in the second decade or later and cardiac lesions are also late.

Neurological complications result from compression of the spinal cord and medulla. Aplasia or hypoplasia of the odontoid process is probably invariable in MPS IV with spinal cord compression developing sooner or later in most patients from atlanto-axial subluxation. This results in a combination of lower motor neuron weakness in the arms with spastic paraplegia and is very difficult to manage surgically, though a collar to stabilize the neck is of some help.

The carpal tunnel sydrome may result from compression of the median nerve.

Radiological features

The lumbar vertebrae may show beaking as early as the first year of life. This may suggest MPS IH at that stage, but somewhat later the thoracic vertebrae in MPS IV are typically ovoid in shape while in adult life the vertebral bodies are flattened and rectangular with widened disc spaces. The odontoid process is absent or hypoplastic. In the hips the ilia are flared and later the femoral heads often disappear. The long bones are short and poorly tubulated, especially in the arms where the short ulnae contribute to ulnar deviation of the hands. The carpal centres of ossification are small and delayed in development and the metacarpals and phalanges short and wide, though retaining their normal 'waist', unlike those in MPS IH. The ribs may be spatulate and a dorsal kyphosis be seen on X-rays.

MPS VI (Maroteaux-Lamy syndrome)
(Maroteaux et al 1963)

This syndrome has features resembling those of

MPS IH, including dwarfism, but differs from the other MPS disorders, except for MPS IS and IV, in showing normal intelligence and urinary excretion of dermatan sulphate. It exists in severe (A) and milder (B) forms.

The mild form was first described by Alder (1939) who studied two siblings with a Perthes-like disorder. Alder granulation was present in the neutrophils of both but was not seen in their parents or normal siblings.

Growth retardation is noted at 2 or 3 years of age with lumbar kyphosis and sternal bulging. The face is abnormal and suggestive of a MPS disorder. Joint limitation is seen and the carpal tunnel syndrome also occurs. Inguinal herniae are commom. Cardiac defects similar to those in MPS I may be present. Corneal clouding (Fig. 5.38) may develop in the first decade and vision may also be impaired by retinopathy and optic nerve or chiasmal compression by arachnoid cysts. Deafness occurs in some patients and may be partly due to recurrent ear infections. Obstructive hydrocephalus may result from meningeal thickening and require shunting. Odontoid hypoplasia, as in MPS IV, may cause atlanto-axial dislocation, spinal cord compression. spastic paraplegia and upper limb weakness and wasting.

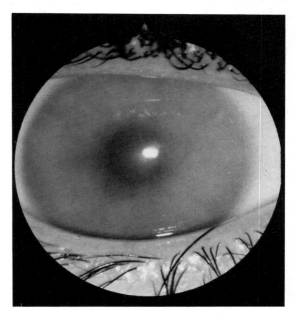

Fig. 5.38 Maroteaux-Lamy syndrome (MPS VI) 8-year-old girl: eye showing corneal clouding

The bony abnormalities shown on X-rays may be as severe as those in MPS IH. The vertebral bodies often have convex upper and lower borders. The first and second lumbar vertebrae are commonly hypoplastic with anterior beaking. Changes in the hand bones are variable making a distinction from MPS IH and IV difficult on these criteria. The skull may show identical changes to those in MPS IH, but many emissary vessels are often seen, especially near the torcular Herophili.

Death may occur from chest infections, cardiac defects, spinal cord compression or the effects of hydrocephalus. The retention of intelligence in the presence of such severe defects means that affected patients have insight into their plight making this syndrome one of the saddest among these tragic disorders.

MPS VII (β-glucuronidase deficiency)

Patients with a condition having some resemblances to MPS IH and IV and a deficiency in β-glucuronidase have been proposed as examples of a further MPS disorder, number VII (Pfeiffer et al 1977).

Diagnostic biochemical tests

The commonest method used for the diagnosis of the MPS is measurement of the type and quantity of acid MPS in urine. They may also be measured in the CSF. White blood cells or cultured fibroblasts may be used to detect deficiency of the enzymes shown in Table 5.4, obviating the need for more cumbersome methods of cell culture, isolation of soluble corrective factors and cross-correction. Fibroblast culture may also be used for prenatal diagnosis.

Haematological findings

Granulations and inclusions occur in leucocytes in peripheral blood and bone marrow in the various MPS disorders and these have been found to vary in their distribution and frequency in the different members of the group. These haematological findings, which can provide helpful confirmation of the diagnosis, have been reviewed by Hansen (1972).

The most striking changes were found in MPS VI in which granulations (Alder granulations) occurred in all neutrophils. Occasional large inclusions may be seen in the neutrophils in MPS IV but the changes are subtle and may not be consistent.

Lymphocytes are the most useful indicators of the MPS with numerous prominent cytoplasmic inclusions which stain metachromatically with toluidine blue (Muir et al 1963) in MPS III. Less numerous metachromatic inclusions occur in MPS I and II (Plate 6). In MPS IS and I H/S these inclusions are rarely found.

Treatment of the MPS disorders

This is at present symptomatic. Orthopaedic and neurosurgical intervention may be helpful in the carpal tunnel syndrome, in hydrocephalus and in some cases of spinal cord compression. There is at present no effective treatment for the corneal clouding, since corneal grafts quickly become opacified. The severe contractures causing flexion deformities at knees and elbows are difficult to influence and surgical manoeuvres are usually only temporarily helpful.

Arachnoid cysts which threaten vision by distorting or compressing the optic nerves or chiasm can sometimes be dealt with surgically.

More specific treatment is at present at the experimental stage. In MPS I H and MPS II infusions of plasma and leucocytes have been given in the hope of producing biochemical and clinical improvement, but the benefits reported (Di Ferrante et al 1971, Knudson et al 1971) have not been found by other workers (Dekaban et al 1972, Erickson et al 1972).

Another possible approach is by the use of implanted normal fibroblasts and bone marrow, but the results of such attempts are not yet clear.

THE MUCOLIPIDOSES

These disorders combine features of the mucopolysaccharidoses and the sphingolipidoses, with clinical resemblances to the former but with no excess of MPS in the urine.

Four main types of mucolipidosis (ML) are recognized by most authors, ML I, II, III and IV. All but type IV have Hurler-like features and are inherited as autosomal recessives.

ML I (lipomucopolysaccharidosis, sialidosis II)

Mild Hurler-like manifestations are combined with moderate progressive mental retardation, skeletal changes and peculiar inclusions in cultured fibroblasts. Although there is no excess of MPS in the urine, the cytoplasmic inclusions show the staining properties of both sphingolipids and MPS.

ML II (I-cell disease) (Leroy et al 1971)

This is a Hurler-like disorder with severe clinical and radiological features, striking inclusions in cultured fibroblasts ('I-cells') and no excess of MPS in urine. The condition is evident from birth, the clinical features being gradually accentuated to become fully expressed between the ages of 6 and 18 months. Most children have by then learned to sit with support and some to stand or walk with help, but motor development remains at this stage and social and speech skills are severely retarded. Respiratory infections and nasal discharge are common and growth in height slows down at about one year of age to cease before the age of two. The face becomes progressively coarser and more Hurler-like. The corneae are clear or faintly hazy. A slight kyphosis in the lower dorsal or upper lumbar region is seen with progressive limitation of joint mobility. Systolic murmurs are common after one year of age. Death has often occurred between 2 and 8 years of age from pneumonia and congestive heart failure.

The radiological bony changes resemble those in type 1 G_{M1}-gangliosidosis and the later stages of MPS IH. Lymphocytes show marked cytoplasmic vacuolation.

ML III (pseudo-Hurler polydystrophy)

Children with many features of Hurler's syndrome but with a much slower clinical evolution and no mucopolysacchariduria were reported by Maroteaux & Lamy (1966). Presentation is usually at about 3 years of age with stiff joints. Corneal

clouding and aortic valve disease, usually with regurgitation, also occur.

ML IV

A 7-year-old Ashkenazi Jewish boy reported by Tellez-Nagel et al (1976) showed clinical and ultrastructural findings suggesting a new variant of the mucolipidoses, ML IV. Severe retardation and corneal clouding were present early. Biopsy of cornea, conjunctiva and brain, and fibroblast cultures suggested the storage of material resembling lipid and mucopolysaccharide. Membranous lamellar structures were found in the cornea, brain and lymphocytes reminiscent of those in the gangliosidoses. Further cases of this type have been reported by Goutières et al (1979). A milder variant has been described by Lake et al (1982).

The cherry-red spot-myoclonus syndrome (Sialidosis I)

Rapin and her colleagues (1978) have reported the cases of three young women, 2 of them sisters, who were found to have cherry-red spots at the macula in childhood and developed severe myoclonus and insidious visual loss in adolescence. They had normal intelligence and showed no Hurler-like features. Various lysosomal inclusions were seen in cortical neurons in a biopsy from one patient in childhood, while a liver biopsy 15 years later showed mucopolysaccharide-like inclusions in Kupffer cells and hepatocytes. The patients excreted sialic-containing oligosaccharides not found in normal urine, suggesting a defect in glycoprotein degradation. The specific enzyme defect is one of lysosomal neuraminidase. The authors believe that more than 24 previously reported patients may have been example of this disorder including a child classified as having mucolipidosis I.

An inherited disorder of anabolism

The neurometabolic disorders so far considered are due to deficiencies of catabolic hydrolytic enzymes. An example has now been recognized of a disease due to lack of a *synthetic* enzyme (Max et al 1974, Brady 1976, Maclaren et al 1976). The child was abnormal from birth and died at $3\frac{1}{2}$ months. Post-mortem showed extreme vacuolation in the cerebral hemispheres, cerebellum, brain stem, optic nerves and spinal cord with large unmyelinated tracts. A grossly abnormal ganglioside pattern was found in the brain, with a 3.5-fold increase in ganglioside G_{M3} (hematoside), which is only a minor component of normal brain. This was due to a deficiency of the synthetic enzyme needed for the formation of ganglioside G_{M2} from G_{M3}. The discovery of this disorder of ganglicoside catabolism suggests that there may be other such disorders to be recognized.

Mannosidosis

Among patients bearing a superficial resemblance to that of some children with mucopolysaccharide disorders and suspected of having Hurler's syndrome a small number have been shown to have an entirely different disorder, an inborn error of metabolism due to deficiency of the lysosomal enzyme α-mannosidase.

The first patient to be reported (Öckerman 1967, Bjellman et al 1969) was dysmature and hypotonic at birth and in infancy had hepatosplenomegaly which disappeared at $2\frac{1}{2}$ years. He was developmentally retarded with coarse features, a large tongue, a lumbar kyphosis, and frequent infections. The corneae were clear but small cloudy opacities were seen on the anterior surfaces of the lenses. From the age of $2\frac{1}{2}$ he showed pyramidal features, became progressively more retarded and died at the age of 4 years and 4 months. Biopsy of bone marrow showed vacuolated lymphocytes and inclusion bodies in granulocytes. At autopsy the brain showed diffuse loss of myelin in the white matter and diffuse loss of nerve cells in the cerebral cortex and of Purkinje cells and neurons in the cerebellum. Throughout the cortex, brain stem and spinal cord nerve cells showed ballooning of their cytoplasm with PAS-positive material later found to be oligosaccharides rich in the sugar mannose. High levels of mannose were also found in the liver. The lysosomal enzyme α-mannosidase was found to be decreased in the brain, liver and spleen. Deficiency of this enzyme appears to impair the normal degradation of glycoproteins causing mannose to accumulate in the brain and other tissues.

More recently several further cases have been reported including two sisters of the first Swedish patient (Norden et al 1973), three Finnish patients including two brothers (Autio et al 1973) and two unrelated British patients (Milla et al 1977). Coarse features, retardation, kyphosis or kyphoscoliosis, conductive deafness and frequent infections have been the main features. Most have not been as severely handicapped as the original patient of Öckerman.

Radiological abnormalities of vertebrae vary from one case to another but include 'beaking' of lumbar vertebrae, as in the mucopolysaccharidoses, erosions and partial collapse.

The diagnosis is strengthened by the finding of vacuolated lymphocytes (though these are seen in other conditions) and is confirmed by assay of α-mannosidase in leucocytes or cultured skin fibroblasts.

Inheritance is as an autosomal recessive trait. Prenatal diagnosis is possible from cultured amniotic cells.

The condition may be commoner than the paucity of reports suggests. Some patients may have been wrongly diagnosed as suffering from one or other of the mucopolysaccharide disorders and confusion is possible with cases of late-onset G_{M1}-gangliosidosis. Screening of retarded deaf children might result in more cases being detected.

Fucosidosis

A condition with variable but mainly progressive neurological features with some resemblances to Hurler's syndrome is associated with deficiency of the enzyme α-L-fucosidase which, like α-mannosidase, is involved in glycoprotein degradation. Fucose-containing compounds accumulate in many organs including the brain. (Durand et al 1968, Van Hoof 1973).

THE CHOICE OF INVESTIGATION IN PROGRESSIVE DEGENERATIVE NEUROMETABOLIC DISEASE IN CHILDHOOD

From what has been said about these varied diseases it should be clear that careful assessment of the clinical data will often point towards a particular diagnosis, or at least towards the *type* of disorder. This should suggest the tests which are most likely to be helpful. The approach to investigation should be selective and a blunderbuss attack should be avoided. The routine use of neural biopsies, whether of brain, nerve, rectum or appendix, without due regard to the use of less drastic methods of making a diagnosis, is quite inexcusable; still less is it defensible when the clinical evidence suggests that the underlying pathology is of a static rather than a progressive nature.

Clearly the choice of investigation must be partly determined by the availability and reliability of diagnostic methods. Measurement of lysosomal enzymes is still limited to certain centres, and when the investigation is not available biopsy may still be needed. Care should be taken to exploit the less

traumatic before resorting to the more drastic tests. Thus when metachromatic leucodystrophy is suspected electrical evidence for peripheral neuropathy should be sought, the urine examined for intracellular metachromatic material and the aryl-sulphatase A activity assayed. The diagnosis can usually be so readily made by such methods that resort to more drastic techniques should be regarded as a failure. It should always be remembered that the physician must justify the investigation to the parents of the affected child, and is morally obliged to explain that the chances of their leading to the discovery of a curable disorder are very remote. Genetic and prognostic considerations are usually quoted, correctly in most cases, as the main indications for vigorous investigation in these diseases, but it should be remembered also that most of them are recessively inherited so that when

Table 5.5 The choice of investigation in some progressive neurometabolic diseases in childhood

Disease	Brain biopsy positive	Rectal or appendix biopsy positive	Other simpler, or more reliable diagnostic methods available	Preferred investigation
G_{M2}-gangliosidoses (all types)	Yes	Yes	Yes	Hexosaminidase assay in leucocytes or serum
G_{M1} gangliosidoses (both types)	Yes	Yes	Yes	β-galactosidase assay in leucocytes; bone marrow biopsy. Vacuolated lymphocytes in Type 1. X-rays may be helpful especially in Type I
Batten's disease — infantile, late infantile and juvenile varieties	Yes	Yes	Electron microscopy (EM) of lymphocytes is probably very reliable	Rectal biopsy. Electron microscopy of skin biopsy, except in juvenile form, EEG, ERG and visual evoked responses. EM of lymphocytes
Gaucher's disease	No	No	Yes	Glucocerebrosidase assay in leucocytes of fibroblasts. Biopsy of bone marrow, liver or lymph node
Niemann-Pick disease	A. Yes B Not applicable	Yes Yes	Yes Yes	Bone marrow biopsy. Sphingomyelinase assay in leucocytes if possible, otherwise liver biopsy. X-rays of chest and long bones
Neurovisceral storage disease with vertical supranuclear ophthalmoplegia	Yes	Yes	Not yet	Bone marrow biopsy Rectal biopsy

contd on p. 172

Table 5.5 (cont'd)

Disease	Brain biopsy positive	Rectal or appendix biopsy positive	Other simpler, or more reliable diagnostic methods available	Preferred investigation
Fabry's disease	Not applicable	Not applicable	Yes	Urine chromatography for ceramide trihexoside. Leucocyte assay for α-galactosidase activity
Mucopolysaccharidases	Unjustifiable	Yes, but not diagnostic of type	Yes	Urine mucopolysaccharides. Metachromasia in leucocytes. Enzyme assay in leucocytes and cultured fibroblasts. X-rays.
Metachromatic leucodystrophy (late infantile and juvenile varieties)	Yes	Yes — but only through changes in included nerves	Yes	Urine for intracellular metachromatic material. Aryl-sulphatase assay in urine and leucocytes. Nerve conduction studies. Sural nerve biopsy diagnostic but should not be necessary
Krabbe's globoid body leucodystrophy (infantile and later onset varieties)	Yes	No	Yes	Galactocerebrosidase activity in leucocytes or fibroblasts. Nerve conduction studies in commoner infantile variety
Adrenal leucodystrophy	Yes	No	Yes	Adrenal function tests (electron microscopy of adrenal biopsy is used by some). Serum long chain fatty acids.
Spongiform leucodystrophy	Yes	No	No	Brain biopsy
Alexander's leucodystrophy	Yes	No	No	Brain biopsy

one of them is strongly suspected a *provisional* assessment of the risks of recurrence in future pregnancies can be given, and the clinical course of the illness in many cases points all too clearly towards a fatal outcome. When the child's condition has deteriorated so far that he is unlikely to live for long, the use of invasive investigations is harder to justify. In such a situation the physician may feel that the chances of the parents agreeing to an autopsy are good, and this may also influence him in his approach.

In Table 5.5, we have listed the relevant and preferred investigations in many of the diseases considered in this chapter.

DIAGNOSTIC PITFALLS IN PROGRESSIVE DEGENERATIVE BRAIN DISEASE IN CHILDREN

More diagnostic errors are made through inadequate history-taking than through faults in examination. This is particularly true of degenerative brain disease in childhood.

The commonest error is the basic one of failing to appreciate that a child has a progressive disease rather than a static condition. This is less frequent, and less excusable, in older children who have lived long enough to have passed sufficient milestones to show that their development is or is not progressing normally and, if not, to show whether it has always been abnormal or has started normally and shown slowing or regression. A child of seven years who did not walk alone until the age of 4 or speak sentences until the age of 6 is unlikely to have a progressive degenerative brain disease.

The younger the child the greater the difficulty may be. It is quite common for children with Tay-Sachs disease and Krabbe's leucodystrophy to be regarded for a time as suffering merely from retardation perhaps with cerebral palsy, but a careful history should show that development was normal for some months before the onset of slowing and regression. Disorders presenting slightly later tend to cause less difficulty; metachromatic leudodystrophy and the infantile and late infantile types of Batten's disease give clear indications of loss of skills to alert the doctor to their progressive nature.

The later the age of onset, in general, the more insidious the deterioration, and confusion is particularly likely to occur with degenerative diseases coming on in older children with symptoms of a psychiatric nature. Learning difficulties, behaviour disorders and aggressive conduct in the early stages of juvenile metachromatic leucodystrophy, adrenal leucodystrophy and juvenile Batten's disease commonly lead to psychiatric referral with resultant delay in the correct diagnosis since the psychiatric label lessens the chances of underlying organic disease being considered. In a series of 12 children with organic neurological disease presenting as psychiatric disorder (Rivinus et al 1975) the interval between application of the psychiatric label and the correct organic diagnosis was up to 6 years. The patterns of intellectual change in the dementing school child are discussed by Lobascher & Cavanagh (1980).

When seizures are a prominent symptom it is common for regression of development and dementia to be overlooked or to be attributed to the fits themselves or to the large doses of anticonvulsant drugs which may be given in an attempt to control them. This is most likely to occur in the late infantile form of Batten's disease in which intractable seizures are common and in which cerebellar ataxia may be wrongly attributed to the effects of phenytoin or other drugs. Careful history and observation and measurement of drug blood levels should prevent these errors.

THE EFFECTS OF PROGRESSIVE DEGENERATIVE BRAIN DISEASE ON THE FAMILY

The impact of these tragic diseases upon the families of the affected children is immense. Only the parents themselves can experience this, but it is essential for the doctor concerned to have some understanding of what they mean to the family as a whole, if he is to be able to feel sympathy with (in the sense of 'suffering with') the parents and to help them as much as possible to come to terms with their lot.

There are few guidelines available. MacKeith (1973) has written helpfully of the feelings and behaviour of parents of handicapped children. His analysis refers to those with non-progressive conditions, but provides a useful starting point for those with progressive diseases and an inevitably fatal outcome. The feelings of bereavement experienced by the parents of the child with a non-progressive handicap relate to the normal child whom they expected but never had; if the disorder is evident at birth, as with Down's syndrome or spina bifida, the normal process of 'bonding' or 'falling in love' with the child may not occur, and partial or complete rejection by the parents may result. When the child has been clearly normal and became an integral part of the family, the deterioration and eventual recognition of the diagnosis, a diagnosis amounting in most cases to a death sentence, can have profound and variable effects on his parents. Rejection is rare. Often the child is seen by the parents as already dead. Guilt is often prominent; they have caused the child's condition by passing it on to him. Parents will often try to blame one another for the disease and quote in support of this the occurrence of seizures or psychiatric disorder in remote relatives. When the disease is X-linked there is a risk of the father holding the mother responsible, and the greatest tact, patience and sensitivity are required from the doctor to overcome this. Many families are split as a result of these illnesses, though in some cases it may be that the marriage was unstable before the tragedy arose, and that some other issue might have resulted in its breakdown had the illness not occurred. The help of an experienced medical social worker to assist the doctor in his supporting role to the family is invaluable.

It must be remembered that the making of a diagnosis, often the culmination of a prolonged process during which the parents may have lost confidence in their medical advisers, is not the end of the case, but in some sense the beginning of a new phase. The readjustments in living pattern of the entire family during the period varying from months to many years which will pass before the death of the child, the changing needs, physical, educational, emotional and social, of the child himself, and the compounded difficulties when two or more siblings are affected require constant, thoughtful, close and practical support. How is this to be achieved? Often the hospital at which the diagnosis has been made is far distant from the patient's home. It is essential for the local hospital and paediatrician with his staff to be in close touch with the family, ready to help in practical ways at periods of crisis, such as episodes of status epilepticus, chest infections, increased difficulties with feeding, and the understandable feeling of parents from time to time that they must have a respite from the constant onerous task of looking after their deteriorating child.

REFERENCES

Aguilar M J, O'Brien J S, Taber P 1967 The syndrome of familial leukodystrophy, adrenal insufficiency and cutaneous melanosis. In: Aronson S M, Volk B W (eds) Inborn errors of sphingolipid metabolism. Pergamon Press, Oxford

Alder A 1939 Uber konstitutionell bedingte granulations veränderungen der leucocyten. Deutsch Archiv für Klinische Medizin 183: 372

Alexander W S 1949 Progressive fibrinoid degeneration of fibrillary astrocytes associated with mental retardation in a hydrocephalic infant. Brain 72: 373–381

Alpers B J 1931 Diffuse progressive degeneration of the cerebral grey matter. Archives of Neurology and Psychiatry 25: 469

Alpers B J 1960 Progressive cerebral degeneration of infancy. Journal of Nervous and Mental Diseases 130: 442

Armstrong D, Dimmit S, Van Worner D E 1974 Studies in Batten disease. I. Peroxidase deficiency in granulocytes. Archives of Neurology 30: 144

Autio S, Norden N E, Ockerman P A, Riekkinen P, Rapola J, Louhimo T 1973 Mannosidosis: clinical, fine-structural and biochemical findings in three cases. Acta paediatrica scandinavica 62: 555–565

Batten F E 1903 Cerebral degeneration with symmetrical changes in the maculae in two members of a family. Transactions of the Ophthalmological Society of the United Kingdom 23: 386

Batten F E 1914 Family cerebral degeneration with macular changes (so-called juvenile form of family amaurotic idiocy). Quarterly Journal of Medicine 7: 444

Bielschowsky M 1913 Über spät-infantile familiäre amaurotische idiotie mit kleinhirnsymptomen. Deutsche Zeitschrift für Nervenheilkunde 50: 7–29

Bjellman B, Gamstorp I, Brun A, Öckerman P-A, Palmgren B 1969 Mannosidosis: a clinical and histopathologic study. Journal of Pediatrics 75: 366–373

Blackwood W, Buxton P H, Cumings J H 1963 Diffuse cerebral degeneration in infancy (Alper's disease). Archives of Disease in Childhood 38: 193–204

Blackwood, W, Corsellis J A N (eds) 1976 Greenfield's neuropathology, 3rd. edn. Edward Arnold, London

Boltshauser E, Wilson J 1976 Value of brain biopsy in neurodegenerative disease in childhood. Archives of Disease in Childhood 51: 264–268

Brady R O 1976 Biochemical genetics in neurology. Archives of Neurology 33: 145

Brady R O, Pentchev P G, Gal A E 1975 Investigations in enzyme replacement therapy in lipid storage diseases. Federation Proceedings 34: 1310

Brady R O, Pentchev P G, Gal A E, Hibbert S R, Dekaban A S 1974 Replacement therapy for inherited enzyme dificiency: use of purified glucocerebrosidase in Gaucher's disease. New England Journal of Medicine 291: 989

Brady R O, Tallman J F, Johnson W G, Gal A E, Leahy W R, Quirk J M, Dekaban A S 1973 Replacement therapy for inherited enzyme deficiency: use of purified ceramidetrihexosidase in Fabry's disease. New England Journal of Medicine 289: 9

Brett E M, Ellis R B, Haas L, Ikonne J U, Lake B D, Patrick A D, Stevens Rosemary 1973 Late onset G_{M2}-gangliosidosis. Clinical, pathological and biochemical studies in eight patients. Archives of Disease in Childhood 48: 775–785

Canavan M 1973 Schilder's encephalitis periaxialis diffusa. Report of a child of sixteen and one half months. Archives of Neurology and Psychiatry 25: 229

Conzelmann E, Sandhoff K 1979 AB Variant of Infantile G_{M2}- gangliosidosis: deficiency of a factor necessary for stimulation of Hex A-Catalysed degradation of ganglioside-G_{M2} and glycolipid G_{A2}. Proceedings of the National Academy of Sciences, USA 75: 3979

Crocker A C 1961 The cerebral defect in Tay-Sachs disease and Niemann-Pick disease. Journal of Neurochemistry 7: 69

Crocker A C, Farber S 1958 Niemann-Pick disease: a review of 18 patients. Medicine (Baltimore) 37: 1

Crome L, Hanefeld F, Patrick D, Wilson J 1973 Late onset globoid cell leucodystrophy. Brain 96: 841

Dawson G, Tsay G C 1976 Chemical diagnosis of inborn lysosomal storage diseases involving the eye. In: The eye and inborn errors of metabolism. Birth defects: Original Article Series, Vol 12, A R Liss, New York

Dekaban A S, Holden K R, Constantopoulos G 1972 Effects of fresh plasma or whole blood transfusions on patients with various types of mucopolysaccharidosis. Pediatrics 50: 688

De Long G R, Halperin J J, Richardson E P 1982 A 15-year-old boy with slowly progressive dementia. New England Journal of Medicine 306: 286–293

Di Ferrante N, Nichols B L, Donnelly P V, Neri G, Hrgovic R, Berglund R K 1971 Induced degradation of glycosaminoglycans in Hurler's and Hunter's syndromes by plasma infusions. Proceedings of the National Academy of Science 68: 303

Dreborg S, Erikson A, Hagberg B 1980 Gaucher disease — Norrbottnian type. European Journal of Pediatrics 133: 107–118

Dunn H G, Dolman C L, Farrell D F et al 1976 Krabbe's leucodystrophy without globoid cells. Neurology (Minneapolis) 26: 1035–1049

Dunn H G, Lake B D, Dolman C L, Wilson J 1969 The neuropathy of Krabbe's infantile cerebral sclerosis (globoid cell leucodystrophy). Brain 92: 329–344

Durand P, Borrone C, Della Cella G, Philippart M 1968 Fucosidosis (letter) Lancet 1: 1198

Elfenbein I B 1968 Dystonic juvenile idiocy without amaurosis. Johns Hopkins Medical Journal 123: 205

Ellis R (ed) 1980 Inborn errors of metabolism. Croom Helm, London

Erickson R P, Sandman R, Robertson W van B, Epstein C J 1972 Inefficacy of fresh frozen plasma therapy of mucopolysaccharidosis II. Pediatrics 50: 693

Fullerton P M 1964 Peripheral nerve conduction in metachromatic leucodystrophy (sulphatide lipidosis). Journal of Neurology, Neurosurgery and Psychiatry 27: 100–105

Gaucher P C E 1882 De l'épithéliome primitif de la rate. Thèse de Paris

Goutières F, Arsenio-Nunes M-L, Aicardi J 1979 Mucolipidosis IV. Neuropädiatrie 10: 321–331

Gray A M 1969 Addison's disease and diffuse cerebral sclerosis. Journal of Neurology, Neurosurgery and Psychiatry 32: 344

Greene H L, Hug G, Schubert W K 1969 Metachromatic leucodystrophy: treatment with arylsulfatase-A. Archives of Neurology (Chicago) 20: 147–153

Groth C G, Hagenfeldt L, Dreborg S, Löfstrom B, Öckerman P A, Samuelson K et al 1971 Splenic transplantation in a case of Gaucher's disease. Lancet 1: 1260

Hagberg B, Haltia M, Sourander P, Svennerholm L, Eeg-Olofsson O 1974 Polyunsaturated fatty acid lipidosis. Infantile form of so-called neuronal ceroidlipofuscinosis. I. Clinical and morphological aspects Acta paediatrica scandinavica 63: 753

Hagberg B, Sourander P, Svennerholm L 1968 Late infantile progressive encephalopathy with disturbed polyunsaturated fat metabolism. Acta paediatrica scandinavica 57: 495

Halliday A M 1967 The electrophysiological study of myoclonus in man. Brain 90: 241

Halliday A M, Halliday E 1970 Cortical evoked potentials in patients with benign myoclonus and progressive myoclonic epilepsy. Electroencephalography and Clinical Neurophysiology 29: 104

Haltia M, Rapola J, Santavuori P 1973 Infantile type of so-called neuronal ceroid lipofuscinosis. Acta neuropathologica (Berlin) 26: 157

Hansen H G 1972 Hematologic studies in mucopolysaccharidoses and mucolipidoses. Birth Defects: Original Article series, vol VIII, no 3 (June 1972) National Foundation-March of Dimes, Williams and Wilkins, Baltimore

Harden A, Pampiglione G, Picton-Robinson N 1973 Electroretinogram and visual evoked response in a form of 'neuronal lipidosis' with diagnostic EEG features. Journal of Neurology, Neurosurgery and Psychiatry 36: 61

Herg H G, Van Hoof F 1973 (eds) Lysosomes and storage diseases. Academic Press, New York

Herrlin K M, Hillborg P D 1962 Neurological signs in the juvenile form of Gaucher's disease. Acta paediatrica (Uppsala) 51: 137

Hoefnagel D, Van Den Noort S, Ingbar S H 1962 Diffuse cerebral sclerosis with endocrine abnormalities in young males. Brain 85: 553

Hogan G R, Richardson E P 1965 Spongy degeneration of the nervous system (Canavan's disease). Report of a case in an Irish-American family. Pediatrics 35: 284

Hunt J R 1921 Dyssynergia cerebellaris myoclonica. Brain 44: 490

Hunter C 1917 A rare disease in two brothers. Proceedings of the Royal Society of Medicine 10: 104

Hurler G 1919 Ueber einen typ multiplier abartungen vorwiegend am skelettsystem. Kinderheilkunde 24: 220

Huttenlocher P R, Solitare G B, Adams G 1976 Infantile diffuse cerebral degeneration with hepatic cirrhosis. Archives of Neurology 33: 186

Jansky J 1908 Dosud nepopsany pripad familiarni amaurotické idiotie komplikovane hypoplasii mozeckovou. Sborn Lek 13: 165

Johnson W G, Chutorian A, Miranda A 1977 A new juvenile heoxsaminidase deficiency disease presenting as cerebellar ataxia. Neurology 27: 1012–1018

Karpati G, Carpenter M D, Wolfe L S, Andermann F 1977 Juvenile dystonic lipidosis. An unusual form of neurovisceral storage disease. Neurology 27: 32

Klenk E 1939 Beiträge zur chemie der lipoidosen, Niemann-Picksche krankheit und amaurotische idiotie. Hoppe-Seylers Zeitschrift Für Physiologische Chemie 262: 128–143

Knudson A G, Di Ferrante N, Curtis J E 1971 Effect of leukocyte transfusion in a child with type II mucopolysaccharidosis. Proceedings of the National Academy of Science 68: 1738

Kocen R S, Thomas P K 1970 Peripheral nerve involvement in Fabry's disease. Archives of Neurology 22: 81–88

Krabbe K 1916 A new familial infantile form of diffuse brain-sclerosis. Brain 39: 73–114

Kufs H 1925 Über eine spätform der amaurotischen idiotie unde ihre heredofamiliären grundlagen. Zentralblatt für Die Gesamte Neurologie und Psychiatrie 95: 169

Kuritzky A, Berginer V M, Korczyn A D 1979 Peripheral neuropathy in cerebrotendinous xanthomatosis. Neurology 29: 880–881

Lake B D, Cavanagh N P C 1978 Early juvenile Batter's disease — a recognisable sub-group distinct from other forms of Batten's disease. Journal of Neurological Sciences 36: 265

Lake B D, Milla P J, Taylor D S I, Young E P 1982 A mild variant of mucolipidosis type 4 (ML4) In: Berman E, Merin S (eds) Genetics in ophthalmology. Alan R Liss, New York

Leroy J G, Spranger J W, Feinggold M, Opitz J M, Crocker A C 1971 T-cell disease: a clinical picture. Journal of Pediatrics 79: 360

Lobascher M E, Cavanagh N P C 1980 Patterns of intellectual change in the dementing school child. Child Care Health and Development 6: 255–265

Long R G, Lake B D, Pettit J E, Scheuer F J, Sherlock S 1977 Adult Niemann-Pick disease. Its relationship to the syndrome of the sea-blue histiocyte. American Journal of Medicine 62: 627

MacFaul R, Cavanagh N, Lake B D, Stephens R, Whitfield A E 1982 Metachromatic leucodystrophy: review of 38 cases. Archives of Disease in Childhood 57: 168–175

Mackeith R C 1973 The feelings and behaviour of parents of handicapped children. Developmental Medicine and Child Neurology 15: 524–527

McKusick V A 1972 Heritable disorders of connective tissue, 4th edn. C V Mosby Company, Saint Louis

Maclaren N K, Max S R, Cornblath M, Brady R O, Ozand P T, Campbell J et al 1976 G$_{M3}$: a novel human sphingolipodystrophy.

Maroteaux P, Leveque B, Marie J, Lamy M 1963 Une nouvelle dysostose avec élimination urinaire de chondroitin-sulfate B. Presse Médicale 71: 1849

Mastropaolo C, Pampiglione G, Stephens R 1971 EEG studies in 22 children with sulphatide lipidosis (metachromatic leucodystrophy). Developmental Medicine and Child Neurology 13: 20

Max S R, Maclaren N K, Brady R O, Bradley R M, Rennels M B et al 1974 G$_{M3}$ (hematoside) sphingolipodystrophy. New England Journal of Medicine 291: 929–931

Mayou M S 1904 Cerebral degeneration with symmetrical changes in the maculae in three members of a family. Transactions of the Ophthalmological Society of the United Kingdom: 24: 142

Melchior J C, Clausen J 1968 Metachromatic leucodystrophy in early childhood: treatment with a diet deficient in vitamin A. Acta paediatrica scandinavica 57: 2–8

Milla P J, Black I E, Patrick A D, Hugh-Jones K, Oberholzer V 1977 Mannosidosis: clinical and biochemical study. Archives of Disease in Childhood 52: 937–942

Miller J D, McCluer R, Kanfer J N 1973 Gaucher's disease: neurologic disorder in adult siblings. Annals of Internal Medicine 78: 833

Moosa A, Dubowitz V 1971 Late infantile metachromatic leucodystrophy. Archives of Disease in Childhood 46: 381–383

Morquio L 1929 Sur une forme de dystrophie osseuse familiale. Archives de Médecine des Enfants. 32: 129–140

Moser H W, Moser A B, Frayer K K, Winston C, Schulman J D, O'Neill B P et al 1981 Adrenoleukodystrophy: increased plasma content of saturated very long chain fatty acids. Neurology 31: 1241–1249

Muir H, Mittwoch U, Bitter T 1963 The diagnostic value of isolated urinary mucopolysaccharides and of lymphocyte inclusions in gargoylism. Archives of Disease in Childhood 38: 358

Neville B G R, Lake B D, Stephens R, Sanders M D 1973 A neurovisceral storage disease with vertical supranuclear ophthalmoplegia and its relation to Niemann-Pick disease. Brain 96: 97–120

Niemann A 1914 Ein unbekanntes krankheitsbild. Jahrbuch für kinderheilkunde 79: 1

Norden N E, Öckerman P A, Szabo L 1973 Urinary mannose in mannosidosis. Journal of Pediatrics 82: 686–688

Öckerman P A 1976 A generalized storage disorder resembling Hurler's syndrome. Lancet 2: 239–241

O'Neill B P, Marmion L C, Feringa E R 1981 The adrenoleukomyeloneuropathy complex: expression in four generations. Neurology 31: 151–156

Pampiglione G, Harden A 1973 Neurophysiological identification of a late infantile form of 'neuronal lipidosis'. Journal of Neurology, Neurosurgery and Psychiatry 36: 68

Pampiglione G, Privett G, Harden A 1974 Tay Sachs disease: neurophysiological studies in 20 children. Developmental Medicine and Child Neurology 16: 201

Pfeiffer R A, Kresse H, Bäumer H, Sattinger E 1977 Beta-glucuronidase deficiency in a girl with unusual clinical features. European Journal of Pediatrics 126: 155

Pilz H, Goebel H H, O'Brien J S 1976 Isoelectric enzyme patterns of leukocyte. Peroxidase in normal controls and patients with neuronal ceroid-lipofuscinoses. Neuropädiatrie 7: 261–270

Poser C M, Van Bogaert L 1956 Natural history and evolution of the concept of Schilder's diffuse sclerosis. Acta psychiatrica et neurologica scandinavica 31: 285

Powers J M, Schaumburg H H 1974 Adrenoleukodystrophy (sex-linked Schilder's disease). American Journal of Pathology 76: 481–492

Proops R, Green S H 1981 Neuronal ceroid lipofuscinosis and arthropathy: a family study. Journal of Medical Genetics 18: 101–104

Rapin I, Goldfischer S, Katzman R, Engel J, O'Brien J S 1978 The cherry-red spot-myoclonus syndrome. Annals of Neurology 3: 234

Rees L H, Grant D B, Wilson J 1975 Plasma corticotrophin levels in Addison-Schilder's disease. British Medical Journal 3: 201–202

Rivinus T M, Jamison D L, Graham P J 1975 Childhood organic neurological disease presenting as psychiatric disorder. Archives of Disease in Childhood 50: 115–119

Sachs B 1887 On arrested cerebral development with special reference to its cortical pathology. Journal of Nervous and Mental Diseases 14: 541

Sanfilippo S J, Podosin R, Langer L O, Good R A 1963 Mental retardation associated with acid mucopolysacchariduria (heparitin sulfate type). Journal of Pediatrics 63: 837

Santavuori P, Haltia M, Rapola J, Raitta C 1973 Infantile type of so-called neuronal ceroid-lipofuscinosis. I. A clinical study of 15 patients. Journal of the Neurological Sciences 18: 257

Schaumburg H H, Powers J M, Raine C S, Suzuki K, Richardson E P 1975 Adrenoleukodystrophy. A clinical and pathological study of 17 cases. Archives of Neurology 33: 577–591

Scheie H G, Hambrick G W, Barness L A 1962 A newly recognized forme fruste of Hurler's disease (gargoylism). American Journal of Ophthalmology 53: 753

Schilder P 1912 Zur Kenntnis der sogeanten diffusen sklerose (uber encephalitis periaxialis diffusa). Zeitschrift für Die Gesamte Neurologie Und Psychiatrie 10: 1

Schilder P 1913 Zur Frage der Encephalitis diffusa. Zeitschrift für die Gesamte Neurologie und Psychiatrie 15: 358–376

Schilder P 1924 Die Encephalitis periaxialis diffusa. Archiv für Psychiatrie und Nervenkrankheiten 71: 327–356

Schneck L, Maisel J, Volk B 1964 The startle response and serum enzyme profile in early detection of Tay-Sachs disease. Journal of Pediatrics 65: 749

Schutta H S, Pratt R T C, Metz H, Evans K A, Carter C O 1966 A family study of late infantile and juvenile forms of metachromatic leucodystrophy. Journal of Medical Genetics 3: 86

Seitelberger F, Jacob H, Schnabel R 1967 The myoclonic variant of cerebral lipidosis. In: Aronson S M, Volk B W (eds) Inborn disorders of sphingolipid metabolism. Pergamon Press, Oxford

Sjögren T 1931 Die juvenile amaurotische idiotie. Klinische und erblichkeitsmedizinische untersuchungen. Hereditas (Lund) 14: 197

Spielmeyer W 1905 Über familiare amaurotische idioten. Neurologisches Zentralblatt 24: 620–621

Stanbury J B, Wyngaarden J B, Fredrickson D S 1978 The metabolic basis of inherited disease, 4th edn. McGraw Hill, New York

Stock W 1908 Über eine bis Jetzt noch night beschriebene form der familiär auftretenden netz haut degeneration bei gleichzeitiger verblödung und über pigmentdegeneration der netzhaut. Klinische Monatsblatter für Augenheilkunde 5: 225–244

Svennerholm L 1962 The chemical structure of normal human brain and Tay-Sachs gangliosides. Biochemical and Biophysical Research Communications 9: 436–441

Svennerholm L 1964 The gangliosidoses. Journal of Lipid Research 5: 145

Tay W 1881 Symmetrical changes in the region of the yellow spot in each eye of an infant. Transactions of the Ophthalmological Society of the United Kingdom 1: 55

Tellez-Nagel I, Rapin I, Iwamoto T, Johnson A B, Norton W T, Nitowsky H 1976 Mucolipidosis IV. Clinical, ultrastructural, histochemical and chemical studies of a case, including a brain biopsy. Archives of Neurology 33: 828

Terry R D, Korey S R 1960 Membranous cytoplasmic granules in infantile amaurotic idiocy. Nature (London) 188: 1000

Tripp J H, Lake B D, Young E, Ngu J, Brett E M 1977 Juvenile Gaucher's disease with horizontal gaze palsy in three siblings. Journal of Neurology, Neurosurgery and Psychiatry 40: 470–478

Ulrich J, Herschowitz N, Heitz Ph, Sigrist Th, Baerlocher P 1978 Adrenoleukodystrophy. Preliminary report of a connatal case. Light- and electron microscopical, immunohistochemical and biochemical findings. Acta neuropathologica (Berlin) 43: 77–83

Unverricht H 1891 Die Myoklonie. Franz Deuticke, Leipzig

Van Bogaert L, Bertrand I 1949 Sur une idiotie familiale avec dégénerescence spongieuse du nevraxe. Acta neurologica belgica 49: 572

Van Bogaert L, Scherer H J, Epstein E 1937 Une forme cérébrale de la cholesterinose generalisée. Masson, Paris

Van Hoof F 1973 Fucosidosis. In: Hers H G, Van Hoof F (eds) Lysosomes and storage diseases. Academic Press, London

Vogt H 1905 Über familiäre amaurotische idiotie und verwandte krankheitsbilder. Monatschrift für Psychiatrie und Neurologie 18: 161–171 and 310–357

Von Specht B U, Geiger B, Arnon R, Passwell J, Keren G, Goldman B et al 1979 Enzyme replacement in Tay-Sachs disease. Neurology 29: 848–854

Warner J O 1975 Juvenile onset metachromatic leucodystrophy. Archives of Disease in Childhood 50: 735–737

Wefring K W, Lamvik J D 1967 Familial progressive poliodystrophy with cirrhosis of the liver. Acta paediatrica scandinavica 56: 295

Wiesmann U N, Rossi E E, Herschowitz N 1972 Correction of the defective sulfatide degradation in cultured fibroblasts from patients with metachromatic leucodystrophy. Acta paediatrica scandinavica 61: 296–302

Weiss G M, Nelson R L, O'Neill B P, Carney J A, Edis A J 1980 Use of adrenal biopsy in diagnosing adrenoleukomyeloneuropathy.

Willner J E, Grabowski G A, Gordon R E, Bender A N, Desnick R J 1981 Chronic G_{M2} gangliosidosis masquerading as atypical Friedreich ataxia: clinical, morphologic and biochemical studies in nine cases. Neurology 31: 787–798

Wilson J, Manners B T B, Robins D G, Erdohazi M 1981 Persistent hiccups as a presenting feature of Alexander's leucodystrophy. Developmental Medicine and Child Neurology 23: 660–661

Wolfe L S, Ng Ying Kin N M K, Baker R R, Carpenter S, Andermann F 1977 Identification of retinoyl complexes as the autofluorescent component of the neuronal storage material in Batten disease. Science 175: 1360

Zeman W 1970 Historical development of the nosological concept of amaurotic familial idiocy. In: Vinken P J, Bruyn G W (eds) Handbook of clinical neurology. Leucodystrophies and poliodystrophies. North Holland, Amsterdam, American Elsevier, New York, vol 10, p 212–233

Zeman W 1974 Studies in the neuronal ceroid-lipofuscinoses. Journal of Neuropathology and Experimental Neurology 33: 1–12

Zeman W, Alpert M 1963 On the nature of the 'stored' lipid substances in juvenile amaurotic idiocy (Batten-Spielmeyer-Vogt). Proc. I. International Congress of Histochemistry and Cytochemistry (Paris) 1960

Zeman W, Donahue S 1963 Fine structure of the lipid bodies in juvenile amaurotic idiocy. Acta neuropathologica (Berlin) 3: 144

6

Phenylketonuria and its variants, and some other amino-acid disorders

E. M. Brett

PHENYLKETONURIA (PKU) DUE TO PHENYLALANINE HYDROXYLASE DEFICIENCY

Despite its relative rarity, phenylketonuria (PKU) is of great importance practically and historically as the first inborn error of metabolism shown to cause mental retardation and as a condition in which dietary treatment, if started early enough, can prevent retardation. Its discovery has acted as a stimulus to the recognition of other inborn metabolic errors causing subnormality and other neurological deficits and has helped partially to dispel the aura of hopelessness surrounding the subject, leading to world-wide programmes of neonatal screening to prevent handicap.

It is now known that there are a number of different disorders which may lead to the typical chemical picture of PKU, i.e. elevation of blood phenylalanine levels and an excess of phenylketones in the urine. Some of these are due to deficiency of phenylalanine hydroxylase and others to tetrahydrobiopterin deficiency.

In 1934 the mother of two mentally retarded Norwegian children commented on the musty smell of their napkins (diapers). This clue was followed up by Folling who identified phenylpyruvic acid in their urine leading to recognition of the disorder which soon came to be called phenylketonuria. Jervis (1953) showed that the liver in affected patients cannot convert phenylalanine to tyrosine. This conversion depends on the enzyme phenylalanine hydroxylase and occurs in the liver, kidney and pancreas in mammalian tissues. Tyrosine, the product of hydroxylation, is essential for several purposes, as a precursor of dopamine and norepi-

nephrine in the CNS, as a substrate for melanin and thyroxine synthesis and also for the synthesis of proteins.

PKU is inherited as an autosomal recessive disorder, and the carrier rate is estimated as about 1 in 50 in people of Caucasian stock with a frequency of the disease in newborns of about 1 in 12 000 in South-East England and in Massachusetts, but as high as 1 in 4000 in Northern Ireland and in Eire. In the mentally defective population the frequency previously was estimated at about 1 in 200 (Jervis 1954).

The main clinical features relate to the nervous system and to reduction of skin pigmentation and are seen — happily more and more rarely — in untreated patients. In the first year of life there are few clues to point to the possibility of PKU and, as with all cases of developmental retardation, time is needed for the gap between the expected and actual performance to widen sufficiently to attract attention. Thus, in the fortunately rare cases which escape the net of neonatal screening (in areas where this is universal or frequent) it may not be until the child is a year old that advice is sought and the diagnosis made, by which time untreated patients are estimated to have lost some 50 points of IQ.

Seizures occur in about 25% of cases, often with infantile spasms at about 5 or 6 months of age and grand mal convulsions later. The occurrence of these attacks should always prompt a search for PKU or other neurometabolic disorders.

The facial appearance of the affected children is normal but they are classically fair-haired and blue-eyed, with a rough, dry skin often with eczema after the first year. The growth of the head circumference often slows down so that microcephaly develops. Cerebral palsy is not often associated with PKU and the children tend to be hyperkinetic and restless. A musty smell, due to phenylacetic acid, is often present and may suggest the diagnosis, as in Følling's first cases.

Detection and screening

At birth the blood levels of phenylalanine in the child with PKU are usually within the normal range, but when the baby ingests protein the absence of phenylalanine hydroxylase activity causes this amino-acid to accumulate in serum and CSF and to be excreted in the urine in large amounts. Instead of being degraded in the normal way phenylalanine is converted to phenylpyruvic and phenylacetic acids and to phenylacetylglutamine. A simple means of detecting phenylpyruvic acid is the ferric chloride test in which three to five drops of 10% ferric chloride are added to 1 ml of urine. Phenylpyruvic acid causes an emerald green colour to develop which fades in 20 to 40 minutes. A simple 'dip-stick' test (Phenistix) is available for use in urine and on wet napkins (diapers). In the first few weeks of life phenylpyruvic acid may not be formed from phenylalanine and these tests may therefore give false negative results, with potentially devastating consequences for the child's development (MRC Working Party on PKU, 1968). (It is never safe, when faced with an older retarded child, to assume that screening in the newborn period has reliably excluded PKU. Many paediatricians have had the sad experience of diagnosing it at 2 or 3 years of age in child who had been tested as a neonate with false-negative results).

A reliable screening test based on detecting raised *blood* levels of phenylalanine and applicable to the whole newborn population is therefore needed. The Medical Research Council (MRC) Working Party on PKU (1968) found that three alternative screening procedures were more efficient than Phenistix for detecting the disorder at an early age. These were a paper chromatography test for O-hydroxyphenylacetic acid in urine, the Guthrie test for phenylalanine in blood and a modified Guthrie test for phenylalanine in urine. Mass screening programmes based on these various methods are now in use throughout the developed nations with generally satisfactory results but with occasional false-positives and more serious false-negatives.

The experience of screening in the United Kingdom has been reviewed by Hawcroft & Hudson (1974). Since 1964 new cases of PKU have been reported to the MRC-Department of Health and Social Security PKU Register Office. Most laboratories use the Guthrie test. A smaller number examine blood samples by paper or thin layer chromatography or by fluorimetry. Blood is collected from the newborn infant by the midwife or health-visitor, usually between the 6th and 14th day of life. Most of the blood tests require blood dropped on to absorbent paper, as originally described by Guthrie. In a few areas blood is collected in heparinized microcapillary tubes. The average age of collection of blood and of diagnosis of PKU was found by Hawcroft and Hudson to be 10 and 17 days compared with 41 and 47 days in 1964 and 1965, when urine testing was the only method of screening. The main benefit of improved screening organization has been the trend towards earlier diagnosis, shown in the numbers of cases reported to the Register Office since 1964. Late diagnosis, with cases presenting after the age of one year with established mental retardation, was fairly frequent in earlier years but has become progressively more rare. The percentage of infants tested in the United Kingdom is very high, and approaches 100% if allowance is made for deaths in the first week of life (about 1% of live births) in which a screening test will usually not be done. During the 3-year period 1974–1976 over 90% of infants judged to need treatment had their first screening test before 14 days of age. Some 80% had started the diet before 3 weeks of age, and in over half of those in whom treatment was delayed beyond this age the reason was doubt about the diagnosis (MRC/DHSS Phenylketonuria Register Newsletter No. 5, February 1978).

Treatment

The basis of treatment is a diet low, but not totally lacking, in phenylalanine. Over-restriction of phenylalanine intake is associated with blood levels below the normal range and may cause iatrogenic problems, such as poor growth, delayed bone age, hypoglycaemia, neurological symptoms and repeated infections. The daily requirement for phenylalanine varies with age and decreases from a maximum in the newborn period of 60 to 70 mg per kg. The aim of treatment is usually to maintain a blood level of between 3 and 10 mg per 100 ml (181.5 to 605 μmol/l). The safe upper limit is still uncertain, but levels over 20 mg per 100 ml (1210 μmol/1) are considered undesirable. An artificial feed with low phenylalanine content is the primary source of protein; many commercial protein-substitute preparations low in phenylalanine are available. (Minafen, Albumaid XP, Lofenelac, Aminogran, PK Aid) High-protein foods, such as eggs, meat, fish and cheese, are usually omitted; milk, cereals, potatoes and some other protein-containing foods are given in measured amounts. Fruit and vegetables are usually allowed freely. The diet is monotonous and unnatural and can occasionally cause serious psychological problems for the child and his parents, but the stakes involved are so great that — at least in young children — every effort must be made to ensure conformity and to keep the blood levels in the desired range. Much time and patience are demanded of the team (physician, psychologist, dietitician, biochemist, social worker etc.) who are supporting the family. The management of PKU is a very specialized subject which should be handled by special centres with experience and expertise. The monitoring and supportive role of the psychologist is particularly important.

With early and effective treatment in classical PKU mental retardation can be avoided and normal growth achieved. However, preliminary analysis of the United Kingdom Register data on 157 early treated cases aged 4 years or more in 1975 showed that the mean IQ of these children was 95. 90% of cases fell within the range 70–129, while 3% were above and 7% below this range. This small shift downwards from the general population mean IQ of 100 is statistically significant. Similar results were obtained in an American study of 111 four-year old children (Dobson et al 1977).

Without treatment most PKU patients will have an IQ below 50, although a London survey of sibling pairs (Smith & Wolff 1974) suggested that approximately 1 in 6 or 7 untreated patients achieve an IQ above 70, but with evidence of intellectual impairment. In the same study the highly significant difference in intellectual outcome between the early treated and late or untreated second siblings of index cases showed the beneficial effect of early treatment on the intelligence of affected children.

The optimum duration of diet has still to be decided. There has been a tendency to lower the age at which it is stopped to 5 or 6 years, and emotional gains have been noted when it was discontinued at 8 years. However, a Polish study (Cabalska et al 1977) of 22 classical PKU patients treated for a mean of 4 years 8 months and 10 treated for 2 years four months showed a decrease in IQ in most of these children with difficulties in adaptation and school achievements and many EEG abnormalities after stopping diet. It was concluded that 5 years dietary treatment was too short to be effective. Similar findings emerged from a British study (Smith el al 1978) of 47 patients put on a normal diet between the ages of 5 and 15 years. Significant falls in mean IQ of about 6 points were noted. By contrast 22 similar patients in Germany placed on a relaxed low-phenylalanine diet rather than a normal diet showed smaller and non-significant falls in mean IQ. At present therefore it seems advisable to persist with diet at least until the age of 10 years.

MATERNAL PHENYLKETONURIA

Pregnancy in women with phenylketonuria raises special problems. Abnormalities are common in their children, with microcephaly and intrauterine growth retardation almost universal and with mental retardation in over 90% (Mabry et al 1966). Congenital heart disease is also common. Spontaneous abortion during the first trimester is another complication. The detrimental effects of maternal PKU on embryogenesis and fetal development were considered by Fisch et al (1969) who reviewed the clinical features in 37 cases. Brown and Waisman (1971) reported four infants of hyperphenylalaninaemic mothers who had various congenital anomalies and decreased head size at birth which later approached normal. It seemed likely that the high blood phenylalanine levels in the mothers, averaging 16 mg per 100 ml, were responsible for these abnormalities in the children, who escaped from this harmful milieu after delivery. The implications are that women with PKU should be on a strict diet in pregnancy and that the diet should be introduced before conception. The importance of this is shown by the contrasting results in the British case (Smith et al 1979) in which severe fetal damage occurred despite introduction of diet 5 weeks after conception and the Danish case (Nielsen et al 1979) in which a phenylketonuric woman who had had a previous microcephalic infant had a normal child when diet was started before conception. It is also shown by a recent international survey of the results of untreated and treated pregnancies (Lenke & Levy 1980). 524 pregnancies in 155 women were involved and only in 34 pregnancies was a low phenylalanine diet begun after or shortly before pregnancy was established. Among the untreated pregnancies mental retardation, microcephaly and congenital heart disease were much commoner than in the normal population and the increase could be related to maternal blood levels of phenylalanine. 95% of mothers with blood levels of 20 mg per 100 ml or higher had at least one mentally retarded child.

Maternal PKU should be considered in the differential diagnosis of microcephaly and intrauterine growth retardation, and the finding of a phenylketonuric member in a family justifies investigation of all its members, especially the females. It has been suggested that breast-feeding is inadvisable for the infants of mothers with PKU unless the mothers are on a low phenylalanine diet, since their milk will otherwise contain increased amounts of phenylalanine.

Girls with PKU who were treated early and successfully are now reaching adult life with normal intelligence and the problems of managing their diets both before and during pregnancy will become increasingly important. The harmful effects of the disorder operate very early in pregnancy, so that diet must be started early to be effective. In some cases PKU had not been diagnosed in the mothers previously. Women who are of below normal intelligence are likely to be less cooperative and successful in keeping to their diet. These problems are discussed by Komrower et al (1979) in relation to the management of four pregnancies. The authors point out that the number of women at risk will reach a peak in 10 years' time so that a well-planned prospective study of this problem is needed.

VARIANTS OF PHENYLKETONURIA

It was in the course of screening for PKU that certain other rare disorders were detected with raised phenylalanine levels in the newborn period. Among 300 patients with PKU seen at The Hospital for Sick Children, Great Ormond Street, were 3 children, 2 of them siblings, with a progressive neurological illness unlike the classical condition and quite unresponsive to phenylalanine restriction (Smith et al 1975). Swallowing difficulty was their first and most persistent symptom, developmental delay was obvious at 5 months of age and no progress occurred after this. Seizures developed early with bouts of myoclonic attacks and occasional grand mal. They showed hypotonia of the trunk at 5 months with rigidity in the limbs, and choreiform movements appeared at 8 or 9 months. These clinical features and their failure to respond to a low phenylalanine diet suggested that the block in the conversion of phenylalanine to tyrosine was due to a defect in the metabolism of biopterin.

Between 1 and 3% of babies with positive results to the Guthrie test are examples of what has been called 'malignant hyperphenylalaninaemia' (MHPA) because of the severity of the symptoms and the lack of response to dietary treatment. These patients all have a deficiency of L-erythro-5, 6, 7, 8 tetrahydrobiopterin which is the cofactor of the apoenzymes phenylalanine-4-hydroxylase, tyrosine-3-hydroxylase and tryptophan-5-hydroxylase. Since the last two are key enzymes in neurotransmitter biosynthesis, deficiency of tetrahydrobiopterin will reduce neurotransmitter synthesis and could account for the progressive neurological illness in these children. The good results of treatment with L-dopa and 5-hydroxytryptophan reported by Bartholomé & Byrd (1975) support this hypothesis. The deficiency of tetrahydrobiopterin in one patient with atypical PKU was found to be due to lack of the enzyme 7, 8-dihydrobiopterin synthetase (Niederweiser et al 1979). In another case of atypical PKU a deficiency of dihydropteridine reductase was found (Butler et al 1975). This enzyme is needed for the regeneration of tetra-hydrobiopterin.

At present the neurological illness of patients with defects of biopterin metabolism is probably best treated, or prevented, by a combination of tetrahydrobiopterin therapy (Niederweiser et al 1979) and supplements of 5-hydroxytryptophan, dopa and carbidopa (Bartholomé et al 1977).

The distinction between PKU due to phenylal-anine hydroxylase deficiency and that due to tetrahydrobiopterin deficiency may be made by measuring the level of phenylalanine hydroxylase in liver biopsy material combined with measuring the blood level of phenylalanine after a protein load. Bartholomé et al (1979) found that in classical PKU the enzyme level was usually less than 1%, but in hyperphenylalaninaemia was over 5%. Blood phenylalanine values showed an inverse relation-ship to the enzyme level. Danks et al (1979) rec-ommend systematic testing of all babies with persistently raised levels of serum phenylalanine by measuring the response to a single oral dose of tetrahydrobiopterin. This should be done before diet is started, the serum phenylalanine levels being measured before and 6 hours after the dose. 'MHPA' is recognised by a fall in phenylalanine to normal levels, while patients with classical PKU show no response. The result can be known at once. Adequate supplies of tetrahydrobiopterin should be obtainable from the laboratories which synthesize it.

HOMOCYSTINURIA (CYSTATHIONINE-SYNTHETASE DEFICIENCY)

This recessively-inherited inborn error of amino acid metabolism was first discovered in the course of a survey of mentally retarded patients in an institution in Northern Ireland. (Carson & Neill 1962), and soon afterwards cases were reported from the United States. Many systems are involved apart from the CNS and there is great clinical var-iation between cases, although untreated affected siblings tend to show similar features. Milder cases may well be missed, especially if intelligence is normal or only slightly reduced.

The basic enzyme defect is one of cystathionine-synthetase, which is absent from liver and brain and which is normally responsible for the conver-sion of homocysteine to cystathionine. The bio-chemical results of the block are an accumulation of homocystine and other sulphur-containing metabolites, low cystine and cystathionine levels, and usually a rise in plasma methionine. There is evidence for genetic heterogeneity in that patients in some sibships respond biochemically to treat-ment with pyridoxine, while others do not. Both groups show abnormally high levels of homocystine and methionine in plasma, the former being unde-tectable in normal individuals by the usual meth-ods. In the urine homocystine and methionine may be detected, but the latter is less often found since its renal tubular reabsorption is very efficient. Homocystinuria is most easily detected by the uri-nary cyanide-nitroprusside test which gives a deep red or magenta colour. Other disulphides, such as cystine, may be detected by this reaction, but can be distinguished from homocystine by thin-layer chromatography or electrophoresis.

Clinical features

Four main systems are involved in homocystinuria: the eye, skeletal, central nervous and vascular sys-tems. These are well reviewed by Stanbury et al (1978).

Ocular

The most frequent features are ectopia lentis, a dislocation of the lens, usually posteriorly, and iridodonesis, with myopia. The lens dislocation is due to disruption of the zonular fibres which sus-pend it from the ciliary body. A ragged fringe of zonular remnants can sometimes be seen round the periphery of the lens. (Lens dislocation also occurs in Marfan's syndrome, which has sometimes been wrongly diagnosed in cases of homocystinuria, but is more often anterior in that condition.) Ectopia lentis in homocystinuria usually develops by the age of 10 years, though rarely under 3. A bizarre quivering or wobbliness of the iris, known as iri-dodonesis, is seen, especially when the head is moved, due to the lack of the stable support which the lens normally provides for the iris. If the lens dislocates anteriorly glaucoma may result. Progres-sive myopia and astigmatism also occur. Optic atrophy, degeneration and detachment of the retina and cataracts have also been described.

Skeletal

Osteoporosis is very frequent, most often affecting the spine, with scoliosis, kyphosis or vertebral collapse as complications. Less often the long bones are affected. They may show pathological fractures and are often thin and abnormally long in older children. Biconcave, 'codfish' vertebrae are commonly seen on X-rays, and may be due to vascular occlusion of vertebral arteries rather than to osteoporosis. Arachnodactyly is present in less than half the patients and the same is true of pectus excavatum or carinatum. Pes cavus and a high-arched palate are frequent. Genu valgum is common with widened tibial and femoral condyles, and radiologically growth arrest lines and metaphyseal spicules.

CNS

Mental retardation is the commonest and often the first symptom. It is usually less severe than in untreated PKU, though often evident in the first or second year. Walking and speech are delayed and the gait is often waddling, sometimes prompting orthopaedic referral, with delay in recognition of the diagnosis until the extent of the retardation and other stigmata become obvious. The IQ has varied between under 30 and 75, but about 20% of reported patients have had normal or near-normal intelligence. This is probably an under-estimate as judged by the finding of McKusick et al (1971) that about half of 84 patients, ascertained largely on the basis of ectopia lentis, had at least average intelligence.

Convulsions have been reported in 10 to 15% of cases. They may be generalized or focal and occasionally followed by a hemiplegia, suggesting a cerebrovascular occlusion. Specific neurological abnormalities, such as hemiplegia and other deficits, are rare and often associated with cerebrovascular disease.

Vascular

Vascular occlusions with thrombosis and embolism in large and small arteries and veins are common in homocystinuria and are an important cause of death, from carotid, coronary or venous sinus thrombosis or pulmonary embolism. Renal infarcts may lead to hypertension.

These vascular episodes can occur at any age and are often precipitated by surgery or intravenous injection, which should be avoided when possible. Arteries, even at a young age, may show gross intimal thickening with fibrosis, and fraying and splitting of muscle and elastic fibres are seen in the media. A further factor contributing to vascular occlusion is an increased degree of platelet stickiness or adhesiveness which has been shown in many homocystinuric patients; homocystine and methionine added to normal blood have been reported to cause increased adhesiveness of normal platelets.

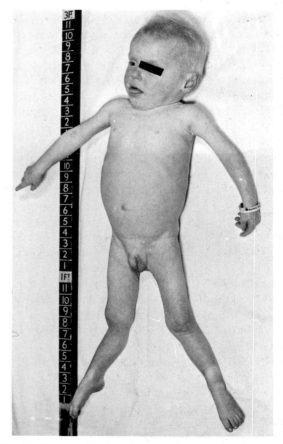

Fig. 6.1 Homocystinuria — boy aged 2 years. Note the hypotonic posture, fair brittle hair, malar flush and mottling over shins.

Two other vascular features of the disease, which vary from one time to another but provide helpful diagnostic clues, are a malar flush and livedo reticularis, an erythematous mottling of the limbs, most marked over the shins.

The patients often have fair, brittle hair and a thin skin as further clinical pointers (Fig. 6.1).

The relationship between the enzyme deficiency and the very varied clinical features of the disease, and the reason for its variable severity remain obscure. The improvement in the biochemical abnormality brought about in some patients by large doses of pyridoxine has not helped to explain the pathophysiology.

Management

A diet low in methionine started in the newborn period prevents the clinical features of homocystinuria from developing. Experience of dietary treatment is less abundant than with the commoner but analogous condition, PKU. However, encouraging results have been reported from Britain (Komrower 1971) and the United States (Perry 1974) in children given low methionine diets with added L-cystine from the neonatal period. In children treated later the results have been less good, but if the severe thrombo-embolic complications could be prevented by later diet the outlook would be improved.

In rather more than half of reported patients large doses of pyridoxine have produced partial or complete biochemical remission (Brenton & Cusworth 1971). The effective doses used have ranged from 50 to 500 mg daily. Patients with homocystinuria have an increased requirement for folate since the disposal of excess homocysteine consumes methyltetrahydrofolate. Folate deficiency has been precipitated by pyridoxine treatment, and folate supplements should probably be given to homocystinuric infants treated with pyridoxine. There are grounds for optimism with regard to preventing clinical deterioration in treated cases, but time is needed to assess the results.

Drug treatment has been used in an attempt to prevent thromboembolic episodes. Régimes with dipyramidole alone or alternating with acetylsalicylic acid have given promising results. (Harker et al 1974)

Effective treatment depends on early diagnosis, which in turn depends on detection in siblings of a known case or neonatal screening. The incidence of homocystinuria in the general population is still uncertain: it has been estimated variously as 1 in 3 million and 1 in 200 000. It varies from one area to another, being highest in Northern Ireland (1 in 35 000) on routine neonatal screening compared with 1 in 120 000 in London. These figures may well be underestimates due to false negative results. Prenatal diagnosis is possible.

Rarer forms of homocystinuria

Two other rare inherited disorders of methionine degradation are recognized in which there is homocystinuria, but low or normal blood levels of methionine (Scriver & Rosenberg 1973). In one of these there is a defect of the synthesis of methyl and adenosyl B12, the co-factors for the conversion of homocysteine to methionine and of methylmalonic acid to succinate. This is associated with methylmalonic aciduria. The disorder responds to vitamin B12 in a dose of 250 to 1000 μg per day. In the other disorder there is a block in the synthesis of methyltetrahydrofolate and treatment with folic acid (10 to 15 mg per day) is effective.

HISTIDINAEMIA

This rare metabolic disorder, usually inherited as an autosomal recessive, was recognized in 1961. It is due to lack of the enzyme histidase which normally converts histidine to urocanic acid so that increased blood levels and urinary excretion of this amino-acid are found. The results of the urine screening programme of newborn babies in Massachusetts suggested that histidinaemia may have a similar incidence in that population to that of PKU.

There is still some doubt about the significance of the clinical abnormalities which have been described in association with the chemical defect. The reported features are very variable but in over half the cases have included mental retardation often with defective or retarded speech. A prospective study of British infants diagnosed on neonatal screening (Neville & Lilly 1973) suggested that mental retardation is not an inevitable or even a likely outcome. Speech defects, when present, may be due to cultural deprivation, mental subnormality or hearing loss rather than to a specific effect (Lott et al 1970).

Diets low in histidine have been tried with biochemical improvement but no obvious clinical benefit (Corner et al 1968).

REFERENCES

Bartholomé K, Byrd D J 1975 L-Dopa and 5-hydroxytryptophan therapy in phenylketonuria with normal phenylalanine hydroxylase activity. Lancet 2: 1042–1043

Bartholomé K, Byrd D J, Kaufman S, Milstien S 1977 Atypical phenylketonuria with normal phenylalanine hydroxylase and dihydropteridine reductase activity in vitro. Pediatrics 59: 757–761

Bartholomé K, Schmidt H, Lutz P 1979 Phenylalanine hydroxylase and protein loading test in phenylketonuria and hyperphenylalaninaemia. European Journal of Pediatrics 130: 206

Brenton D P, Cusworth D C 1971 The response of patients with cystathionine synthase deficiency to pyridoxine. In: Carson N A J, Raine D N (eds) Inherited disorders of sulphur metabolism. Churchill Livingstone, Edinburgh, p 264

Brown E S, Waisman H A 1971 Mental retardation in four offspring of a hyperphenylaninemic mother. Pediatrics 48: 401–410

Butler I J, Holtzman N A, Kaufman S, Koslow S, Krumholz A, Milstien S 1975 Phenylketonuria due to deficiency of dihydropteridine reductase. Pediatric Research 9 (551): 348

Cabalska B, Duczyńska, Borzymowska J, Zorska Z, Kośłacz-Folga A, Bożkowa K 1977 Termination of dietary treatment in phenylketonuria. European Journal of Pediatrics 126: 253–262

Carson N A J, Neill D W 1962 Metabolic abnormalities detected in a survey of mentally backward individuals in Northern Ireland. Archives of Disease in Childhood 37: 505–513

Corner B D, Holton J B, Norman R M, Williams P M 1968 A case of histidinaemia controlled with a low histidine diet. Pediatrics 41: 1074–1081

Danks D M, Cotton R G H, Schlesinger P 1979 Diagnosis of malignant hyperphenylalaninaemia. Archives of Disease in Childhood 54: 329–330

Dobson J C, Williamson M, Azen C, Koch R 1977 Intellectual assessment of 111 four-year-old children with phenylketonuria. Pediatrics 60: 822–827

Fisch R O, Doeden D, Lansky L L, Anderson J A 1969 Maternal phenylketonuria. American Journal of Diseases of Children 118: 847–858

Folling A 1934 Uber Ausscheidung von Phenylbenztraubensäure in Verbindung mit imbezzillität Hoppe Seylers Zeitschrift für Physiologie und Chemie. 277: 169

Harker L A, Slichter S J, Scott C R, Ross R, 1974 Homocystinaemia: vascular injury and arterial thrombosis. New England Journal of Medicine 291: 537–543

Neville B G R, Lilly P M 1973 Histidinaemia: its significance in neonatal screening. Archives of Disease in Childhood 48: 325–326

Niederweiser A, Curtius H-Ch, Bettoni O, Bieri J, Schircks B, Visconti M 1979 Atypical phenylketonuria caused by 7-8-dihydrobiopterin synthetase deficiency. Lancet 1: 131–133

Nielsen K B, Wamberg E, Weber J 1979 Successful outcome of pregnancy in a phenylketonuric woman after low-phenylalanine diet introduced before conception. Lancet 1: 1245

Perry T L 1974 Homocystinuria. In: Nyhan W L (ed) Heritable disorders of amino acid metabolism. Wiley, New York, p 395

Scriver C R, Rosenberg L E 1973 Vitamin responsive amino-acidopathies. In: Amino acid metabolism and its disorders. Saunders, Philadelphia Ch. 3, p. 42

Smith I, Erdohazi M, Macartney F J, Pincott J R, Brenton D P, Biddle S A, Fairweather D V I, Dobbing J 1979 Fetal damage despite low-phenylalanine diet after conception in a phenylketonuric woman. Lancet 1: 17–19

Smith I, Lobascher M E, Stevenson J E, Wolff O H, Schmidt H, Grubel-Kaiser S et al 1978 Effect of stopping low-phenylalanine diet on intellectual progress of children with phenylketonuria. British Medical Journal 2: 723–726

Smith I, Wolff O H 1974 Phenylketonuria and influence of early treatment. Lancet 2: 540–544

Stanbury J B, Wyngaarden J B, Fredrickson D S 1978 The metabolic basis of inherited disease, 3rd edn. McGraw Hill, New York

Hawcroft J, Hudson F P 1974 Screening for phenylketonuria in the United Kingdom. Health Trends 6: 72–74

Jervis G A 1954 Phenylpyruvic oligophrenia (phenylketonuria). Association for Research in Nervous and Mental Disease 33: 259

Komrower G M, Sardharwalla I B, Coutts J M J, Ingham D 1979 Management of maternal phenylketonuria: an emerging clinical problem. British Medical Journal 1: 1383–1387

Lenke R R, Levy H L 1980 Maternal phenylketonuria and hyperphenylalaninemia: an international survey of the outcome of untreated and treated pregnancies. New England Journal of Medicine 303: 1202–1208

Lott I T, Wheelden J A, Levy H L 1970 Speech and histidinaemia. Methodology and evaluation of four cases. Developmental Medicine and Child Neurology 12: 596–603

Mabry C C, Denniston J C, Coldwell J G 1966 Mental retardation in children of phenylketonuric mothers. New England Journal of Medicine 275: 1331–1336

7

Inherited disorders of the urea cycle and organic acidaemias

J. V. Leonard

1. INHERITED DISORDERS OF THE UREA CYCLE

General introduction

Ammonia is a major product of the catabolism of nitrogenous compounds and is highly toxic if allowed to accumulate. In man it is detoxified by synthesis to urea: the steps are shown in Figure 7.1. Disorders of each step have been described.

Clinical presentation — introduction

The clinical features of each of the inherited disorders of the urea cycle are broadly similar and symptoms may develop at almost any age. (Hsia 1974, Shih 1978).

Those most severely affected present in the neonatal period. At birth they appear normal but within the first week there is a gradual onset of lethargy, poor feeding, vomiting, tachypnoea (often with grunting), seizures and alterations in tone eventually progressing to loss of all reflex activity and apnoea. Liver failure may develop with a bleeding diathesis and a pulmonary or intracranial haemorrhage may be the terminal event.

In patients with less severe disease symptoms develop later. Persistent vomiting and failure to thrive with developmental retardation are common, and often it is possible to elicit a history of protein intolerance. During acute exacerbations neurological symptoms and signs such as headaches, irritability, ataxia, slurring of speech, confusion, alterations in consciousness and seizures may predominate but the severity of all symptoms is remarkably variable. Behavioural problems are also frequent. The pattern of the illness may have a rather characteristic episodic or fluctuating course with symptoms often being precipitated by a protein load or by intercurrent infection. A urea cycle disorder should always be considered in a child who is thought to have 'encephalitis', particularly if the child has more than one episode.

The most mildly affected patients have no symptoms at all or just a dislike of protein-rich foods.

1. *Carbamyl phosphate synthetase deficiency (CPSD)* (Freeman et al 1964)

The clinical and biochemical features of CPSD are varied (Shih 1978) but patients have usually developed symptoms with evidence of protein intolerance during the early weeks of life.

2. *Ornithine carbamyl transferase deficiency (OCTD)* (Russell et al 1962)

Ornithine carbamyl transferase deficiency is one of the commoner disorders of the urea cycle and has an X-linked mode of inheritance. Affected males usually have little enzyme activity and develop symptoms soon after birth. Even with energetic treatment most boys will die in the early weeks or months of life (McReynolds et al 1978, Donn et al 1979, Wiegand et al 1980). The female heterozygotes are less severely affected and symptoms are very variable. Those most severely affected develop symptoms in early infancy whereas those least affected remain asymptomatic although they may still have mild protein intolerance and a slight reduction in IQ (Batshaw et al 1980a).

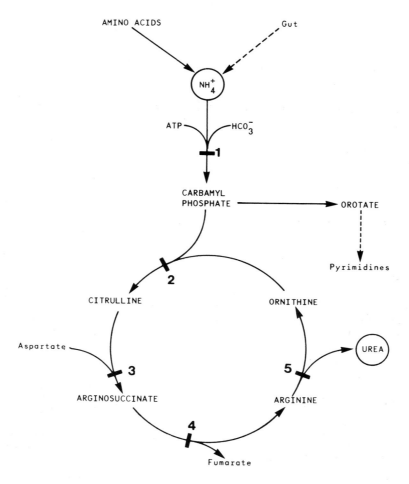

Fig. 7.1 Inherited disorders of the urea cycle
1. Carbamyl phosphate synthetase deficiency (CPSD)
2. Ornithine carbamyl transferase deficiency (OCTD)
3. Citrullinaemia (ASSD)
4. Arginosuccinic aciduria (ASLD)
5. Arginase deficiency

3. *Citrullinaemia (arginosuccinate synthetase deficiency — ASSD)* (McMurray et al 1962)

The age of presentation of this condition is variable although symptoms most commonly develop in the neonatal period or in early infancy.

4. *Arginosuccinic aciduria (arginosuccinate lyase deficiency — ASLD)* (Allan et al 1958)

The majority of the patients with this condition present with neurological problems including fits, intermittent ataxia, irritability and delayed devel-

opment. About half the patients have friable short hair with the characteristic microscopic appearance of trichorrhexis nodosa. Patients may present in the neonatal period or early infancy. Asymptomatic forms of ASLD also exist (Shih 1978).

5. *Arginase deficiency*

This is a rare disorder characterised by recurrent vomiting, fits, mental retardation and spastic diplegia (Terheggen et al 1969). One child treated from birth has developed normally (Snyderman et al 1979).

Diagnosis

a. Physical examination

There are no diagnostic physical signs. Short friable hair in a mentally retarded child suggests the diagnosis of ASLD but it is not specific. In all urea cycle disorders hepatomegaly may be present, and is more likely to be found during acute attacks.

b. Biochemical tests

i. Blood urea. The blood urea is normal or only slightly reduced in all but the severest neonatal forms.

ii. Liver function tests. The aminotransferases (alanine and aspartate) are commonly raised during acute exacerbations but jaundice is unusual.

iii. Ammonia. Reliable and simple methods for measuring plasma ammonia are now available. In infants and older children, the concentrations in plasma do not usually exceed 40 μmol/l but levels are higher in preterm infants (Batshaw & Brusilow 1978). Blood samples must be separated quickly and the plasma deep frozen if not analysed immediately to prevent breakdown of nitrogenous compounds to form more ammonia. Haemolysed specimens give falsely high values because the ammonia concentration in red blood cell is more than twice that in plasma (Colombo 1971). Plasma ammonia levels are closely related to protein and calorie intake and in order to interpret plasma ammonia results satisfactorily it is often necessary to have an assessment of the recent diet.

Children with urea cycle disorders usually have raised ammonia values but levels are very variable and may be normal on a low protein diet. When being screened for these disorders the children should be receiving adequate protein ($>$ 2.5 g/kg per day). Patients in coma due to ammonia intoxication usually have very high values ($>$ 400 μmol/l) but this is not invariable.

iv. Plasma and urine amino acids. The plasma and urine amino acid abnormalities of the urea cycle disorders are shown in Table 7.1. The results of these investigations are diagnostic in ASSD, ASLD and arginase deficiency, but there are no specific changes in CPSD and OCTD.

Arginine levels are often reduced except in arginase deficiency (Shih 1972, Hartlage et al 1974), but ornithine levels are normal.

v. Urine orotic acid. Carbamyl phosphate (CP) is a precursor of pyrimidines as well as of urea. If reactions in the urea cycle distal to the formation of CP are blocked then CP is diverted to the synthesis of orotic acid and pyrimidines (Fig. 7.1). The excess orotic acid is excreted in the urine and can be estimated in a random specimen. The result is most conveniently expressed as an orotic acid/creatinine ratio. The ratio is elevated in all the urea cycle defects except CPSD (Table 7.1) (Bachmann & Colombo 1980). This investigation is useful for the detection of OCTD carriers as it is more

Table 7.1 Biochemical findings in inherited disorders of the urea cycle. Abnormalities of plasma and urine amino acids, urine orotic acid excretion and the tissues in which enzyme defect is expressed.

Disorder	Amino acids		Urine orotic acid excretion	Tissues in which enzyme defect is expressed
	plasma	urine		
Carbamyl phosphate synthetase deficiency	↑ glutamine ↑ alanine	as in plasma	normal	liver jejunal mucosa
Ornithine carbamyl transferase deficiency	↑ glutamine ↑ alanine	as in plasma	increased	liver jejunal mucosa
Citrullinaemia	↑ ↑ citrulline	↑ citrulline homocitrulline and other metabolites	increased	liver skin fibroblasts
Arginosuccinate lyase deficiency	arginosuccinic acid (not normally present)	↑ arginosuccinic acid and other metabolites	increased during acute attacks	liver red blood cells skin fibroblasts
Arginase deficiency	↑ ↑ arginine	↑ Arginine ↑ Ornithine ↑ Cystine ↑ Lysine	increased	liver red blood cells ? skin fibroblasts

sensitive for this purpose than the plasma ammonia (Batshaw & Brusilow 1978).

vi. Enzyme assay. The diagnosis of a urea cycle disorder should always be confirmed by measurement of enzyme activity in suitable tissue (see Table 7.1) although in difficult or atypical cases a needle biopsy of the liver should be obtained. The activity of the enzymes in white blood cells is generally lower than those in liver and it is doubtful that the results of such assays are satisfactory for the diagnosis of these disorders (Snodgrass et al 1978.)

c. Histology

i. Liver. The liver in children with urea cycle defects may be normal microscopically or may show mild fatty infiltration and focal changes (Labrecque et al 1979). These changes cannot be reliably distinguished from those found in Reye's syndrome (J. R. Pincott: personal communication) (Chapter 22).

ii. Post-mortem histology of the brain. At autopsy the brain may appear normal microscopically or it may be congested and oedematous. Cerebral atrophy and ventricular dilatation have also been reported (Bruton et al 1970). Microscopically many changes have been described (Hsia 1974) but the most consistent finding in patients dying after the neonatal period is glial proliferation of Alzheimer type II cells (Hopkins et al 1969, Solitaire et al 1969). This appearance may be mistaken for an infiltrating glioma.

Treatment

The mainstay of the treatment of the urea cycle disorders is the restriction of dietary protein to approximately 0.75–1.5 g/kg per day (depending on age and protein tolerance) with a generous energy intake. The protein should be spread throughout the day in frequent small meals. Many affected patients spontaneously select a low protein diet as they have discovered that their symptoms improve. The effect of the diet should be monitored by measurement of plasma ammonia, amino acids and growth. However the protein restriction necessary to control the plasma ammonia may be insufficient to support normal growth but, by giving supplements of essential amino acids, the natural protein intake may be reduced and the requirements of essential amino acids for growth still be met (Snyderman et al 1976). Alternatively keto-analogues of the essential amino acids may be used (Thoene et al 1977). A small percentage of the administered dose is transaminated to form the respective amino acid, thereby both providing additional amino acids for growth and further reducing the nitrogen load to be excreted (Brusilow et al 1979).

Since arginine is normally synthesised in the urea cycle it is not an essential amino acid, but in urea cycle disorders it may become semi-essential or essential because of the metabolic block. Arginine deficiency may be one factor responsible for the growth retardation and poor intellectual development of patients with these disorders (Danks et al 1974, Hartlage et al 1974). As it is difficult to estimate requirements we routinely give arginine supplements giving 3–12 mmol/d (0.5–2 g/d). In ASSD and ASLD the removal of ammonia is limited by the supply of ornithine and supplements of arginine up to 5 mmol/kg per day may be needed to control the ammonia levels (Brusilow & Batshaw 1979).

If these measures fail to control hyperammonaemia, other forms of treatment may be used. By promoting the excretion of nitrogenous compounds other than urea the load on the urea cycle can be reduced (Brusilow et al 1979). If sodium benzoate is administered it is conjugated with glycine to form hippuric acid which has a high renal clearance. Phenylacetic acid is coupled to glutamine to form phenylacetylglutamine which is also rapidly excreted. When these compounds are given to patients with urea cycle defects urinary nitrogen excretion increases and plasma ammonia falls. Although doubts about their use have been expressed (Woolf 1980), in the short term both compounds appear to be safe and effective. Oral citrate has been given to increase the supply of Krebs cycle intermediates and in some patients it reduces post-prandial elevation of ammonia (Levin et al 1969, Sunshine et al 1971).

In many patients ammonia levels can be satisfactorily controlled for much of the time but all patients are liable to develop episodes of severe hyperammonaemia. These may be precipitated by infection, a protein load or surgery but are often unexplained. In the acute episodes the protein intake should be stopped and a high energy intake, as fat and carbohydrate, given orally or intravenously (See organic acidaemias). Ammonia levels may still rise rapidly and if simple measures are not quickly effective peritoneal or haemodialysis should be performed (Donn et al 1979, Wiegand et al 1980). More recently the use of intravenous sodium benzoate has been shown to be effective (Batshaw & Brusilow 1980).

Outcome

Even with the most vigorous treatment the outlook for the majority of affected babies who present in the neonatal period is poor (McReynolds et al 1978, Donn et al 1980). However, not all patients with severe hyperammonaemia in the neonatal period have an inborn error of metabolism. Preterm babies may develop a clinical syndrome indistinguishable from those with urea cycle defects (Ballard et al 1978) but with active treatment they make a complete recovery without any persistent biochemical abnormalities. No explanation has yet been found.

Delayed development and failure to thrive are common problems in those who are less severely affected, but with careful management normal growth and development are possible.

Acute hyperammonaemia may develop in all patients, including those with apparently mild disease and despite active treatment patients may sustain a severe cerebral insult and die with evidence of raised intracranial pressure. Plasma ammonia is not a good predictor of outcome since although high levels carry a bad prognosis, severe encephalopathy may occur with moderate levels (~ 250 μmol/l). Bessman & Bessman (1955) have suggested that depletion of Krebs cycle intermediates by the synthesis of glutamine from 2-oxoglutarate is responsible for hepatic encephalopathy. In two infants with OCTD hyperammonaemic coma was preceded by a fall in plasma 2-oxoglutarate and it was suggested that this might be of predictive value (Batshaw et al 1980b).

Genetic considerations

All the conditions are inherited as autosomal recessives except OCTD which is X-linked. Prenatal diagnosis of ASLD and other disorders in which the enzyme deficiency is expressed in fibroblasts should be possible (see Table 7.1, ASSD, arginase deficiency).

Detailed family studies of those with OCTD are indicated to detect the female carriers whose symptoms vary widely because of the genetic implications. At any early stage of fetal development there is random inactivation of one X chromosome within each cell (the Lyon hypothesis). As a result the liver contains two populations of cells, one with OCT and one without (Ricciuti et al 1975). The relative proportions of the two populations will determine the total OCT activity and hence the individual's symptoms. Most, but probably not all, carriers can be identified by using a standardised protein load and measuring plasma ammonia and the urinary orotic acid excretion. When counselling parents it is important to note that mild disease in the mother does not imply mild disease in her offspring.

2. THE ORGANIC ACIDAEMIAS

Introduction

By convention the term 'organic acidaemias' is used to refer to the inborn errors of the metabolism of methylmalonate and propionate and of the catabolism of the essential amino acids leucine, isoleucine and valine (Gompertz 1975). Disorders of 9 enzymes (Fig. 7.2) are now recognised but the individual enzyme deficiencies are not easily or reliably distinguished on clinical grounds. Several more inborn errors of metabolism of other pathways that present in a similar manner have now been described, including glutaric aciduria (Goodman et al 1975) and multiple acyl CoA dehydrogenase deficiency (Przyrembel et al 1975).

Clinical presentation

These disorders may present in several ways and should be considered in neonates with severe unex-

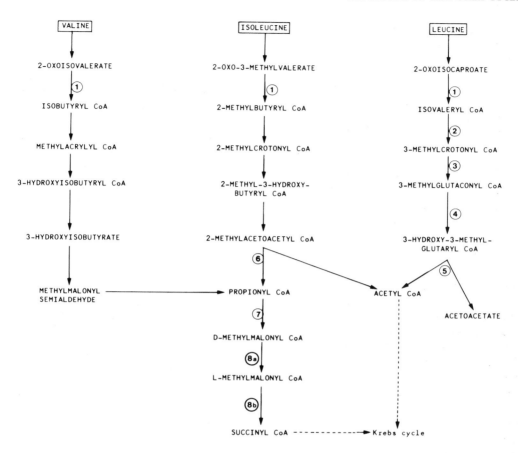

Fig. 7.2 The catabolic pathways of leucine, isoleucine, valine and propionate. The inborn errors of these pathways are:

1. Maple syrup urine disease (Dancis et al 1959)
2. Isovaleric acidaemia (Tanaka et al 1966)
3. 3-methylcrotonylglycinuria (Eldjarn et al 1970)
4. 3-methylglutaconic aciduria (Robinson et al 1976)
5. 3-hydroxy-3-methylglutaryl CoA lyase deficiency (Faull et al 1976)
6. 2-oxothiolase deficiency (Daum et al 1971)
7. Propionic acidaemia (Childs et al 1961)
8. Methylmalonic acidaemia (Oberholzer et al 1967, Stokke et al 1967)

plained metabolic acidosis, in infants with failure to thrive and in children with a variety of neurological symptoms and signs. A small number of children are healthy but have episodes of metabolic acidosis.

a. Neonatal

At birth these babies are normal but within the first few days they commonly develop an unexplained severe metabolic acidosis (base deficit > 15 mmol/l) and progressively deteriorate with lethargy, poor feeding, vomiting, tachypnoea and neurological signs. The babies may become gradually more hypotonic and less responsive with loss of all reflex activity. It is common for them to develop apnoea and to need respiratory support. Less often hypertonia with 'fisting' and abnormal movements are seen.

The majority of babies are initially thought to

have an overwhelming infection or an intracerebral catastrophe. A useful diagnostic clue can be persistent ketosis which is otherwise unusual in the neonatal period.

b. Failure to thrive

Affected infants may present during the first year of life with failure to thrive. Commonly these children are generally unwell with persistent vomiting and hypotonia, and they make poor developmental progress. Symptoms are usually worse during intercurrent infections. Persistent metabolic acidosis or ketosis is often present.

c. Neurological

The organic acidaemias may present with a wide variety of neurological symptoms and signs (Table 7.2). Mental retardation is common, particularly when the children are untreated.

d. Intermittent

Rarely these children have a mild form of the illness so that they grow and develop normally or have only mild developmental delay (Goedde et al 1970). However at times of stress (for example intercurrent infections or following surgical oper-

Table 7.2 Neurological symptoms with which organic acidaemias may be present

Presenting feature	Organic acidaemia
Infantile spasms	3-methylcrotonylglycinuria (Finnie et al 1976)
Seizures resistant to anticonvulsants	3-methylcrotonylglycinuria (Lehnert et al 1979)
Hypotonia	3-methylcrotonylglycinuria (Keeton & Moosa 1976)
A syndrome resembling Reye's syndrome	3-hydroxy-3-methylglutaric aciduria (Faull et al 1976)
Progressive neurological deterioration	3-methylglutaconic aciduria (Greter et al 1978) Glutaric aciduria (type I) (Goodman et al 1975)
Dystonia and abnormal movements	Glutaric aciduria (type I) (Gregersen et al 1977)
Pseudo-tumour cerebri	Maple syrup urine disease (Mantovani et al 1980)
Intermittent ataxia	Maple syrup urine disease (Morris et al 1961)

ations) severe metabolic acidosis often with neurological signs (confusion, ataxia, coma) may develop. These episodes may be fatal (Kiil & Rokkones 1964).

Diagnosis

The first step to making the diagnosis is to think of the possibility. Since all these disorders are inherited as autosomal recessives, a history of parental consanguinity, unexplained deaths of siblings in the neonatal period or later in childhood should increase the clinician's suspicions.

a. Clinical examination

There are no specific physical signs. During the acute illness hepatomegaly is common but not invariable. The neurological signs have already been discussed. Occasionally the baby or the urine may have an unusual smell which can alert the clinician but this is not a reliable physical sign.

b. Biochemical tests

Care must be taken to collect specimens under the right conditions, that is either during an acute illness or whilst the child has a metabolic acidosis. If neither of these conditions is fulfilled then the child must be receiving an adequate protein intake (> 2.5 g/kg per day) since otherwise the diagnosis may be missed, particularly in the milder variants.

 i. Plasma. Metabolic acidosis is usually present in those whose symptoms develop in the neonatal period but may be mild or absent in children who present later. Plasma lactate levels are often raised during the acute episode; this may cause diagnostic difficulties as the acidosis may be attributed wholly to a lactic acidosis, without organic acids being examined (Leonard et al 1981). During the acute attack concentrations of the plasma amino acids will be diagnostic in maple syrup urine disease (marked elevation of leucine, isoleucine, valine and allo-isoleucine) but in all other conditions the amino acid levels are variable and may indeed be normal. Occasionally mildly raised levels of the branched chain aminoacids may be found. Plasma glycine and plasma ammonia concentrations are frequently raised in methylmalonic acidaemia and propionic acidaemia (Rosenberg 1978).

In propionic acidaemia plasma propionate concentrations are diagnostic but examination of the urine organic acids is generally preferred for establishing the diagnosis of an organic acidaemia. Plasma organic acid concentrations are useful for monitoring the effect of treatment.

ii. Urine. Persistent ketonuria is often present during acute attacks and a heavy precipitate may form with 2–4 dinitrophenylhydrazine (DNP) demonstrating the presence of keto-acids. However these tests are non-specific and only indicate the need for more detailed studies. Although methylmalonic acid can be detected rapidly by a specific colour reaction (Gutteridge & Wright 1970), the diagnosis of an organic acidaemia can usually only be made by using gas-liquid chromatography which enables the complete pattern of urine organic acids to be identified. Mass spectrometry may be needed to confirm the identity of some metabolites. If possible urine should not be collected whilst a child is receiving sodium valproate as this drug is metabolised to a variety of propionate derivatives which may cause diagnostic difficulties.

The biochemical and genetic basis

The decreased enzyme activity may arise because of an abnormality of the apoenzyme or in the metabolism of its cofactor (e.g. biotin, vitamin B_{12}). In some children the activity of the enzyme may be increased by giving pharmacological doses of the cofactor or its precursor. Disorders that have cofactor-responsive variants are listed in Table 7.3. The precise nature of the biochemical abnormality should always be confirmed by measuring the enzyme activity in cultured fibroblasts.

Table 7.3 Cofactor-responsive organic acidaemias

Organic acidaemia	Vitamin (daily dosage)
Methylmalonic acidaemia (Hsia et al 1970)	Cyanocobalamin (1 mg)
3-Methylcrotonylglycinuria (Gompertz et al 1971) Propionic acidaemia (Barnes et al 1970)	Biotin (10 mg)
Maple syrup urine disease (Scriver et al 1971)	Thiamine (10 mg)

The organic acidaemias (listed in Fig. 7.2) are inherited as autosomal recessives. The recurrence risk for subsequent children is 1 in 4 and provided the enzyme deficiency is expressed in fibroblasts, prenatal diagnosis is possible.

Treatment

a. Acute illness

During acute illness, which may be precipitated by intercurrent infection or following surgical operations, endogenous protein catabolism will release large quantities of amino acids which may precipitate serious metabolic acidosis. One aim of treatment is to suppress the protein catabolism by giving protein-free energy as carbohydrate and fat. Dietary protein is reduced to less than 0.5 g/kg per day with an energy intake up to 200 kcal/kg per day (800 kJ/kg per day).

If oral fluids are not tolerated 10% glucose should be given intravenously. Fat emulsions may be also given to increase energy intake. Metabolic acidosis should be controlled with sodium bicarbonate either orally or intravenously. If the child fails to respond to this therapy, peritoneal dialysis, exchange transfusion or haemodialysis should be used to remove organic acids and to correct acidosis (Russell et al 1974, Sandubray et al 1980). Since acute episodes of acidosis are often precipitated by infection this should always be sought carefully and treated vigorously. Leucopenia and thrombocytopenia may complicate these episodes particularly in the neonatal period.

Parents should be taught an emergency regime for use at home in which dietary protein is reduced and a plentiful energy intake given in a form that is palatable and easily assimilated (e.g. soluble glucose polymers). Some patients may need sodium bicarbonate in addition. Hospital treatment will be needed if the child does not respond quickly.

When the diagnosis is first established pharmacological doses of the cofactor should be given to test for cofactor-responsiveness. Those children who are responsive rapidly improve clinically although it may be possible to detect some persistent biochemical abnormalities.

b. Long-term management

Children who are fully cofactor-responsive will need no treatment other than to continue the cofactor idefinitely. All other patients will need restriction of dietary protein combined with generous energy intake (Francis 1974). The dietary management is difficult, and it requires considerable skill to nurture these patients over long periods. Close co-operation between the paediatrician, dietitian and biochemist is essential.

In some conditions it is possible to increase the excretion of toxic metabolites thereby improving control of the disease. The administration of glycine in isovaleric acidaemia increases the formation of isovalerylglycine which is relatively non-toxic and rapidly excreted by the kidney (Yudkoff et al 1978).

The effect of the therapy must be monitored by measurement of urine or plasma organic acids and the plasma amino acids. In the long term the child's growth in height and weight and his developmental progress are important indices of health. The diet will need to be continued indefinitely.

Prognosis

Untreated, most children will die and those who survive usually do not thrive and are often mentally retarded. Children who are cofactor-responsive have a good prognosis for growth and mental development provided the disease is diagnosed before serious neurological damage has occurred.

For those patients who are not cofactor-responsive the prognosis both for life and for mental development is guarded. Despite treatment affected children may die during an acute attack. Most children will thrive but there may be some in whom the degree of protein restriction necessary to control their symptoms is insufficient for normal growth. The prognosis for mental development depends on many factors and varies with each condition. Two factors of particular importance are the age and the neurodevelopmental status at the time of diagnosis. However the outlook for children with propionic acidaemia seems particularly poor. Patients frequently die in the early years of life and the developmental progress of the survivors is often delayed.

NON-KETOTIC HYPERGLYCINAEMIA

Non-ketotic hyperglycinaemia is an inherited disorder of glycine metabolism. The primary defect is thought to be the failure of decarboxylation of glycine in the liver and the brain (Perry et al 1975, Nyhan 1978).

Presentation

The majority of children present in the neonatal period. They appear normal at birth but then develop lethargy and marked hypotonia with loss of normal reflex activity and seizures. Respiratory support is often required. Those children who survive the neonatal period make little or no developmental progress and usually have frequent episodes of fits which are resistant to anticonvulsants. Metabolic acidosis and ketosis are noticeably absent.

Some children have a less severe form of the disease and present later with convulsions or developmental retardation (Holmgren & Blomquist 1977).

Investigations

Plasma glycine concentrations are usually raised (> 500 μmol/l) but levels vary considerably as they are affected by the protein intake and other factors. CSF glycine concentrations are increased (normal < 15 μmol/l) and so is the ratio of the concentration of glycine in CSF and plasma (Normal < 0.025) (Perry et al 1975, Steinmann & Gitzelmann 1979). There is massive excretion of glycine in the urine.

Hyperglycinaemia may also be secondary to one of the organic acidaemias which can present with similar symptoms so plasma and urine organic acids should always be examined to exclude these conditions. The collective term 'ketotic hyperglycinaemia' has been used to describe them but it is now known that it is caused by several inborn errors including propionic acidaemia and methylmalonic acidaemia. (See organic acidaemias.)

Treatment

Reduction of the plasma glycine concentration

with a low-protein diet or sodium benzoate has no effect on the course of the disease (Nyhan 1978), nor has the administration of 1-carbon donors such as N^5 formyl tetrahydrofolate (Spielberg et al 1976) or methionine (De Groot et al 1970). It seems that the high plasma glycine levels are probably of little consequence but that the high CSF and brain glycine levels are likely to be responsible for the symptoms. Gitzelmann et al (1977) have proposed the use of strychnine. This alkaloid is a potent inhibitor of glycine-mediated neurotrans-

mission and it is suggested that the high glycine concentrations are responsible for excess post-synaptic inhibition which may be blocked by the drug. Although some patients may have improved when given strychnine (Gitzelmann et al 1977) the majority have not (Steinmann & Gitzelmann 1979, von Wendt et al 1980). Thus for most patients the prognosis remains very poor. The condition is inherited as an autosomal recessive and it has recently been suggested that prenatal diagnosis is feasible (Garcia-Castro et al 1982).

REFERENCES

Allan J D, Cusworth D C, Dent C E, Wilson V K 1958 A disease, probably hereditary, characterised by severe mental deficiency and a constant gross abnormality of amino acid metabolism. Lancet 1: 182–187

Bachmann C, Colombo J P 1980 Diagnostic value of orotic acid excretion in heritable disorders of the urea cycle and in hyperammonemia due to organic acidurias. European Journal of Paediatrics 134: 109–113

Ballard R A, Vinocur B, Reynolds J W, Wennberg R P, Merritt A, Sweetman L et al 1978 Transient hyperammonemia of the preterm infant. New England Journal of Medicine 299: 920–925

Barnes N D, Hull D, Balgobin L, Gompertz D 1970 Biotin responsive propionicacidaemia. Lancet 2: 244–245

Batshaw M L, Brusilow S W 1978 Asymptomatic hyperammonemia in low birth weight infants. Pediatric Research 12: 221–224

Batshaw M L, Brusilow S W 1980 Treatment of hyperammonemic coma caused by inborn errors of the urea synthesis. Journal of Pediatrics 97: 893–900

Batshaw M L, Roan Y, Jung A L, Rosenberg L A, Brusilow S W 1980 Cerebral dysfunction in asymptomatic carriers of ornithine transcarbamylase deficiency. New England Journal of Medicine 302: 482–485

Batshaw M L, Walser M, Brusilow S W 1980b Plasma α-ketoglutarate in urea cycle enzymopathies and its role as a harbinger of hyperammonemic coma. Pediatric Research 14: 1316–1319

Bessman S P, Bessman A N 1955 The cerebral and peripheral uptake of ammonia in liver disease with an hypothesis for the mechanism of hepatic coma. Journal of Clinical Investigation 34: 622–628

Brusilow S W, Batshaw M L 1979 Arginine therapy of arginosuccinase deficiency. Lancet 1: 124–127

Brusilow S, Batshaw M, Walser M 1979 Use of keto acids in inborn errors of urea synthesis. In: Myron Winik (ed) Nutritional management of genetic disorders. John Wiley, New York, ch 4, p 65–75

Brusilow S W, Valle D W, Batshaw M L 1979 New pathways of nitrogen excretion in inborn errors of urea synthesis. Lancet 2: 452–454

Bruton C J, Corsellis J A N, Russell A 1970 Hereditary hyperammonaemia. Brain 93: 423–434

Childs B, Nyhan W L, Borden M, Bard L, Cooke R W 1961 Idiopathic hyperglycinemia and hyperglycinuria: new disorder of amino acid metabolism. Pediatrics 27: 522–538

Colombo J P 1971 Congenital disorders of the urea cycle and ammonia detoxication. Karger, Basel

Dancis J, Levitz M, Miller S, Westall R G 1959 Maple syrup urine disease. British Medical Journal 1: 91–93

Danks D M, Tippett P, Zentner G 1974 Severe neonatal citrullinaemia. Archives of Disease in Childhood 49: 579–581

Daum R S, Lamm P H, Mamer O A, Scriver C R 1971 A 'new' disorder of isoleucine catabolism. Lancet 2: 1289–1290

De Groot C J, Troelstra J A, Hommes F A 1970 Non-ketotic hyperglycinaemia: an in vitro study of the glycine-serine conversion in the liver of three patients and the effect of dietary methionine. Pediatric Research 4: 238–243

Donn S M, Swartz R D, Thoene J G 1979 Comparison of exchange transfusion, peritoneal dialysis and hemodialysis for the treatment of hyperammonemia in an anuric newborn infant. Journal of Pediatrics 95: 67–70

Eldjarn L, Jellum E, Stokke O, Pande H, Waaler P E 1970 β-hydroxyisovaleric aciduria and β-methylcrotonylglycinuria. A new inborn error of metabolism. Lancet 2: 521–522

Faull K, Bolton P, Halpern B, Hammond J, Danks D M, Hähnel R et al 1976 Patient with defect in leucine metabolism. New England Journal of Medicine 294:1013

Finnie M D A, Cottrall K, Seakins J W T, Snedden W 1976 Massive excretion of 2-oxo-glutaric acid and 3-hydroxyisovaleric acid in a patient with deficiency of 3-methylcrotonyl CoA carboxylase. Clinica chimica acta 73: 513–519

Francis D E M 1974 Diets for sick children, 3rd edn. Blackwell Scientific Publications, Oxford

Freeman J M, Nicholson J F, Masland W S, Rowland L P, Carter S 1964 Ammonia intoxication due to a congenital defect in urea synthesis. Journal of Pediatrics 65: 1039–1040

Garcia-Castro J M, Isales-Forsythe C M, Levy H M, Shih V E, Lao-Velez C R, Gonzalez-Rios M del C et al 1982 Prenatal diagnosis of non-ketotic hyperglycinaemia, New England Journal of Medicine 306: 79–81

Gitzelmann R, Steinmann B, Otten A, Dumermuth G, Herdan M, Reubi J C et al 1977 Nonketotic hyperglycinaemia treated with strychnine, a glycine receptor antagonist. Helvetica paediatrica acta 32: 517–525

Goedde H W, Langenbeck V, Brackertz D, Keuer W, Rokkones T, Halvorsen S et al 1970 Clinical and biochemical-genetic aspects of intermittent branched chain ketoaciduria. Acta paediatrica scandinavica 59: 83–87

Gompertz D 1975 The organic acidaemias. In: Raine D N (ed) The treatment of inherited metabolic disease. MTP, Lancaster, ch 8, p 191–217

Gompertz D, Draffan G H, Watts J L, Hull D 1971 Biotin responsive β-methylcrotonylglycinuria. Lancet 2: 22–24

Goodman S I, Markey S P, Moe P G, Miles B S, Teng C G 1975 Glutaric aciduria: a new disorder of amino acid metabolism. Biochemical medicine 12: 12–21

Goodman SI. 1981 Antenatal diagnosis of defects of ureagenesis. Pediatrics 68: 446–447

Gregersen N, Brandt N J, Christensen E, Gron I, Rasmussen K, Brandt S 1977 Glutaric aciduria: clinical and laboratory findings in two brothers. Journal of Pediatrics 90: 740–745

Greter J, Hagberg B, Steen G, Soderhjelm U 1978 3-methylglutaconic aciduria: report on a sibship with infantile progressive encephalopathy. European Journal of Pediatrics 129: 231–238

Gutteridge J M C, Wright E B 1970 A simple and rapid thin layer chromatographic technique for the detection of methylmalonic acid in urine. Clinica chimica acta 27: 289–291

Hartlage P L, Coryell M E, Hall W K, Hahn D A 1974 Arginosuccinic aciduria: perinatal diagnosis and early dietary management. Journal of Pediatrics 85: 86–88

Holmgren G, Blomquist K H 1977 Non-ketotic hyperglycinaemia in two sibs with mild psychoneurological symptoms. Neuropädiatrie 8: 67–72

Hopkins I J, Connelly J F, Dawson A G, Hird F J R, Maddison T G 1969 Hyperammonaemia due to ornithine transcarbamylase deficiency. Archives of Disease in Childhood 44: 143–151

Hsia Y E 1974 Inherited hyperammonaemic syndromes. Gastroenterology 67: 347–374

Hsia Y E, Lilljeqvist A Ch, Rosenberg L E 1970 Vitamin B12-dependent methylmalonic aciduria: amino acid toxicity, long chain ketonuria and protective effect of B12. Pediatrics 46: 497–507

Kang E S, Snodgrass P J, Gerald P S 1972 Methylmalonyl CoA racemase defect: another cause of methylmalonic aciduria. Pediatric Research 6: 875–879

Keeton B R, Moosa A 1976 Organic aciduria. Treatable cause of floppy infant syndrome. Archives of Disease in Childhood 51: 636–638

Kiil R, Rokkones T 1964 Late manifesting variant of branch chain ketoaciduria (maple syrup urine disease). Acta paediatrica scandinavica 53: 356–364

Labrecque D R, Latham P S, Riely C A, Hsia Y E, Klatskin G 1979 Heritable urea cycle enzyme deficiency — liver disease in 16 patients. Journal of Pediatrics 94: 580–587

Lehnert W, Niederhoff H, Junker A, Saule H, Frasch W 1979 A case of biotin responsive 3-methyl crotonylglycin- and 3-hydroxyisovaleric aciduria. European Journal of Pediatrics 132: 107–114

Leonard J V, Seakins J W T, Bartlett K, Hyde J, Wilson J, Clayton B 1981 Inherited disorders of 3-methylcrotonyl CoA carboxylation. Archives of Disease in Childhood 56: 53–59

Levin B, Abraham J M, Oberholzer V G, Burgess E A 1969 Hyperammonaemia: a deficiency of liver ornithine transcarbamylase. Archives of Disease in Childhood 44: 152–161

Mantovani J F, Naidich T P, Prensky A L, Dodson W E, Williams J C 1980 MSUD: Presentation with pseudotumor cerebri and CT abnormalities. Journal of Pediatrics 96: 279–281

McMurray W C, Mohyuddin F, Rossiter R J, Rathbun J C, Valentine W G, Koegler S J et al 1962 Citrullinuria: a new aminoaciduria associated with mental retardation. Lancet 1:138

McReynolds J W, Mantagos S, Brusilow S, Rosenberg L E 1978 Treatment of complete ornithine transcarbamylase deficiency with nitrogen-free analogues of essential amino acids. Journal of Pediatrics 93: 421–427

Morris M D, Lewis B D, Doolan P D, Harper H A 1961 Clinical and biochemical observations on an apparently non-fatal variant of branch chain ketoaciduria (maple syrup urine disease). Pediatrics 28: 918–923

Morrow G, Barness L A, Cardinale G J, Abeles R H, Flaks J G 1969 Congenital methylmalonic acidemia: enzymatic evidence for two forms of the disease. Proceedings of the National Academy of Sciences (USA) 63: 191–197

Nyhan W L 1978 Non-ketotic hyperglycinemia. In: Stanbury J B, Wyngaarden J B, Fredrickson D S (eds) The metabolic basis of inherited disease, 4th edn. McGraw Hill, New York, ch 26, p 518–527

Oberholzer V G, Levin B, Burgess E A, Young W F 1967 Methylmalonic aciduria: an inborn error of metabolism leading to chronic metabolic acidosis. Archives of Disease in Childhood 42: 492–504

Perry T L, Urquart N, MacLean J, Evans M E, Hansen S, Davidson A G F et al 1975 Non-ketotic hyperglycinemia. New England Journal of Medicine 292: 1269–1273

Przyrembel H, Wendel U, Becker K, Bremer H J, Bruinvis L, Ketting D et al 1976 Glutaric aciduria type II. Report on a previously undescribed metabolic disorder. Clinica chimica acta 66: 227–239

Ricciuti F C, Gelehrter T D, Rosenberg L E 1975 X-chromosome inactivation of human liver: confirmation of X-linkage of ornithine transcarbamylase (OTC). American Journal of Human Genetics 27: 77A

Robinson B H, Sherwood W G, Lampty M, Lowden J A 1976 β-Methylglutaconic aciduria: a new disorder of leucine metabolism (abstract). Pediatric Research 10: 371

Rodeck C R, Patrick A D, Pembrey M E, Tzannatos C, Whitfield A E 1982 Fetal liver biopsy for prenatal diagnosis of ornithine carbamyl transferase deficiency. Lancet 2: 297–299

Rosenberg L 1978 Disorders of propionate, methylmalonate and cobalamin. In: Stanbury J B, Wyngaarden J B, Fredrickson D S (eds) The metabolic basis of inherited disease, 4th edn. McGraw-Hill, New York, ch 21, p 411–429

Russell A, Levin B, Oberholzer V G, Sinclair L 1962 Hyperammonaemia; a new instance of an inborn enzymatic defect of the biosynthesis of urea. Lancet 2: 699–700

Russell G, Thom H, Tarlow M J, Gompertz D 1974 Reduction of plasma propionate by peritoneal dialysis. Pediatrics 53: 281–283

Saudubray J-M, Amèdèe-Manesme O, Lavaud J, Mselati J C, Besson-Leaud M, Ogier H et al 1979 Traitement d'urgence des aminoacidopathies à rèvèlation nèonatale. Archives francaises de Pèdiatrie 36: 969–980

Scriver C R, Mackenzie S, Clow C L, Devlin E 1971 Thiamine-responsive maple syrup urine disease. Lancet 1: 310–312

Scriver C R, Rosenberg L E 1973 Amino acid metabolism and its disorders W B Saunders, Philadelphia, ch 22, p 453–478

Shih V E 1972 Early dietary management in an infant with arginosuccinase deficiency: preliminary report. Journal of Pediatrics 53: 281–283

Shih V E 1978 Urea cycle disorders and other congenital hyperammonemic syndromes. In: Stanbury J B, Wyngaarden J B and Fredrickson D S (eds) The metabolic basis of inherited disease, 4th edn. McGraw-Hill, New York, ch 18, p 362–386

Snodgrass P J, Wappner R S, Brandt I K 1978 White cell ornithine transcarbamylase activity cannot detect the liver enzyme deficiency. Pediatric Research 12: 873

Snyderman S E, Sansaricq C, Phansalkar S V, Schacht R G, Norton P M 1976 The therapy of hyperammonemia due to ornithine transcarbamylase deficiency in a male neonate. Pediatrics 56: 65–73

Snyderman S E, Sansaricq C, Norton P M, Goldstein F 1979 Argininemia treated from birth. Journal of Pediatrics 95: 61–63

Solitaire G B, Shih V E, Nelligan D J, Dolan T F 1969 Arginosuccinic aciduria: clinical, biochemical, anatomical and neuropathological observations. Journal of Mental Deficiency Research 13: 153–170

Spielberg S P, Lucky A W, Schulman J D, Kramer L I, Hefter L, Goodman S I 1976 Failure of leucovorin therapy in nonketotic hyperglycinemia. Journal of Pediatrics 89: 681–682

Steinmann B, Gitzelmann R 1979 Strychnine treatment attempted in newborn twins with severe ketotic

hyperglycinaemia. Helvetica paediatrica acta 34: 589–599

Stokke O, Eldjarn L, Norum K R, Steen-Johnsen J, Halvorsen S 1967 Methylmalonic aciduria. A new inborn error of metabolism which may cause fatal acidosis in the neonatal period. Scandinavian Journal of Clinical and Laboratory Medicine 20: 313–328

Sunshine P, Lindenbaum J E, Levy H L, Freeman J M 1971 Hyperammonemia due to a defect in hepatic ornithine transcarbamylase. Pediatrics 50: 100–111

Tanaka K, Budd M A, Efron M L, Isselbacher K J 1966 Isovaleric acidemia: a new genetic defect of leucine metabolism. Proceedings of National Academy of Science (USA) 56: 236–242

Terheggen H G, Schwenk A, Lowenthal A, Van Sande M, Colombo J P 1969 Argininaemia with arginase deficiency. Lancet 2: 748–749

Thoene J, Batshaw M, Spector E, Kulovich S, Brusilow S, Walser M et al 1977 Neonatal citrullinemia: treatment with ketoanalogues of essential amino acids. Journal of Pediatrics 90: 218–224

Von Wendt L, Similä S K, Saukkonen A L, Koiviko M 1980 Failure of strychnine treatment during the neonatal period in three Finnish children with non-ketotic hyperglycinemia. Pediatrics 65: 1166–1169

Wiegand C, Thompson T, Bock G H, Mathis R K, Kjellstrand C M, Mauer S M 1980 The management of life-threatening hyperammonemia: a comparison of several therapeutic modalities. Journal of Pediatrics 96: 142–144

Woolf L I 1980 Toxicity of phenylacetic acid used in treating hyperammonemia (letter). Journal of Inherited Metabolic Disease 3: 61

Yudkoff M, Cohn R M, Puschak R, Rothman R, Segal S 1978 Glycine therapy in isovalericacidemia. Journal of Pediatrics 92: 813–817

8

The spinocerebellar degenerations and some related conditions

E. M. Brett

INTRODUCTION

The term 'abiotrophy' was proposed by Sir William Gowers in 1893 for certain familial progressive neurological diseases as 'a convenient designation for the cases in which certain systems of structure have an essential defect of vital endurance, in consequence of which their life slowly fails. The termination of life of the isolated structures is to us what we call disease'. Gowers believed that these defects might be due to 'deranged chemical processes in the vital laboratory of the human frame'. The nature of this presumed chemical defect in most of the diseases regarded as examples of abiotrophy is still unknown, and the understanding of this group of disorders is less advanced than that of the conditions described in the previous chapter. The term 'system disease' is perhaps a more suitable name for these disorders though their nomenclature and classification are still far from satisfactory.

The spinocerebellar ataxias were classified by Greenfield (1967) into the *spinal* forms, of which Friedreich's ataxia is the commonest, and the *spinocerebellar* and *cerebellar* varieties. In his revision of this review Oppenheimer (1976) classified the diseases under discussion as *primary neuronal degenerations* or diseases in which for unknown reasons nerve cells of a particular type or in a particular region successively shrivel and die. The common characteristics of these disorders are their selective nature, affecting one or more 'systems' of neurons in a more or less symmetrical manner, the fact that they are steadily progressive, though not necessarily fatal, and their variable clinical and pathological features often overlapping with one another so that accurate classification may be difficult. Some have a clear genetic basis and others not.

Previously no consistent biochemical abnormality was recognised in these disorders, but recent studies have shown evidence of reduced activity of the pyruvate dehydrogenase and oxoglutarate dehydrogenase enzyme complexes in some patients with Friedreich's ataxia and in other disorders. (Blass et al 1976, Cavanagh 1978).

The classification of these diseases in childhood is indeed difficult and, though Oppenheimer logically includes the spinal muscular atrophies among his primary neuronal degenerations, these conditions are discussed elsewhere in this book in the chapter on neuromuscular diseases.

FRIEDREICH'S ATAXIA (Friedreich 1863)

This disorder, the prototype of Gowers' abiotrophies, is among the commonest of the primary neuronal degenerations and occurred in one in 10 000 of the Swedish population in the study by Sjögren (1943). Inheritance is as an autosomal recessive character; though dominant inheritance was described previously, this is now known to be incorrect.

The condition was first described by Friedreich in 9 members of 3 sibships in a series of five papers between 1863 and 1877.

The largest series of patients with Friedreich's ataxia reported is the very recent one of Harding (1981). She reviewed 115 patients from 90 families (53 male and 62 female) seen at The Hospital for Sick Children, Great Ormond Street, the National Hospitals for Nervous Diseases and other neurological centres in London between 1966 and 1980.

Most patients in this series developed symptoms between the ages of 2 and 16 years, and only 4 did

Table 8.1 Friedreich's ataxia: presenting symptoms. (From Harding A E 1981 Brain 104: 589–620, reproduced with permission)

	No. of cases	%
Ataxia	72	62.6
Generalized clumsiness	29	25.2
Tendency to trip	5	4.3
Scoliosis	6	5.2
Tremor	1	0.9
Cardiac symptoms	2	1.7

so after the age of 20. The mean age of onset was 10.52 ± 7.4 years.

The presenting symptoms of Harding's patients are shown in Table 8.1. Ataxia was the commonest but in a few patients scoliosis and cardiac symptoms were the earliest features.

Ataxia of the limbs and trunk and absent tendon reflexes in the legs appeared to be the only consistent early features present within five years of presentation. Dysarthria, signs of pyramidal tract dysfunction in the legs and loss of joint position and vibration sense were not necessarily present in the first five years after onset, but appeared to develop eventually in all cases. Scoliosis and ECG evidence of cardiac involvement were found in over two-thirds of cases. Less frequent features were pes cavus, distal amyotrophy, optic atrophy, nystagmus and deafness. In all cases the course of the disease was gradually progressive. The mean age

of losing the ability to walk was 25.14 ± 15.5 years, and 95% of patients were chair-bound by the age of 44 years.

Unsteadiness in walking is most often the presenting symptom. This may develop insidiously after a period of normal walking. In a few cases the gait may never have improved from its initial toddler unsteadiness and occasionally the onset of walking is delayed. There is progressive ataxia due to a combination of cerebellar dysfunction and loss of kinaesthetic sensation. The child loses the ability to run, if he has gained it, and staggers increasingly as he walks, with a wide-based, reeling, 'drunken' gait.

Ataxia in the upper limbs develops, with intention tremor impairing the performance of fine tasks, and he may become unable to drink from a cup without spilling the contents unless it is held in both hands or only partly filled. There may be truncal ataxia. Later speech may become progressively affected with a scanning, slurring type of dysarthria which makes communication difficult and distresses the child.

Skeletal deformities are common, especially scoliosis, present in about 80% of cases, and pes cavus, seen in about 55% (Fig. 8.1). Harding found that scoliosis was commoner in those who developed symptoms below the age of 12 years and often progressed rapidly during growth spurts; it is very difficult to control. Pes cavus may have been present,

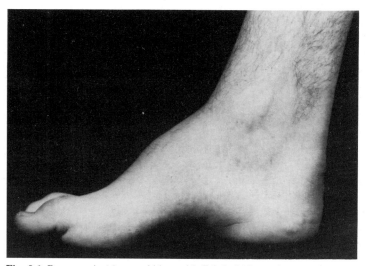

Fig. 8.1 Pes cavus in 14-year-old boy with Friedreich's ataxia

but unrecognized, from an early age, and I suspect that it is sometimes the presenting clinical feature. Contractures at the knees and fingers were relatively rare.

Examination confirms the inco-ordination of gait and in the arms. The tendon reflexes are usually absent or, at least, reduced. In Harding's series there was complete areflexia in over 70% of patients, but in 29 cases one or both biceps jerks were just detectable. They were never brisk. The plantar responses were extensor in 102 patients, absent in 12 and flexor in only one.

An interesting finding in Harding's series was the presence of amyotrophy, a feature not usually considered typical of Friedreich's ataxia. Distal wasting was noted in the small muscles of the hands in 48.6%, sometimes associated with weakness. Distal weakness in the legs was also quite common. Pyramidal weakness was found in all but the earlier cases, but upper limb weakness of pyramidal type was confined to severely disabled patients. In most cases muscle tone was normal.

Sensory testing in the legs showed impairment of joint position sense in 78.3% of cases and of vibration sense in 73%. Sensory loss in the arms was rarer and tended to occur in the later stages of the disease. Abnormalities of pain and light touch were found in a few patients, but some of these were diabetic and might have had a diabetic neuropathy as an additional complication; this is probably rare in childhood. Romberg's sign may be positive, with the child becoming much more unsteady when he stands with his eyes closed (this explains why tabes dorsalis or locomotor ataxia was previously confused with Friedreich's ataxia in an age when tabes was much commoner than it is today).

Nystagmus was found in 20% of Harding's cases, and slow, broken-up pursuit eye movements were seen in 12.2%. Similar movements are seen in ataxia-telangiectasia. Optic atrophy was found in about one-third of cases and varied from mild disc pallor to virtual blindness. It showed significant clustering with diabetes and with deafness in individual patients. Dysarthria of cerebellar type was present in nearly all cases and was absent only in the early stages of the disease. A titubatory tremor of the head was present in a very few patients. Deafness occurred in 9 patients.

CARDIOMYOPATHY IN FRIEDREICH'S ATAXIA

Cardiac involvement is very common in Friedreich's ataxia and is often of major clinical importance. Strangely enough, although Friedreich reported severe fatty degeneration of the myocardium in two patients at necropsy, this was probably due to the typhoid fever of which they died while in hospital for investigation of their neurological disease. In 16 cases reported by Hewer (1969) all the hearts examined pathologically were abnormal showing muscle fibre hypertrophy and interstitial fibrosis. Changes in the electrocardiograph (ECG), with inversion of the T wave, sometimes with signs of left ventricular hypertrophy, occur in about one third of all patients with Friedreich's ataxia and are usually the first sign of cardiac involvement, often appearing several years before the development of cardiomegaly and heart failure. The symptoms of cardiac involvement are those of progressive congestive heart failure or of cardiac arrhythmias, particularly atrial fibrillation or frequent extrasystoles. In a few patients such symptoms precede neurological symptoms. More often they develop some years after neurological deterioration has started and there is a risk that their cardiac origin may be overlooked.

The nature of the cardiac involvement, its relation to the neurological illness and the reason why cardiomyopathy occurs, and is severe, in some patients but not in others, are questions which remain to be answered. Several recent reports have suggested a similarity between the findings in the cardiac involvement of Friedreich's ataxia and in hypertrophic obstructive cardiomyopathy (idiopathic hypertrophic subaortic stenosis). In two siblings with Friedreich's ataxia who were investigated by echocardiography in addition to the other methods, van der Hauwaert and Dumoulin (1976) showed gross thickening of the interventricular septum and evidence of left ventricular outflow tract obstruction.

It has been suggested (van der Hauwaert & Dumoulin 1976) that most patients with Friedreich's ataxia die from cardiac complications, mainly from intractable cardiac failure or disturbances of cardiac rhythm which may rarely cause sudden death. Hewer's (1968) study of 82 fatal cases showed that over half died of heart failure, while nearly three quarters had evidence of cardiac dysfunction during life. Death from cardiac causes is uncommon in childhood and usually occurs in the third or fourth decade. However, 5 patients in Hewer's (1969) series died between the ages of 10 and 16 years, 3 of them with heart failure, one suddenly on exercise and one from a subarachnoid haemorrhage.

Diabetes mellitus

Diabetes is a well recognised association of Friedreich's ataxia. It was present in 10% of Harding's patients, often associated with optic atrophy and deafness, and also clustering within sibships. The mean age of onset of diabetes was 25.0 ± 10.64 years. Diabetic coma was the cause of death in some of Hewer's (1968) patients but the youngest of these was aged 19.

The rate of progression of the disease varies but eventually, if the cardiac lesions have not outstripped the neurological deterioration, the patient becomes immobile, helpless and bedridden, sometimes with a severe scoliosis causing gross deformity and adding to his cardiopulmonary problems. Death often occurs in the third decade of life.

Differential diagnosis

The differential diagnosis in a typical case is not difficult. It includes other syndromes with progressive ataxia, particularly ataxia-telangiectasia in which the ocular and skin changes of dilated blood vessels, the frequent tendency to infections and the lack of pes cavus and spinal deformity usually point to the diagnosis. Peroneal muscular atrophy, familial spastic paraplegia and other syndromes with cerebellar ataxia and polyneuritis show sufficient differences to prevent confusion, but it is likely that many cases of the syndrome with early onset cerebellar ataxia with retained tendon reflexes (Harding 1981) are misdiagnosed as Friedreich's ataxia. This condition is described below with the clinical and other points of distinction.

Investigation

Investigations are confirmatory rather than conclu-sive. Spine X-rays often show kyphoscoliosis. Chest X-rays may show cardiac enlargement and the ECG confirms the presence of a cardiomyopathy (Fig. 8.2) sometimes with excessive muscle tremor in the limb leads. The contribution of the CT scan is not often of positive value in Friedreich's ataxia, since it rarely shows cerebellar atrophy (Langelier et al 1979); it is of value, however, in excluding cerebellar tumours and hydrocephalus.

Nerve conduction studies in Friedreich's ataxia must be detailed if they are to be of value, since measurement of the motor nerve conduction velocity alone may fail to show evidence of a peripheral neuropathy. Dunn (1973) in a study of nine patients with the disease aged between $2\frac{1}{2}$ and $21\frac{1}{2}$ years found only normal or slightly slow conduction velocity in the motor fibres of the median and lateral popliteal nerves, contrasting with marked reduction or absence of sensory action potentials in the median and ulnar nerves and of the ascending nerve action potentials in the lateral popliteal nerves. He found that this pattern of results in motor and sensory nerves was helpful in the early diagnosis of Friedreich's ataxia and was not found in peroneal muscular atrophy, or in other diseases in which cerebellar ataxia and polyneuropathy might co-exist. Harding (1981) found the mean motor nerve conduction velocity in the median nerve to be slightly reduced in 22 patients. Sensory action potentials (SAP) were abnormal with at least one SAP absent in 24 of 26 patients studied.

No diagnostic biochemical investigations were previously available but Blass and his colleagues (1976) showed low activities of the pyruvate and oxoglutarate dehydrogenase complexes in five patients with Friedreich's ataxia and these studies may have implications for other disorders with ataxia (Cavanagh 1978). Availability of the assay of these enzymes in cultured skin fibroblasts is a limiting factor at present.

Treatment

No effective basic treatment is yet known though a ketogenic diet based on the presumed enzyme defect has been suggested (Falk et al 1976).

Physiotherapy and symptomatic treatment of the cardiac condition may be beneficial.

The role of orthopaedic surgery in Friedreich's

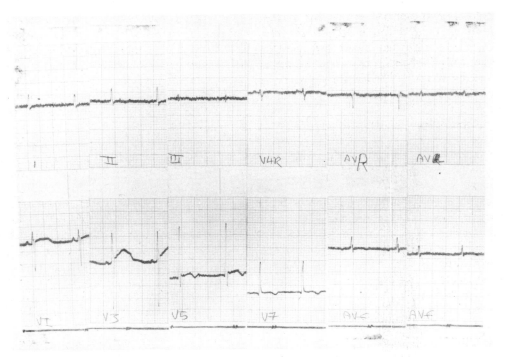

Fig. 8.2 Friedreich's ataxia. ECG in 14-year-old boy showing T wave abnormalities in all leads, leftward axis, and low voltage in limb leads. Note excessive muscle tremor in limb leads.

ataxia is still controversial. Surgical procedures to stabilize the foot have often been associated with avascular necrosis, non-union of the talonavicular joint, and unsatisfactory correction of the deformity. However, Levitt and his colleagues (1973) have reported excellent or good results in three of four patients. All those with satisfactory results had a triple arthrodesis with appropriate soft-tissue procedures when indicated. The aim of their surgery was to prolong the ability to walk for as long as possible, by correcting the existing foot deformity. Clearly the patient's neurological status, particularly the degree of ataxia, is an important factor in selection for operation, but in suitable cases surgery has a contribution to make and should be considered.

Pathology

The most striking pathological changes are seen in the peripheral and central nervous system and in the heart. Motor nerve fibres and anterior horn cells are usually normal, but sensory nerve fibres, posterior roots and ganglion cells show degenera-

tion. The pyramidal tracts are least affected at brainstem level and show progressively greater involvement as they reach lower levels. The spinocerebellar tracts are also affected. Lesions in the brain itself are less constant and less well documented. Loss of nerve fibres has been seen in the optic tracts, sometimes with cell loss in the lateral geniculate bodies.

At necropsy the heart is usually found to be enlarged, sometimes with pericardial adhesions. Microscopically there is interstitial fibrosis with necrosis or granular degeneration of some fibres and hypertrophy of others. Sometimes diffuse or focal cellular infiltration is seen. Intracardiac thrombosis is a common finding. Cerebral complications of the cardiac disease are not uncommon with diffuse hypoxic damage or focal infarcts caused by emboli from mural thrombi in the heart.

FAMILIAL SPASTIC PARAPLEGIA (FSP)

A slowly progressive spastic paraplegia is occasionally seen in a familial setting and may show an autosomal dominant or recessive mode of inheritance. Strümpell (1880), whose name is sometimes linked with the condition, reported two brothers who developed progressive weakness and spasticity mainly affecting the legs in middle age. He later (1886) reported the pathological findings in one of these and in another, unrelated, case.

The condition most often shows an autosomal dominant pattern of inheritance. It may develop in childhood when it presents as a mild spastic paraparesis, usually with a history of normal motor milestones. In some cases the child may be late in walking, but he has not usually been late in achieving independent sitting, and it is unusual for parents to have noticed stiffness of the legs earlier. A history of prematurity or perinatal problems to explain the disorder is usually absent. The affected children show the classical features of pyramidal dysfunction in their lower limbs, with an equinus gait, hyperreflexia, extensor plantar responses, sometimes ankle clonus and a mild increase in tone. Their upper limbs are usually normal, and there are no abonormalities of the cranial nerves, vision, hearing or intelligence. Their disability is usually much milder than in a case of spastic diplegia classed as cerebral palsy (i.e. due to non-progressive disorder of the immature brain, (Ch. 11) and they may be able to take part successfully in competitive games at school. In some cases it is only the tight heel cords with difficulty in getting the heels to the floor which constitute a problem.

The severity of the condition and its rate of progression vary greatly between families and even within a family, so that some patients remain mobile throughout their lives, which are not shortened, while others may become dependent on wheelchairs. This rarely happens in childhood. The upper limbs commonly remain unaffected or are involved only very late in the course of the disease. Sensory changes and sphincter disturbances are not usually seen.

Autosomal recessive forms have been noted to have an earlier onset and a more rapid progression (Bell 1939), usually presenting under the age of 10 years.

In considering the diagnosis meticulous attention to the family history is needed. One should not merely *ask* if both parents and any siblings are normal, but *examine* them for any evidence of the disease. Minor features in relatives may easily be missed. Affected parents may be unaware of any real disability or may explain it away by various misdiagnoses. The situation in this regard is very similar to that with peroneal muscular atrophy (HMSN).

When it is clear that no relative is affected, and the case is an isolated one, it remains possible that it has arisen as a new mutation or has been inherited as an autosomal recessive. In the absence of a family history or of perinatal abnormality it becomes particularly important to exclude other causes, especially treatable and serious ones. Compression of the spinal cord by tumour or other pathology and spina bifida occulta should be excluded by plain X-rays and, when indicated, myelography.

Neuropathological reports on the condition are few, probably because the disease is so often benign and may be unrecognized. Strümpell's two cases (1886, 1904) both showed lesions almost entirely confined to the spinal cord and consisting of degeneration of the lateral pyramidal tracts, increasing from cervical to lumbar region, with less obvious involvement of anterior corticospinal fibres and slight degeneration of the lateral cerebellar tracts and of the columns of Goll. The motor cortex, internal capsule, basal ganglia and medulla were normal. Behan & Maia (1974) studied six families with uncomplicated dominantly-inherited FSP and examined neuropathological material from two patients. They found similar degenerative changes in the corticospinal tracts and posterior columns.

EARLY ONSET CEREBELLAR ATAXIA WITH RETAINED TENDON REFLEXES

In the course of a study of 200 families with progressive cerebellar and spinocerebellar degenerations Harding (1981) found 20 patients with a distinctive clinical syndrome of progressive cerebellar ataxia developing within the first two decades. It was associated with dysarthria of mild to moderate degree, pyramidal signs in the limbs, normal or increased knee jerks and upper limb reflexes with absent ankle jerks and, in some cases, sensory loss. Other important differences from

Friedreich's ataxia are absence of optic atrophy, cardiomyopathy, diabetes mellitus and severe skeletal deformity. Ten patients had pes cavus, but it was severe in only one case. Mild scoliosis was present in 4 patients. Comparison of these 20 patients with a series of 115 patients with Friedreich's ataxia showed that, although the mean age of onset was very similar (9.42 ± 5.23 years and 10.52 ± 7.4 years), the prognosis was better than in Friedreich's ataxia, the patients remaining ambulant, on average, for more than 10 years longer. Parental consanguinity was present in 3 cases and no patient had affected parents or children, so that autosomal recessive inheritance is likely.

Nerve conduction studies were made in 6 patients and were normal in 4. In 2 cases sensory action potentials were reduced in size, but motor conduction velocity was normal. These findings contrast with those in Friedreich's ataxia in which sensory action potentials are usually absent. 9 patients had CT scans which were normal in 4 cases and showed cerebellar atrophy in 5.

Nine of these 20 patients had been diagnosed as suffering from Friedreich's ataxia at some stage of their disease. Some idea of the relative frequency of the condition can be gained from an analysis of Harding's 200 families: in addition to the 20 patients there were 90 families with Friedreich's ataxia, 29 with hereditary spastic paraplegia, 11 with late onset cerebellar ataxia of autosomal dominant inheritance, 36 single cases of late onset cerebellar ataxia, and other syndromes. The better prognosis makes it important to distinguish the condition from Friedreich's ataxia.

OTHER, RARER, SPASTIC-ATAXIC SYNDROMES

Familial spastic ataxia

In childhood this has also been described by Hogan & Bauman (1977). Their five patients showed recessive inheritance with no sex preponderance, and with progressive involvement of the cerebellum, corticospinal tracts and ocular system over a period of 5 to 13 years. These cases resemble those described earlier by Sanger Brown (1892). The onset is often insidious and therefore difficult to date accurately. Death has usually followed between 5 and 20 years from onset. The neuropathological findings have been variable, affecting the cerebellum and spinal cord but usually sparing the cerebrum.

The autosomal recessive spastic ataxia of Charlevoix-Saguenay (Bouchard et al 1978)

This is a syndrome affecting an inbred population in an area of Canada where tyrosinaemia and a familial form of callosal agenesis with sensorimotor neuropathy (Ch. 4) are also found. The patients show a typical picture of spasticity, dysarthria, distal muscle wasting, foot deformities, truncal ataxia, absent of sensory evoked potentials in the legs, retinal striation reminiscent of Leber's atrophy and the frequent presence of a prolapsed mitral value. The ankle jerks may be normal or brisk initially, but are absent after the age of 24 years. Pes cavus, equinus and clawing of the toes are common, but true kyphoscoliosis is never seen. The age of onset is early and none of the patients has ever walked normally, but the course is long and progression slow compared with Friedreich's ataxia, with little deterioration after the age of 20 in many cases.

The Troyer syndrome

This is a recessive form of spastic paraplegia with distal muscle wasting and with mild cerebellar symptoms in many cases. It occurs most notably among a genetic isolate of the Old Order Amish in Holmes country, Ohio. The eponym Troyer refers, not to a physician, but to the family in which it was first identified. The disorder was reviewed by Cross & McKusick (1967) in 20 cases. The onset was in early childhood with dysarthria, muscle wasting and difficulty in learning to walk. Progressive spasticity and contractures made walking impossible by the 3rd or 4th decade.

A spinocerebellar degeneration with X-linked inheritance

This was reported by Spira et al (1979) in a kindred of 64 members with 10 individuals affected in 5 generations. The clinical features were delay in walking, slowly progressive ataxia of gait and incoordination in arms and legs, with slowly progressive wasting of muscles in the legs and minimal distal wasting in the arms. Spasticity was found in younger patients but was later succeeded by hypotonia. Weakness of pyramidal type, increased deep tendon reflexes and extensor plantar responses were present. Sensory changes were found only in two older patients with loss of posterior column sensation. There was also slurring dysarthria, variable nystagmus, pes cavus and scoliosis. No patients showed dementia or visual impairment. A sural nerve biopsy in one patient showed changes similar to those of Friedreich's ataxia, but the results of neurophysiological studies were quite unlike those in that disorder, showing preserved sensory action potentials and reduced motor conduction velocity. An important clinical difference from Friedreich's ataxia, in which the average age of death is 26.5 years (Bell & Carmichael 1939), is the far better prognosis; deterioration was slow, with two older patients in wheelchairs by 30, but life expectation did not seem to be affected, one patient dying at the age of 71.

Adrenomyeloneuropathy

A rare X-linked disease has been recognised with a slowly progressive spastic paraplegia, distal symmetrical polyneuropathy, long-standing primary Addison's disease and variable hypogonadism (Griffin et al 1977). This condition has been called adrenomyeloneuropathy and Schaumburg et al (1977) have presented biochemical and pathological evidence that it is a variant of adrenal leucodystrophy (Addison-Schilder's disease) (Ch. 5). Symptoms of adrenal insufficiency have been present in childhood in some cases, but the onset of neurological problems has been in adult life. A family has been reported (Griffin et al 1977) in which a five-year-old boy suffered from typical adrenal leucodystrophy and his 41-year-old maternal uncle from a progressive spastic paraparesis, suggesting the possible occurrence of adrenal leucodystrophy and adrenomyeloneuropathy within the same family. Adrenal biopsy has been used to diagnose adrenomyeloneuropathy in an adult patient (Weiss et al 1980).

Dyck & Lambert (1968b) reported among their families with 'peroneal muscular atrophy' patients in two kinships with a syndrome of spastic para-plegia, weakness of distal muscles and pes cavus, having its onset in childhood.

G_{M2}-gangliosidosis mimicking Friedreich's ataxia

Chronic G_{M2}-gangliosidosis masquerading as a typical Friedreich's ataxia has been described by Willner et al (1981) in 11 patients from four unrelated Ashkenazi Jewish families in the United States. The patients were aged between 11 and 37 years and their clinical features included early cerebellar dysfunction and, later, upper and lower motor neuron disorder. Three older patients, aged from 26 to 37, had dementia or recurrent psychotic episodes. A motor neuropathy was present in three cases.

The activity of β-hexasaminidase-A was deficient in all patients, while their parents showed somewhat higher levels consistent with the heterozygous state.

The olivopontocerebellar atrophies (OPCA)

This neuropathological term was given by Déjerine & Thomas (1900) to a form of chronic progressive ataxia, beginning in middle age, in which atrophy of the cerebellum, pons and inferior olives are conspicuous findings on post-mortem study.

Konigsmark & Weiner (1970) have reviewed this group of conditions. Their classification, based on neuropathological and clinical features, divides them into five different disorders. These are dominant OPCA I, recessive OPCA II, OPCA with retinal degeneration (OPCA III), the Schut-Haymaker type (OPCA IV) and OPCA with dementia and extrapyramidal signs (OPCA V). All are rare with only a few families reported, and all are inherited as autosomal dominants except for OPCA II. The age of onset of ataxia is very variable, but has been in childhood in a minority of cases in OPCA II, III and V. Many of the sporadic cases may be examples of the recessive type II.

ATAXIA-TELANGIECTASIA (LOUIS-BAR SYNDROME)

This recessively inherited disease of childhood is

another example of a multi-system disorder. Though first described by Syllaba & Henner in 1926, it is usually known by the name of Mme Louis-Bar whose report was published in 1941. Since it combines progressive neurological deterioration with ocular and cutaneous telangiectasia, it is occasionally classified with the neurocutaneous syndromes or 'phakomatases' such as tuberose sclerosis and neurofibromatosis. However, as the critical features are the degenerative neurological symptoms it is more logical to consider it with the spinocerebellar disorders. A good review is provided by Boder (1975).

The name ataxia-telangiectasia refers to the main clinical features. Neurological symptoms are the earliest to develop and most often take the form of cerebellar ataxia. Early development is often normal, but when the child starts to walk, which may be at the usual age or somewhat later, ataxia of gait and truncal ataxia become obvious. These worsen and later ataxia is noted in the arms. The rate of progression is usually slower than the rate at which the child develops his normal motor skills and, as a result, the progressive nature of the disease may be masked in the same way as occurs in Duchenne muscular dystrophy. Later titubation and dysarthria develop. In many cases involuntary movements of extra-pyramidal type are seen, usually starting after the ataxia has developed and sometimes coming to dominate the clinical picture. In rarer cases involuntary movements of athetoid, choreiform or dystonic type are the earliest symptom: in the original report of Syllaba & Henner (1926) the patients were described as showing 'double athetosis'.

The ataxia and movement disorder tend to progress to the stage of enforcing a wheelchair existence by the age of 10 or 12 years as independent walking becomes impossible, after which increasing immobility usually imposes severe limitation on further survival, with death generally before adult life is reached. Chest infections (see below) are frequent and these cause the death of many patients. The neurological course, however, is not invariably progressive and I have seen two mildly affected siblings and a more severely affected boy in whom there has been no deterioration and slight improvement over many years.

Mental retardation is common and sometimes there is progressive dementia.

Retarded growth in height and weight are very common, particularly in the children who are prone to frequent and severe pulmonary infections.

On examination the children often show a facial appearance at rest which is dull and flat, but a smile, when stimulated, which has been described as saccharine and slow-spreading.

An essential part of the disease is the telangiectasia, first noticed in the exposed parts of the bulbar conjunctiva as bright red, symmetrical, horizontal streaks radiating from the inner and outer canthi (Fig. 8.3). These are usually not clearly visible before the age of 3 years and increase with age, so that in suspicious cases the eyes must be examined at intervals before one can be certain that the problem is not merely one of conjunctivitis. Later telangiectases develop in exposed areas of the skin, particularly the pinnae of the ears, the butterfly area of the face, the V area of the neck and the flexures of the elbows and knees.

Almost all patients show a defect of voluntary control of external ocular movements, which is sometimes regarded as a form of oculomotor dyspraxia. The eye movements on attempted following of a visual lure or attempted movement to command have a jerky, broken-up character rather similar to that seen in patients with Huntington's chorea.

Speech is often slurred and dysarthric and tongue movements are impaired.

The degree and character of the motor disorder in the limbs depends on the age of the patient and the stage of the disease, varying degrees of cerebellar ataxia and extrapyramidal involuntary movements being found. At times large range jerky movements of the arms are seen in children with severe cerebellar dysfunction which are reminiscent of myoclonic jerks but are probably of cerebellar origin. Seizures are in fact uncommon in this disorder.

Deep tendon reflexes are normal at first but tend to become reduced or absent later in the course of the disease. The plantar responses usually remain flexor, although occasional extensor responses are seen.

Sensory examination is usually normal in the ear-

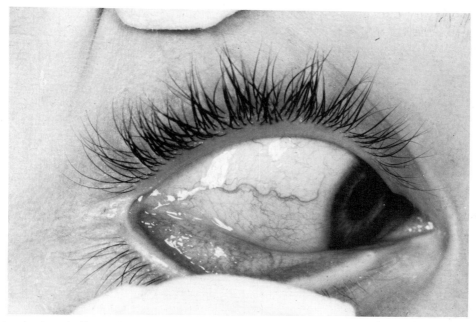

Fig. 8.3 Ataxia-telangiectasia. 7-year-old boy with marked conjunctival telangiectasia.

lier stages but patients surviving for more than 10 to 15 years may develop distal weakness and wasting, with loss of joint position sense and vibration.

Skeletal deformities are less common than in Friedreich's ataxia, and pes cavus is rare. Scoliosis and equinovarus deformity of the feet are seen in a minority of patients.

There may be some variation between the severity of the condition in affected siblings. This was striking in the patient reported by Amronin et al (1979), with the longest recorded survival. She died one day before her 32nd birthday from T-cell leukaemia, whereas her affected sister had died at $10\frac{1}{2}$ years from pneumonia and bronchiectasis.

Involvement of other systems in ataxia-telangiectasia

1. Immunological

Many children with this disease show an increased incidence of infections of the upper and lower respiratory tract. These sino-pulmonary infections, affecting the nasal sinuses and middle ear as well as the lungs, may occur as early as the first year of life but usually only become troublesome after the

age of 3 or 4 years. In severe cases recurrent episodes of lung infection cause structural changes of bronchiectasis, and progressive respiratory insufficiency may lead to death, even when the neurological deficit is relatively mild, since there is no close correlation between the severity of the neurological and infectious problems.

The tonsils are hypoplastic and biopsy shows poor follicular development and failure of secondary crypt formation. Examination of the throat may thus be helpful in this disorder as in the rare Tangier disease.

A series of 18 children with ataxia-telangiectasia was studied in detail from the point of view of infections and immunological abnormalities by McFarlin et al (1972). The children could be divided into three groups of roughly equal size with regard to their infectious problems. Six patients had frequent and severe infections associated with progressive lung disease (Group I), five had an increased incidence of infections not associated with progressive lung disease (Group II) and seven showed only a normal incidence of infections. Humoral immunity was studied by measurement of immunoglobulin levels in serum and saliva studies of immunofluorescence and immunoglobulin metabolism and antibody production. The abnormal findings included reduced synthesis of IgA in 73% of cases, slightly reduced synthesis of IgG in 18% and abnormal IgM in 78%. Cellular immunity was investigated by skin tests to common antigens, allograft survival and study of lymphocyte levels, lymphocyte transformation and morphology of lymphoid tissues. Analysis of the three clinical groups in terms of immunological defects showed that severe defects in both humoral and cellular immune systems were associated with progressive respiratory infection often leading to pulmonary insufficiency and death (Group I). Patients with profound defects in cellular or humoral immunity, but not both, generally had increased respiratory disease which was non-progressive and not life-threatening (Group II). The Group III patients with no increased incidence of infections showed either no detectable immunological defects or mild defects in either system.

Autopsy was performed in three patients in Group I; the thymus was undetectable in one case and very poorly differentiated in two others, showing a stage of development corresponding to that seen in the human fetus by the end of the third month of gestation. Similar findings have been reported by other authors and abnormal histology has also been noted in lymph nodes with severe depletion of lymphocytes. The importance of the thymus in the immunological defects of ataxia-telangiectasia seems clear, but the thymic defect alone cannot explain them and other factors may be involved, since neither congenital absence of the thymus nor thymectomy results in total absence of IgA, and attempts to treat patients with the disease by transplanting fetal thymus have been unsuccessful.

2. Neoplastic disease

Malignant disease of various types has been reported in patients with ataxia-telangiectasia with a significantly increased frequency. The diseases encountered included lymphoma, sarcoma, lymphosarcoma, leukaemia, Hodgkin's disease, cerebellar neoplasms, ovarian dysgerminoma and gastric carcinoma.

3. Haematological features

Lymphocytopenia is common in this disease, the other types of leucocyte being normal.

4. Endocrine disorders

Abnormal carbohydrate metabolism is also common. It occurred in nine of the patients reported by McFarlin and his colleagues, consisting in its severe form of glucose intolerance, raised fasting plasma insulin levels, excessive insulin production in response to glucose and tolbutamide, and failure of insulin to reduce blood sugar levels. These abnormalities were rarely associated with glycosuria and never with ketosis. They were not associated with increased steroid excretion or growth hormone levels and their cause is not clear.

Investigations

Until some years ago the diagnosis was basically a clinical one, since there was no investigation which could be considered pathognomonic. In 1972, Waldmann and McIntire reported the results of estimation of serum-α-fetoprotein in 20 patients with ataxia-telangiectasia and in all cases the levels were above 30 ng per ml. Normal levels were found in the parents and siblings of the patients and in series of normal children and adults and patients with other immunodeficiency states. The measurement of serum-α-fetoprotein provides a valuable test for the disease. The synthesis of this fetal protein of hepatic origin by patients with ataxia-telangiectasia suggests that the liver is not fully developed and that there may be a primary defect in tissue differentiation.

Enhanced in vitro radiosensitivity has been shown in this disease, and this may also be exploited diagnostically. A high frequency of chromosome abnormalities after in vitro irradiation of lymphocytes from patients was shown by Taylor et al (1976). Cultured skin fibroblasts from patients show increased sensitivity to X-ray inactivation (Cox et al 1978) and this is also of diagnostic value.

Neurophysiological studies of peripheral nerve function may be helpful, but as in Friedreich's ataxia, must be detailed if they are to be of value.

Motor nerve conduction velocity may be normal, but in two older patients reported by Dunn (1973) it was slower than in controls and similar to that found in Friedreich's ataxia. By contrast, Dunn found only mild electrical evidence of sensory neuropathy in the same two children, aged 13 and 17 years, so that the sensory neuropathy of ataxia-telangiectasia appears to develop later or more slowly than in the other disease. Biopsy of the sural nerve in three children seen at the Hospital for Sick Children, Great Ormond Street, showed only mild chronic axonal degeneration selectively affecting large diameter fibres with some evidence of regeneration.

Pathology

Changes are most marked in the cerebellum, the vermis often being grossly atrophic with degeneration of granular and Purkinje cells. Degeneration of the posterior columns has also been reported in a few cases. Although dilated meningeal veins have been noted occasionally, there is no constant abnormality of blood vessels comparable to the oculo-cutaneous telengiectasia.

The lungs show the changes of recurrent infections and the thymus is absent or rudimentary and lacks Hassall's corpuscles, while lymphoid tissue generally is reduced. Hypoplasia of the gonads, especially the ovaries, may be seen.

OTHER RARER FORMS OF CEREBELLAR SYSTEM DEGENERATION

There are several other much rarer cerebellar system degenerations, whose clinical and pathological classification is difficult.

Oppenheimer (1976) classifies the cerebellar system degenerations, in addition to the relatively common Friedreich's ataxia, into cerebellar cortical degeneration of the type described by Gordon Holmes (1907) affecting four siblings in their fourth decade, and pontocerebellar or olivopontocerebellar atrophy as described by Menzel (1891) and by Déjèrine and Thomas (1900). Such cases are very rare, and their diagnosis in life is extremely difficult, although it may be suspected when all other progressive cerebellar diseases have been excluded or, a fortiori, when the diagnosis has been established at autopsy in a previously affected sibling. There may be considerable variation in the distribution and severity of the lesions in a single family.

A recessively inherited form of cerebellar ataxia is occasionally seen with early onset and associated optic atrophy, spasticity, posterior column sensory loss and mental retardation. The name 'Behr's syndrome' is sometimes applied to this combination and the condition appears to be relatively non-progressive. Peripheral neuropathy was also present in two sisters with Behr's syndrome reported by Landrigan et al (1973).

Dentatorubral atrophy (Ramsay Hunt syndrome) and progressive myoclonic epilepsy (Lafora Body disease) are considered in Chapter 5.

MENKES' SYNDROME; KINKY OR STEELY HAIR DISEASE; TRICHOPOLIODYSTROPHY

Various names are applied to this X-linked disease with abnormal absorption of copper, which was first described by Menkes and his colleagues in the United States in 1962, and is perhaps still most usefully designated by his name. The first report concerned five boys with severe psychomotor retardation, seizures, abnormal hair, failure to thrive and widespread cerebral and cerebellar degeneration. Progressive deterioration led to death by the age of three years. Similar reports from other areas have all been consistent with an X-linked recessive mode of inheritance and a metabolic error. The nature of this was at first unknown, but the constant finding of abnormal hair led Danks and his colleagues (1972) to investigate copper metabolism in infants with kinky hair disease in Australia (where its frequency in Victoria was estimated at 1 in 35 000 live births) since copper-deficient sheep were known to grow abnormal wool and to show vascular changes similar to those of affected children. These workers found that serum copper and copper oxidase (caeruloplasmin) levels were extremely low in all patients examined. Since no nutritional cause for copper deficiency was present, and oral administration of copper failed to raise serum levels, a defect of copper absorption seemed likely and this was proved by studies using oral radioactive copper with the finding of low copper levels in liver and brain tissues. It now seems probable that all the main features of the disease stem directly or indirectly from copper deficiency due to failure of absorption.

Many affected boys are born prematurely, and these may encounter the normal hazards of premature delivery. Many appear normal in the newborn period, but hypothermia is a common neonatal problem. The earliest developmental milestones such as social smiling, visual following and achieving a degree of head control, are usually normal, but thereafter symptoms begin, often with seizures at 6 or 8 weeks of age followed by slowing in the rate of developmental progress and physical growth. The tempo of slowing varies from one case to another but the infant is usually obviously retarded by a few months of age and his height and weight generally drop towards the third centile by one year (Singh & Bresnan 1973). Careful attention to the child's hair may suggest the diagnosis. The primary fetal-type hair is often normal, but when the secondary hair appears it is clearly abnormal. It is often stubbly and white or the colour of old ivory, stiff, lack-lustre and easily tangled. Danks et al (1973) have suggested that the term 'steely-hair syndrome' is more accurate than the earlier term 'kinky', which suggests the crinkly hair of the African. The hair looks and feels like steel wool. Microscopical examination shows twisting of the hair round its longitudinal axis, like a plaited rope (pili torti), with a frayed, nodular appearance (trichorrhexis nodosa) to the numerous broken ends. It may show a segmental narrowing (monilethrix) at the site of a single twist. It is helpful to examine hair with the naked eye against the background of a black surface, such as a card or book, held beside the child's scalp. Scanning electron-microscopy shows the typical changes more clearly, both in patients and in some carriers (Taylor & Green 1981).

Progressive deterioration continues with the development of increasing spasticity and seizures, failure to thrive, a tendency to frequent infections and often extreme misery and irritability. Subdural haematomas are commoner in affected boys than in other children, and this, together with radiological changes in long bones, may raise the false suspicion of non-accidental injury. (It should be remembered, however, that children who are abnormal are more frequent victims of baby-battering than normal infants.) The seizures, which are mainly grand mal in type but can include typical infantile spasms, are often very resistant to anticonvulsant treatment. Problems with hypothermia may continue beyond the newborn period.

Investigation

The basic investigation is measurement of the serum or plasma copper and copper oxidase (caeruloplasmin) levels which are found to be low. Low copper levels are also found in liver removed at biopsy, but this investigation is not justified as a routine.

Radiological investigations may be helpful. Skull X-rays often show an increased number of Wormian bones in the sagittal and lambdoid sutures. X-rays of long bones and ribs may show widening of the metaphysis with lateral spurs which may become fragmented or fractured. Subperiosteal formation of new bone may also be seen, and these changes resemble those seen in non-accidental injury and scurvy. Arteriography of the cerebral, visceral and limb circulation shows tortuous and elongated arteries with irregular lumen, some of them being occluded.

The EEG is abnormal, and becomes more so as time passed (Friedman et al 1978). Variable discharges are seen and often no normal rhythmic activity is detectable. A hypsarrythmic pattern is sometimes seen, particularly in children with infantile spasms.

Fibroblasts cultured from skin biopsies have shown metachromatically staining granules with toluidine blue in primary culture, but not in serial subcultures, in some patients and heterozygotes.

Treatment

Symptomatic treatment of fits with anti-convulsants is needed, but is often ineffective when seizures are severe and frequent.

Demonstration of abnormal absorption of copper as a constant biochemical finding in Menkes' syndrome, and presumably, as a basic aetiopathogenic factor, led to the hope that the disease could be effectively treated by parenteral copper administration and deterioration prevented. Sadly this hope has not been fulfilled. The chelate, copper EDTA, is known to reverse copper deficiency in the sheep and it has therefore been given regularly by intramuscular injection to many patients. In a 14-month-old boy so treated (Walker-Smith et al 1973) plasma copper and copper oxidase levels rose to normal but there was no improvement in the neurological features and the child died of bronchopneumonia three months later. In theory, the earlier treatment is started the better the chance of benefit resulting, but six children have now been treated at the Hospital for Sick Children, Great Ormond Street, from as early as three months of age, and despite the expected rise in plasma copper and caerulopasmin, no clinical improvement has resulted, with the sole exception that the hair has often become more normal and luxuriant. The latest age at death was six years. One patient starting treatment at 28 days of age showed more encouraging progress at 6 months (Grover & Scrutton 1975). Copper deficiency is probably involved so early in disturbing the normal function of the nervous system (by effects on enzyme systems and blood vessels) that treatment would need to be applied in a pre-symptomatic stage. At present the situation is frustrating since treatment which in theory should be effective is in practice of no value. Further advances are needed and are likely to make treatment possible.

Pathology

At necropsy the brain is usually small and atrophic, often with cystic changes and sometimes with an unsuspected subdural haematoma.

Widespread vascular changes are seen in both the cerebral and general vasculature. Tortuosity, elongation and irregularity of the lumen of cerebral arteries as well as renal, common iliac and lower limb arteries were found on aortography and at necropsy in the patients reported by Danks et al (1972). Microscopically the arterial walls show fragmentation of the internal elastic lamina with thickening of the intima in the most severely affected vessels. The diffuse neuronal damage, gliosis

and cystic changes seen in the brain are probably due, at least in part, to vascular insufficiency.

Barnard et al (1978) have reviewed the neuropathology in three personal cases and in eight previously reported. They emphasise that the pattern of the disease indicates impaired antenatal and postnatal development, complicated by later degenerative changes in the CNS.

Haas et al (1981) have recently described an X-linked neurological disease with disordered copper metabolism and features differing from Menkes' disease. Four cases occurred in two generations of one family. The similarities to Menkes' syndrome were X-linked recessive inheritance, marked retardation with seizures, low serum copper and caeruloplasmin levels, and a block in gut copper absorption. The differences were normal birth weight at term, absence of hypothermia and survival to a later age with static neurological features, including hypotonia and choreo-athetosis. Two boys also had undescended testes and growth retardation.

THE LESCH-NYHAN SYNDROME

(Hyperuricaemia and hyperuricosuria with mental retardation, choreo-athetosis and self-mutilation)

Clinical and biochemical features

This rare and distinctive X-linked disorder, an inborn error of purine metabolism, was first reported in Germany and Britain but described in fuller biochemical and clinical detail by Lesch & Nyhan (1964). The clinical features are progressive retardation of mental and motor development starting in the first six months of life, choreo-athetoid movements and opisthotonic spasms developing usually in the second year and later replaced by spasticity and self-mutilation. The last feature, which is virtually pathognomonic of the disease in the clinical context described, usually appears in the third or fourth year of life. The affected boys appear compelled to bite their fingers, arms and lips and soon inflict horrifying injuries on these parts, often biting their fingers to the bone (Fig. 8.4) and sometimes amputating their finger-

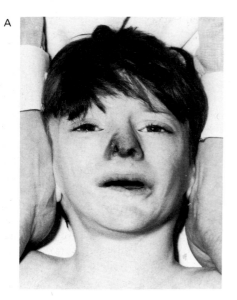

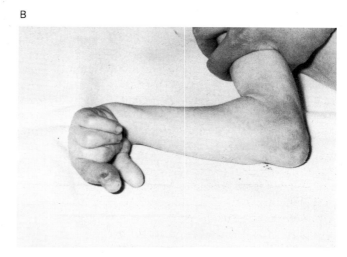

Fig. 8.4 Lesch-Nyhan syndrome. 7-year-old boy: A. showing mutilated nose and lips B. dystonic posture of arm. Note mutilated finger.

tips. Often the lower lip is chewed away and the tongue may be scarred (Fig. 8.4A). Self-injury may also be directed to the nose, which may be scratched and torn away, and to the eyes so that the corneae may be scarred by repeated scratching with the finger-nails. This pattern of self-mutilation is quite different from the common tendency to self-injury shown by many retarded children of either sex in whom head-banging and hair-pulling are particularly common. It more closely resembles the self-mutilation seen in some children of either sex with so-called 'congenital indifference to pain' due to a congenital sensory neuropathy, (Ch. 4) often recessively inherited, although in these the tendency to bite the fingers is often noticed at an earlier age, and the children do not seem to feel pain and often sustain accidental injury such as burns or fractures without any reaction. By contrast the boys with the Lesch-Nyhan syndrome appear to be disturbed and frightened by their compulsion to hurt themselves, and often seem to be happier when restrained from doing so (Berman et al 1969).

The clinical features show clear progression in the successive development of retardation, involuntary movements and self-mutilation, but the patients may survive until the third decade, usually developing haematuria and renal calculi and often dying of renal failure secondary to the persistent hyperuricaemia and hyperuricosuria. Subcutaneous tophi of urates and gouty arthritis may develop, usually late in the illness, although this was present in the report on the first British case, on 'Gout and cerebral palsy in a three-year-boy' (Riley 1960).

Levels of uric acid are grossly raised in serum, urine and cerebrospinal fluid and the turnover rates of uric acid are excessive, being approximately six times that of gouty adult subjects. The formation of uric acid from glycine in affected patients exceeds that of control patients by 200 times. These metabolic disturbances are due to deficiency in brain, liver fibroblasts and red blood cells of the specific enzyme hypoxanthine-guanine-phosphoribosyl-transferase (HG-PRT), which normally catalyses the conversion of hypoxanthine to hypoxanthine ribosylphosphate, so allowing hypoxanthine to be re-used for nucleotide synthesis. As its re-use is prevented hypoxanthine is either excreted or broken down to xanthine and uric acid. Attempts have been made to treat the disease with allopurinol, a xanthine oxidase inhibitor which blocks the last steps of uric acid synthesis. This reduces the high levels of uric acid in blood and urine, causing an equivalent rise in hypoxanthine and xanthine, which carries the risk of replacing uric acid stones by xanthine stones. Clinically the renal tract and gouty problems may be helped, but unfortunately there is no evidence of improvement in any of the neurological features.

Treatment

Apart from allopurinol treatment, drug therapy has recently been directed towards reducing the self-mutilation, a feature which relatives and attendants alike find intensely distressing. Excellent results were reported by Mizuno & Yugari (1975) from the use of L-5 hydroxytryptophan in four boys with the Lesch-Nyhan syndrome, but no such improvement was found by Anderson et al (1976) in four other patients treated with the same drug alone or in combination with Carbidopa when compared with a placebo nor by Anders et al (1978) in their patient. Good results have been obtained with diazepan in some patients.

The judicious use of physical restraints to reduce self-injury is very important (Berman et al 1969) and techniques of behaviour modification may be helpful.

The choreo-athetoid movements are unfortunately not usually influenced by drug treatment.

Pathology

Neuropathological studies of the disease have been limited. In the case reported by Sass and his colleagues (1965) a boy of 11 years who died with uraemia and septicaemia, multiple lesions of vascular and demyelinating type were seen in the cerebral and cerebellar white matter of the brain with discrete focal infarcts of the cerebellar folia and degeneration of its granule cell layer. These changes resemble those seen in various uraemic states. The brains of two brothers aged 11 months and 4 years examined by Crome & Stern (1967) were smaller than usual with cortical neuronal loss and astrocytic hyperplasia in the molecular layer of the cortex.

WILSON'S DISEASE (HEPATOLENTICULAR DEGENERATION)

In 1912 Kinnier Wilson in an article on 'Progressive lenticular degeneration: a familial nervous disease associated with cirrhosis of the liver' published the classic description of the disease that came to be known as Wilson's disease. This is one of the recessively-inherited inborn errors of metabolism (with a carrier rate of about 1 in 140), affecting the handling of copper with resultant accumulation of the metal in the brain, liver, kidneys and cornea. Despite its rarity it is of more importance to the clinician than many commoner neuro-metabolic disorders because it can be simply and effectively treated and its otherwise progressive course halted. The explanation for the accumulation of copper in the tissues, which causes the pathological changes, is not clear, but the available evidence favours a defect in biliary excretion of copper rather than excess intestinal absorption of the metal.

Clinically the presenting symptoms, though variable, can be classified as either hepatic or neurological in type. In the United Kingdom, Walshe (1970) showed in his series of 71 patients that the age of ten years is a watershed, since below this age Wilson's disease always presented as a hepatic illness, with jaundice, failure to thrive, fluid retention or abdominal pain, whereas above this age neurological symptoms predominated and hepatic features were less common. The earlier hepatic form of the disease seems to resemble other types of chronic or subacute liver injury in children except for the common association of a mixed hepatic and haemolytic jaundice. Its early recognition is important so that effective treatment can be started early since without this the hepatic illness progresses and is often rapidly fatal. Occasionally patients have been known to recover spontaneously from their hepatic failure and to present later with neurological symptoms. Other patients give no history of liver disease at all. In a combined series of United Kingdom patients and Chinese patients from Taiwan, Strickland et al (1973) showed a similar association between early onset and hepatic features contrasting with later onset and neurological symptoms, but found that some children under the age of ten did present with CNS dysfunction.

A recent Japanese series of 49 children with Wilson's disease treated under the age of 15 years (Arima et al 1977) did not show this association so clearly. In the 26 patients with cerebral symptoms alone or combined with hepatic symptoms the former began between the ages of 6 years 9 months and 13 years 11 months, in 10 cases under the age of 10.

The neurological features are very variable and Walshe (1970) stresses this by saying that no two patients are ever quite the same and that there is no such thing as a typical case of Wilson's disease. The onset of neurological symptoms is often so insidious, as with many other progressive disorders of the nervous system in childhood, that it cannot be dated with certainty. In school-children there is often a complaint of slowly deteriorating work sometimes attributed to laziness, naughtiness or psychological factors and referral to a psychiatrist may follow. If the child is fortunate, the psychiatrist will quickly recognize the organic nature of the disease when tremor or other movement disorder appears. If he is less lucky he may have deteriorated grossly both physically and intellectually before recognition dawns. The grosser types of movement disorder which follow, in varying degrees and combinations, are tremor, cerebellar ataxia, titubation, dystonia, rigidity and a Parkinsonian-like bradykinesia with immobile face and stooped posture. The facial appearance is commonly of a facile grin, retracted upper lip and drooling mouth (Walshe 1970). Examination of the nervous system shows a variety of cerebellar, extrapyramidal and later pyramidal deficits. Tremor and involuntary movements of dystonic or choreo-athetoid type may be unilateral to start with, but usually become generalised later if treatment is not given. The dystonic movements and postures may (as in dystonia musculorum deformans, from which Wilson's disease must be distinguished) be very variable and brought out by physical effort, as when the patient jumps or runs, or by mental effort, as in attempting calculations, or embarassment. This variability often leads, as with torsion dystonia, to a diagnosis of conversion hysteria. Speech is often grossly affected by an explosive, cerebellar dysarthria with difficulty in control of breathing and of tongue movements; sometimes it is faint and monotonous and heard with great difficulty. As in many neurological disorders, the handwriting and drawings of the patient repay study, and provide a simple permanent record of the progress of the disease. School books may show changes in the writing from normal to a crabbed, tiny hand, as in Parkinsonism, or give evidence of involuntary movements causing the pen to jerk away from its intended course.

The pathognomonic sign of Wilson's disease is the Kayser-Fleischer ring, a brown or greenish-brown layer of pigment in Descemet's membrane on the deep surface of the cornea. The degree of pigmentation increases with the duration of the untreated illness. It starts as a crescent above the pupil, later appearing as a lower crescent and eventually forming a complete circle which is always broadest in the upper segment. The ring is seen most easily with a blue iris and less easily when it is brown. It is best looked for by examining the eye with a strong light obliquely from above. In doubtful cases the eye should be examined under a slit-lamp microscope or a gonioscope. Without this examination a Kayser-Fleischer ring cannot be confidently excluded.

Investigations

The simplest and best of these (Walshe 1970) are estimation of the urinary excretion of copper, the concentration of copper in the serum and the oxidase activity of the serum which gives an approximate estimate of the serum copper protein caeruloplasmin. In Wilson's disease increased urinary copper excretion is found with low levels or absence of serum copper and caeruloplasmin. These tests can sometimes fail to give a definite diagnosis and there may be difficulty in distinguishing between a pre-symptomatic patient and a heterozygote for the disease. In such doubtful cases a clear answer can usually be obtained from a liver biopsy with estimation of its copper content or from serial radio-active copper studies on serum after an intravenous injection. Occasionally a test dose of penicillamine with measurement of copper excretion in the next six hours will help to resolve the difficulty.

Differential diagnosis

In view of the varying neurological features mentioned this includes many diseases in which tremor, involuntary movements, ataxia, dystonia, rigidity and bradykinesia occur. Thus Sydenham's and Huntington's chorea, cerebellar syndromes, progressive and non-progressive, dystonia musculorum deformans, and juvenile Parkinsonism must be considered. Drug-induced dyskinesia and metachromatic leucodystrophy, in which extrapyramidal features are sometimes seen, also need to be borne in mind.

Treatment

The aim of treatment is to deplete the body stores of copper by establishing and maintaining a negative copper balance. Excellent results can be anticipated in most patients, provided irreparable tissue damage has not occurred before diagnosis, and a return to normal life is possible even for those totally disabled by tremor or involuntary movements (Walshe 1967). The chelating agent penicillamine is widely used. The dose in children depends on age and size, but is not usually less than 0.5 g daily. Toxic reactions are unfortunately not uncommon, and are likely to occur at some stage of treatment, which must be life-long. The most serious complication is the nephrotic syndrome. Thrombocytopenia and purpura are rather commoner and sensitivity rashes may develop soon after starting treatment. Biochemical values should be followed regularly on treatment in order to confirm that the desired 'decoppering' process takes place and is maintained. The aim of treatment should be to reduce the serum copper concentration below 10 μg/100 ml and the serum oxidase activity to near zero, while the basal urine copper excretion should return to the normal range. Neurological signs will disappear slowly when these results have been achieved, but they may take two or three years to do so. The liver abnormalities, clinical and biochemical, will also return slowly to normal and renal tubular defects will also resolve.

Temporary deterioration in neurological symptoms is sometimes seen after starting treatment. It is important to document as fully as possible the neurological deficit before starting treatment as a guide to progress. Thus records of handwriting, ciné films of selected movements, and tape recordings of speech should be made. Walshe (1970) also uses a simple method of recording involuntary movements involving a photographic record of the patient maintaining a posture or making certain simple movements with coloured lights attached to the tips of his fingers.

Few large series of children with Wilson's disease are available but the results obtained in the Japanese series of 49 children treated under 15 years of age (Arima et al 1977) show the importance of early treatment. The prognosis seemed to depend on their clinical condition before starting penicillamine treatment. All 10 asymptomatic children, found on routine examination of the siblings of known patients, remained symptom-free. Twelve of the 13 patients with hepatic symptoms only were apparently normal. The results when treatment began after the onset of cerebral symptoms were less good and depended on the delay in starting therapy, being best when this was under one year. Children with combined hepatocerebral symptoms had a poorer prognosis, not always related to delayed tretreatment, the cerebral symptoms responding less well and more slowly to penicillamine. Maximum recovery was seen 1 to 3 years after the start of treatment.

HUNTINGTON'S CHOREA IN CHILDHOOD

Clinical, genetic and epidemiological aspects

When Dr George Huntington in 1872 described the condition which bears his name, he stressed that one of the features distinguishing this type of chorea from that described by Sydenham was the onset in adult life, other features being its hereditary nature, chronicity and invariable mental deterioration. It is now well recognized, however, that the disease can present in childhood and varying figures are quoted from different series, from Julia Bell's (1934) estimate of 5% of patients presenting under 14 years of age to that of Dewhurst & Oliver (1970) of an incidence of juvenile and adolescent forms between 10.7 and 12.7%.

In adults Huntington's chorea is a rare but well recognized disease with an incidence of about 1 in 25 000 of the normal population, inheritance as a dominant and presentation usually between the ages of 30 and 50 years. It is commonly misdiagnosed and the recognized incidence is probably only a fraction of total cases, since careful family studies will often show relatives in affected pedigrees, dead or alive, in whom the diagnosis can either be established or strongly suspected.

There are many reasons why the diagnosis may be missed in adults and therefore, a fortiori, in children. Often the family history, though well known to relatives of the patient, is concealed from him through mistaken kindness or fear of the effect the knowledge would have on him. Other more respectable and less terrifying labels may be applied by relatives, such as Sydenham's chorea, Parkinson's disease or feeble-mindedness. Sometimes an affected parent has committed suicide or has died from natural causes. Doctors have often failed to recognize the disease, deceived perhaps by suppression or falsification of the family history. Paediatricians, not accustomed to thinking of the disease as occurring in children, are often insufficiently rigorous in their pursuit of the family history, and may fail to insist on seeing a parent who is said to have a neurological illness. A healthy scepticism about the accepted diagnosis in a neurologically abnormal parent is essential. The diagnosis of Parkinson's disease is often made initially in adult patients with Huntington's chorea by neurologists from whom the history of disease in a child is deliberately concealed. In one such personal case when a girl with epilepsy and rapidly progressive dementia was being investigated, it was only the belated appearance of her allegedly 'Parkinsonian' father with typical involuntary choreiform movements and grimaces which allowed the correct diagnosis to be made.

The clinical picture in childhood is so variable that the term 'Huntington's *chorea*' is far from ideal in this age group and phrases such as 'Huntington's disease' or 'striato-cortical degeneration of children in families with Huntington's chorea' have been suggested by some writers. Chorea and choreo-athetosis are much less common in affected children than adults. The clinical picture in childhood is more often dominated by dementia, seizures, reduced movement and rigidity. Epilepsy is common as an early feature. It was a prominent symptom, often with episodes of status epilepticus, in three of 5 cases seen recently at the Hospital for Sick Children, Great Ormond Street. It occurred in five of twenty-four childhood cases in four other series (Markham & Knox 1965, Byers & Dodge 1967, Oliver & Dewhurst 1969, Dewhurst & Oliver 1970), making a total of 27% in the five series. Cerebellar ataxia is also common, and hemiplegia of subacute onset has been seen in one affected child without seizures. In the earlier stages disturbed, withdrawn behaviour and loss of interest in games and lessons may be the only symptoms, and these may understandably be attributed for a time to psychological causes, particularly if an affected parent has recently died of the disease or as happens quite often, committed suicide or has been sent to prison for a criminal offence. Sometimes the child's development has appeared retarded from an early age, perhaps partly in response to the environmental and emotional deprivation in families with this disease, and in such cases a label of non-progressive mental subnormality may be applied and may not be revised for some years, especially if the child is admitted to an institution. Violence is often endemic in affected families, and gross examples of 'non-accidental injury' may be seen in children, as well as more subtle damaging influences. Oliver & Dewhurst (1969) have reported on six generations of ill-used children in a Huntington's pedigree, showing that even when children did not carry the gene themselves the consequences of their unhappy upbringing often resulted in psychiatric and antisocial sequelae.

The hypothesis of 'anticipation' has often been invoked to explain the phenomenon of progressively earlier onset in succeeding generations of families with Huntington's chorea. Doubt has been cast on this concept, however, partly because of the artefact of more diligent observation of the children of a known patient leading to earlier diagnosis, and partly because no doctor's professional life-time is long enough to allow him to study the disease through three or more generations

The size and cost of the problem in Britain are well reviewed in a recent report on Huntington's chorea from the Office of Health Economics (1980). Over 4000 people suffer the symptoms of the disease and another 20 000 or more stand a one in two or one in four chance of developing the condition in later years. It is an extremely expensive disease for the health and social services. For the estimated 500 patients in Britain in institutions such as psychiatric hospitals it has been calculated that the NHS hospital costs imposed by the disease are at least £2.5 million.

Differential diagnosis and diagnostic investigations

For the reasons mentioned above, many incorrect diagnoses are made in children with Huntington's chorea — and their parents. These are well illustrated by the initial diagnoses made in the thirteen patients under 21 in two series (Dewhurst & Oliver 1970). These diagnoses were subnormality (five cases), Friedreich's ataxia (3), Sydenham's chorea (2) and abnormal personality (3). Detailed attention to the family history will in most cases exclude these diagnoses, either as being non-genetically determined or as showing a different clinical picture. There is still uncertainty about the diagnosis of Huntington's chorea in a child when both parents are found normal on careful examination. Features of the disease may not yet have appeared in a parent but may do so later [only 52% of patients had developed chorea by the age of 45 years in a series of 762 patients (Bundey 1973)]. It is also possible that the disease may appear in a child as a new mutation.

When choreiform movements are prominent the possibility that they are caused by phenothiazine drugs should be considered. Care should be taken to exclude Wilson's disease when movement disorder or chorea are prominent, since this is one of the few treatable disorders likely to be confused and, if untreated, carries a grim prognosis.

Laboratory and X-ray investigations in general, however, are not of great value in children with Huntington's chorea, which is basically a clinical diagnosis. Skull X-rays show no specific changes, although the bones of the vault may appear thickened. Atrophy of the caudate nucleus, often regarded as very suggestive in air encephalograms and CT of adults, is not often seen in children with the disease. No constant biochemical test has yet been devised which will confirm the diagnosis. The EEG may be of some value in older patients, showing a 'low-voltage' pattern (Scott et al 1972) but is less useful in children, whose EEGs often show paroxysmal features in keeping with the common occurrence of seizures.

Brain biopsy should not, in my opinion, be considered when the diagnosis is suspected, since it is unlikely to be diagnostic, as the main histological abnormalities are found in the caudate nucleus and

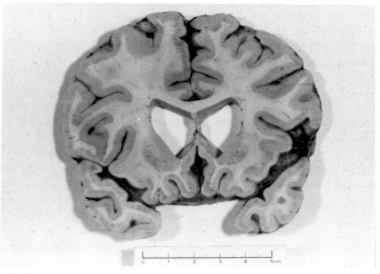

Fig. 8.5 Coronal slice of brain through the striate body showing marked atrophy of the caudate nucleus and putamen. Note enlargement of the lateral ventricles.

putamen (areas which no neurosurgeon is likely to attempt to biopsy). In both these areas extensive loss of small nerve cells is seen with relative preservation of large cells, accompanied by a variable degree of astrocytic proliferation. Other parts of the basal ganglia and the cerebral cortex may also be affected. Grossly the brain shows symmetrical enlargement of the lateral ventricles and atrophy of cerebral gyri, especially in the frontal region (Fig. 8.5).

No basically effective treatment is available and symptomatic treatment is limited to the control of seizures as far as possible with anticonvulsants and the use of drugs such as Reserpine and phenothiazine to reduce the choreiform movements.

Presymptomatic detection

The detection of presymptomatic cases of Huntington's chorea from among the offspring of patients known to suffer from the disease has been attempted in recent years. Klawans et al (1972) have used L-dopa for this purpose in 28 subjects genetically at risk, with 24 control subjects. Chorea developed in the form of facial movements or limb dyskinesia or both in 10 of the 28 adolescents and adults who were candidates for the disease and in none of the controls. The movements always disappeared on stopping the L-dopa. Clearly a long follow-up period is needed to assess how many of those showing transient drug-induced chorea later develop the disease, but it seems likely that a positive response is a useful prognostic sign. The individuals involved were aged between 17 and 32 years. Most of them had sought help in preclinical detection because of their desire for genetic counselling. Increased prognostic accuracy of this kind has eugenic advantages, but these must be balanced against the implications for the individual child or adolescent of the certainty of developing the parental disease with its familiar horrors. Suicide is a common event in these families.

Debatable cases of childhood Huntington's disease

The nosological position of certain cases of striatal degeneration in childhood with neuropathological features similar to those of childhood Huntington's disease is still debated. Roessman & Schwartz (1973) reported two brothers with progressive neurological problems dying at 22 months and $2\frac{1}{2}$ years. The lateral ventricles in both brains were much enlarged due to shrinking of the basal ganglia, especially the caudate nucleus, in which small neurons had almost disappeared while large neurons were preserved. The health of these boys' parents is not mentioned.

Erdohazi & Marshall (1979) reported 3 unrelated children with striatal degeneration. The problem of age of onset are illustrated by one patient whose father developed chorea one year after the child's death. Pathologically all 3 cases showed progressive degeneration of the striate body, both caudate nucleus and putamen being severely affected in 2 cases while only the caudate was badly affected in the third. The authors reasonably concluded that their case with a (later) affected father was an example of juvenile Huntington's disease. It seems likely that their other 2 cases and those of Roessman and Schwartz may be other examples, despite the absence of a positive family history.

DYSTONIA MUSCULORUM DEFORMANS
(Idiopathic torsion dystonia)

Clinical features

The word 'dystonia' and the title 'dystonia musculorum deformans' were both introduced by Oppenheim (1911) who used 'dystonia' to imply abnormal muscle tone without pyramidal deficit. Some neurologists apply the word only to the abnormal postures produced by the disorder of tone and others to the involuntary movements between the postures, but in the context of torsion dystonia it refers to abnormal postures.

Although many different brain diseases can give rise to this type of movement disorder, idiopathic torsion dystonia is now well recognized. The severity and age of onset of this syndrome can vary greatly and there appear to be several genetically distinct types. An autosomal recessive form with onset between four and sixteen years of age is frequent in the United States among Ashkenazi Jews. Another form with dominant inheritance shows a slower evolution and affects a wider ethnic spectrum. Paediatricians in the United Kingdom, by contrast, rarely encounter genetically determined cases, and only exceptionally meet families with more than one affected child. This was the experience in a series of forty-two British patients seen between 1955 and 1970 and reported by Marsden & Harrison (1974) and in a small series of seven personal cases. The sex distribution in Marsden and Harrison's series was almost equal. Six patients came from Jewish families, three were Asian and 33 of 'Caucasian' extraction. No cases of dominant inheritance were seen, and there were only two pairs of affected siblings, suggesting recessive inheritance.

Twenty-five (60%) of the patients developed symptoms under the age of 15 years. The presenting symptoms were strikingly different in those with onset under 15 and at later ages. Although the commonest initial symptoms in the whole series was difficulty in the use of one or both arms, this occurred in only 32% of those presenting under 15, compared with 59% of those presenting later. With younger age of onset symptoms most often started in the legs (52%), whereas this happened in only 12% of those with later onset. Disorders of arm function included writer's cramp (always with impairment of other actions besides writing), dystonic postures of the arm noted when lifting a glass or cup, pouring from a teapot, doing up buttons or carrying out other fine actions, and occasionally spontaneous contractions of the muscles of one arm causing it to jerk and twist and grossly hampering its actions.

The initial disorder of gait was often an abnormal posture of the foot with plantar flexion and inversion as it approached the ground in walking. In many cases the gait disorder was bizarre, producing patterns of walking so strange that conversion hysteria was strongly suspected. In some cases the gait is so peculiar that words are inadequate to describe it, and even when analysed in slow motion by ciné-film, it may still defy description. It is easy to understand how such patients are suspected of 'putting it on' or of imitating the gait of a neuro-logically handicapped relative. The patient may walk sideways like a crab, be able to walk backwards, but not forwards, and to run but not to walk. He may hop on one leg in an attempt to avoid the abnormal posturing of the affected foot induced by walking.

Less common than disordered leg or arm function in children with torsion dystonia are distortion of the neck or trunk with torticollis or tortipelvis. Speech may be affected with a 'strangled' quality when dystonia affects the muscles of articulation.

Examination fails to show neurological signs other than the abnormal postures or movements. In particular the cranial nerves are normal apart from involuntary movements of the face, jaw, tongue and eyelids seen in a few patients, and pyramidal and cerebellar dysfunction are not seen. The patient's intelligence is unimpaired, though his mood may be understandably depressed by realisation of his plight and by the sometimes punitive and usually uncomprehending reactions of family and medical advisers towards it.

Initially the abnormal postures and movements are intermittent, tending to be increased by emotional stress or physical effort. Attempts to write will often increase the jerky movements of an affected arm and in time may force the patient to change to using the good hand, an adaptation which is often made with remarkable ease (Fig. 8.6). Sometimes the child learns to minimise abnormal arm movements by holding his arm against his chest when manipulating a toy or threading beads on to a stick. Later spread to involve other limbs, often with generalised dystonia, is common.

The course of the disease varied greatly in Marsden and Harrison's 42 patients, in half of whom it progressed to involve all the limbs and trunk, as generalized torsion dystonia, the maximum progression usually occurring in the first 5 or 10 years from onset. In over three quarters of patients followed up to the age of 35 or more the disability seemed to become static. In 50% of the patients the disease was confined to one portion of the body and never became generalized (segmental dystonia). The main factors related to outcome in this series of patients were the age and site of onset of dystonia. A younger age of onset and an onset in the legs were associated with the development of generalized dystonia, but a later age of onset and initial involvement of the arms with the condition remaining segmental. However, with onset in the arms progression was also more likely in children than in adults. Analysis of the final disability of the 42 patients showed that only two had died (one by

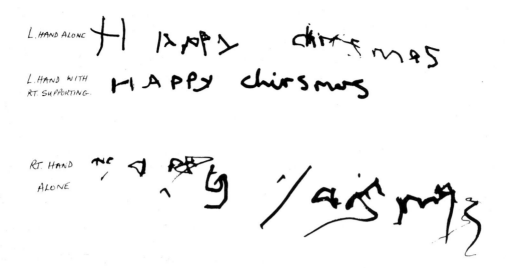

Fig. 8.6 Dystonia musculorum deformans. Writing of 11-year-old boy with severe dystonia in arms, more marked on right than left.

suicide and one of carcinoma of the bladder), approximately a third were bed- or chair-bound, a third were moderately disabled, and a third were mildly disabled but independent. Of 25 patients with onset under 15, 11 were bed- or chair-bound, compared with only 3 or the 17 adult-onset cases. Similar findings were noted in a larger series by Marsden et al (1976).

Investigations

The most important, because treatable, differential diagnosis is Wilson's disease, and this should be excluded in all patients who develop movement disorder, including those who have been referred to psychiatrists. (Hysteria had initially been diagnosed in 43% of Marsden and Harrison's patients, many of whom had had prolonged psychotherapy, while one had been subjected to leucotomy.) Radiological and biochemical investigations are not diagnostic, although raised blood levels of the enzyme dopamine-β-hydroxylase have been reported in some genetically determined cases.

Treatment

Many drugs have been tried and none has proved consistently helpful. Clonazepam has recently been noted to give good results in reducing the more rapid jerky movements. Artane (Benzhexol) has helped some patients. Tetrabenazine, Carbamazepine and Phenothiazines have produced varying degrees of improvement, usually at the expense of a degree of drug-induced pseudo-Parkinsonism. Levadopa has been reported by some workers to be of value, but others have not found it helpful, and it has even been suggested that it may aggravate torsion dystonia (Cooper 1972).

Surgical treatment with stereotactic thalamotomy has greatly helped some patients, particularly those with dystonia confined to an arm or arm and neck. Most patients with progressive generalized dystonia derive at least temporary benefit from bilateral stereotactic surgery. The timing of surgery is important, since it should not be considered until a carefully planned trial of medical treatment with available drugs has been made and found unhelpful. It should be remembered also that occasional remissions lasting some years are seen. There have been impressive developments in stereotactic surgery in recent years, and improved results are likely with further refinements.

Hereditary progressive dystonia with diurnal variation

A variant of idiopathic torsion dystonia has been described in Japan (Segawa et al 1976). Nine patients with hereditary progressive dystonia showing marked diurnal variation were seen, 6 of them from 3 families. The onset of symptoms was between 16 months and 9 years of age. The dystonia spread gradually from its site of origin in one limb to involve other limbs following the pattern of the letter 'N', i.e. if it started in one leg, it would spread to the ipsilateral arm, and then successively to the contralateral leg and arm. All limbs were affected within 4 or 5 years, the legs being more severely involved than the arms, often asymmetrically. The bulbar muscles were either spared or only mildly affected, and axial torsion was rare and slight. There was no pyramidal, cerebellar or sensory disorder and no intellectual deterioration. A striking feature was marked diurnal fluctuation of the symptoms with worsening over the course of the day and remarkable improvement after sleep. The dystonia was relieved for a time after a daytime sleep, but not by a rest without sleep. Levadopa produced dramatic improvement in the movement disorder. The disorder may be inherited as an autosomal dominant with low penetrance.

Although torsion dystonia may vary greatly from one time to another, such gross short-term fluctuation is unusual among patients seen in the West, and this disorder may be a distinct entity. It will be interesting to see whether cases are recognised in other countries.

JUVENILE PARKINSONISM

For neurologists concerned with adults, Parkinson's disease and Parkinsonian syndromes are among the commoner disorders encountered, but Parkinsonism in childhood is an uncommon condition and most paediatricians have probably never seen a case. The rarity of the juvenile form of the disease was commented on by Ramsay Hunt in 1917 in his report of four patients with 'progressive astrophy of the globus pallidus', two of whom had the onset of symptoms in their early teens. Tremor and rigidity were the main clinical features, as described one hundred years earlier by James Parkinson himself in his 'Essay on the Shaking Palsy'. Hunt regarded the condition as a system disease, or abiotrophy, in the sense in which Gowers used this term.

Juvenile Parkinsonism was not always so rare. After the 1917–1926 pandemic of encephalitis lethargica, Parkinsonism was often seen as a sequela in adults and sometimes in children or adolescents. 80% of all the cases of post-encephalitic Parkinsonism had developed their symptoms within 10 years of the infection (Duvoisin & Yahr 1965) and this resulted in a 15 years reduction in the mean age of onset of Parkinsonism in general (Dimsdale 1946). Sacks (1971) pointed out that post-encephalitic cases were occurring long before 1917. Europe in 1580 had been swept by a severe febrile and lethargic illness, or Schlafkrankheit, which led to Parkinsonism and other neurological sequelae. Sydenham described a 17th century epidemic in London, and Albrecht of Hildesheim in 1495 described oculogyric crises and Parkinsonian symptoms following an attack of 'febre lethargica' in a 20-year-old girl. It is probable that cases of juvenile Parkinsonism described by Charcot were also post-encephalitic.

Rare cases of juvenile Parkinsonism are still seen in which a post-encephalitic aetiology is suspected from the history and the occurrence of oculogyric crises (which are not seen in idiopathic Parkinsonism). A benign early onset of Parkinson's disease was described by Scott & Brody (1971) with a possible post-encephalitic causation. They regarded it as a syndrome distinct from classic post-encephalitic Parkinsonism, having an age of onset intermediate between that in several post-encephalitic series and that generally accepted for the idiopathic disease. The youngest age at onset of Parkinsonian symptoms was 14 years, five years after the febrile illness considered responsible. The symptoms of these patients responded particularly well to thalamic surgery. Such cases must be rare in the experience of most paediatricians and paediatric neurologists, but it is wise to be alert to the possibility of the syndrome complicating a viral encephalitis and to realise that this could again become a common occurrence.

At present, however, the clinical picture of juvenile Parkinsonism is more likely to be due to certain rare diseases in which striatal features may occur. These include Wilson's disease, Huntington's chorea and certain forms of olivopontocerebellar degeneration. Some patients with subacute sclerosing panencephalitis (Ch. 22) may show rigidity and hypokinesia of Parkinsonian type as a transient stage of their illness, but the clinical, EEG and other features should allow the diagnosis to be made. Parkinsonian features may also be seen in some patients with juvenile Batten's disease and metachromatic leucodystrophy. Iatrogenic Parkinsonism may follow the use of many drugs, particularly the phenothiazines, reserpine and tetrabenazine, but these cases will not usually cause much diagnostic difficulty. In adults treated with prolonged and massive doses of psychotropic drugs, an irreversible syndrome of drug-induced Parkinson-like disease is sometimes seen, known as tardive dyskinesia, but fortunately this seems to be rare in children.

Wilson's disease is the only one of the progressive diseases giving a Parkinsonian picture for which effective treatment is available, and every effort much therefore be made to exclude it as a cause.

Symptomatic treatment should be tried in other cases of juvenile Parkinsonism with anti-Parkinsonian drugs. Benzhexol (Artane) may be helpful and benefit has been reported from treatment with Levodopa of two brothers in their twenties whose symptoms began in childhood. (Martin et al 1971) and in a younger boy with presumed post-encephalitic Parkinsonism with oculogyric crises reported by Kilroy et al (1972). In general hypokinesia is the feature most improved by Levodopa. The same side-effects of treatment can occur in children as in adults, including distressing involuntary movements and the 'on-off phenomenon' or 'oscillation in performance' with episodes of rapid transient deterioration in the Parkinsonian motor deficit. These oscillations are commonest in patients who have been treated with levodopa for over a year and seem less common when the drug carbidopa is used. Other side-effects include postural hypotension, cardiac arrhythmias and psychological disturbances, of which the commonest are depression, confusion, delirium, agitation and restlessness.

LEIGH'S SUBACUTE NECROTIZING ENCEPHALOMYELOPATHY (Leigh's disease)

Clinical features

In 1951 Denis Leigh of the Maudsley Hospital published the case of a seven month-old-boy who died within six weeks of the onset of a neurological illness with somnolence, blindness, deafness and spasticity. At autopsy he found focal, symmetrical subacute necrotic lesions or softenings in scattered areas from the thalamus to the pons, the inferior olives and posterior columns of the spinal cord. Intense capillary proliferation was present in some of these lesions and in many ways the pathology resembled the changes seen in Wernicke's encephalopathy so that the role of thiamine deficiency in its aetiopathogenesis came to be suspected.

Since then many cases have been reported. The disease is inherited as an autosomal recessive character and appears to affect males and females in a ratio of 3 to 2. A review of 86 reported cases (Pincus 1972) has shown wide variation in the clinical features, which are partly related to the age of onset. In 52 cases this was under 12 months of age and in 78 under 2 years. Only 8 patients had an onset over the age of 2 years. Rare cases with onset in adult life have also been reported, but these need not concern us here.

In cases starting in the first year of life the presenting symptoms were fairly uniform and often insidious. In 45 of the 52 cases weight loss, weakness and psychomotor retardation were prominent, alone or in combination. Vomiting and anorexia were also common. Eight patients had periodic unexplained fevers, often accompanied by acute neurological symptoms such as fits, which occurred in 15 cases. Microcephaly has been reported in several cases, suggesting an onset in very early life, perhaps even prenatally. In 14 children becoming ill after 18 months of age the presenting complaints were much more variable. Six of these showed some form of movement disorder, which included clumsiness, ataxia, falling and loss of ability to walk. Four children showed some degree of mental retardation, mild in some cases and amounting to frank dementia in others. Seizures occurred in 3 cases, vomiting in 2 and hemiplegia in 2.

Disturbances of respiration occurred in over 75% of cases, usually later in the course of the illness, and were the main terminal problem in 60 of the 86 patients. They took the form of dyspnoea, tachypnoea, apnoea, Cheyne-Stokes breathing and ataxic respiration. Episodes of intermittent hyperventilation, sobbing or sighing are useful diagnostic clues and are probably commoner than is realized (de Villard 1970). These can often be provoked by blowing in the child's face or startling him in some way.

The findings on examination depend on the stage the disease has reached. In the earlier phases, there may be few striking neurological symptoms and signs, but in the later stages there is obvious regression, often with disordered respiration, and hypotonia is also often a prominent feature. Reduced or absent deep tendon reflexes were recorded in 21 of 86 cases in the literature and this finding is probably commoner than is reported. Evidence of peripheral neuropathy on nerve conduction studies or sural nerve biopsy has been found in several cases (Reye 1960, Namiki 1965, Robinson et al 1967, Clayton et al 1967, Dunn & Dolman 1969, Moosa 1975). The neuropathy is of demyelinating type. A child reported by Dunn & Dolman (1969) with the disease had clinical and electrical evidence of a relapsing polyneuropathy with two episodes of severe weakness and loss of tendon reflexes, from which he made a fairly good recovery before progressive deterioration began. In some cases tone in the limbs is increased and tendon reflexes may be exaggerated, with other evidence of pyramidal disorder sometimes present in the form of extensor plantar responses and ankle clonus and occasionally a hemiplegia. Varying degrees of cerebellar ataxia may also occur.

Ocular features are sometimes prominent (Montpetit et al 1971). Bizarre involuntary nystagmoid eye movements may be seen episodically and optic atrophy has been noted at a late stage in some cases. Pigmentary changes in the maculae and retinae are not seen.

Seizures, which occur in a minority of cases of Leigh's disease, are usually generalised, but focal and myoclonic attacks and infantile spasms have also been seen.

The course of the illness is usually chronic and relentlessly progressive over at least 6 months, but occasionally its tempo has been subacute or even acute with death within two weeks of onset. Spontaneous remissions occurred in about a quarter of the 86 cases of Pincus, but were usually brief, lasting only a few weeks and often limited to improvement in mood or the ending of an episode of hyperventilation. Exacerbations of the illness

occurring in a step-wise fashion, often in relation to mild intercurrent infections, are very characteristic of Leigh's disease, which may account for some of the previously reported cases of relapsing encephalomyelitis.

More than half of the reported patients have lived for less than a year from the onset of their symptoms, but 30% have survived for more than two years. The longest reported survival has been 15 years (Namiki 1965), but it is possible that milder degrees of the disease, which are not recognised, are compatible with longer life. The lack of a simple, readily available diagnostic test for Leigh's disease makes it possible that statistics are misleading, depending on the severity of the condition and on whether an autopsy is performed or enzymatic studies are arranged.

There seems to be little variation in the age of onset within families with more than one affected child, which seldom varies by more than six months. This is helpful in considering the prognosis for the normal siblings of the affected children. This situation is different for the duration of the illness which has varied by more than $2\frac{1}{2}$ years in five families, so that assessment of any therapeutic measures must take this into account. Sometimes a family history is obtained of a sibling having died acutely in circumstances suggesting that he too may have been a victim of the same disease.

Sipe (1973) has suggested that the term 'Leigh's disease' be confined to the classical infantile cases with recessive inheritance and onset under 2 years of age, and that the much rarer childhood cases with onset between 7 and 14 and adult cases with onset between 21 and 43, both of which are sporadic, should be referred to as 'Leigh's syndrome'. The neuropathological findings are the same in all 3 groups but the course of the illness is more chronic in the older cases in contrast to the subacute course of the infantile form. There is neuropathological evidence that some cases of Leigh's syndrome may be examples of mitochondrial cytopathy (Ch. 3) (Crosby & Chou 1974, Egger et al 1982).

Investigations and treatment

In the past these have not been helpful and the

diagnosis could only be suspected in life, and proved at autopsy, unless a sibling was known to have died of the disease.

The findings of clinical and electrical signs of a peripheral neuropathy will increase the index of suspicion of the diagnosis in the context of a progressive disorder of the central nervous system. Other diseases in which peripheral neuropathy is associated with CNS disease, such as metachromatic and Krabbe's leucodystrophy, neuroaxonal dystrophy and ataxia-telangiectasia, can be excluded by clinical and laboratory findings.

The EEG has not shown any specific abnormalities.

Air encephalography has usually given normal results, but it is not without risk and one patient is known to have died after the procedure. The CT scan is a safer alternative. In some cases it has shown low density areas in the basal ganglia, especially in the lentiform nuclei, with generalized atrophy.

The finding of an elevated protein level and lymphocytic pleocytosis in a few cases is not diagnostically helpful and could lead to a misdiagnosis of encephalitis.

Reports of a few cases with raised blood levels of lactate and pyruvate have led to speculation that there may be a deficiency of pyruvate dehydrogenase or one of its co-factors in some cases of the disease. Some patients diagnosed as having Leigh's disease have been shown to be deficient in pyruvate carboxylase or decarboxylase (Grover et al 1972, Farmer et al 1973). (It is possible that Leigh's disease is a syndrome resulting from deficiency of different enzymes in different cases rather than of one alone).

Investigations of various enzymes requiring thiamine pyrophosphate (TPP) as a cofactor have given equivocal results. The activity of TPP-dependent erythrocyte transketolase in cases of Leigh's disease was studied by McBurney et al (1980). They found no alteration in its activity and concluded that it was unlikely to be of value for the diagnosis of the disorder.

Thiamine triphosphate, which may be the neurophysiologically active form of thiamine, was found to be absent or greatly reduced in the brains of six children dying of Leigh's disease and Pincus (1972) believes that this may be due to a substance which inhibits the enzyme which normally catalyzes the formation of thiamine triphosphate (TTP) from thiamine pyrophosphate (TPP). This inhibitor substance has been found by Pincus in the blood, urine and CSF of patients with the disease, and it is suggested that this can provide a specific diagnostic test. These results have not been confirmed by other workers, however.

If they were confirmed, the logical treatment would be to eliminate the inhibitor substance. At present, however, treatment is based on attempts to restore biochemical normality by giving large doses of thiamine and related substances. Lipoic acid, biotin, thiamine and the pyrophosphate, propyldisulphide and tetrafurfuryldisulphide of thiamine have been used for this purpose, but so far without clinical success. It is certainly justified to try these substances serially or in combination in the hope of obtaining benefit and throwing more light on a lethal and poorly understood disorder.

INFANTILE NEUROAXONAL DYSTROPHY

Spheroid bodies in axons have been reported in various pathological conditions, thought by Seitelberger, (1971) to form a spectrum of related disorders, the neuroaxonal dystrophies, ranging from infantile neuroaxonal dystrophy, [first described by Seitelberger (1952) and sometimes known as 'Seitelberger's disease'] to Hallervorden-Spatz disease. In typical cases of infantile neuroaxonal dystrophy (INAD) spheroid bodies are widely distributed throughout the CNS but are also found in peripheral nerves, especially in nerve endings in intramuscular nerves and in skin and cunjunctiva (Arsenio-Nunes & Goutiéres 1978). In Hallervorden-Spatz disease spheroids are less widespread and are more abundant in the basal ganglia, brainstem and spinal cord, with cortical involvement lacking or less marked. The presence of an iron-containing pigment in the basal ganglia was earlier considered specific for Hallervorden-Spatz disease, but is now known to occur in INAD.

The clinical features of INAD have been reviewed by Huttenlocher and Gilles (1967), Gordon (1978) and Aicardi & Castelein (1979). Aicardi and Castelein have emphasized the clinical picture which they believe is at least as important a criterion for the diagnosis as the neuropathology. They reviewed 50 cases (8 personal and 42 well documented cases from the literature) with pathological proof in 45. There was a characteristic clinical course starting between 6 months and two years of age with slowing, and later loss, of motor and mental milestones, early visual involvement, symmetrical pyramidal tract signs but marked hypotonia, and often evidence of peripheral motor involvement of anterior horn cell type. Seizures and extrapyramidal features were usually lacking. Deterioration progressed with dementia, a decerebrate state and death before the age of 10 years. The CSF protein is usually normal and electromyography often shows signs of denervation with normal nerve conduction velocity. The latter is an important point of distinction from metachromatic and Krabbe's leucodystrophy and indeed from most degenerative CNS disorders. The EEG often shows high voltage fast rhythms, the ERG is preserved, and the visual evoked responses are reduced or absent.

INAD is inherited as an autosomal recessive, with an increased incidence of parental consanguinity, and with the age of onset and clinical course varying little within affected sibships.

Pathologically the diagnosis can be made by electron-microscopy of cortical biopsy material, but peripheral biopsies containing terminal axons, as in muscle end-plate biopsies or biopsies of skin or conjunctiva, provide a reliable and less drastic alternative in experienced hands. The spheroid bodies in axonal endings are not specific to INAD, however, and both clinical and pathological features are needed to make a firm diagnosis.

Juvenile cases of neuroaxonal dystrophy with a later age of onset, a more protracted course, very slow intellectual deterioration and myoclonic epilepsy show the same pathological features as INAD (Scheithauer et al 1978).

Vakili et al (1977) have reported the clinical and neuropathological features of two siblings with the insidious onset of symptoms in the second year of life and inexorable progression to a state of continuous dystonic and athetoid movements with complete loss off speech and death after six years. Radio-active iron studies showed an increase in the uptake of iron in the basal ganglia in one sibling and in another patient. The authors regard these

children as examples of a late infantile form of Hallervorden-Spatz disease.

DISSEMINATED SCLEROSIS IN CHILDHOOD

For most adult neurologists the term 'demyelinating disease' is almost synonymous with disseminated sclerosis. The array of white matter disorders considered in Chapter 5 in which demyelination is prominent and a genetically determined metabolic defect is probable makes the situation very different for the paediatric neurologist.

Disseminated sclerosis is not common in childhood although it certainly occurs. The evidence from the literature is conflicting on the question of how common it is (Wilson 1955, Low & Carter 1956). Kinnier Wilson (1955) reported two examples in 9-year-old girls, and in 1107 cases of disseminated sclerosis in the literature he found an incidence of 2.2% under the age of 10 years, but expressed scepticism about the figure, feeling that many earlier reported cases were not acceptable. He was probably correct in this view, since there is room for doubt about many reports; the case of a 9 year old boy with supposed disseminated sclerosis reported by Westphal in 1888 was a premature report and was withdrawn a year later because the patient was shown to have died of a thalamic tumour. The first autopsy-proved case in a child was reported in 1896 by Eichhorst in an 8 year old boy, and the youngest documented case may be that of Nobel (1911), a child who died at the age of $2\frac{1}{2}$ years.

The problem with many potential cases in childhood is that not enough time has passed for the criteria of dissemination in time and in space to be met, or to be seen not to be met. The paediatrician, who often loses contact with his patient in his teens, is not in a good position to see the later evolution of an illness with relapses and exacerbations which may be spread over many years.

In the series of 40 cases with childhood onset reported by Gall (1958) the peak age of onset was 12 to 13 years. 15 patients had suffered only one episode during childhood and the fully developed picture did not appear until the later teens. In the other 25 cases more than one episode with varied symptoms had occurred by the age of 14.

A common presentation of disseminated sclerosis in adults is with optic or retrobulbar neuritis. Such neuritis in childhood, which is not uncommon, is therefore potentially a harbinger of the disease. Experience varies on how often optic neuritis in childhood proves to be the first sign of disseminated sclerosis. A series of 30 children with optic neuritis of unknown cause with onset between 5 and 15 years was followed up by Kennedy & Carter (1961) and 8 of these were found to have developed disseminated sclerosis at varying times after their original illness. In 6 cases children had developed evidence of dissemination within $2\frac{1}{2}$ years of the optic neuritis, but the other 2 did not do so until 12 and 16 years later. There appeared to be nothing characteristic about the ocular findings to indicate those who would later develop evidence of the disease, but it was noted that bilateral involvement and papillitis were more frequent in children than in adults who later developed disseminated sclerosis. Our own experience of children with unexplained optic neuritis has been different from that of Kennedy and Carter, in that few have so far developed signs of dissemination. Careful follow-up over many years is needed, however, to observe the outcome.

Disorder of gait, with ataxia or spasticity, is also a common presenting feature in children who later prove to have disseminated sclerosis. Seizures are rare as in the adult disease.

The differential diagnosis in childhood includes a host of varied diseases of infectious, para-infectious, toxic, metabolic, vascular and neoplastic type. A relapsing and remitting course may be seen in many of these (for example, relapsing encephalomyelitis, Leigh's subacute necrotizing encephalomyelopathy, Moya Moya disease, homocystinuria, various forms of hyperammonaemia, etc.) but clinical and laboratory features usually indicate the correct diagnosis. Examination of the cerebrospinal fluid in disseminated sclerosis is often of value, showing a moderate pleocytosis with increased protein content and a first or mid-zone colloidal gold curve. More recent advances in the diagnosis of disseminated sclerosis have come with the use of the CT scan which may show areas of low attenuation sometimes enhancing with contrast, which decrease during remission of the disease and probably represent areas of demyelination. These features were seen, for example, in a two-year old boy with multiple sclerosis reported by Brandt et al (1981) in whom the Active-E-rosette test was also positive. This test with the patient's lymphocytes also indicates demyelination. The results of nuclear magnetic resonance imaging of the brain in multiple sclerosis appear to be very promising indeed (Young et al 1981).

NEUROMYELITIS OPTICA: DEVIC'S DISEASE

The simultaneous occurrence of optic neuritis and spinal cord symptoms in children was recognized from 1879 onwards and came to be associated with the name of Devic in 1895. Devic himself considered that the disseminated foci found at autopsy in the brains of patients represented an acute stage of disseminated sclerosis, but his name was nonetheless adopted as the eponym for what came to be regarded as a distinct though rare clinical entity. Whether it is distinct is rather doubtful. The overlap with disseminated sclerosis in childhood is a possible source of confusion and some authorities (e.g. Oppenheimer 1976) frankly regard Devic's disease as a subgroup of 'multiple sclerosis'. There is also no doubt that transverse myelitis and optic neuritis can occur simultaneously as part of a post-infectious encephalomyelitis.

A healthy scepticism therefore seems appropriate when the diagnosis of Devic's disease in childhood is mooted.

REFERENCES

Aicardi J, Castelein P 1979 Infantile neuroaxonal dystrophy. Brain 102: 727–748

Amromin G D, Boder E, Teplitz R 1979 Ataxia-telangiectasia with a 32-year-survival. A clinicopathological report. Journal of Neuropathology and Experimental Neurology 38: 621–643

Anders Th F, Cann H M, Ciaranello R D, Barchas J D, Berger Ph A 1978 Further observations on the use of 5-

hydroxytryptophan in a child with Lesch-Nyhan syndrome. Neuropädiatrie 9: 157–165

Anderson L T, Herrmann L, Dancis J 1976 The effect of L-5-hydroxy-tryptophan on self-mutilation in Lesch-Nyhan disease: a negative report. Neuropädiatrie 7: 439–442

Arima M, Takeshita K, Yoshino K, Kitahara T, Suzuki Y 1977 Prognosis of Wilson's disease in childhood. European Journal of Pediatrics 126: 147–154

Arsenio-Nunes M L, Goutières F 1978 Diagnosis of infantile neuroaxonal dystrophy by conjunctival biopsy. Journal of Neurology, Neurosurgery and Psychiatry 41: 511–515

Barbeau A, Melançon S, Butterworth R, Filla A, Izumi K, Ngo T T 1978 Pyruvate dehydrogenase complex in Friedreich's ataxia. In: The inherited ataxias. Biochemical, viral, and pathological studies. In: Kark R A P, Rosenberg R N, Schut L J (eds), Advances in Neurology vol 21, Ch. 14

Barnard R O, Best P V, Erdohazi Magda 1978 Neuropathology of Menkes' disease. Developmental Medicine and Child Neurology 20: 586–597

Behan W M H, Maia M 1974 Strümpell's familial spastic paraplegia: genetics and neuropathology. Journal of Neurology, Neurosurgery and Psychiatry 37: 8–20

Bell Julia, Carmichael EA 1939 On hereditary ataxia and spastic paraplegia. In: Treasury of human inheritance. Cambridge University Press, London, vol 4, p 141–28

Berman P H, Balis M E, Dancis J 1969 Congenital hyperuricemia: an inborn error of purine metabolism associated with psychomotor retardation, athetosis, and self-mutilation. Archives of Neurology 20: 44–53

Blass J P, Kark P, Menon N K 1976 Low activities of the pyruvate and oxoglutarate dehydrogenase complexes in five patients with Friedreich's ataxia. New England Journal of Medicine 295: 62–67

Boder E 1975 Ataxia-telangiectasia: some historic, clinical and pathologic observations. Birth Defects: original article series, vol XI, no 1, p 255–270 Bouchard J P, Barbeau A, Bouchard R, Bouchard R W 1978, Autosomal recessive spastic ataxia of Charlevoix-Saguenay. Canadian Journal of Neurological Sciences, 5: 61–69

Brandt S, Gyldensted C, Offner H, Melchior J C 1981 Multiple sclerosis with onset in a two-year-old boy. Neuropediatrics 81: 75–82

Brown S 1892 On hereditary ataxia, with a series of 21 cases. Brain 15: 250–282

Bundey S 1973 Basic principles of human genetics. 9. Problemsencountered in genetic counselling clinics. Modern Medicine March 1973: 130–133

Bundey Sarah, Harrison M J G, Marsden C C 1975 A genetic study of torsion dystonia. Journal of Medical Genetics 12: 12–19

Byers R K, Dodge J A 1969 Huntington's chorea in children. Neurology 17: 587–596

Cavanagh N P C 1978 Cerebellar ataxia in infancy and childhood related to a disturbance of pyruvate and lactate metabolism (annotation). Developmental Medicine and Child Neurology 20: 672–

Clayton B E, Dobbs R H, Patrick A D 1967 Leigh's subacute necrotizing encephalopathy: clinical and biochemical study with special reference to therapy with lipoate. Archives of Disease in Childhood 42: 467–478

Cox R, Hosking G P, Wilson J 1978 Ataxia telangiectasia: evaluation of radiosensitivity in cultured skin fibroblasts as a diagnostic test. Archives of Disease in Childhood 53: 386–390

Crome L C, Stern J 1967 The pathology of mental retardation. J and A Churchill, London

Crosby T W, Chou S M 1974 'Ragged-red' fibers in Leigh's disease. Neurology 24: 49–54

Cross H E, McKusick V A 1967 The Troyer syndrome. A recessive form of spastic paraplegia with distal muscle wasting. Archives of Neurology 16: 473–485

Danks D M, Campbell P E, Stevens B J, Mayne Valerie, Cartwright Elizabeth 1972 Menkes' kinky-hair syndrome. An inherited defect in copper absorption with widespread effects. Pediatrics 50 188–201

Danks D M, Cartwright E, Stevens B J 1973 Menkes' steely-hair (kinky-hair) disease. Lancet 1: 891

Déjerine J, Thomas A 1900 L'atrophie olivo-ponto-cérebelleuse, Nouvelle Iconographie de la Salpetrière, Clinique des maladies du Système nerveux, 13: 330–370

Devic E 1895 Myélite aiguë dorso-lombaire avec névrite optique. Cong. franç. méd 1: 434

Déjerine J, Thomas A 1900 L'atrophie olivo-ponto-cérebelleuse.

Dewhurst K, Oliver J 1970 Huntington's disease of young people. European Neurology 3: 278–289

Dimsdale H 1947 Changes in the Parkinsonian syndrome in the 20th century. Quarterly Journal of Medicine 15: 155–170

Dunn H G 1973 Nerve conduction studies in children with Friedreich's ataxia and ataxia-telangiectasia. Developmental Medicine and Child Neurology 15: 324–337

Dunn H G, Dolman C L 1969 Necrotizing encephalomyelopathy. Report of a case with relapsing polyneuropathy and hyperalaninemia and with manifestations resembling Friedreich's ataxia. Neurology (Minneapolis) 19: 536–550

Duvoisin R C, Yahr M D 1965 encephalitis and Parkinsonism. Archives of Neurology 12: 227–239

Egger J, Wynne-Williams C J E, Erdohazi M 1982 Mitochondrial cytopathy or Leigh's disease. Neuropediatrics 13: 219–224

Eichhorst H 1896 Ueber infantile und hereditäre multiple sklerose. Virchow's Arch. Path. Anat. 146: 173

Erdohazi Magda, Marshall P 1979 Striatal degeneration in childhood. Archives of Disease in Childhood 54: 85–91

Falk R E, Cederbaum S D, Blass J P, Gibson G E, Kark R A P, Carrel R E 1976 Ketogenic diet in the management of pyruvate dehydrogenase deficiency. Pediatrics 58: 713–721

Farmer T W, Veath L, Miller A L, O' Brien J S, Rosenberg R M 1973 Pyruvate decarboxylase deficiency in a patient with subacute necrotising encephalomyelopathy. Neurology 23: 429 (abstract)

Friedman E, Harden A, Koivikko M, Pampiglione G 1978 Menkes' disease: neurophysiological aspects. Journal of Neurology, Neurosurgery and Psychiatry 41: 505–510

Friedreich N 1863 Ueber degenerative atrophie der spinalen hinterstrange. Virchow's Archiv für Anatomie und Physiologie 26: 391 & 433, 27: 1

Gall J C et al 1958 Multiple sclerosis in children. Pediatrics 21: 703–709

Gordon N 1978 Infantile neuroaxonal dystrophy and related disorders (annotation). Brain 20: 497–500

Gowers W 1893 A manual of diseases of the nervous system, 2nd. edn. P. Blakiston, Philadelphia, vol 1

Greenfield J G 1967 System degenerations of the cerebellum, brain stem and spinal cord. In: Blackwood W, McMenemey W H, Meyer A, Norman R, Russell D S (eds) Greenfield's neuropathology, 2nd edn. Edward Arnold, London

Griffin J W, Goren E, Schaumburg H, Engel W K, Loriaux L 1977 Adrenomyeloneuropathy: a probable variant of adrenoleukodystrophy. 1. Clinical and endocrinologic aspects. Neurology 27: 1107–1113

Grover W D, Auerbach V H, Patel M S 1972 Biochemical studies and therapy in subacute necrotising encephalopathy (Leigh's syndrome). Journal of Pediatrics 81: 39–44

Grover W D, Scrutton M C 1975 Copper infusion therapy in trichopoliodystrophy. Journal of Pediatrics 86: 216–220

Haas R, Robinson A, Evans K, Lascelles P T, Dubowitz V 1981 An X-linked disease of the nervous system with disordered copper metabolism differing from Menkes' disease. Neurology 31: 852–859

Harding A E 1981a Early onset cerebellar ataxia with retained tendon reflexes: a clinical and genetic study of a disorder distinct from Friedreich's ataxia. Journal of Neurology, Neurosurgery and Psychiatry 44: 503–508

Harding A E 1981b Friedreich's ataxia: a clinical and genetic study of 90 families with an analysis of early diagnostic criteria and intrafamilial clustering of clinical features. Brain 104: 589–6201

Hewer R L 1968 Study of fatal cases of Friedreich's ataxia. British Medical Journal 3: 649–652

Hewer R L 1969 The heart in Friedreich's ataxia. British Heart Journal 31: 5–14

Hogan G R, Bauman M L 1977 Familial spastic ataxia: occurrence in childhood. Neurology 27: 520–526

Holmes G 1907 Familial spastic paralysis associated with amyotrophy. Review of Neurology and Psychiatry 3: 256–263

Hunt J R 1917 Progressive atrophy of the globus pallidus. Brain 40: 56–148

Huntington G 1872 On chorea. Medical and Surgical Reports 26: 317

Huttenlocher P R, Gilles F H 1967 Infantile neuroaxonal dystrophy. Clinical, pathologic and histochemical findings in a family with three affected siblings. Neurology (Minneapolis) 17: 1174–1184

Jason J M, Gelfand E W 1979 Diagnostic considerations in ataxia-telangiectasia. Archives of Disease in Childhood 54: 682–689

Kark R A P, Rodriguez-Budelli Maria, Blass J P 1978 Evidence for a primary defect of lipoamide dehydrogenase in Friedreich's ataxia. In: Kark R A P, Rosenberg R N, Schut L J (eds) The inherited ataxias. Biochemical, viral and pathological studies Advances in Neurology vol 21, Ch. 11, p. 163–181

Kennedy C, Carter S 1961 Relation of optic neuritis to multiple sclerosis in children. Pediatrics 28: 377–387

Killroy A W, Paulsen W A, Fenichel G M 1972 Juvenile Parkinsonism treated with levodopa. Archives of Neurology 27: 350–353

Konigsmark B W, Weiner L P 1970 The olivoponto cerebellar atrophies: a review. Medicine 49: 227–241

Klawans H L, Paulson G W, Ringel S P, Barbeau A 1972 Use of L-dopa in the detection of presymptomatic Huntington's chorea. New England Journal of Medicine 286: 1332–1334

Landrigan P, Berenberg W, Bresnan M 1973 Behr's syndrome: familial optic atrophy. Spastic diplegia and ataxia. Developmental Medicine and Child Neurology 15: 41–47.

Langelier R, Bouchard J P, Bouchard R 1979 Computed tomography of posterior fossa in hereditary ataxias. Canadian Journal of Neurological Sciences 6: 195–198

Leigh D 1951 Subacute necrotizing encephalomyelopathy in an infant. Journal of Neurology, Neurosurgery and Psychiatry 14: 216–221

Lesch M, Nyhan W L 1964 A familial disorder of uric acid metabolism and central nervous system function. American Journal of Medicine 36: 561–570

Levitt R L, Canale S T, Cooke A J, Cartland J J 1973 The role of foot surgery in progressive neuromuscular disorders in children. Journal of Bone and Joint Surgery 55A: 1396–1410

Louis-Bar D 1941 Sur un syndrom progressif comprenant des télangiectasies capillaires cutanées et conjunctivals symétriques à disposition adenoide et des troubles cérébelleux. Confinia neurologica 4: 32–42

Low N L, Carter S 1956 Multiple sclerosis in children. Pediatrics 18: 24–30

McBurney A, Leigh D, McIlwain H 1980 Erythrocyte transketolase activity in suspected cases of Leigh's disease, or subacute necrotising encephalomyelopathy. Archives of Disease in Childhood 55: 789–794

McFarlin D E, Strober W, Waldmann T A 1972 Ataxia-telangiectasia. Medicine 51: 281–314

Markham C H, Knox J W 1965 Observations on Huntington's chorea in childhood. Journal of Pediatrics 67: 46–57

Marsden C D, Harrison M J G 1974 Idiopathic torsion dystonia (DMD). A review of 42 patients. Brain 97: 793–810

Martin W E, Resch J A, Baker A B 1971 Juvenile Parkinsonism. Archives of Neurology 25: 494–500

Menkes J H, Alter M, Steigleder G K, Weakley D R, Sung J H 1962 A sex-linked recessive disorder with retardation of growth, peculiar hair, and focal cerebral and cerebellar degeneration. Pediatrics 29: 764–779

Menzel P 1891 Beitrag zur kenntnis der hereditären ataxie und kleinhirnatrophie. Archiv für Psychiatrie 22: 160–190

Mizuno T, Yagari Y 1975 Prophylactic effect of L-5-hydroxytryptophan on self-mutilation in the Lesch-Nyhan syndrome. Neuropädiatrie 6: 13–23

Montpetit V J A, Andermann F, Carpenter S, Fawcett J S, Zborowska-Sluis D, Giberson H R 1971 Subacute necrotizing encephalomyelopathy. A review and a study of two families. Brain 94: 1–30

Moosa A 1975 Peripheral neuropathy in Leigh's subacute necrotising encephalomyelopathy. Developmental Medicine and Child Neurology 17: 621–640

Namiki H 1965 Subacute necrotizing encephalomyelopathy. Case report with special emphasis on associated pathology of peripheral nervous system. Archives of Neurology 12: 98–107

Nobel E 1911 Histologischer befun in einem Falle von akuter multiplier Sklerose. Wiener Medizinische Wochenschrift 62: 2632

Office of Health Economics 1980 Huntington's chorea. London

Oliver J E, Dewhurst K E 1969a Six generations of ill-used children in a Huntington's pedigree. Postgraduate Medical Journal 45: 757–760

Oliver J, Dewhurt K 1969b Childhood and adolescent forms of Huntington's disease. Journal of Neurology, Neurosurgery and Psychiatry 32: 455–459

Oppenheim H 1911 Uber eine eigenartige Krampfkrankheit des kindlichen und jugendlichen Alters (Dysbasia lordotica progressiva. Dystonia musculorum deformans). Neurologisches Zentralblatt 30: 1090–1107

Oppenheimer D R 1976 Diseases of the basal ganglia, cerebellum and motor neurons. In: Blackwood W, Corsellis J A N (eds) Greenfields neuropathology, 3rd edn. Edward Arnold, London

Pincus J H, 1972 Subacute necrotizing encephalomyelopathy (Leigh's disease): a consideration of clinical features and etiology. Developmental Medicine and Child Neurology 14: 87–101

Reye R D K 1960 Subacute necrotizing encephalomyelopathy. Journal of Pathology and Bacteriology 79: 165–173

Riley I D 1960 Gout and cerebral and palsy in a 3-year-old boy. Archives of Disease in Childhood 35: 293–295

Robinson F, Solitaire G B, Lamarche J B, Levy L L 1967 Necrotizing encephalomyelopathy of childhood. Neurology (Minneapolis) 17: 472–484

Roessmann U, Schwartz J F 1973 Familial striatal degeneration. Archives of Neurology 29: 314–317

Sacks O W 1971 Parkinsonism — a so-called new disease. British Medical Journal 4: 111

Sass J K, Itabashi H H, Dexter R A 1965 Juvenile gout with brain involvement. Archives of Neurology 13: 639–655

Schaumburg H H, Powers J M, Raine C S, Spencer P S, Griffin J W, Prineas J W, Boehme D M 1977 Adrenomyeloneuropathy: a probable variant of adrenoleukodystrophy. II. General pathologic, neuropathologic and biochemical aspects. Neurology 27: 1114–1119

Scheithauer B W, Forno L S, Dorfman L J, Kane C A 1978 Neuroaxonal dystrophy (Seitelberger's disease) with late onset, protracted course and myoclonic epilepsy. Journal of the Neurological Sciences 36: 247–258

Scott D F, Heathfield K W G, Toone B, Margerison J H 1972 The EEG in Huntington's chorea: a clinical and neuropathological study. Journal of Neurology, Neurosurgery and Psychiatry 35: 97–102

Scott R M, Brody J A 1971 Benign early onset of Parkinson's disease: a syndrome distinct from classic postencephalitic Parkinsonism. Neurology 21: 366–368

Seitelberger F 1952 Eine unbekannte Form von infantiler Lipoid Speicher Krankheit des Gehirns. In: Proceedings of the First International Congress of Neuropathology, Rome, Torino. Rosenberg and Sellier 1956, vol III, p. 323–333

Seitelberger F 1971 Neuropathological conditions related to neuroaxonal dystrophy. Acta neuropathologica, Berlin, supplement 5: 17–29

Singh S, Bresnan M J 1973 Menkes' kinky hair syndrome (trichopoliodystrophy). American Journal of Diseases in Children 125: 572–578

Sipe J 1973 Leigh's syndrome: the adult form of subacute necrotizing encephalomyelopathy with predilection for the brainstem. Neurology 23: 1030–1038

Sjögren T 1943 Klinishche und erbbiologische Untesuchungen über die Heredoataxien. Acta psychiatrica scandinavica suppl. 27

Spira P J, McLeod J G, Evans W A 1979 A spinocerebellar degeneration with X-linked inheritance. Brain 102: 27–41

Strickland G T, Frommer D, Leu M-L, Pollard R, Sherlock S, Cumings J N 1973 Wilson's disease in the United Kingdom and Taiwan. I. General characteristics of 142 cases and prognosis. II. A genetic analysis of 88 cases. Quarterly Journal of Medicine 42: 619–638

Strümpell A 1880 Beiträge zur Pathologie des Rückenmarks. Archiv Für Psychiatrie und Nervenkrankheiten 10: 676–717

Strmpell A 1886 Ueber eine bestimmte Form der primären kombinierten Systemerkrankung des Rckenmarks. Archiv für Psychiatrie und Nervenkrankheiten 17: 227–238

Strümpell A 1904 Die primäre Seitenstrangsklerose (spastische Spinalparalyse). Deutsche Zeitschrift für Nervenheilkunde 27: 291–339

Syllaba L, Henner K 1926 Contribution à l'indépendance de l'athetose double idiopathique et congenitale. Revue neurologique 33: 541–562

Taylor A M R, Metcalf J A, oxford J M, Harnden D G 1976 Is chromatid-type damage in ataxia-telangiectasia after irradiation at G_o a consequence of defective repair? Nature 260: 441–443

Taylor C J, Green S H 1981 Menkes' syndrome (trichopoliodystrophy). Use of scanning electron-microscope in diagnosis and carrier identification. Developmental Medicine and Child Neurology 23: 361–368

Vakili S, Drew A L, von Schuching S, Becker D, Zeman W 1977 Hallervorden-Spatz syndrome. Archives of Neurology 34: 729–738

Van der Hauwaert L G, Dumoulin M 1976 Hypertrophic cardiomyopathy in Friedreich's ataxia. British Heart Journal 38: 1291

Villard R de 1970 L'Encéphalomyélopathie Subaiguë Infantile. MD thesis, University of Lyons

Waldmann T A, McIntire K R 1972 Serum-alpha-fetoprotein levels in patients with ataxia-telangiectasia. Lancet 2: 1112–1115

Walker-Smith J A, Turner B, Blomfield J, Wise G 1973 Therapeutic implications of copper deficiency in Menkes' steely-hair syndrome. Archives of Disease in Childhood 48: 958 –962

Walshe J M 1967 The physiology of copper in man and its relation to Wilson's disease. Brain 90: 149–176

Walshe J M 1970 Wilson's disease: its diagnosis and management. British Journal of Hospital Medicine 4: 90–98

Weiss G M, Nelson R L, O'Neill B P, Carney J A, Edis A E 1980 Use of adrenal biopsy in diagnosing adrenoleukomyelopathy. Archives of Neurology 37: 634–636

Westphal A 1888 Ueber multiple Sklerose bei zwei Knaben. Charité-Ann 13: 459

Willner J E, Grabowski G A, Gordon R E, Bender A N, Desnick R J, 1981 Chronic GM2 gangliosidosis masquerading as atypical Friedreich ataxia: Clinical, morphologic and biochemical studies of nine cases. Neurology 31: 787–798

Wilson S A K 1912 Progressive lenticular degeneration: a familial nervous disease associated with cirrhosis of the liver. Brain 34: 295

Wilson S A K 1955 Neurology, 2nd edn. Williams and Williams, Baltimore

Young I R, Hall A S, Pallis C A, Legg N J, Bydder G M, Steiner R E 1981 Nuclear magnetic resonance imaging of the brain in multiple sclerosis. Lancet 2: 1063–1067

9

Ataxia

E. M. Brett

INTRODUCTION

Although ataxia has been discussed in other chapters in several different contexts, the importance of this disorder as a symptom of many different diseases entitles it to more detailed consideration.

The word is used for both a *sign* and a *symptom*. As a symptom it is sometimes regarded as synonymous with unsteadiness, but this is incorrect, since unsteadiness can result from weakness, epileptic attacks and vertigo, as well as from the inco-ordination of movement and impairment of balance which specifically determine ataxia. The paediatrician sometimes uses the word ataxia for cerebellar disorder alone but cases of sensory ataxia are also seen in which unsteadiness and poor co-ordination result from sensory loss, especially of joint position sense, rather than cerebellar dysfunction. This type of sensory ataxia was often seen when syphilis of the nervous system, in the form of tabes dorsalis, was common. Sensory ataxia is now most often seen in patients with acute polyneuropathy of the Guillain-Barré type (Ch. 22) in whom the inco-ordination due to sensory loss and/or to weakness may be confused with cerebellar ataxia.

Ataxia (i.e. inco-ordination due to cerebellar dysfunction or to sensory loss) may be generalized or focal, unilateral or bilateral, and may affect upper and lower limbs equally or differentially. It may be acute or intermittent, subacute or chronic, progressive or non-progressive. Its distribution and natural history help to indicate its probable cause.

PITFALLS IN THE RECOGNITION OF ATAXIA

The problems of chronic ataxia in childhood differ in several ways from those of adult life, since the disorder must be judged against the background of a rapidly developing individual. Development in the early years of life proceeds at a rapid rate with dramatic acquisition of motor and social skills. The recognition of all disorders of movement requires the passage of time. The newborn baby or slightly older infant is expected only to feed, evacuate and show some degree of social responsiveness. He is not yet expected to perform such motor tasks as sitting, crawling, standing, walking, reaching and grasping which require co-ordination. Only when he achieves an age and a stage of development at which these functions form part of his repertoire can inco-ordination in his performance be detected.

The motor difficulty imposed by ataxia usually delays the motor milestones, and these may be further delayed by any degree of mental retardation which accompanies it. The child who is destined to become ataxic is often severely hypotonic in his early months (so much so that at times a neuromuscular disease is wrongly suspected). The difficulty is compounded by the fact that other motor deficits, such as the spastic and extrapyramidal forms of cerebral palsy, may show themselves initially by a similar picture of delayed motor development, so that ataxia can only be clearly recognized later when movement and posture are *quantitatively* adequate for accurate *qualitative* analysis of the type of movement disorder.

Ataxia is first detectable as the child begins belatedly to achieve sitting balance. He is noticed to be abnormally unsteady in the balance of his head and body. His attempts to reach and grasp for objects are jerky and abortive. The fact that they remain so and fail to show the steady improvement seen in the efforts of the normal child helps to distinguish the situation from the normal 'physiological ataxia' of limited duration shown by the healthy infant. Difficulty may also be encountered when the child begins, again later than usual, to stand and to walk, and allowance must be made for the impressive unsteadiness of the normal toddler phase with its frequent tumbles. This phase is usually fairly short, and its prolongation should raise the suspicion of ataxia of non-progressive or progressive type. Titubation (wobbling of the head on the neck), truncal instability, and a wide-based reeling gait will confirm the suspicion of ataxia. This may be strengthened by the finding of nystagmus and of a scanning dysarthria, features often, but not invariably, present with cerebellar lesions. In some mentally retarded children who eventually outgrow their motor problems the normal stage of 'physiological ataxia' may also be unduly prolonged, but its eventual termination will clarify the situation. Many mentally retarded children who are labelled 'ataxic' come in time to develop normal co-ordination.

In the older ataxic child, whose failure to perform actions and to walk in smooth and co-ordinated fashion is obvious, the problem may be to distinguish between ataxia and other motor deficits, including involuntary movements. Many older children will co-operate well in the conventional neurological examination, but younger children and older retarded children cannot be expected to perform to order, and are best examined by the use of toys and games. Attempts to reach for and to grasp sweets (candy) or toys, to build with bricks, to thread beads on to a stick or string, and to touch various parts of dolls or teddy-bears or play at feeding them or even hitting them (or the doctor) with the doctor's reflex hammer will readily bring out ataxia and usually allow it to be distinguished from athetoid or choreiform movements, dystonia, other forms of tremor (e.g. benign familial tremor) or myoclonus. The same terminal exaggeration of the inco-ordinate movements of the hands is seen in such actions as in the older patient's performance of the finger-nose test. Hand-writing and drawing are impaired by ataxia (Fig. 9.1). Assessment of gait in those who can walk will show ataxia, which can be more clearly demonstrated on attempts to walk heel to toe (the child is asked to walk along an

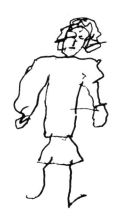

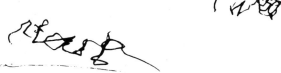

Just a note to give you a sample of my typing.
I forgot to tell you that I have resently joined
the local scout troop, and i am getting along very well.
Also next week I am starting rifle shooting with them.

Fig. 9.1 Ataxic cerebral palsy in an intelligent boy of 9 years. Characteristic ataxic handwriting contrasts with results on electric typewriter.

imaginary tight-rope represented by a line on the floor perhaps with an imaginary crocodile in a river below), to run, to hop and to jump. Tone is usually reduced in children with ataxia, and tendon reflexes are often depressed, but with an associated pyramidal tract defect they may be exaggerated. Pendular knee jerks can often be shown if the child sits with his legs dangling loosely over the side of the bed or chair. Instead of swinging through only a short arc and quickly coming to rest, the lower legs swing freely through a wider arc several times before halting.

The problems of acute ataxia are considered below, both with regard to the disorders causing true cerebellar ataxia and to those which may simulate it by causing other disturbances.

ACUTE ATAXIA

Acute ataxia in a previously normal child presents dramatically and may result from a wide variety of disorders, particularly infections and intoxications.

Direct infections of the cerebellum such as bacterial cerebellar abscess (less common than cerebral abscess), hydatid cysts or cerebellar tuberculoma and the post-infectious complications of virus diseases (Ch. 22) may all cause ataxia, though they may also give rise to other symptoms due to raised intracranial pressure and disorder of other parts of the brain. The encephalitis which may complicate chicken-pox, usually following the exanthem but sometimes preceding or simultaneous with its onset, shows a predilection for the cerebellum so that the clinical picture is often dominated by ataxia; other features of encephalitis such as disordered consciousness, seizures and pyramidal signs are commonly associated.

Two conditions with acute unsteadiness and inco-ordination often preceded by a virus infection deserve special mention. These are acute cerebellar ataxia of childhood and 'the dancing eye syndrome'.

ACUTE CEREBELLAR ATAXIA OF CHILDHOOD

This term is used for a dramatic disorder, probably first described by Batten (1907), in which a previously normal child shows the startlingly sudden onset of ataxia, tremor and hypotonia, often with nystagmus and dysarthria. These features are usually bilaterally symmetrical. An upper respiratory infection may precede the onset by one to three weeks, suggesting a viral aetiology. The condition has been noted in the course of influenza and poliomyelitis epidemics and Echo, Coxsackie and other viruses have been implicated in individual cases.

Fever, headache, meningism and seizures are uncommon so that the picture is unlike that in most cases of encephalitis. The physical signs are mainly those of acute cerebellar dysfunction. Hypotonia may be gross and contrasts with normal or increased tendon reflexes. Other signs of pyramidal involvement sometimes seen are ankle clonus and extensor plantar responses.

A survey by Cottom (1957) of 7 personal cases and 33 considered acceptable from the literature showed that half the patients had the onset of the illness under 3 years of age and only 6 out of 40 over 5. The prognosis was good, the average duration of the disease being 2 months and some children recovering within a week. Sequelae were rare, unlike the post-infectious (exanthematous) encephalitides, and all but 2 patients had recovered fully, though some had taken up to a year to do so.

Investigations

In Cottom's series the white blood cell count averaged 10 000 per cu mm with a normal differential and the erythrocyte sedimentation rate was usually normal. The CSF, examined in 30 cases, showed up to 90 cells per cu mm but only 6 patients had over 10 cells. The CSF protein was usually normal when first examined, but on re-examination a few weeks later the cell count had often fallen and the protein had risen. Sugar and chloride levels were normal. Skull X-rays and ventriculograms were also normal. The EEG was normal in 8 of 14 cases examined, while in 4 patients a slow 4 to 5, c/s rhythm was seen, especially over the occipital region.

Differential diagnosis

In many cases the children are referred to hospital

with the diagnosis of a cerebellar tumour, but the speed of onset of the ataxia in acute cerebellar ataxia is seldom seen with a neoplasm in which the presentation is usually more insidious and features of raised intracranial pressure are often present. Post-infectious encephalitis, such as with varicella, may be distinguished by the occurrence of a preceding exanthem, by the presence of fever, headache, altered consciousness, meningeal irritation and sometimes by the finding of raised intracranial pressure, pyramidal or extrapyramidal signs. A history of drug ingestion should always be sought, and may suggest that the ataxia is due to phenytoin, piperazine or other drugs. A picture of 'pseudo-ataxia' may be produced by continuous seizures (myoclonic or minor epileptic status), by weakness and/or sensory loss as in the Guillain-Barré syndrome and by the 'dancing-eye syndrome' (see below.) Acute vertigo may also be confused with ataxia.

Treatment

Spontaneous improvement is the rule. ACTH and cortical steroids have been used in some cases, but the results in this self-limited condition are more difficult to assess than in the other neurological diseases for which they may be given.

THE 'DANCING EYE SYNDROME' (MYOCLONIC ENCEPHALOPATHY OF INFANCY)

This bizarre condition may be confused with acute cerebellar ataxia with which it has some affinities, but the two can usually be distinguished by a careful analysis of the movement disorder.

First recognized by P. H. Sandifer at The Hospital for Sick Children, Great Ormond Street, it was first described by Kinsbourne (1962) in six children in whom myoclonic jerking produced a consistent and distinctive clinical picture unlike that seen in any other disorder. The condition presents, often soon after an upper respiratory virus infection, with chaotic, rapid, irregular, jerking movements involving the extra-ocular muscles and the limbs, so that cerebellar nystagmus and ataxia are simulated. The movements vary from one time

to another and differ from those of acute cerebellar ataxia, being present at rest and usually not aggravated by attempted movement. The EEG fails to show discharges accompanying the movements and evidence of encephalitis is lacking, though a form of brain-stem encephalitis or auto-immune disease has been postulated. The course of the illness may be brief with rapid recovery, or protracted with remissions and exacerbations over months or even years, the latter often provoked by intercurrent infections. Anticonvulsant treatment is unhelpful and the best results have been obtained with ACTH or steroids. A prolonged maintenance dose of the latter may be needed as patients often relapse when the treatment is stopped or the dose reduced. The irregular, jerky eye movements may be seen at times even when the eyes are closed, and show no constant relationship to the direction of gaze, unlike the nystagmus of cerebellar dysfunction. Although the condition eventually resolves completely in most cases leaving no motor deficit, a number of children who were of normal intelligence premorbidly are left mentally retarded. In a few cases the movement disorder at the start shows features both of 'the dancing eye syndrome' and of cerebellar ataxia.

The striking clinical picture is easily recognized and, once it has been seen, is usually readily distinguished from other disorders. Concern about a cerebellar tumour is understandable and, when there is doubt, this should be resolved by appropriate radiological investigations, preferably the CT scan. There is a well recognized association between 'the dancing eye syndrome' and neuroblastoma, which is usually occult, and care should be taken to exclude this by urinary assay of vanillyl-mandelic acid (VMA), chest X-rays, intravenous pyelography and sometimes by bone marrow biopsy. In such cases the prognosis for survival seems to be much better than in neuroblastoma in general, suggesting that the neurological dysfunction in these patients may be related to an unknown factor (possibly auto-immune) which also controls growth and spread of the tumour (Altman & Baehner 1976). In our experience of many cases of the dancing eye syndrome at The Hospital for Sick Children, Great Ormond Street, evidence for neuroblastoma has rarely been found.

A confusing array of different names has been

suggested for the disorder ('Dancing eyes, dancing feet: infantile polymyoclonia', Dyken & Kolar 1968; opsoclonus-myoclonus Syndrome; Syndrome of rapid irregular movements of eyes and limbs in childhood, Pampiglione & Maia 1972). The latter emphasized the value of polyelectromyography (poly-EMG) with single or multiple spikes as electrical accompaniments of the brief myoclonic phenomena occurring at irregular intervals and independently in different muscles, and of electro-oculographic (EOG) studies showing variable, irregular jerky eyeball movements without rhythmicity. These studies help to distinguish the disorder from myoclonic epilepsy, gross cerebellar ataxia, tremor and choreiform movements.

A fluctuating condition of 'pseudo-ataxia' due to the intrusion of very frequent myoclonic attacks or status myoclonicus is seen in some children with 'minor epileptic status' (Ch. 12). This is clinically distinguished from 'the dancing eye syndrome' by the fact that the eye movements are seldom so striking and that the EEG is usually grossly abnormal with multifocal discharges.

TOXIC CAUSES OF CEREBELLAR ATAXIA

Anticonvulsant drugs

Excessive dosage of these drugs is a fairly common cause of ataxia in children with epilepsy. Phenytoin (Dilantin) is the commonest offender since the principle of careful assessment of the dose based on weight or surface area is still too often neglected. Adult doses of the drug were often given to children when the only suspension available was of adult strength and required dilution. Errors of prescribing and dispensing, the interactions of various drugs (Ch. 12) and renal or hepatic insufficiency are still common causes of ataxia in the child with epilepsy. The widespread availability of measurement of anticonvulsant blood levels makes this less excusable than in the past, and should make it rarer. The ataxia is usually reversible but occasional cases of its persisting have been reported in children (Selhorst et al 1972) and adults (Kokenge et al 1965). Studies by the latter authors on rats and cats intoxicated with diphenylhydantoin blood levels between 30 and 61 μg per ml showed that animals kept intoxicated for 14 days or more developed gross histological changes in the cerebellum, whereas shorter periods produced only minimal changes.

Piperazine toxicity ('worm wobble')

Piperazine, in use for many years as a vermifuge, may cause neurological, gastrointestinal and allergic side-effects. Of the former, cerebellar ataxia and hypotonia are the commonest, so that the condition is well described as 'worm wobble'. It is seen with overdosage, accidental or deliberate, with renal insufficiency and more rarely after normal therapeutic dosage. This was the case in the child reported by Parsons (1971) who became ataxic about 48 hours after a 750 mg dose of the drug on several occasions. Rapid and complete recovery occurs in almost all cases. The more soluble the salt of piperazine used the higher the incidence of side-effects, and this may partly explain their greater frequency in Europe where the small molecule hexahydrate is commonly used.

A past history of neurological symptoms, especially convulsions, should be taken as a contraindication to the use of piperazine, for which safer alternatives such as viprynium embonate are available.

Thallium

Pesticides containing thallium may be accidentally swallowed by children causing severe neurological effects and even death in renal or cardiac failure. Cerebellar ataxia is one symptom but seizures, drowsiness and neuritis are also seen. Loss of hair is a common symptom which may suggest the diagnosis.

METABOLIC CAUSES OF ACUTE OR INTERMITTENT ATAXIA

Ataxia may occur episodically in association with other features, such as drowsiness, coma, vomiting and convulsions, in certain rare neurometabolic diseases, including arginosuccinic acidaemia, maple syrup urine disease, Hartnup disease and hyperalaninaemia (Ch. 7). The severe associated symptoms usually suggest a more widespread disorder than that of the cerebellum alone.

CHRONIC CEREBELLAR ATAXIA

Cerebellar ataxia is a feature of many neoplastic, neurometabolic and developmental disorders. It may be progressive or non-progressive and be accompanied by a host of other neurological features or occur as the sole neurological deficit.

Its recognition and distinction from other disorders in the young child have been discussed earlier in this chapter.

Cerebal palsy of the ataxic and spastic-ataxic varieties has been referred to in Chapter 11 with the problems of differentiation from other causes of ataxia. Hydrocephalus in the older child, in whom growth of the head circumference may be limited, may present with disordered gait and manipulation due mainly to ataxia but often with a pyramidal component especially with aqueduct stenosis.

Cerebellar agenesis or dysplasia is often found radiologically in children investigated for chronic, non-progressive ataxia. In most cases this is not genetically determined but a rare syndrome (Joubert's Syndrome) with ataxia, episodic hyperpnoea, abnormal eye movements and mental retardation associated with agenesis of the cerebellar vermis has been recognised (Joubert et al 1969; Boltshauser & Isler 1976). The condition is inherited in autosomal recessive fashion, so that correct diagnosis is important for genetic counselling. The unusual respiratory pattern has been compared to the panting of a dog in one patient of Boltshauser and Isler, who showed intermittent shallow respiration at a rate of up to 180 per minute. The mental retardation is severe and the prognosis poor. The abnormal respiration tends to improve with increasing age. Abnormal jerky eye movements are often seen, with an irregular, conjugate rotary and pendular character. The combination of abnormal eye movements and respiration may raise the suspicion of a metabolic disorder such as Leigh's subacute necrotizing encephalomyelopathy (Ch. 8), but this is easily distinguished clinically and radiologically.

Tumours in the posterior fossa are important causes of progressive ataxia and must rank high in the list of diagnostic suspects. The clinical features of the medulloblastoma, astrocytoma, ependymoma and cerebellar haemangioblastoma have been considered in Chapter 18. The clinical picture, especially the association with features of raised intracranial pressure, point towards the diagnosis, which is easily made in most cases by the CT scan.

Among the progressive degenerative neurometabolic diseases (Ch. 5) ataxia is a common symptom, especially in the infantile and late-infantile forms of Batten's disease and metachromatic leucodystrophy of early onset. The association with particular constellations of neurological deficits helps to suggest the diagnosis. For example, seizures, dementia and visual failure are prominent accompaniments to ataxia in late infantile Batten's disease. Reduced or absent tendon reflexes suggesting peripheral neuropathy point to the diagnosis of metachromatic leucodystrophy in the young child with progressive ataxia.

In marked contrast to these degenerative disorders in which ataxia is associated with other progressive neurological deficits was a remarkable case reported by Johnson et al (1977) of an unusual form of Sandhoff's disease G_{M2}-gangliosidosis (Ch. 5). The patient, a boy, was normal until the age of $2\frac{1}{2}$ years when he developed a slight intention tremor in the arms. At the age of 4 years 4 months this was accompanied by mild truncal ataxia, slight clumsiness of gait, pale optic discs and bilateral cherry red spots, but there was no evidence of dementia, seizures, nystagmus, dysarthria or pyramidal signs. Thus the clinical picture was unlike that in most cases of Sandhoff's disease or other forms of G_{M2}-gangliosidosis.

Other progressive disorders with a probable or proven metabolic basis causing ataxia are Friedreich's ataxia, ataxia-telangiectasia, Wilson's disease, abetalipoproteinamia, Refsum's syndrome, mitochondrial cytopathy and early onset cerebellar ataxia with retained tendon reflexes (Harding 1981). The natural history of these diseases with their associated features point to the correct diagnosis. Thus the stigmata of pes cavus, ocular and cutaneous telangiectasia and a Kayser-Fleischer ring suggest respectively the first three conditions in this list while pigmentary retinopathy and peripheral neuropathy occur in abetalipoproteinaemia and Refsum's Syndrome associated with other features.

Non-progressive developmental syndromes of clumsiness and poor co-ordination are seen in which the deficit, though often difficult to define, seems to be other than cerebellar. Such cases need careful assessment and will sometimes be found to be examples of a mild congenital peripheral neuropathy, a choreiform syndrome, a benign familial tremor or a defect of eye movement such as Cogan's oculomotor apraxia. An interesting group of children showing many of the features of the so-called 'clumsy boy syndrome' or 'minimal cerebral dysfunction' (Ch. 15) is found among children of both sexes treated for hypothyroidism from early life. The minor motor disorder of these patients is difficult to classify. In one series of 30 patients (MacFaul et al 1978) clumsiness was found in 33%, but did not conform to the pattern of any of the forms of cerebral palsy, while only two showed definite signs of cerebellar disorder. The verbal IQ exceeded the performance IQ by 15 points or more in 42%, an incidence three times higher than in the general population.

REFERENCES

Altman A J, Baehner R L 1976 Favorable prognosis for survival in children with coincident opso-myoclonus and neuroblastoma. Cancer 37: 846–852

Batten F E 1907 Transactions of the Clinical Society of London 40: 276

Cavanagh N P C 1978 Cerebellar ataxia in infancy and childhood related to a disturbance of pyruvate and lactate metabolism (annotation). Developmental Medicine and Child Neurology 20: 672–674

Boltshauser E, Isler W 1976, Joubert Syndrome: episodic hyperpnoea, abnormal eye movements, retardation and ataxia, associated with dysplasia of the cerebellar vermis. Neuropädiatrie 8: 57–66

Cottom D G 1957 Acute cerebellar ataxia. Archives of Disease in Childhood 32: 181

Dyken P, Kolař O 1968 Dancing eyes. Dancing feet: infantile polymyoclonia. Brain 91: 305–320

Harding A E, 1981, Early onset cerebellar ataxia with retained tendon reflexes: a clinical and genetic study of a disorder distinct from Friedreich's ataxia Journal of Neurology, Neurosurgery and Psychiatry 44: 503–508

Johnson W G, Chutorian A, Miranda A 1977 A new juvenile hexosaminidase deficiency presenting as cerebellar ataxia. Neurology 27: 1012–1018

Joubert M, Eisenring J-J, Robb, J P, Andermann F, 1969, Familial agenesis of the cerebellar vermis. A syndrome of episodic hyperpnoea, abnormal eye movements, ataxia and retardation. Neurology 19: 813–825

Kinsbourne M 1962 Myoclonic encephalopathy of infancy. Journal of Neurology, Neurosurgery and Psychiatry 25: 271–276

Kokenge R, Kutt H, McDowell F 1965 Neurological sequelae following Dilantin® overdose in a patient and in experimental animals. Neurology (Minneapolis) 15: 823–829

MacFaul R, Dorner S, Brett E M, Grant D B 1978 Neurological abnormalities in patients treated for hypothyroidism from early life. Archives of Disease in Childhood 53: 611–619

Pampiglione G, Maia M 1972 Syndrome of rapid irregular movements of eyes and limbs. British Medical Journal 1: 469–473

Parsons A C 1971 Piperazine neurotoxicity: 'worm wobble'. British Medical Journal 4: 792

Selhorst J B, Kaufman B, Horwitz S J 1972 Diphenylhydantoin-induced cerebellar degeneration. Archives of Neurology 27: 453

10

Some syndromes of involuntary movements

E. M. Brett

Involuntary movements may occur in neurological disorders of many kinds, and some of these are described in the chapters on cerebral palsy and on progressive neurometabolic brain diseases. In some disorders, however, involuntary movements of a dramatic sort constitute the main, if not the only, clinical abnormality. Some of these syndromes are considered together in this chapter for convenience of discussion of the unwanted movements and of their differential diagnosis.

SYDENHAM'S CHOREA (ST. VITUS' DANCE)*

The rapid, jerky movements of chorea may be seen as a form of cerebral palsy or in certain progressive disorders such as Wilson's disease and Huntington's chorea (Ch. 8). They are also seen in the condition first described by Thomas Sydenham in 1684.

---

* The story of St. Vitus (Coulson 1958) is, briefly, that he was the son of a Sicilian senator and was converted to Christianity in his boyhood in about the year 300. To escape persecution and his father's displeasure, he fled with his tutor and an attendant to southern Italy where they preached the gospel. They then went on to Rome where Vitus cured the son of the Emperor Diocletian, but afterwards he and his companions were cruelly tortured because they would not sacrifice to the gods. Set free by an angel, they returned to southern Italy, where they died as a result of their sufferings. That Vitus and his companions were martyrs probably in southern Italy is supported by the early veneration paid to them in that region and persisting until modern times, since he is apparently still prayed to in Sicily for the relief of the insane. How he became the protector of sufferers from what later came to be known as St Vitus' dance and from epilepsy is uncertain. He was also invoked for protection against over-sleeping (narcolepsy comes to mind and would make him something of a specialist in neurological disorders). It is of interest that he is also the patron of *dancers* and actors.

The disorder presents insidiously or acutely in childhood or adolescence, most cases occurring between the ages of 5 and 15 years, with girls affected more often than boys. There is often a family history of chorea or of acute rheumatic fever and frequently an antecedent streptococcal infection. The first complaint is often that the child becomes clumsy and drops things. He is described by his parents and teachers as fidgety, restless and unable to keep still. The involuntary movements of chorea are of a high order and quasi-purposive, of a type which in a different context could be regarded as appropriate and normal but which, in their disorderly and unpredictable sequence, are quite inappropriate and so are often misunderstood and invite sanctions. Bilateral facial movements reproduce the facial representation of emotion with smiles, frowns, grimaces, pursings of the lips and movements of the tongue and mouth pursuing one another rapidly across the child's face in the absence of the feelings which these movements normally reflect. The eyes, head and limbs are also involved. The arms are most active, with movements at all joints, exaggerated on voluntary effort and on emotion, so that co-ordination is impaired and the child may have great difficulty in writing, feeding and dressing and may be punished for this and for the breakages that may occur in the course of household chores, such as washing and drying crockery. Thomas Sydenham himself in 1686 described the arm movements as follows: 'then it is seen in the hand on the same side. The patient cannot keep it a moment in its place, whether he lay it upon his breast or any other part of his body. Do what he may it will be jerked elsewhere convulsively. If any vessel filled with drink be put into his hand, before it reaches his mouth he will exhibit a thousand gesticulations like a mountebank. He holds the cup out straight as if to move it to his mouth, but has his hand carried elsewhere by sudden jerks. Then perhaps he contrives to bring it to his mouth. If so, he will drink the liquid off at a gulp, just as if he were trying to amuse the spectators by his antics'.

In severe cases the speech is dysarthric, with a slurred or explosive character. With more severe involvement, chewing and swallowing are affected so that artificial feeding may be needed. Breathing may be jerky and irregular and interupted by sudden trunk movements. The legs are less involved, the feet being more affected than the proximal parts of the limbs. In some cases the movements are entirely unilateral, 'hemichorea'. They always disappear during sleep. The associated movements normally seen during strong muscular contraction are exaggerated in chorea. In severe cases muscle power is reduced, though not totally lost. Movement are carried out abruptly; when asked to stretch out his arms the patient does this suddenly as if flinging them away from him. Hypotonia is always present and is associated with abnormal postures such as that of the outstretched hands with flexion at the wrist and hyperextension at the metacarpophalangeal joints and of the arms extended above the head showing excessive pronation. The tendon reflexes are usually normal and the plantar responses flexor. Sensory and sphincter disturbances do not occur and intellect is intact, though emotional lability is common. Seizures are rare in Sydenham's chorea but EEG abnormalities were found in many cases by Chien et al (1978), who suggested that minor seizures might be masked by the choreic movements.

The relationship between Sydenham's chorea and rheumatic fever has been recognized for two hundred years. There is often a recent history of a streptococcal infection or rarely of rheumatic fever before the onset of chorea. Often Group A β-haemolytic streptococci are grown from throat swabs and the antistreptolysin-O titre is raised. In some cases rheumatic heart disease or other features of rheumatic fever follow the onset of the chorea. With improvement in the health of children in the developed nations rheumatic fever and Sydenham's chorea have both become much rarer in the past 20 years.

Opportunities for neuropathological studies have been few since the prognosis is usually good, but mild perivascular infiltration with lymphocytes and plasma cells and diffuse loss of neurons have been described in some patients coming to autopsy.

Prognosis and treatment

Most patients recover completely from the neurological symptoms in two or three months. The condition may recur and in some cases two to four attacks are recorded. Recurrences are less likely after a period of 2 years' freedom.

Penicillin treatment is advisable to eradicate streptococci. Rheumatic fever and heart disease require appropriate treatment. Drugs used in the treatment of chorea include phenobarbitone, chlorpromazine and, more recently, haloperidol. The latter was found by Shenker and his colleagues (1973) to abolish the movements rapidly in 4 children with daily doses of between 1 and 3 mg. In one patient the movements recurred when treatment was stopped after two months, but improved again when it was resumed.

The differential diagnosis from Huntington's chorea, Wilson's disease of neurological type (both rare in childhood), tics, and various other movement disorders is described below. Clinically the distinction is seldom difficult.

TICS OR HABIT SPASMS

These abrupt, repetitive and stereotyped movements are common in children, and not rare in adults. The movements themselves are not abnormal but are of a kind which though frequent in all of us in our normal activities and social behaviour, become pathological by their inappropriate repetition. They most often affect the face, head or upper limbs. Blinking of one or both eyes, twitching of the face, raising of an eyebrow, tossing of the head, shrugging the shoulders, sniffing, grunting and clearing the throat are among the commonest patterns seen. It is usual for the patient to display one particular movement at any one time, but the pattern may then change and another movement replace it. Sometimes a movement may be determined by a normal movement in response to a transient disorder, for example a blinking tic may follow conjunctivitis or a throat-clearing tic tonsillitis. The movements are worse when under emotional stress and tend to diminish when the child's attention is distracted. Thus when he is asked to draw a picture the tics often cease completely, only to recur when he is spoken to. In this they differ from the movements of Sydenham's chorea. They differ also in their stereotyped nature, contrasting with the rich repertoire of quasi-purposive movements of chorea.

It is remarkable how much anxiety tics can engender in the minds of parents, who probably also find them very irritating. It can be a source of quiet amusement for the doctor, as he takes the history or examines the child, to observe very similar movements in the distressed parent. [Abe & Oda (1980) suggest that there may be a genetic basis for the tendency to develop tic.] Tactful reference to this fact and explanation that this is one of the commonest ways in which tension is expressed can help to reduce anxiety. Strong reassurance that the child is healthy and does not have chorea, with advice to ignore the movements, is usually followed by improvement. Certainly the more they are commented on, especially if the child is ridiculed or punished, the worse the tics will be. Medication is usually not required in simple tics, except occasionally by persistently anxious parents. In severe cases psychiatric help is needed by the whole family to help them to understand and cope with their psychopathology. Often the child is having difficulties at school and help in this area may relieve the symptom.

GILLES DE LA TOURETTE'S SYNDROME

The euphoniously named syndrome of Gilles de la Tourette encompasses rarer, more complex types of tic often associated with compulsive verbal obscenities and sometimes also with echolalia and echopraxia (imitation of movements). The socially embarrassing nature of the motor and verbal tics,

sometimes with grunting and barking animal noises, may necessitate drug treatment with haloperidol or tetrabenazine. Corbett et al (1969) have reviewed tics and Gilles de la Tourette's syndrome and found the prognosis generally to be good. Two-thirds of all those followed up for 8 years or more were fully recovered from their tics and the outcome was best when the age of onset of the tics was between 6 and 8 years.

In a review of 81 patients with this syndrome and their relatives Eldridge et al (1977) found that males predominated among those with persistent symptoms, but females among those with spontaneous improvement. 12 propositi had troublesome sexual and aggressive impulses, but these differed only quantitatively from the normal. No evidence of any biochemical abnormality was found.

BENIGN FAMILIAL TREMOR (ESSENTIAL TREMOR)

A rhythmic tremor increased by voluntary movement, absent in sleep and usually affecting the upper limbs is seen in some families with a pattern of autosomal dominant inheritance. The tremor rarely seriously impairs co-ordination, unlike a tremor of cerebellar origin, but it may cause embarrassment at the tea-table, and later the cocktail party, when the beverages are spilled. The tremor may increase in childhood but does not usually worsen in adult life. It is sometimes markedly reduced by alcohol and this may constitute a danger for the older patient. Movement disorders of progressive type and non-progressive chorea can usually be distinguished from benign familial tremor by the history, including that of an affected parent, and by the lack of other neurological deficits. In all cases of tremor in childhood it is essential to examine both parents carefully.

In an interesting report Vanasse et al (1976) have described shuddering attacks in children as an early clinical manifestation of essential tremor. These attacks began in infancy or early childhood, were brief and could be as frequent as several hundred daily or be absent for two weeks. They were graphically described by parents in the following terms: 'as if water was poured down the child's back,' 'as if he had gone into the cold' and 'as if he needed to move his bowels'. There were flexion movements of the head, elbows, trunk and knees with adduction of elbows and knees, and, less often, head turning, arm extension, raising of one arm or sympathetic changes. During the attacks the children would normally stop walking and would sometimes fall or sink to the floor. The episodes became less frequent or remitted in the later part of the first decade. In two patients they ceased at 4 and $7\frac{1}{2}$ years of age. Recognition of these strange attacks as precursors of essential tremor (easier if a parent is known to have the disorder) is important in preventing undue concern and saving the child from unnecessary investigations.

The pathology of the disorder is unknown. Treatment with propranolol is often helpful.

BENIGN FAMILIAL CHOREA WITH INTENTION TREMOR

Pincus & Chutorian (1967) have reported three cases of familial chorea with associated intention tremor in two families. In one child the movement disorder was noted as early as two years of age. It continued unchanged, in some cases into adult life. Autosomal dominant inheritance seemed likely.

FAMILIAL PAROXYSMAL CHOREO-ATHETOSIS

Many families and some sporadic patients have been reported in whom paroxysmal involuntary movements of choreo-athetoid and dystonic type occur in the absence of any progressive disease.

In the family reported by Mount & Reback (1940) prolonged episodes occurred in the propositus and in 28 other members in 5 generations, the onset of symptoms always dating back to infancy and the life-span being normal. Briefer episodes have been reported in many other families.

These disorders have been reviewed by Lance (1977), who described 4 generations of an Austra-lian family in which 7 of 8 affected members suffered from prolonged dystonic attacks while the eighth members had attacks of paroxysmal choreo-athetosis. These attacks lasted up to 4 hours and were precipitated by alcohol, emotion or fatigue. They responded poorly to phenytoin and barbitu-rates but were controlled by clonazepam. In most cases the onset was in infancy or childhood. Lance believes that this family has the same condition as that described by Mount and Reback for which the name *paroxysmal dystonic choreoathetosis* seems most appropriate.

These cases should be distinguished from a commoner syndrome in which much shorter episodes of paroxysmal choreo-athetosis occur, often precipitated by sudden movement or startle. The term *paroxysmal kinesigenic choreoathetosis* is often applied to this condition and is preferable to the earlier term 'seizures induced by movement' since the evidence for an epileptic origin is unconvincing.

Lance's analysis of 100 reported cases showed that the attacks last less than 5 minutes and usual-ly respond well to phenytoin or barbiturates. 72 of the cases were familial, usually with autosomal dominant inheritance, and 28 sporadic. In some cases an autosomal recessive pattern seemed likely. The age of onset in the familial cases was 5 to 15 years but the range was wider in the sporadic cases. The maximum frequency of attacks was 100 per day. The attacks always lasted less than 5 mi-nutes and usually under one minute. Conscious-ness was usually preserved. The commonest pre-cipitating factor was sudden movement after rest as on standing up and walking after lengthy sit-ting. In a few cases epileptic phenomena were seen including tonic-clonic seizures, but the EEG was normal in most patients, even when recorded dur-ing attacks.

DRUG-INDUCED EXTRAPYRAMIDAL REACTIONS

Many psychotropic drugs commonly used in paediatric practice, the phenothiazines and the butyrophenones such as haloperidol, and drugs used to control vomiting (prochlorperazine and metoclopramide) or enuresis (imipramine), may give rise to involuntary movements. These disorders are well reviewed by Mowat (1973). The commonest is an acute dystonic reaction or acute dyskinesia. The onset is usually abrupt with facial grimacing and contortions, bizarre tongue and jaw movements, dysarthria, torticollis, retrocollis, scoliosis, lordosis, opisthotonos and sinuous writhing movements. Trismus, catatonic postures and oculogyric crises may also occur. These features can be very baffling and worrying if the drug history is not known. Sometimes the drugs have been swallowed by the child unknown to his parents or fed to him by an older sibling. The symptoms are dose-related and are especially liable to follow intramuscular injection. Liver disease and pre-existing brain disorder are thought to predispose to these effects. (I have seen severe dyskinesia persisting for a month after a single intramuscular injection of 25 mg of a phenothiazine in a girl with juvenile metachromatic leucodystrophy wrongly diagnosed as schizophrenic.) The differential diagnosis of these reactions is lengthy. It includes meningitis and encephalitis, tetanus, strychnine poisoning and cerebrovascular accidents. Clearly a history of drug ingestion is all-important and should be sought in all unexplained acute neurological disorders of childhood. It should include a search of the household medicine bottles for any source of drugs. The diagnosis of a drug-induced reaction is strongly supported by a rapid response to an intramuscular injection of diphenhydramine (benadryl) or cogentin. In some cases these agents may need to be given by continuous intravenous infusion for some days to counteract continuous release of the culpable drug from an intramuscular injection.

Phenytoin-induced involuntary movements are discussed in Chapter 12.

CONTORTIONS OF THE NECK AND ABNORMAL POSTURES IN CHILDREN WITH HIATUS HERNIA (SANDIFER'S SYNDROME)

Complex contortions of the head and neck and sometimes of the upper part of the trunk were observed by Sandifer in children with hiatus hernia and reported by his colleague Kinsbourne (1964) and later by Sutcliffe (1969). The movements had previously been regarded as involuntary and one patient had been referred for consideration of stereotactic surgery with the mistaken diagnosis of torsion dystonia. The contortions appear to be voluntarily performed with the aim of relieving discomfort. Radiological investigations showed that the movements tended to coincide with paradoxical descent of the left leaf of the diaphragm and with subsequent transient elevation of the gastro-oesophageal junction.

The movements usually consist primarily of a sudden extension of the head and neck into an opisthotonic position. The head may be twisted continuously from side to side. The upper part of the trunk may become bent acutely to one side. The child may seem to be trying to turn himself upside down. Some children will habitually be supine with head and neck hyperextended over the side of the bed pointing to the floor. Others will hold their heads inclined to one side for long periods so that it is more appropriate to speak of abnormal postures rather than movements. The contortions sometimes continue no matter what activity the child is engaged in, but cease during sleep. They may increase during and immediately after meals. Gastro-intestinal symptoms of a kind conventionally associated with hiatus hernia are common, including vomiting, which may decrease with age, haematemesis and anaemia. Dysphagia is not common. Upper adominal discomfort may be complained of and some older children will report relief of this symptom obtained by the movements. This is difficult to understand since they often promote gastro-oesophageal reflux.

The rarity of the association between these bizarre movements and hiatus hernia is shown by the fact that only 7 of the 900 children with hiatus hernia seen at the Hospital for Sick Children, Great Ormond Street, over a 15-year period have demonstrated them. (Sutcliffe 1969). However many cases probably go unrecognized since the syndrome is not widely known (Werlin et al 1980) and the radiological diagnosis of hiatus hernia may be difficult, especially in departments with limited experience of children.

SYNDROME WITH TREMOR IN CHILDREN RECOVERING FROM KWASHIORKOR

Severe malnutrition is common in children from many parts of the world due to diets composed mainly or entirely of cereals and lacking in milk or other foods of animal origin. The name 'kwashiorkor' (meaning 'red child' in the Ga language of the Gold Coast) is widely used and refers to the change in colour of the skin of the affected Negro child from dark to light brown. His scalp hair, normally black, thick and curly, becomes greyish-brown, thin and straight. Dietary treatment with milk or other protein foods usually brings rapid improvement in a few weeks and neurological symptoms are rare in these children apart from irritability.

In recent decades a rare syndrome has been recognized in children with its onset from 6 days to several weeks after the faulty diet has been corrected. It consists of coarse tremors, rather Parkinsonian in type, affecting most commonly the arms and less often the legs, neck, tongue, face and abdominal muscles. In severe cases the whole body is shaken by the tremors, which cease, though not always completely, during sleep. The children are usually rather irritable but remain fully conscious. The arms may show abnormal postures, being abducted at the shoulders and flexed at the elbows with the hands in pronation and ulnar deviation and the thumbs flexed in the half-closed palms. The limbs may show rigidity and the tendon reflexes are usually exaggerated. In severe cases myoclonus is seen in one or more limbs at a rate of about one per second and may continue during sleep.

In a series of 8 South African Bantu children, 3 girls and 5 boys, (Kahn & Falcke 1956) with this syndrome the ages were from $7\frac{1}{2}$ months to 3 years. Symptoms began some days or weeks after the physical condition of the malnourished children had improved on a high-protein diet. Before the onset of the tremors these children differed in no way from the average severe case of malnutrition, so that it was not possible to predict which patients would develop it. The tremors ceased entirely after a few weeks or months.

Investigations were unhelpful with results similar to those in other malnourished children who did not develop the syndrome. The EEG was normal in the two children examined.

The cause of the syndrome remains obscure. It is not due to electrolyte imbalance or to hepatic dysfunction.

Similar cases have been reported from other parts of the world where childhood malnutrition occurs and the prognosis for recovery from the neurological disorder seems to be excellent. It is important to distinguish the syndrome from other disorders, such as encephalitis, cerebellar tumour, acute cerebellar ataxia, the dancing-eye syndrome, and drug effects.

MIRROR MOVEMENTS IN THE KLIPPEL-FEIL SYNDROME

Mirror movements, in which voluntary movements initiated in one limb, usually an arm, are also executed involuntarily by the opposite limb, are common in young children. The dominant hand tends to show these synkinetic movements more than the non-dominant. These movements normally decrease with maturation.

Occasionally abnormally prominent and persistent mirror movements are transmitted as an isolated autosomal dominant disorder from parent to offspring. They are also seen sporadically in some patients with the Klippel-Feil syndrome, a rare malformation of the cervical spine in which the vertebrae are reduced in number and sometimes completely fused (Ch. 17).

The patient may be unable to dissociate the movements of his two hands so that every movement of his right hand is closely imitated by the left. This may constitute a grave handicap and make climbing a ladder, for example, a hazardous task since the patient cannot release his grip on the rung with one hand without the other hand also following suit. The movements are present from birth and persist, but may decrease with age.

The patient reported by Gunderson & Solitare (1968) showed mirror movements in his legs as well as his arms and had progressive dementia for the four years before his death at the age of 11 years. Autopsy disclosed lack of fusion of the dorsal halves of the neural plate in the upper cervical spinal cord. No pyramidal tract decussation could be identified and this may have been the basis for the pathological mirror movements. There was also a third ventricular cyst with enlargement of the lateral and third ventricles.

DELAYED-ONSET DYSTONIA WITH 'STATIC' ENCEPHALOPATHY

The disorders of movement and posture constituting the classical forms of cerebral palsy due to perinatal problems or to post-natal brain injury usually show themselves within a relatively short period of time after the insult responsible. Thus most children with post-icteric cerebral palsy of dyskinetic or choreo-athetoid type develop the characteristic involuntary movements towards the end of the first year of life.

However a small number of cases have been reported in which persistent dystonia has appeared one to 14 years after non-progressive cerebral insults. Eight cases of this delayed-onset dystonia were recently reported (Burke et al 1980). Five were due to perinatal anoxia, one to trauma, and two to cerebral infarction. In each case a non-progressive cerebral insult was followed by a period of one to 14 years during which the patients had mild or no neurological deficit. They then developed abnormal dystonic movements which increased in severity over a period of months or years, but then stabilized. The dystonic movements persisted in all cases. This confusing clinical picture may raise the suspicion of a progressive disorder, particularly of dystonia musculorum deformans, Wilson's disease or Huntington's chorea, but the evolution of the clinical features makes these unlikely. Burke et al suggest that some cases reported in the literature as dystonia musculorum deformans were actually examples of delayed dystonia.

BENIGN PAROXYSMAL TORTICOLLIS IN INFANCY

A benign and self-limited form of paroxysmal torticollis in infancy has been described by Snyder (1969) and Deonna & Martin (1981). The episodes start in the first months of life and show frequent and often regular recurrence, but tend to remit spontaneously and to disappear after a few months or years of life. During the attacks, which usually occur without obvious provoking factors, the head is tilted to one side, (usually either side) and may be slightly rotated. Associated symptoms include pallor, vomiting, irritability and general malaise; unsteady gait may also be present. No other abnormalities are noted on general and neurological examination apart from the head posture and gait. EEGs and neuroradiological investigations give normal results. Snyder (1969) found a lack of vestibular responses to caloric testing in many of his patients, with decreased hearing in some, and postulated a peripheral vestibular disorder (a form of labyrinthitis) as the cause of the disorder, but these findings were not noted by other authors.

In two of Thierry and Martin's five cases the attacks ceased between $2\frac{1}{2}$ and 3 years of age, but in two others they were replaced by episodes of typical migraine. The occurence of migrainous symptoms and a family history of migraine in many patients suggest a relationship to basilar migraine.

Two familial cases of paroxysmal torticollis of infancy affecting siblings have been reported by Lipson & Robertson (1978).

REFERENCES

Abe K, Oda N 1980 Incidence of tics in the offspring of childhood tiquers: a controlled follow-up study. Development Medicine and child Neurology 22: 649–653

Avery L N, Rentfro C C 1963 The Klippel-Feil syndrome: a pathologic report. Archives of Neurology and Psychiatry 36: 1068–1076

Bauman G I 1932 Absence of the cervical spine: Klippel-Feil syndrome. Journal of the American Medical Association 98: 129–132

Burke R E, Fahn S, Gold A P 1980 Delayed-onset dystonia in patients with 'static' encephalopathy. Journal of Neurology, Neurosurgery and Psychiatry 43: 789–797

Chien L T, Economides A N, Lemmi H 1978 Sydenham's chorea and seizures, clinical and electroencephalographic studies, Archives of Neurology 35: 382–385

Corbett J A, Matthews A M, Connell P H, Shapiro, D A 1969 Tourette tics and Gilles de la Tourette's Syndrome: a follow-up study and critical review, British Journal of Psychiatry 115: 1229

Coulson J (ed). 1958 The saints. A concise biographical dictionary, Burns Oates, London

Deonna T, Martin D, 1981 Benign paroxysmal torticollis in infancy. Archives of Disease in Childhood 56: 956–959

Eldridge R, Sweet R, Lake CR, Ziegler M, Shapiro A K, 1977 Gilles de la Tourette's syndrome: clinical genetic, psychologic, and biochemical aspects in 21 selected families. Neurology 27: 115–12

Gunderson C H, Solitare G B 1968 Mirror movements in patients with the Klippel-Feil syndrome. Archives of Neurology 18: 675–679

Kinsbourne M 1964 Hiatus hernia with contortions of the neck. Lancet 1: 1058–1061

Lance J W 1977 Familial paroxysmal dystonic choreoathetosis and its differentiation from related syndromes. Annals of Neurology 2: 285–293

Larsson T Sjögren T 1960 Essential tremor — a clinical and population study. Acta psychiatrica et neurologica scandinavica (suppl 144) 36: 1–176

Lipson E H, Robertson W C 1978 Paroxysmal torticollis of infancy: familial occurrence. American Journal of Diseases of childhood 132: 422–423

Mount L A, Reback S 1940 Familial paroxysmal choreoathetosis. Archives of Neurology and Psychiatry 44: 841

Mowat A P 1973 Dystonic reactions to drugs. Developmental Medicine and Child Neurology 15: 654–662

Pincus J H, Chutorian A 1967 Familial benign chorea with intention tremor: clinical entity. Journal of Pediatrics 70: 724–729

Pryles C V, Livingston S, Ford F R 1952 Familial paroxysmal choreoathetosis of Mount and Reback. Study of a second family in which this condition is found in association with epilepsy. Pediatrics 9: 44–47

Shenker D M, Grossman H J, Klawans, H L 1973 Treatment of Sydenham's chorea with haloperidol. Developmental Medicine and Child Neurology 15: 19–24

Sidaway M 1965 Torsion spasm and hiatus hernia. Annals of Radiology 8: 15–19

Snyder C 1969 Paroxysmal torticollis in infancy: a possible form of labyrinthitis. American Journal of Diseases of Childhood, 117: 458–460

Sutcliffe J 1969 Torsion spasms and abnormal postures in children with hiatus hernia. Sandifer's syndrome. Progress in Pediatric Radiology 2: 190–197

Sydenham T 1686 Schedula monitoria. Latham's translation. Sydenham Society's Edition, Vol II, p 198

Tierney R C, Kaplan S 1965 Treatment of Sydenham's chorea. American Journal of Diseases of Childhood 109: 408–411

Vanasse M, Bedard P, Andermann F 1976. Shuddering attacks in children: an early clinical manifestation of essential tremor. Neurology 26: 1027–1030

Walshe J M 1976 Wilson's disease (Hepatolenticular degeneration). In: P J Vinken, G W Bruyn, (eds) Handbook of clinical neurology. North Holland, Amsterdam, American Elsevier, New York, vol 27, ch 16, 379–414

Werlin S L, D'Souza B J, Hogan W J, Dodds W J, Arndorfer R C 1980 Sandifer syndrome: an unappreciated clinical entity. Developmental Medicine and Child Neurology 22: 374–378

Williams J, Stevens S 1963 Familial paroxysmal choreo-athetosis. Pediatrics 31: 656–659

11

Cerebral palsy, perinatal injury to the spinal cord and brachial plexus birth injury

E. M. Brett

CEREBRAL PALSY

DEFINITION

Cerebral palsy has been variously defined, but the best working definition is probably 'a persistent, but not unchanging, disorder of movement and posture due to non-progressive disorder of the immature brain'. It may also be defined as 'the name given to the motor manifestations of non-progressive brain damage sustained during infancy and childhood'.

The concept of cerebral palsy is in some ways an artificial one since it groups together conditions which are widely disparate but have in common an early age of onset, a non-progressive motor disorder and shared problems of management and requirements, therapeutic and educational. The definition quoted includes the essential ingredients of aetiology in an early and static disorder at cerebral level (excluding progressive pathology and lesions at spinal cord and brachial plexus level). Previous definitions have included arbitrary age limits, such as the first two or three years of life, but these seem unjustified since, for example, an acute hemiplegia produces similar problems whether it presents before or after the third birthday. The definition of the motor disorder as persistent but not unchanging recognizes the fact that the clinical picture is an evolving one. This evolutionary component figures in all neurological problems of childhood, but is particularly important in the field of cerebral palsy in which a changing balance is struck between the positive factors of normal development and growth and the negative effects of disordered brain function and in which this balance can be favourably influenced by therapeutic interventions, with physiotherapy, drug treatment and orthopaedic manoeuvres.

INCIDENCE

The incidence of cerebral palsy has varied in different series according to the criteria for selection, time and community studied. A figure of between one and three cases per 1000 live births has been quoted. Accurate figures are only obtainable for the more developed nations, in which a trend has been noted towards a progressive reduction in incidence in recent decades. Thus in Denmark the incidence figures were about 3 per 1000 in the early 1950s but had fallen to about 2 per 1000 in the mid-sixties (Glenting 1973). In Sweden over the years 1954 to 1970 a progressive decrease in four successive four-year periods has been noted from 2.24 to 1.34 per 1000. Analysis of types of cerebral palsy has shown the reduction to be greater in some syndromes than others (Hagberg et al 1975), being most marked in diplegia and dyskinetic syndromes, while hemiplegia has come to contribute a higher proportion of the total.

CLASSIFICATION OF CEREBRAL PALSY

It is understandable that in such a diverse collection of disorders many attempts at classification should be of limited value. The history of these attempts has been well reviewed by Ingram (1964, 1966) whose book *Paediatric Aspects of Cerebral Palsy* is especially useful.

The earlier attempts at classification were made by pathologists who were interested in different forms of 'cerebral atrophy' related to inflammatory disease, old haemorrhagic lesions and loss of cerebral substance (porencephaly). For a time clinical syndromes were thought to be closely correlated with specific pathological findings in the brain, but the limitations of this correlation were exposed by Freud who pointed out the complexity of the late pathological changes in which processes of repair may co-exist with, and sometimes conceal, the nature of the original brain lesions. The very limited opportunities for autopsies in patients with cerebral palsy today make a classification based on pathology of mainly theoretical interest. The series of 69 autopsied Danish cases reported by Christensen & Melchior (1967) is one of the largest in recent years but it has the inevitable disadvantages that many years had passed between the brain insult responsible for the crebral palsy and death and that it included a high proportion of severe cases (of tetraplegia). Volpe (1976) has described the four main types of neuropathological sequelae of hypoxic — ischaemic encephalopathy in the newborn and their commoner clinical correlates (Chapter 1).

Attempts at a clinical classification probably began with Sachs (1891) who suggested a grouping of cases according to timing of aetiological factors (intra-uterine onset, birth palsies and acute (acquired) palsies) and according to distribution and type of clinical disorder (diplegia, paraplegia, hemiplegia, ataxia, choreic and athetoid disorders).

Little (1843, 1862) had described three categories of paralysis as 'hemiplegic rigidity, paraplegia or generalized rigidity' and a condition with 'disordered movement. His 'hemiplegic rigidity' referred to congenital hemiplegia but his use of the term 'rigidity' made it difficult for some physicians to equate the two. Little's second category of 'paraplegia or generalized rigidity' became known as Little's disease and later as 'diplegia'. His category of 'disordered movement' attracted little attention for some years, but in 1871 Hammond coined the word 'athetosis' to describe the involuntary movements of the fingers seen in some hemiplegic patients. Involuntary movements of 'choreoid' and 'dystonic' type were distinguished from these by Gowers (1876) but the term 'athetosis' came to be applied by many workers to an entire category of cerebral palsy — that in which involuntary

movements are prominent (for which the term 'dyskinesia' was later introduced).

Freud introduced the term 'cerebral diplegia' for conditions with bilateral impairment of motor function, contrasting these with hemiplegia, and including among them generalized and paraplegic rigidity (Little's disease), bilateral hemiplegia, generalized chorea and double athetosis. His group of Little's disease was distinguished from bilateral hemiplegia by the latter's greater involvement of the arms compared with the legs and greater frequency and severity of mental defect, epilepsy and pseudobulbar palsy. The further category of ataxic cerebral palsy was defined by Batten (1903).

The various ways in which movement and posture may be disordered in patients with cerebral palsy (spasticity, rigidity, athetosis, tremor and ataxia) together with the distribution of the disorder form the basis of the classifications of Phelps (1950) and Perlstein (1952) and their modifications. These have some advantages but share the drawback, pointed out by Ingram, that muscle tone may vary with environmental and other factors and that in the evolution of cerebral palsy a hypotonic stage may precede the development of hypertonia, so that reclassification may be needed. The same criticism can be applied to the classification of Minear (1956) in which similar motor variables are listed with topographical and aetiological categories and additional factors such as psychological and physical status, epilepsy, visual, auditory and speech disorders, 'neuroanatomical basis', functional capacity and therapy also being considered.

Spastic forms of cerebral palsy were contrasted with 'extrapyramidal' forms and with mixed types by Crothers and Paine (1959) in their classification. Mixed types, which are quite common, are mentioned also in the classification suggested by the Little Club (1959), together with spastic forms (hemiplegia, diplegia and double hemiplegia), choreoathetoid, ataxic and dystonic forms and 'atonic diplegia'. In neither of these classifications are the changing features of cerebral palsy in the young child sufficiently recognized.

Another group of physicians involved with cerebral palsy met at Oxford in 1964 under the auspices of the Spastics Society in order to discuss classification, but found great difficulty over the basic word 'spastic', which was recognized to have rather different meanings for British and American neurologists, on the one hand, and for Continental physicians on the other.

Ingram has attempted to overcome some of these difficulties in his classification with its six categories of hemiplegia, bilateral hemiplegia, diplegia, ataxia, dyskinesia and 'other'. He uses the word 'diplegia' in the sense of Freud, for a condition with bilateral involvement of the limbs, whether a paraplegia, triplegia or tetraplegia. His diplegic category is further subdivided into rigid or spastic, hypotonic or dystonic groups and an ataxic diplegic group which is contrasted with pure ataxia. Ingram adopted the term 'dyskinesia' (literally 'difficulty with movement') suggested by Perlstein (1952) for the syndromes with involuntary movements: this category comprises dystonic, choreoid, athetoid, tension and tremor as subdivisions. Unfortunately these terms are subject to widely differing interpretation by various writers, and to define in words precisely what the first three terms mean is harder than to recognize them clinically or to imitate them. Many patients show more than one type of involuntary movement and these may vary from one time to another. Some movements may appear intermediate between two types and their classification may be arguable.

An important element in the motor problems of cerebral palsy is the presence of primitive postural reactions or reflexes, such as the tonic neck reflexes, asymmetrical and symmetrical, the Moro and automatic walking and placing reactions. The persistence and severity of these reactions is to some extent related to the severity and type of the cerebral palsy and to the stage of its evolution. In some cases they may constitute a major disability in their own right.

A further important factor in classifying children with cerebral palsy is the presence and severity of associated handicaps caused by the condition responsible for the motor disorder. Thus mental retardation and epilepsy are common in children with cerebral palsy and these added handicaps may in some cases be more critical than the motor defect itself in limiting potential for improvement in function. Hearing loss, common in athetoid cerebral palsy, may profoundly affect speech and communication if not recognised early and compensated for. Visual problems of many kinds, optic atrophy, field defects, squints and nystagmus may contribute to a child's problems and need careful assessment and appropriate management (Black 1980). Psychological problems and specific learning disorders due to perceptual motor difficulties may occur in cerebral palsy and constitute additional stumbling blocks in management and education. Orthopaedic deformities secondary to disordered tone may, despite adequate physiotherapy, compound the motor problems and require skilled management. All these added factors in classification need careful assessment by the appropriate specialists, who should be members of a 'multidisciplinary' team. It is important to remember that the purpose of accurate classification of children with cerebral palsy is not as an academic exercise but to achieve a full assessment and understanding of their problems in order to provide the most appropriate help.

The final element in classification is aetiology, where this is known. Often it is not known or merely suspected. (Even detailed neuropathological studies in those few patients who come to autopsy may throw little light on the aetiology, since in the many years that may have passed between the occurrence of the insult responsible and death the original lesion may have been hidden by later processes of repair). In many cases of cerebral palsy, particularly of congenital hemiplegia, the history gives no clues as to causation, since no adverse factors can be recognized in the pregnancy, delivery or newborn period. In some of these cases special X-rays, such as the CT scan, may show the presence of porencephalic cysts or old infarcts, suggesting a vascular aetiology, though rarely defining the exact cause. In some severely handicapped children with rigid or spastic diplegia, epilepsy, microcephaly and gross retardation, a major cerebral malformation may be suspected and demonstrated by special X-rays, or an intrauterine infection may be proved by serological and other tests. Certain clear correlations do exist between specific insults and the type of cerebral palsy resulting. Neonatal jaundice with kernicterus commonly gives rise to a dyskinetic syndrome of athetoid cerebral palsy with high tone deafness and a defect of upward gaze, but a rather similar syndrome may occur in children who have suffered from neonatal anoxia without jaundice. Prematurity, often without recognized neonatal problems, is commonly noted in the past history of children with spastic diplegia. Ataxia may occur as a sequel to neonatal hypoglycaemia or other insults and the syndrome of ataxic diplegia is quite common in children with hydrocephalus. The diagnosis of cerebral palsy implies a non-progressive and non-genetic pathology and it is clearly important to satisfy oneself on these scores before applying the label. The same considerations of careful history and examination and judicious investigation apply as with all other neurological problems of childhood, particularly mental retardation and epilepsy.

Lastly the element of time is an important factor in the classification and assessment of cerebral palsy. When the child is first seen it may be difficult to be certain whether there is a persisting disorder of movement and posture or whether one is dealing with a transient alteration of tone. When such a disorder is clearly present it may be difficult to decide into which category it falls.

Careful follow-up is needed before the picture becomes clear. In the hypotonic stage which occurs early in several forms of cerebral palsy, it may be difficult to predict whether a hypertonic stage will succeed this and what form the eventual motor deficit will take. The passage of time also allows fuller appreciation of additional handicaps which may not be evident in the younger child and which cannot be accurately assessed until he is older. It is necessary to keep an open mind in many cases and this need not preclude the provision of physiotherapy and other forms of treatment. Assessment is, in any case, a continuous process, and it may be harmful for the doctor to see the diagnosis at an early stage as fixed and immutable. No system of classification yet devised is ideal but that of Ingram provides a good basis.

THE DIAGNOSIS OF CEREBRAL PALSY

Developmental diagnosis is particularly important in the recognition of cerebral palsy, as in that of mental retardation. The milestones of development are reached unduly late in both conditions and careful study will help to distinguish the child whose delay in motor milestones is due to mental subnormality from another in whom cerebral palsy, alone or in association with subnormality, is responsible. Comparison is made not only between the patient's development and that of a normal child, but also between the function of right and left limbs, and of arms and legs. In this way hemiplegic and diplegic cerebral palsy may be suspected.

In the earlier stages of many forms of cerebral palsy hypotonia is prominent and the more specific features of hypertonia and involuntary movements appear only later. Persistence of primitive automatic responses such as the Moro, automatic walking and palmar grasp reflexes beyond the age at which they normally disappear is seen in some cases in this early stage when it provides a valuable clue.

With older children parents may be vague as to the ages at which milestones were achieved and documentary evidence such as photographs, ciné-films or baby books may help.

A careful family history is essential. A history of a motor deficit in a sibling or parent or of parental consanguinity will raise the suspicion of a genetically determined disorder and the relatives concerned should be examined. In this way cases of Friedreich's ataxia, ataxia-telangiectasia, peroneal muscular atrophy, familial spastic paraplegia and other diseases may be recognised. The outcome of other pregnancies is often relevant to the diagnosis of cerebral palsy: prematurity, neonatal jaundice and stillbirths are common occurrences in the family history.

In the field of cerebral palsy even more than with other neurological deficits, observation of the child at play and moving around the room is more informative than the more formal approach of conventional neurological examination. Though this should not be neglected it must take its place as a second phase of the examination, especially in the younger child in whom the approach of a white-coated figure wielding a patellar hammer may destroy rapport so that the occasion becomes a battle in which there are no winners instead of a pleasant and informative exercise.

THE VARIOUS FORMS OF CEREBRAL PALSY

In the account that follows, Ingram's classification will be used with some modifications. Since cerebral palsy is a 'persistent but not unchanging disorder of movement and posture', it is clearly inadequate and inaccurate to describe only the final, classical clinical picture in the various syndromes. Instead it is essential to review the stages in the evolution of this picture.

HEMIPLEGIA

Congenital hemiplegia

In most series of hemiplegic cerebral palsy the condition is congenital in from 70 to 90% of the affected children and acquired in a minority. In Perlstein & Hood's (1954) series of infantile spastic hemiplegia, with a mean age of 6.5 years, one third were of postnatal origin compared with one tenth of the total cerebral palsy population.

Congenital hemiplegia is of varied aetiology. Its incidence in Sweden over the years 1954 to 1970 (Hagberg et al 1975b) showed no significant reduction. In this it resembles congenital ataxia and tetraplegia and differs from spastic and ataxic diplegia. In many cases of congenital hemiplegia brain damage in the perinatal period seems responsible. The certainty or probability of this causal relationship will depend on the severity of the documented adverse factors. The history often shows many abnormalities in the last trimester of pregnancy, labour, delivery and neonatal period. There may be antepartum haemorrhage, pre-eclamptic toxaemia, premature delivery, postmaturity, prolonged labour, fetal distress, apnoea in the newborn period, and sometimes neonatal seizures and/or 'cerebral irritation'. Their relative importance when many such factors are present is hard to assess. In the series of Hagberg et al (1975b) perinatal factors were involved in 41%. The cause was unknown in 30%, a proportion second only to that in congenital ataxia, suggesting that prenatal factors are important in both these forms of cerebral palsy. Ingram's (1964) series of congenital hemiplegia also included about one

third of unknown aetiology. Developmental malformations of the brain with hypoplasia or even agenesis of one hemisphere account for a minority of cases of congenital hemiplegia. Some cases in which a porencephalic cyst is shown by special X-rays may be of prenatal origin, though many are probably postnatally acquired (a pre-existing brain abnormality of this kind may well predispose to breathing difficulties in the newborn period so that the problem may be compounded by anoxia).

A preponderance of cases of right hemiplegia over left has been noted by many authors (Perlstein 1954, Crothers & Paine 1959, Ingram 1964). Perlstein suggested that this might be due to the fact that 70% of deliveries occur in a left occipito-anterior position, so that the left side of the skull is more vulnerable to trauma in the maternal pelvis than the right.

Clinical features

Congenital hemiplegia is rarely diagnosed at birth, although it can be demonstrated by careful examination including the exploitation of primitive neonatal responses such as the Moro, 'passage des bras', automatic walking and placing reactions (Ch. 1) to provoke movements of the limbs and allow comparison between the two sides. In only 10 of 93 cases in the series of Crothers & Paine (1959) (in which the age of recognition was accurately known) was the condition diagnosed in the newborn period — and this proportion seems higher than in most series. Byers (1941) in considering the evolution of hemiplegia in infancy found that a brachial plexus palsy was often mistakenly diagnosed because the hemiplegic arm was relatively flaccid, unused and often hyporeflexic compared to the normal limb. (The face may also show poverty of movement to the same side at an early stage, but this is seldom noticed.) It is rare for parents to notice anything amiss with the arm before the baby is three months old but from that age onwards, and especially between 6 and 9 months, his mother, or sometimes his grandmother, usually becomes aware that he does not move the affected arm as much as the normal one and that the hand is held clenched and does not open up as it should by that age. Often the arm is held for some of the time in a typical hemiplegic posture, with the elbow flexed. A clear preference for using the normal hand to reach and grasp may be present from an early age. A definite hand preference under twelve months of age is usually abnormal and should always alert one to the possibility of a hemiplegia. Left-handedness in a child with no family history of this may also suggest a right-sided hemiplegia.

In severer cases there is delay in all activities needing balance of the trunk and the use of both hands for support. Sitting balance is late in developing and the child tends to fall towards the affected side since he lacks saving and balance reactions on that side. Later the intelligent hemiplegic child will learn to fall towards his sound side so that he can protect his face and head.

He progresses along the floor at first by moving his normal limbs in the prone position and dragging his hemiplegic limbs passively behind him. In severer cases he often fails to learn to crawl on hands and knees and instead hitches along taking his weight on the hand and the buttock on the sound side in a kind of unilateral bottom-shuffle, while the hemiplegic arm stiffens and its hand clenches in associated movements provoked by the effort.

The parachute reaction (Ch. 2), which normally appears at about seven months of age, is asymmetrical in the child with a hemiplegia and may provide valuable confirmation of arm dysfunction when other observations are limited by lack of co-operation. The test may upset the child and should not be performed at an early stage of the examination.

Children with milder degrees of congenital hemiplegia show the same variation in pre-walking motor patterns as that described in normal children by Robson (1970). Robson (1978) in a survey of 79 selected hemiplegic children seen in the first year of life without obvious aetiological factors or additional disabilities, found that they could be divided into a fast development group (those who crawled and those who just stood up and walked) and a slow group (those who moved by shuffling on their buttocks, creeping or rolling before walking). In the fast group the mean ages for sitting and first moving did not differ significantly from normal, but standing was 4 months and walking 6

months later. The slow hemiparetic group walked on average only 2.5 months later than normal and their earlier attainments were no different from those of normal shufflers, creepers and rollers.

Spasticity is rarely present in the hemiplegic arm under the age of three months and hyperreflexia may only become evident still later.

Since the leg is less severely affected than the arm it is usually only noticed to be abnormal much later, although a sensitive early sign of hemiplegia is an externally rotated posture of the leg in the supine position (Paine 1960). In retrospect the parents may remember that the affected leg kicked less well than the normal limb. In Crothers and Paine's (1959) series parents had rarely noticed anything wrong with the leg until the child was twelve months old. Often it is only when the child starts to walk that attention is drawn to the defect in the leg, and parents may then be very distressed when it is recognized.

Sometimes the defect in the leg is so mild that the condition masquerades as a 'monoplegia' for some years: most children referred to hospital with the diagnosis of spastic monoplegia affecting one arm turn out to have a hemiplegia. Hemiplegic children rarely walk under the age of one year, but most walk by 3 years, and delay beyond this age is usually due to associated mental subnormality rather than to the hemiplegia itself.

The physical signs in the older child with a hemiplegia are of 'pyramidal' type, with spasticity, increased tendon reflexes, weakness particularly of anti-gravity muscles and difficulty with discrete finger movements. Associated movements are seen, particularly in the arm, when the normal limbs are active. Thus when the sound hand is clenched or when the child walks, runs or tries to jump, flexor tone is increased in the hemiplegic arm which becomes more strongly flexed. The plantar response on the affected side is often, but not invariably, extensor. The abdominal reflexes are usually normal in a congenital hemiplegia, a helpful point of distinction from an acute hemiplegia. Contractures tend to develop, especially at the elbow, wrist and shoulder, sometimes producing a severe 'folded wing' deformity. The arm is held adducted, flexed and internally rotated at the shoulder, with the elbow flexed, wrist flexed and ulnar-deviated, the forearm pronated and the

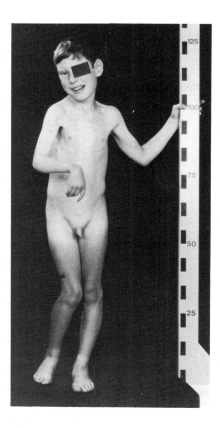

Fig. 11.1 Congenital right hemiplegia — boy aged 9 years

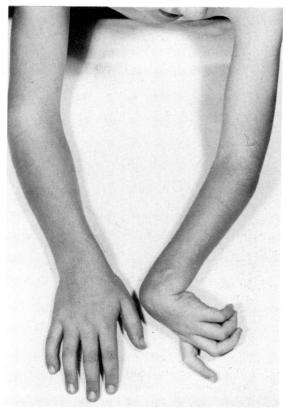

Fig. 11.2 Congenital left hemiplegia — boy aged 7 years. Note small size of left arm and flexed left wrist. The left hand had little useful function.

thumb adducted (Figs. 11.1 and 11.2). The leg is often held adducted, semiflexed at the knee and plantar-flexed at the ankle with equinovarus (Fig. 11.3) or equinovalgus deformity. Scoliosis may also develop. Regular physiotherapy is believed to prevent the severer deformities from developing.

Sensory defects of cortical type affecting two-point discrimination, appreciation of texture and shape and, to some extent, joint position sense can be shown in many co-operative children with hemiplegia. The hand in patients with severe hemiplegia is denied the normal opportunities to develop these finer sensory skills, but there is some evidence that the '**main vierge**' can be educated by deliberate exposure to appropriate stimuli to achieve discriminatory ability.

A visual field defect of homonymous hemianopic type can be shown on the affected side in many children with congenital hemiplegia, yet it rarely seems to constitute a disability. Hemianopia was found in under 25% of 106 hemiplegic patients (Tizard et al 1954) and when present was invariably associated with sensory defects in the limbs on the same side. The hemiplegic limbs are commonly smaller than the normal ones, particularly when the paresis is severe. This dwarfing tends to be more marked in the hand than the foot, and its presence constitutes evidence of a longstanding abnormality, which may be helpful in trying to decide whether a recently noticed hemiplegia is indeed of recent onset or has been present previously but overlooked. Vasomotor changes are also common in the affected limbs which are colder than normal and may show cyanosis distally, sometimes with oedema. Ingram (1964) has noted that the motor disability of the hand in some patients may be much increased in cold weather.

Cranial nerve involvement is seen quite com-

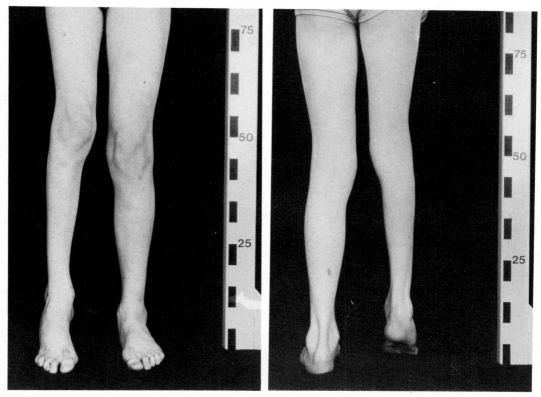

Fig. 11.3 Congenital right hemiplegia. 11-year-old boy. Note small size of right leg, with equinovarus deformity of foot

monly in children with hemiplegia. The face is most often involved with ipsilateral weakness of mild degree, often shown only as slight asymmetry at rest or on movement and seldom consituting a practical handicap. Rarely the facial weakness may be contralateral to the hemiplegia and this may raise suspicion of a brain-stem glioma. Tongue involvement has been reported in some cases. Strabismus is common and is usually convergent in type. Optic atrophy, bilateral or unilateral, is occasionally seen and is presumably related to the cause of the hemiplegia. Rarely ophthalmoscopy shows stigmata of the causative disease, e.g. a phakoma in tuberose sclerosis, retinal haemorrhages in non-accidental injury, or choroido-retinopathy suggesting particular intra-uterine infections.

Mental retardation is less common in hemiplegic cerebral palsy than in double hemiplegia and diplegia of tetraplegic distribution. Approximately 41% of 68 tested patients in one series had IQs below 70, and only 33% above 85 (Ingram 1964).

The IQ does not seem to be correlated well with the severity of the motor handicap. Perceptual motor problems are common in children with hemiplegia, often causing severe educational difficulties even in those of apparently good intelligence. There is some evidence that the body image of hemiplegic children is disturbed.

The prevalence of speech defects in congenital hemiplegia varies in different surveys. Retarded speech development and defects in speech are commoner in hemiplegic children with severe mental impairment than in those in whom it is slight. Experience in Boston (Crothers & Paine 1959) showed no significant difference in the rate of speech development in children with right and left hemiplegia. Of 12 hemiplegic patients with specific language difficulties in Ingram's (1964) series only three had a congenital hemiplegia, whereas eight had an acquired hemiplegia and one a hemiplegia of unknown origin.

The problems of epilepsy in children with hemi-

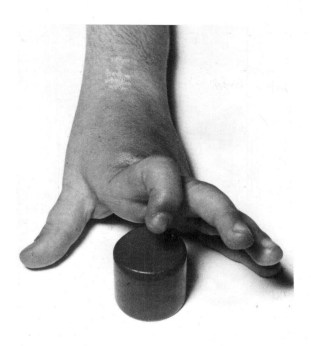

Fig. 11.4 Left hemiplegia. Spastic approach of hand. 10-year-old boy

plegia have been discussed (Ch. 12). Fits are commoner in acquired hemiplegia than in the congenital form.

Acquired hemiplegia

These cases constitute between a tenth and a third of most series of hemiplegic cerebral palsy. In some cases it may be difficult to be sure whether the condition is congenital or acquired. The dramatic onset of the deficit in the average case makes it clear that the condition is acquired, but the delayed recognition of congenital hemiplegia may result in the condition being wrongly regarded as acquired when it is first recognized after a convulsion or an intercurrent illness.

The many causes, vascular, inflammatory, epileptic, traumatic and migrainous, of acute hemiplegia in childhood will not be considered here as they are discussed in other sections (Ch. 19). Like the causes of congenital hemiplegia, they often give rise to associated neurological problems (epilepsy, mental retardation, visual dif-

ficulties) which may profoundly affect the child's functional level and which must be carefully assessed.

The early stages in the evolution of hemiplegia of acute onset are often dominated by the features of the causative illness with coma, seizures and other signs of disturbed brain function. Weakness of the affected limbs is usually maximal immediately after the onset with poverty of movement and flaccidity. Spasticity, increased reflexes and an extensor plantar response develop after a variable interval. Movement returns first in the more proximal parts of the limbs and gradually spreads distally. The degree and rate of recovery vary. In mild cases it is the finer movements, the last to be acquired during normal development, such as thumb abduction and forearm supination, which are lost. Severe cases show virtually no active use of the hand. Intermediate cases show loss of movements which are normally acquired early, such as voluntary extension of the fingers.

Involuntary movements of athetoid or choreoathetoid type are much commoner in the affected hand in acquired hemiplegia of childhood than in congenital cases and in acquired hemiplegia in adult life. These unwanted movements may constitute the major handicap, giving a picture of hemi-athetosis. Epilepsy is roughly twice as common in children with acquired hemiplegia as in those with the congenital type (Crothers & Paine 1959, Ingram 1964). The intelligence level has not differed significantly in most series in cases of acquired hemiplegia compared with those of congenital origin. Dysphasia is commoner in acquired than in congenital hemiplegia and increases in frequency the later the age at which the hemiplegia develops. Less specific speech defects are also seen such as simple retardation of speech development due probably to mental subnormality.

BILATERAL HEMIPLEGIA (TETRAPLEGIA)

Though the former term is not universally accepted, it is appropriate for that type of cerebral palsy in which there is tetraplegia with the upper limbs more severely affected than the lower. In some ways it is as if a hemiplegia were doubled, but the situation is worse than this since, as

Ingram (1964) has pointed out, it amounts to more than the summation of two hemiplegias because the bulbar muscles, spared in hemiplegia, are involved to a greater or less degree and severe mental subnormality and microcephaly are very common. Epilepsy is also common, often taking the form of infantile spasms in younger children.

Aetiology

Perinatal abnormalities figure commonly in the past histories of children with bilateral hemiplegia. Prolonged and difficult or precipitate delivery, foetal distress and antepartum haemorrhage may be recorded. Apnoea and convulsions are often noted in the newborn period with lethargy and feeding difficulty. Recurrent seizures commonly develop in the first year of life. Most cases are clearly of congenital origin, but a few are acquired following a variety of cerebral insults such as meningitis, encephalitis, trauma, asphyxia and cardiac arrest.

Developmental abnormalities of the brain may be shown by air-encephalography or CT scan, hydranencephaly (Ch. 17) being the severest form. Holoprosencephaly, polygyria, agyria or macrogyria may also be found. Porencephalic cysts, usually bilateral and often multiple, (polyporencephaly) may be demonstrated, probably indicating an ischaemic episode affecting the brain during fetal life. Sometimes serology gives evidence of intra-uterine infection with cytomegalovirus, toxoplasma or rubella in such cases, but more often no clues to the cause are found.

Clinical features

This form of cerebral palsy accounts for only about 5% of all cases, but includes the most severely handicapped children since the degree of mental subnormality is usually very gross. Most children remain at a neonatal stage of development as shown by their primitive motor performance, lack of social development and retention of early automatisms (Moro, automatic walking and tonic neck reflexes). Feeding difficulties are often severe with choking, nasal escape and inhalation of food. The resultant pneumonia may cause death.

The neurological signs are those of a 'double hemiplegia' with spasticity and hyperreflexia and with the addition of mental subnormality, often with microcephaly, cranial nerve palsies, optic atrophy, nystagmus and strabismus. The IQ is usually under 50. Speech rarely develops and when it does is often dysarthric. The prognosis for improvement and for any degree of quality of life is poor. Even though the lower limb involvement is milder than that of the upper limbs, independent walking is rarely achieved, and if it develops very late, since the intellectual level of these children and their motivation to become mobile are usually very limited. Physiotherapy is clearly of restricted value in this severe form of cerebral palsy (Fig. 11.5) but can contribute by preventing the grosser patterns of 'windswept' deformity and facilitating the management and so helping the morale of the parents of these tragic children (Fig. 11.6). It is important that false hopes should not be raised by over-optimistic claims for the results of any treatment. In the earlier stages it is hard for parents, as with severe mental subnormality without motor deficit, to appreciate how limited is the future for their child and delicate judgement is needed by the doctor concerned in assessing how ready they are for a frank appreciation. Tactically and humanly speaking, a brutally gloomy prognosis given very early may be inadvisable, especially if no attempt is made to provide any treatment. Acceptance of the situation comes gradually and with less bitterness when time has shown the lack of progress and when it is seen that attempts have been made to help. The doctor may need to let himself be swayed by the dictates of his heart rather than of his head.

Probably the greatest insight into the problems of the families of these maximally handicapped children is given, not by a medical writer, but by the playwright Peter Nichols in his tragicomedy, *A Day in the Death of Joe Egg* (1967). In this work, in which comedy outweighs the tragedy, the parents of the 'vegetable' child are shown coping with their 'unacceptable' predicament by a continuous charade in which they relive their experiences since the child's delivery and their contacts with professional advisers. The work should be required reading or viewing for all paediatricians. Caricatures though many of the characters are, the honest doctor cannot fail to see glimpses of himself in them as they attempt the impossible task of ex-

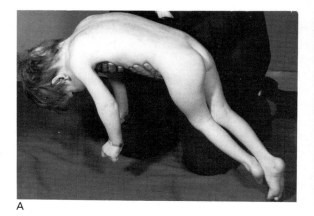

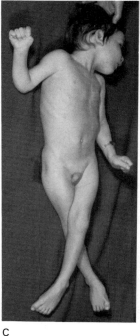

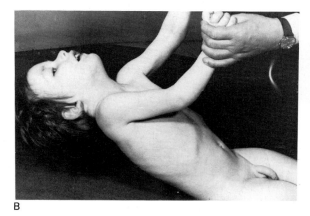

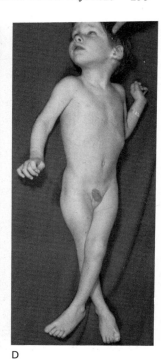

Fig. 11.5 Double hemiplegia, 4½-year-old boy
A. ventral suspension
B. Poor head control
C & D. Severe obligatory asymmetric tonic neck reflex

plaining the inexplicable and making acceptable the intolerable. To see ourselves occasionally as others see us in this way is a rare and salutary experience.

DIPLEGIA

This term suggested by Freud is used for a form of cerebral palsy (formerly often called Little's disease) in which the limbs on both sides of the body are affected, with the legs more severely affected than the arms in contrast to the situation in bilateral hemiplegia. In some cases the upper limb involvement may be fairly severe; in many cases it is mild and in a very few cases upper limb function is normal so that the term 'paraplegia' is appropriate. The evolving nature of the motor disorder in diplegia means that the qualifying terms

rigid, spastic, hypotonic or dystonic are only applicable at a particular stage.

Locomotor development is more impaired than manipulative skills. Mental subnormality may coexist, but is less common and severe than in bilateral hemiplegia. When present it causes retardation in social, language and other fields of development. The more severely physically handicapped children with diplegia tend to be more severely subnormal mentally, though the correlation is incomplete. Epilepsy, visual and ocular problems, deafness and other associated defects may compound the child's difficulties.

Aetiology

Diplegia is almost always congenital in origin and all series have included a high proportion (between a third and a half) of affected children who were

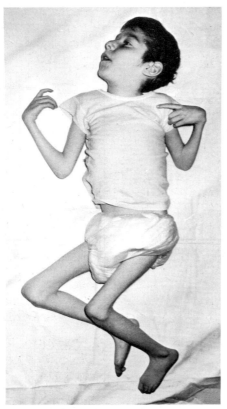

Fig. 11.6 Double hemiplegia in 15-year-old boy, showing severe 'windswept' posture

antepartum haemorrhage, occurring in 40%, usually between the twenty-eighth and thirty-second week of gestation. In most of both the mature and premature children with last trimester abnormalities other complications of pregnancy, labour and delivery were recorded.

Over half of the diplegic children had a history of abnormal labour or delivery or both. This occurred in about 44% of the mature and 65% of the premature patients. About 55% of the children appeared normal immediately after delivery and 36% (apart from prematurity in the premature group) during the neonatal period. Neonatal apnoea and later neonatal complications did not seem likely to be either a cause or a result of diplegia in Ingram's study.

The mothers of the diplegic children in this survey tended to be less fertile than normal with high fetal and infant mortality among their other conceptions through abortion, still birth, neonatal and perinatal death. Drillien (1964) has shown that the surviving siblings of diplegic children have a higher than expected incidence of mental retardation, seizures and other CNS disorder.

The aetiology of diplegia remains uncertain in many cases and the gratifying and impressive reduction in its incidence in low birth weight premature children (Davies & Tizard 1975, Hagberg et al 1975b) which may be related in some way to improvements in care of the newborn, have not been fully explained. This reduced incidence can be correlated with a decreased incidence of periventricular leukomalacia (Ch. 1). Avoidance of birth injury, early feeding and prevention of neonatal hypothermia have all been considered as possible factors, and of these the last may be most relevant. The finding of a lower haematocrit level on the second day of life in premature babies who later developed diplegia compared with those who did not may possibly indicate that haemorrhage had occurred into the brains of those in the former group.

A survey of 669 children in the West Midlands (Bundey & Griffiths 1977) showed a recurrence risk in siblings of children with symmetrical spastic cerebral palsy and a normal birth history of approximately 1 in 9, suggesting that about half of them may have had a recessively inherited condition.

born prematurely, with low birth weight consistent with short gestation. Twin and other multiple births are common, often in association with prematurity.

Ingram's (1964) series of 78 children with congenital diplegia contained 43 who were mature and 34 who were premature (by birth weight). Abnormalities in the pregnancy, labour, delivery and neonatal period were common in both groups. In early pregnancy incomplete abortion, accidental or induced, was the commonest recorded abnormality but seemed unlikely to be important as a cause of the diplegia, since it was almost always accompanied by disorders in later pregnancy, labour or delivery. In the last trimester of pregnancy about 44% of patients had apparent abnormalities. The commonest disorder in the mature diplegic patients was pre-eclamptic toxaemia, occurring in 25%, whereas in the premature children it was

The clinical evolution of diplegia

In children with moderate and severe degrees of diplegia several fairly clear-out stages are seen in the evolution of the motor disorder (Ingram 1955).

In the immediate postnatal period many infants show features suggesting perinatal brain damage. They may be lethargic, difficult to feed and hypotonic or, by contrast, overactive, hypertonic and 'jittery'. Neonatal seizures may occur.

These dramatic neonatal abnormalities usually subside and there follows a latent period of some 6 to 12 weeks in which the infant's behaviour causes little concern to his parents, and all seems to be well. However, examination at this stage may show a lethargic baby lying in a semiflexed position with little spontaneous movement, especially of the legs. The child has poor head control, hypotonia and abnormally easily provoked neonatal automatisms, especially the Moro reflex, automatic walking and tonic neck reflexes.

Gradually this hypotonic stage is replaced by the 'dystonic' stage with involuntary mass movement and generalized increase in tone whenever the child's position is altered. He stiffens up when handled, his legs taking up a 'scissored' posture, while his back extends and his arms may adopt a hemiplegic position or be held extended at the elbows. Primitive automatisms may still persist, the asymmetric tonic neck reflex being much brisker than normal. Palmar and plantar grasp reflexes may be abnormally strong. The parachute reaction may be abnormal. Tone is still decreased rather than increased in the prone position, but tendon reflexes are now usually increased, especially in the legs.

The rigid-spastic stage follows the dystonic stage with hypertonia present not only in the erect position, but also in prone, though more evident when held upright. At first the hypertonia is of rigid type with the legs held extended at the knees and plantar-flexed at the ankles, as in the attacks of stiffening seen in the dystonic phase. Later the final spastic phase of the rigid-spastic stage ensues, with flexor hypertonus gradually replacing the underlying rigidity and with all tendon reflexes increased. In the erect posture the position is similar to that seen in bilateral hemiplegia, except that the abnormality is more marked in the legs than in

the arms. The child stands with hips and knees flexed, taking his weight on his toes often with legs internally rotated (Fig. 11.7). Walking is precarious and unsteady with support needed from parents' hands or mechanical aids such as 'clumpers', crutches or sticks. When independent walking is achieved the child often walks much too fast and, if he can be persuaded to slow down, shows a more normal pattern of gait, with the heels down further and less crossing of the legs. The arms may be held adducted at the shoulders and flexed and pronated at the elbows. The back is often curved in sitting. The condition may be asymmetrical so that one arm functions almost normally and the other is much less useful. Contractures are common with limited abduction and sometimes with dislocation of the hips, short heel cords with equinus deformity of the feet and restricted movement at elbows and wrists.

A few severely affected children do not reach the final rigid-spastic stage but remain dystonic

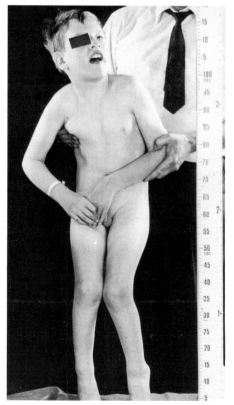

Fig. 11.7 Spastic diplegia. 8-year-old boy

while a very small proportion may live for some years in the hypotonic state. Most children reach the rigid-spastic stage by the age of two or three years. The rate of early evolution through these various stages allows an estimate of the prognosis, since children who pass rapidly through the stages of hypotonia and dystonia to reach the rigid-spastic stage of diplegia have a relatively good prognosis. Those who remain hypotonic for a long time, and dystonic for years with the final stage long delayed have a poor outlook. Those who are still in the dystonic stage by the age of 3 rarely walk unsupported in later childhood.

The 'bottom-shuffling' trait, (Robson 1970) shown by some normal children as a familial alternative to crawling may occur in children who are developing spastic diplegia. This may mask the signs of cerebral palsy in milder cases. Robson and MacKeith (1971) found that the average age of diagnosis of diplegia in 27 non-shufflers was 17.2 months, but in 6 shufflers it was 32 months. Shortening of the hamstrings with limited extension of the knees, brisk tendon reflexes and persistent ankle clonus may help to indicate the true situation.

Additional problems in diplegic cerebral palsy may result from associated athetoid movements such as may occur in hemiplegia, from persistence of dystonic movements into the rigid-spastic stage and from contractures. Some dwarfing of the legs and pelvis occurs in most diplegic patients and is roughly proportional to the severity of the weakness.

Further difficulties may arise from associated mental subnormality, visual and ocular problems, hearing loss and epilepsy. As in all cases of cerebral palsy comprehensive assessment of these problems is needed to ensure optimal progress for the child.

ATAXIC CEREBRAL PALSY AND ATAXIC DIPLEGIA

When the motor disorder is cerebellar ataxia due to a non-progressive lesion of the immature brain, it is classified as 'ataxic cerebral palsy' (semantic accuracy might suggest that it should be classed as *cerebellar* palsy, and indeed Batten (1903) used the term 'cerebellar diplegia', but custom and euphony outweigh logic and the shorter name is preferred). This form of cerebral palsy has been recognized from the time of Freud onwards. Though relatively uncommon, it is less rare than has been suggested and accounts for up to 10% of cases in many series. Most cases are congenital and tend to be diagnosed late because the recognition of ataxia in infancy is difficult and a certain stage of motor development is needed before the cerebellar deficit can be easily seen, in sitting, reaching and grasping and later walking (Ch. 9). These motor milestones are almost invariably delayed in ataxic cerebral palsy and this delay and the frequently associated hypotonia may be wrongly attributed to mental retardation, which may co-exist, to other forms of cerebral palsy or to neuromuscular disease (ataxic cerebral palsy is one of the many causes of the 'floppy baby syndrome' (Ch. 3).

The condition occurs in a pure form with ataxia alone and in a mixed form associated with the development of spasticity in the legs, often known as 'ataxic diplegia' (though it might be better named 'spastic-ataxic diplegia'). Both forms may be either congenital or acquired and due to a wide variety of insults at different epochs of life. Idopathic cases are seen as with other forms of cerebral palsy. Hydrocephalus in early life is often associated with ataxia or ataxic diplegia whether the lesion giving rise to the hydrocephalus itself be congenital or acquired and whether due to developmental malformation, prenatal or postnatal infection, subarachnoid bleeding or even tumour.

The definition of cerebral palsy as due to *non-progressive* disorder must be kept constantly in mind when the diagnosis of ataxic cerebral palsy is mooted, since it is notoriously easy to overlook progressive diseases of degenerative or neoplastic type as a cause of ataxia in young children. The diagnosis of cerebral palsy often has the effect of preventing for all time any consideration of another diagnosis and the clinician should be alert to alternative possibilities. Hydrocephalus should especially be borne in mind as it is usually surgically remediable. So too are many cerebellar tumours. The same is not true of the progressive degenerative diseases, such as metachromatic leucodystrophy, ataxia-telangiectasia, or Friedreich's ataxia, but their recognition is vital for prognostic and genetic reasons. A careful scrutiny (visual as well as verbal) of the family history may indicate a familial and genetic condition.

Aetiology

Experience in Sweden (Hagberg et al 1975b) has shown that the number of children with congenital ataxia remained unchanged over the years 1954–1970 whereas ataxic diplegia showed an impressive reduction parallel to that of spastic diplegia. The same aetiological factors were involved in ataxic and spastic diplegia (prematurity, low birth weight for gestation and perinatal problems). Hydrocephalus was also a common association of ataxic diplegia. In the children with congenital ataxia the distribution of birth weight was the same as for the general population. Prenatal factors were thought to be involved in 25% and no cause could be found in 41%, so that the opportunities for prevention are less in this group than in ataxic diplegia.

Clinical features

The patients are often floppy in infancy with slow motor development and poverty of movement. In some cases hydrocephalus is obvious at birth or become evident in the early months of life. In the early weeks there is little to distinguish those children who will later become ataxic from those who will show ataxic diplegia, though seizures are rather commoner in the latter. In ataxic diplegia the early hypotonia often starts to decrease by about 3 months of age and the legs may soon become spastic and their tendon reflexes increased.

Reaching for objects is delayed and when it develops is seen to be hampered by obvious intention tremor. Sitting is also delayed and it too is accompanied and impaired by truncal ataxia and by tremor of the head (titubation), neither of which has usually been detectable previously while the child spent his time in prone or supine. The recognition of these features may lead the parent and the less experienced doctor to suspect a progressive disorder. The ataxia may be asymmetrical and sometimes seems to spare one arm. The relative severity of the ataxia and the spastic paresis varies from one case to another. In some children with ataxic diplegia the upper limbs are spared from spastic involvement, while in others a motor deficit of pyramidal type compounds the ataxia of manipulation. There is delay in walking and contrasting gait disorders are seen with, on the one hand, a wide-based ataxic gait with no 'spastic' element and, on the other, a spastic and ataxic gait with severe adductor spasm, scissoring and equinovarus. The more ataxic children tend to use their arms to help their balance. Contractures of variable severity occur in ataxic diplegia, as they do in spastic diplegia, but are less than in the pure spastic syndrome.

Intellectual impairment and epilepsy may occur in ataxic diplegia and pure ataxia. Speech disorders including scanning cerebellar dysarthria may occur in either type, as may strabismus and nystagmus. Squint is commoner in ataxic diplegia.

Acquired ataxia and ataxic diplegia may result from a wide variety of disease, including meningitis, pyogenic or bacterial, the hydrocephalus which may complicate these, viral encephalitis (especially varicella), trauma, surgical lesions of the cerebellum and the effects of their surgical treatment.

THE DYSEQUILIBRIUM SYNDROME

A case has been made for separating off from the main body of children with ataxic cerebral palsy a subgroup in which the condition seems sometimes to be inherited as an autosomal recessive character. These children show severe retardation in motor development, seldom walking independently under nine years of age. Spasticity, mental retardation and various sensory deficits may coexist (Hagberg et al 1972, Sanner & Hagberg 1974).

DYSKINETIC (ATHETOID) CEREBRAL PALSY

Involuntary movements in the limbs of patients with cerebral palsy were described in the nineteenth century, by Little (1862), Hammond (1871) and Gowers (1876), among others. The confusingly varied description and interpretation of the movements are well reviewed by Ingram (1964). Gowers' (1876) classification of post-hemiplegic disorders of movement includes the term 'slow, mobile spasm of remitting type' applied to Hammond's category of athetosis. In later accounts terms such as athetosis, athetoid, chorea, choreiform, dystonia and dystonic are applied to unwanted movements of various types, sometimes with different meanings. The finding in the nineteenth century of kernicterus or nuclear jaundice with widespread yellow staining of the brain by bilirubin, particularly affecting the caudate and lenticular nuclei in the basal ganglia, in babies dying with icterus gravis and the much later recognition of the role of rhesus incompatibility in its aetiology led eventually to the prevention of this form of brain damage by exchange transfusion and, more recently, to the prevention of sensitization of the mother by the baby's incompatible red cells. Hyperbilirubinaemia due to ABO incompatibility, to prematurity and to other causes, such as congenital familial non-haemolytic jaundice and glucose-6-phosphate dehydrogenase deficiency, was shown to produce the same neurological sequelae, also preventable by exchange transfusion. The role of anoxia in conjunction with hyperbilirubinaemia in the aetiology of kernicterus has been debated; it is probably most important in the premature infant with moderate jaundice.

A classic account of the 'neurological sequelae of Rhesus sensitization 'was given by Evans & Polani (1950) based on 79 cases. A stormy neonatal period with jaundice, difficulty in feeding, drowsiness, opisthotonos and respiratory disturbances was followed by a silent period between the ages of 1 and 3 months. Thereafter rigidity or intermittent opisthotonos and sometimes involuntary movements became obvious. In the period from one to two or three years the children were often hypotonic, when diagnostic errors could result, but the later appearance of involuntary movements indicated the diagnosis. The same evolution of clinical features has been noted by many workers including Crothers & Paine (1959) and Ingram (1964).

Clinical features

The typical extrapyramidal movements of dyskinetic or athetoid type, which give the condition its names, are not seen in the newborn period, but appear in the course of a prolonged evolution usually many months after birth. The final clinical picture is usually not seen until the child is aged two years or more.

Certain clear-cut stages can be seen in the evolution of dyskinetic cerebral palsy, as in that of diplegia. The first stage in the newborn period was often the most dramatic, although the highest levels of hyperbilirubinaemia can nowadays usually be prevented so that the neonatal features of kernictures are less often seen in centres with adequate facilities. The infant may be jaundiced due to Rhesus or ABO incompatibility, prematurity or glucose-6-phosphate dehydrogenase deficiency. With higher bilirubin levels he is often irritable, hypertonic and opisthotonic with head retraction and sometimes with a high-pitched cry. These features are non-specific, indicating merely the possibility of brain damage, and usually disappear within a few days. With lower bilirubin levels the child may show only lethargy and slowness in feeding. There follows a latent or hypotonic stage usually lasting four to ten months during which feeding difficulties, vomiting and regurgitation are common. In this stage examination shows generalised hypotonia with poverty of movement and persistence of neonatal automatic responses, particularly the asymmetric tonic neck reflex, but also the Moro reflex and automatic walking. Towards the end of this latent period involuntary movements appear. They resemble those seen in the development of diplegia; 'dystonic' movements with extension of trunk and limbs occur especially when the child is moved or when his neck is extended. Gradually they become less wide-spread and more discrete, coming to involve individual limbs. (The 'dystonic' phase of dyskinetic cerebral palsy may lead to a wrong diagnosis of diplegia just as the hypotonic phase may be confused with mental retardation or neuromuscular disease. The evolution of clinical features helps to make the distinction in each case.) Persistence of the Moro response and asymmetric tonic neck reflex is often seen. The final picture, seen after the age of two, is dominated by the involuntary movements of athetoid, choreoid or dystonic type less evident in the prone position than in the supine. These terms are sometimes used with different meanings and in some cases the movement disorder is so complex that its analysis is difficult. Athetosis is the form of dyskinesia most often seen, whence the use of the term 'athetoid' cerebral palsy as an alternative to the more general expression 'dyskinetic'. The movements in athetosis mainly affect the distal part of the limbs; they are slow and purposeless involving both agonist and antagonist muscle groups, and are increased by attempted voluntary movement, which they impede, and by emotional factors. Choreic and choreo-athetoid movements refer to quicker, more jerky movements (chorea = a dance) most marked in the proximal parts of the limbs. The term 'dystonia' is sometimes used for slow, writhing movements involving the trunk muscles and sometimes for abnormal postures which are maintained briefly (Fig. 11.8). In some feet in contact with the floor show the

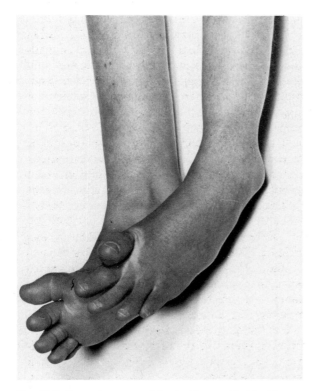

Fig. 11.8 Dystonic posture of feet in 11-year-old girl with dyskinetic (athetoid) cerebral palsy

so called 'athetoid dance', which may be due to a tactile avoiding reaction.

The rate and extent of evolution of the clinical picture along the path described above varies from one patient to another. The most severely affected patients become arrested in the hypotonic stage and remain helpless and immobile throughout their lives. The more severe generalized movements seen in the dystonic stage persist in some dyskinetic children and constitute a severe handicap preventing all but the crudest of willed actions. In the least severely affected children a fairly rapid evolution occurs through hypotonia and dystonia to a stage in which involuntary movements have decreased in extent and degree so as to allow a reasonable range of voluntary movement, with independent walking and some manipulative skills so that dressing, feeding and writing may be possible.

Muscle tone in the limbs is usually normal at rest, though it may be difficult to assess since attempts at handling a limb often provoke an increase in tone with stiffening ('tension athetosis') not only in that limb but also in the trunk and other limbs. Occasionally some spasticity is found, especially in children with a history of perinatal hypoxia. Tendon reflexes also are usually normal though their elicitation can be hampered by tension. Fixed contractures and deformities are less common than in the spastic disorders, but scoliosis and dislocation of the hips may occur in the more immobile patients. Affected children are often very thin and lacking in subcutaneous fat, due probably to their almost continuous involuntary movements.

High-tone deafness is very common in dyskinetic cerebral palsy due to neonatal jaundice. Even a minor degree may constitute a serious handicap and it must be carefully looked for.

Speech is usually impaired to some extent, even if hearing is perfect. A combination of dysarthria from difficulty in controlling the muscles of articulation, difficulty in co-ordinating breathing with speaking and impaired phonation produces speech which is slow, lacking in modulation and at times explosive or 'strangled'. Some children cannot speak at all or at best can utter only a few syllables. It is only too easy to regard such children as mentally subnormal, though intelligence in most patients with dyskinetic cerebral palsy is within the normal range. Careful psychological assessment is vital; this requires a psychologist familiar with the problems of assessing the severely physically handicapped. The child's 'eye-pointing', indicating the answer by whatever limb or head movement is possible, or grunting will allow the experienced psychologist to form a reasonably accurate assessment of his intellectual level and give useful guidance on his potential for education and the appropriate teaching methods, including the use of mechanical aids such as the 'POSSUM' and the Bliss symbol board.

A defect of upward gaze is characteristic of posticteric cases of dyskinetic cerebral palsy, but not of post-anoxic cases. Another clue to the role of neonatal jaundice in its aetiology is given by the common finding of green discolouration of the dental enamel and poor formation of the teeth.

The dyskinetic child often has great difficulty in controlling his head, which may loll about, even when he can sit steadily. Facial grimacing and drooling are common. These features added to the difficulty in communication and the involuntary movements produce a picture which conforms most closely to the sterotyped image which the less instructed members of the public have of the 'spastic' and retarded child. Thus feelings of repugnance and rejection are generated in those on whose tolerance and acceptance these very handicapped children depend in all aspects of living. While still attending school they are to some extent protected, but on leaving school and attempting to compete for employment they become fully aware of how little life has to offer them.

MIXED FORMS

Mixed forms of cerebral palsy are seen with combinations of two or more types. Ataxic diplegia is one example. Dyskinetic and spastic features may co-exist in some tetraplegic and hemiplegic patients. In some cases the motor disorder is so complex as to defy classification. Failure to classify is not of great practical importance, frustrating though it may be to the clinician, since it does not prevent analysis of the *functional* deficit on which to base a plan of treatment.

DIFFERENTIAL AND AETIOLOGICAL DIAGNOSIS OF CEREBRAL PALSY

The recognition of the motor deficit, its classification and the assessment of the associated problems have been discussed. The basic question to be asked at the onset and repeatedly later on is whether the condition is indeed non-progressive, conforming to the definition of cerebral palsy, or whether it may be due to a progressive disorder such as a degenerative CNS or neuromuscular disease. Ataxic and dyskinetic syndromes are particularly liable to cause confusion. Ataxia-telangiectasia, Friedreich's ataxia, Wilson's disease, the Lesch-Nyhan syndrome, torsion dystonia, some cases of hydrocephalus, dystrophia myotonica and other dystrophies may all be mistaken for cerebral palsy, though a careful clinical analysis should prevent this. Degenerative brain diseases with very early onset, such as Tay Sachs disease and the early onset forms of Krabbe's and metachromatic leucodystrophy, are often mistaken for cerebral palsy until progressive deterioration shows this to be incorrect.

This important distinction between a progressive and a non-progressive disorder is made on clinical grounds, particularly on the history, but specific progressive diseases should be excluded by appropriate biochemical, neurophysiological and other tests when they are suspected.

As with non-specific mental retardation radiological and electrical investigations in cerebral palsy are of limited value. Plain skull X-rays may show calcification in cases due to intrauterine infection or tuberose sclerosis. Air-encephalograms and CT scans, if abnormal, are most likely to show cerebral atrophy. This may be unilateral or asymmetrical especially in hemiplegia. A porencephalic cyst or cysts or an old infarct may be found, suggesting a previous vascular episode. The EEG is not a very useful test in cerebral palsy. It is often abnormal, especially in those with epilepsy. The abnormality shows some correlation with the severity of the physical handicap, but little with the level of intelligence (Gordon 1966).

THE ASSESSMENT AND MANAGEMENT OF CEREBRAL PALSY

The purpose of assessment and the need for a multidisciplinary approach.

The purpose of assessment in all handicapping conditions of childhood is to plan appropriate treatment of all deficits. Assessment which leads to no treatment is a sterile exercise. Though opinions differ on the value of physiotheraphy in the young cerebral palsied child, and though facilities for it are sadly lacking in some areas, most paediatricians believe that physical therapy is of benefit and the trend today is towards early provision of such treatment rather than late.

The process of assessment should be carried out as soon as possible after the child presents, in order to plan management. Since the motor deficit in cerebral palsy is not an unchanging one but evolves, the assessment must be repeated from time to time. In this way deterioration in function, which might raise the suspicion that progressive pathology is present and that the case is not one of cerebral palsy, can be detected and the plan of treatment can be altered by, for instance, provision of more physiotherapy or speech therapy or consideration of orthopaedic procedures. Re-assessment is needed in considering appropriate school placement and throughout the child's school career to ensure that his educational and treatment needs are being met as fully as possible. Ciné films are helpful in documenting a child's function for comparison with later occasions and methods of gait analysis by means of multiple sequential camera are particularly useful (Holt et al 1974).

The assessment and management of the complex neurological deficits which constitute cerebral palsy and the frequently associated handicaps is beyond the abilities of the individual physician or therapist. The subject is well reviewed by Holt (1965) and Holt & Reynell (1967). Many experts are needed, working together as a team, the so-called 'multi-disciplinary approach'. Associated defects must be detected and treated. It is never safe to assume that no sensory deficit, for example deafness or a visual defect, is present. Such deficits must be looked for and excluded. The skills and experience of a physician (who

may be paediatrician or paediatric neurologist), physiotherapist, speech therapist, occupational therapist, psychologist, teacher, ophthalmologist, audiologist, ear, nose and throat surgeon, orthopaedic surgeon, orthoptist and social worker must be enlisted in order to assess the child's functional capacity in all areas and to improve that capacity. Though this list is headed by a paediatric physician, who is usually well suited to act as a co-ordinator of the team, the experience of physicians in the field of cerebral palsy varies greatly and in many cases the greatest day to day contribution is that of the physiotherapist. Working in a more intimate and continuous way with young physically handicapped childen than is possible for most doctors, she (or he) often has an unrivalled experience of their problems and management. Paediatric specialization within physiotherapy is a desirable trend which can only serve the interests of the child. The importance of the physiotherapist's contribution is recognized by the tendency among doctors involved in cerebral palsy to 'put themselves to school' with some of the acknowledged experts in the field of therapy.

The role of physiotherapy

There is still debate about the value of physiotherapy in cerebral palsy, some physicians taking a negative view on the grounds of lack of scientific proof of its efficacy or of a clear understanding of how it works. Though attempts have been and are being made to overcome these lacks, there are obvious difficulties in the scientific assessment of treatment in view of the tendency towards spontaneous improvement, the 'placebo' effect of treatment, and the problems of finding a control group of cases since it is rare for two patients to have identical problems and difficult to deny treatment to children who may benefit from it.

There is much evidence that physiotherapy in cerebral palsy *is* effective, particularly when started early, not only in preventing severe contractures and deformity, but also in promoting more normal motor development. It is not necessary and may be harmful to delay treatment until the child is old enough to 'co-operate' (an age which with mental retardation and emotional immaturity is likely to be late). The general aim of physiotherapy is to enable to child to attain the greatest possible degree of independence. In the young child it aims at reducing harmful patterns of movement and posture, whose persistence underlies many of the motor problems of cerebral palsy. These abnormal patterns are largely produced by the persistence of certain primitive reflexes, such as the asymmetrical and symmetrical tonic neck, righting and Moro reflexes (Ch. 1). These reflexes are influenced in turn by the child's posture, and exert their greatest effect in certain positions. For example, the tonic labyrinthine reflexes result in extensor tone being maximal in the supine and flexor tone in the prone position and can be made use of in treatment and nursing. The physiotherapist has a valuable rôle in teaching parents how best to handle their child in feeding, washing, toiletting, dressing and all activities of daily life. An excellent simple account of this kind is provided by Finnie (1974). This educational rôle of the therapist is most important since she can usually manage at best to treat the child for some hours each week, and her aim must largely be to teach the parents (father as well as mother) to be their own child's therapists. Harmful postures and patterns of movement permitted at home for six days a week by an uninstructed mother will outweigh the good done by treatment on the seventh day. A useful account of the every-day activities of the cerebral palsied child is given by Egan (1977) who also considers the choice of suitable furniture such as potties, bath seats, chairs and tables for particular conditions.

There are many different schools of physiotherapy each with its enthusiastic supporters. Their multiplicity suggests that no one school can be superior to all others for *all* cases, and a moment's reflexion on the varied forms of cerebral palsy shows how unlikely such a paramount position must be. These methods of treatment have been reviewed by Scrutton & Gilbertson (1975), Gordon (1976) and Egan (1977). Certain methods are much more intensive, in terms of time and labour, than others and may be described as 'not so much a treatment — more a way of life'. Treatment in its widest sense must indeed be incorporated into the pattern of daily life, but for most families there are limitations on the amount of treatment time possible due to considerations of housework, car-

ing for other children (and spouse) and finances. Only a few of the many methods will be mentioned here. The 'neurodevelopmental' system of treatment devised by the Bobaths (Bobath 1967; Manning 1972) aims at guiding the child through the normal sequences of motor development, placing him in such positions that primitive and abnormal reflexes are inhibited, allowing a more normal state of muscle tone, and facilitating movements. This method and modifications thereof are widely used. The Vojta method (Jones 1972), though relatively intensive, is practicable for home use. The Peto technique was developed in Hungary to provide 'conductive education' in a residential setting by one person, a 'conductor', combining the rôles of therapist and teacher. All activities are broken down into their constituent sequences of movements which are then learned individually and finally combined to produce the required activity. The actions are reinforced by speech, the children announcing what they are doing at each stage, the technique of 'rhythmic intention'. Though suitable for the needs of its country of origin, the method has less to recommend it in other areas, where it tends to be used in a modified form. For most Western parents and paediatricians the idea of residential care for young children with cerebral palsy is unacceptable.

Many physicians and therapists find the claims of the various methods confusing and therefore adopt an eclectic approach, empirically choosing items from different systems which seem appropriate to the needs of the patient at the time. The needs of the family must also be considered when planning treatment. Most children must travel with their parents, and sometimes with their normal siblings, to the treatment centre. In large cities the journey may be long and tiring, so limiting the number of visits possible. If domiciliary treatment can be provided, as occurs in some rural areas, the child and his parents benefit since he is likely to be fresh, happy and well-disposed to do what is asked of him. Schemes of treatment which require the whole family drastically to alter their way of life, sometimes at the cost of other children being neglected, and to enlist squads of helpers may meet the emotional needs of worried parents for a time but are less likely to be continued for long. It is sometimes hard for parents to understand that treatment is a continuous process and not a short and intensive phase. The educating and supporting rôle of the therapist and other members of the team is important in this regard also, as it is in maintaining the morale of parents who often find the rate of progress slower than they had hoped and wished. The social worker also has an important part to play in helping the family in periods of stress, and short-term admissions to hospital may be needed from time to time to give the parents a rest.

Vision and hearing

Vision and hearing must be carefully assessed in all children with cerebral palsy by appropriate techniques. Accurate assessment may be difficult in a severely handicapped child and much experience is needed before reliable results can be obtained. The late Mary Sheridan devised the Stycar series of tests (Sheridan Tests for Young Children and Retardates) to meet the needs for testing vision and hearing in normal and handicapped infants and young children (Sheridan 1976a, b, 1977).

Squints, which are very common in cerebral palsy, should be corrected when possible. Errors of refraction should also be treated.

Feeding and speech

The rôle of the speech therapist in cerebral palsy exceeds that of the conventional stereotype, since it starts early, long before the stage of language has developed. His earlier concerns are with the feeding problems which are so common in cerebral palsied (and mentally retarded) children. The bite reflex and tongue thrust are often troublesome barriers to feeding and they can be partly inhibited by appropriate handling. The therapist needs constantly to stress to parents the fact that children need stimulation to learn to speak and that it is a two-way process. Many parents are inhibited about speaking to their handicapped child, just as they are in handling him, and they must be encouraged to do both. Formal speech therapy may not come into its own until several years later, but the therapist should by then have done much of the groundwork on which it can be based.

In the mentally retarded child with cerebral palsy drooling and dribbling are a major problem, being socially unacceptable and involving expense and difficulty in keeping the child clean. (It might be said that drool and stool are the bugbears of the care of the mentally handicapped.) Anything that can be done to reduce the extent of drooling is desirable. Rapp (1980) has reported recently on a long-term follow-up of a group of severely retarded cerebral palsy children at a special school in Hertfordshire. The children were conditioned to control their drooling by means of an electronic device and 'shaping' and 'conditioning' procedures. Improvement in drooling was maintained after 9 months.

Orthopaedic aspects

The orthopaedic contribution is important and happy is the team (and its patients) which includes a surgeon who is interested in the problems of cerebral palsy. The careful planning of orthopaedic procedures is an essential part of management and it is helpful for the surgeon to meet the children early on, so that he can plan ahead for possible future intervention, in close collaboration with paediatrician, physiotherapist and parents.

Orthopaedic splints and calipers have a limited place in cerebral palsy though useful in selected cases. Boots and shoes need careful consideration and the orthopaedic surgeon can contribute much here. It is in the field of actual surgery that he has most to offer. The many procedures available, which are constantly being revised and improved, are described elsewhere (Samilson 1975, Lloyd-Roberts 1976, Fixsen 1979 and will not be considered here. A few points only will be made. The spastic forms of cerebral palsy (hemiplegia and diplegia) are those in which surgery has most to offer. The legs offer far more scope than the arms. Elongation of the Achilles tendon on one or both sides and procedures to reduce adduction of the hips and flexion of the knees are relatively simple procedures which can greatly improve function. A wrist arthrodesis can help to improve function and appearance in the severely flexed wrist seen in the 'folded wing' deformity in some hemiplegic children. Tendon transfer operations can improve supination. In general dyskinetic or athetoid syndromes are unsuitable for surgery since, even if the deformity is corrected, it usually recurs. In general also severe mental subnormality is a contraindication to surgery, although it may be justified in some children with very tight adductor muscles or dislocated hips to facilitate nursing and perineal toilet, even though there is no prospect of independent walking. The timing of surgery is important and it must always be combined with regular physiotherapy. Surgical intervention is rarely indicated under 5 years of age. It must always be seen as an episode in management and parents should not be allowed to regard it as offering a cure.

The treatment of spasticity by injection of dilute alcohol at the motor point of muscles or by the epidural route was developed by Tardieu et al (1968) in France as a clinical extension of an experiment in the decerebrate cat. Good results were obtained in the treatment of children with cerebral palsy. Carpenter & Seitz (1980) reported good but transient results in children with spastic cerebral palsy, using 50% alcohol in normal saline with a light anaesthetic before injection. The gastrocnemius/soleus group was injected in 130 patients (bilaterally in 80). The equinus gait was corrected in all but 2 cases. Although the improvement only lasted from 7–20 days, valuable information was gained during the improved phase by the therapist and orthopaedist as to whether surgery was indicated to eliminate the equinus. In some patients the injection was repeated once or twice, and the period of improvement became progressively shorter. In no case was the equinus permanently eradicated. In a small number of patients injections were made into the medial aspect of the upper third of the thighs with reduction in scissoring in some cases. Injections into the biceps and forearm flexors was helpful in some cases in deciding whether surgical procedures in these muscle groups were indicated.

Neurosurgery in cerebral palsy

Brain surgery in children with cerebral palsy has at present very limited justification. Hemispherectomy has been used in the past in some hemiplegic children with severe epilepsy and behaviour disorder (Ch. 12) but is rarely necessary today and may have serious delayed complications. Thalamotomy by various methods has been tried in some children with athetosis and rigidity, but improvement in surgical techniques and safety are needed before this can be happily recommended. A cerebellar approach with stereotactic dentatotomy and chronic cerebellar stimulation via implanted electrodes is reported to have given encouraging results in relieving spasticity in some patients with cerebral palsy, including some children. More experience is needed, however, before these procedures can be regarded as acceptable.

Drug treatment

Drugs are of limited value for the motor defects of cerebral palsy, but should be considered, especially in the spastic forms. Diazepam is seldom helpful as it tends to cause drowsiness and sometimes gross hypotonia. Lioresal (Baclofen®) has proved very effective in some hemiplegic and diplegic children in reducing spasticity and facilitating physiotherapy (Milla & Jackson 1977). Unfortunately it may provoke convulsions in children with a tendency to these and a history of seizures should probably be taken as a contraindication. Dantrolene sodium suspension has also been used in the treatment of spasticity. In children with spastic cerebral palsy the drug has varied in its results. A recent report on 20 children treated in a double-blind trial suggested that it produced no significant improvement in their function (Joynt & Leonard 1980).

In dyskinetic syndromes diazepam can sometimes reduce involuntary movements, perhaps by a psychotropic effect. Benzhexol, tetrabenazine and L-dopa have sometimes been helpful but may cause troublesome side-effects.

Psychiatric disturbances may occur in cerebral palsied children, who may understandably suffer depression and anxiety. These must be recognized and treated. Referral to a child psychiatrist is sometimes needed and symptomatic treatment may be helpful.

On a more controversial note, acupuncture may possibly be of value in the symptomatic treatment of cerebral palsy. Sanner and Sundequist (1981) found it effective in relieving painful muscle spasms in four young patients with dyskinetic cerebral palsy and it will almost certainly be tried in similar cases.

Education

The child with cerebral palsy is deprived of much of the experience in daily living by which normal children learn. Using his hands to manipulate objects and his mouth as an organ of exploration may be difficult or impossible for him. Moving around, with the experience of the world which the process itself gives, and the goals towards which movement is directed may also be impossible until a much later age than normal. This deprivation of experience must be compensated for by all those in the child's microcosm, especially his parents, his first teachers, but also physiotherapists, occupational and speech therapists and other professionals. Pre-school teaching should be provided whenever possible in a centre with facilities for his physical needs where therapists, teacher and parents can co-operate in his management. Among the many advantages of this not the least is his exposure to a milieu where his disability is accepted as a matter of course and where he is more likely to be 'stretched' by having more demanded of him in terms of effort and independence than in the emotionally more highly charged atmosphere of the home. Social contacts with his own age group are also ensured with benefit to his social adjustment. The simple routine skills of daily living, feeding, dressing, washing etc. are often achieved more rapidly in the setting of a pre-school centre. A continuous process of assessment is possible which helps in planning for education at school age.

In the decision on school placement many factors besides the type and severity of the motor deficit must be considered. Many children with cerebral palsy unfortunately have sub-normal intelligence, others have epilepsy, visual or hearing problems or other handicaps. These, rather than the cerebral palsy itself, may determine the most suitable placement. Detailed assessment of the child's problems should always precede a decision.

Some cerebral palsied children of normal intelligence, especially those with hemiplegia and diplegia, may manage well in a normal school. There are obvious advantages when this is possible, since the child benefits from contact with normal children and often from a better education. Physical problems of moving from one classroom to another, coping with stairs and with going to the toilet, must be considered. The personality of the child, his parents and the teachers are also important. (Some teachers are emotionally unable to cope with a handicapped child.) A robust personality in a child will help him to cope with the knocks and bruises he will suffer in the playground and the more damaging psychological wounds which may result, sometimes from the slights and taunts of other children, but more often from his own inescapable awareness of his difference from them. Sometimes parents will insist on their child attending a normal school against advice, and may only eventually recognize the unsuitability of this when his sufferings and failure underline it. Parents should be told that decisions on school placement are not irrevocable and that changes of school are possible. Physiotherapy and speech therapy are not usually available in normal schools unless they are closely linked with special schools on a common campus, an arrangement as admirable as it is rare.

In the United Kingdom the choice of special school for the cerebral palsied child lies between a school for physically handicapped children and one for the educationally subnormal, moderate or severe [ESN (M), or ESN (S)]. There are also some schools for 'delicate' children suitable for less severe handicaps. The child's physical and educational needs together, it must be admitted, with the availability of facilities, determine the choice. Parents are often very anxious about this and they should always be brought into the discussion about placement. They will inevitably feel disappointment and resentment in some cases, but they should not feel that arbitrary decisions have been imposed on them, and the possibility of periodic review in the light of progress should be offered.

At the two ends of the intellectual spectrum it is often difficult to meet fully both the physical and educational needs of children with cerebral palsy. The needs of the severely subnormal for physiotherapy and speech therapy may be great, but at times of financial stringency and retrenchment they are less likely to be met. Children of superior intelligence may be bored and frustrated in a school for the physically handicapped where the average IQ of the pupils may be 60 or 70. Attempts to cater for the needs of both these groups are made by voluntary bodies such as the Spastics Society in Britain, whose educational and therapeutic efforts supplement the deficiencies in the services available. Further education in residential colleges for the physically handicapped can sometimes be arranged for the 'spastic' school-leaver. Mechanical aids such as electric typewriters and tape-recorders can greatly extend the powers of communication of the physically handicapped. The POSSUM machine, which allows a movement of hand, foot, shoulder or even tongue to be applied to activate an electric typewriter, has enlarged in a marvelous way the horizons of children with severe athetoid cerebral palsy who can neither speak nor write and has disclosed some unsuspected talents. The writings of the severely athetoid Dubliner, Christy Brown, (1970) give valuable insights into the prison world of the child and adult with severe cerebral palsy, as do those of the young spastic boy, Christopher Nolan (1981).

THE PROGNOSIS OF CEREBRAL PALSY

Young children with severe cerebral palsy and mental subnormality, who are often also subject to epilepsy, have a high mortality from chest infections, status epilepticus and other problems. Severe cerebral palsy continues to carry a poor prognosis for mortality in older patients. Ingram (1964) in a follow-up of 144 patients born between 1938 and 1947 found that seven of these had died between the ages of 10 and 20 years. All had severe physical handicaps and associated disabilities with gross mental defect in all but one. Four had bilateral hemiplegia, two dyskinesia and one diplegia. The yearly mortality rate among the original 144 patients was approximately 5 per 1000, and for severely handicapped patients approximately 29 per 1000 compared with a yearly mortality rate of 0.4 per 1000 in the Edinburgh school population over the same period.

The prospects for employment on leaving school are not encouraging and when unemployment in the general population is high the handicapped tend to fare still worse. Ingram (1964) analysed the employment pattern in his follow-up study of cereral palsy patients in Edinburgh, and found that 53 were unemployed. Fifty-seven were employed, of whom 26 were in open employment in competition with non-handicapped people and with no allowances made for their disabilities, 17 in 'niche' employment with allowances made, 4 in sheltered workshops and 10 in sheltered training. Most of those in open employment had mild hemiplegia or diplegia. Apart from the severity of physical and intellectual handicaps and the social adjustment of the patients, their success or failure in holding satisfactory jobs was also determined by their attitudes to their problems and ability to form rewarding social relationships. Not surprisingly the latter were in turn influenced by the stability of their home backgrounds, the attitudes to their being abnormal of their parents and siblings, and their school experiences. The study also showed the need for a more systematic attempt to fit the person to the job, so that unsuitable placements and resultant discouraging failure may be avoided. A more recent and rather gloomy survey of 1513 cerebral palsy patients from the United States (O'Reilly 1971) showed that 33% were mentally normal and self-sufficient, while in 25% the major problem was mental retardation with minimal physical handicap so that a sheltered environment or custodial or institutional care were needed. A further 25% were so handicapped physically or mentally as to be custodial problems at home or in institutions. Five per cent were mentally bright but had severe physical handicaps and 12% had intermediate problems of mental or physical disability. The needs of the adult with cerebral palsy are poorly met, not only in the United States (O'Reilly 1974), but everywhere, and those involved in the care of children with cerebral palsy should be more concerned for their future integration into the community.

An imaginative and encouraging recent venture in Britain has been the setting up under the auspices of the Spastics Society of an agricultural and horticultural residential unit for physically handicapped adults. Its members operate a successful commercial enterprise with benefit not only in mental and physical improvement in the individual, but also in their integration into the local community.

PREVENTION OF CEREBRAL PALSY

The Swedish experience of the changing picture of cerebral palsy and severe mental retardation has already been mentioned in discussion of these handicaps. The data are unusually comprehensive and allow identification of the factors responsible for the marked reduction in some forms of cerebral palsy and of factors which could lead to a further reduction.

Epidemiological studies on the changing pattern of cerebral palsy in Sweden from 1954 to 1970 (Hagberg 1975) suggest that postnatal preventive measures have been largely exploited and that perinatal brain damage syndromes have decreased significantly, while prenatal mechanisms now predominate as still mainly unsolved problems. These studies and similar ones in the United Kingdom and United States have shown the benefits of modern neonatal intensive care with gains not only in

survival but also in undamaged babies.

Active measures to prevent cerebral palsy in Sweden date from the early 1950s when a centralized regional organization was set up for exchange transfusion services to care for all babies at risk of kernicterus from blood group incompatibility. Within a few years severe icterus was virtually eradicated as a brain-damaging factor, and the number of children with dyskinetic cerebral palsy decreased greatly.

From the mid 1950s each Swedish county (with a population of 200 000 to 400 000) centralized deliveries and neonatal care in one or two large county hospitals with excellent obstetric and neonatal services. Though the proportion of low birth weight infants remained constant at 4.3%, the number of low birth weight children with diplegia decreased significantly from 1954–1970 (Hagberg et al 1975a; (Fig. 11.9). This applied particularly to the babies with birth weights of 2000 g or less, whose chances of normal development have become remarkably good. This decline has also been noted in Britain (Davies & Tizard 1975) and elsewhere. It is clearly related to improved neonatal

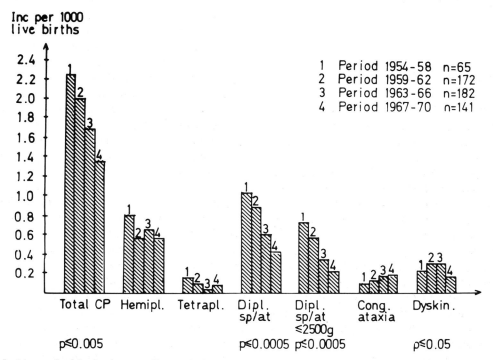

Fig 11.9 Incidence of cerebral palsy according to syndrome. (sp/at spastic/ataxia) from Hagberg et al 1975a

care and due to a systematic campaign to compensate for many adverse factors (acidosis, hypoxia, hypothermia, lack of calories and hypoglycaemia) rather than to any single factor, though early feeding may be particularly important.

After the dramatic fall in the numbers of cases of dyskinetic cerebral palsy which followed the introduction of exchange transfusion this type of cerebral palsy has not shown a further reduction in the years 1954 to 1970. Spastic hemiplegia, spastic tetraplegia and congenital ataxia have also remained fairly constant in numbers over the same period. In these three groups prenatal aetiological factors are thought to be common (Hagberg 1975). These probably accounted for many of the cases of hemiplegia and congenital ataxia in which no obvious cause could be found and also for 42% of the spastic tetraplegias. Low birth weight for gestational age was common in the tetraplegic children and occurred in 10% of the hemiplegias but was not present in those with congenital ataxia (in whom genetic factors may play some part). The years since 1970 have not brought any further decrease in the incidence of cerebral palsy in Sweden (Hagberg et al 1976), despite a further simultaneous reduction in the perinatal and infant mortality figures.

In Sweden, therefore, preventive efforts would seem best directed towards more systematic and reliable screening procedures to detect fetuses at risk, followed by their delivery at the optimal time with the minimum of perinatal trauma and in the best possible condition. Better supervision of the health of pregnant women with education on nutrition and the dangers to the fetus of smoking and alcohol are further fields where preventive efforts should be fruitful. These efforts and others to provide the highest standards of antenatal care, obstetrics and neonatal supervision for all pregnant women are even more necessary in countries whose results in these areas are inferior to those in Sweden and whose standards are less uniform. Recent experience in France has shown the impressive and rapid gains which can result from a nation-wide campaign for improved standards with incentives to encourage the use of antenatal and paediatric facilities (Chapalain 1978, Loring & Holland 1978).

PERINATAL INJURY TO THE SPINAL CORD

Spinal birth injuries have been recognized from the nineteenth century onwards. Crothers (1923) described injuries to the spinal cord in breech extractions as an important cause of fetal death and paraplegia in childhood. Breech presentation is a common feature with excessive longitudinal traction often combined with flexion and torsion of the spinal axis in a difficult delivery. Contributory factors include prematurity, primiparity, intrauterine malposition of the foetus, dystocia and precipitate delivery.

Complete transection of the spinal cord in the cervical region as reported by Byers (1932) was not uncommon in an earlier era when internal podalic version and forceful extraction by the breech was frequently practised. With improvement in obstetric techniques such cases have become much rarer and the spinal cord lesions less severe. Nonetheless Towbin (1969) in a pathological survey of brain and spinal cord in 170 cases found 16 cases with extensive and 14 with less severe cord lesions. The commonest lesions were epidural haemorrhage, dural laceration with subdural and intradural haemorrhage, torn nerve roots with haemorrhage, laceration and distortion of the cord, focal haemorrhage and malacia within the cord substance. Brachial plexus and lower brain stem lesions are often associated.

Clinically three groups of patients are seen (Towbin 1969). In the first the infant dies during labour or soon after birth from damage to the brain stem or cord. The second group is of infants who survive for a period of days with cord or brain stem damage. Respiratory depression is a cardinal sign with relatively good cardiac function. There is often intercostal paralysis and diaphragmatic respiration. The child is hypotonic, often with a frog position, selective segmental weakness in the arms and flaccid weakness and pyramidal features in the legs. In the third group infants survive for long periods, sometimes into adult life, with variable degrees of neurological deficit showing mainly flaccid weakness in the arms and a spastic paraplegia. Localized spinal epidural haematoma may be responsible in some such cases, but occasionally more severe injuries such as fracture-dislocation of vertebrae and cord transection are compatible with long survival. Some cases of milder cord injury with slight neurological deficit are probably wrongly regarded as examples of cerebral palsy. Associated hypoxic brain damage may occur in some infants at birth due to their respiratory depression and this may compound the problem and confuse the clinical picture with the features of spastic cerebral palsy and mental retardation being later superimposed on those due to the original spinal cord injury. Brachial plexus palsy and lower brain stem lesions with bulbar signs also resulting from the traumatic delivery, may further complicate the situation.

Bresnan & Abroms (1974) have drawn attention to the risk of neonatal spinal cord transection secondary to intrauterine hyperextension of the neck in breech presentation. Their review of the literature showed 82 cases of breech presentation with persistent hyperextension of the neck. Of these 56 were delivered vaginally and 14 of them (25%) had transections of the cord. By contrast in 26 infants delivered by caesarean section no case of transection was noted. Radiological detection of the hyperextension ('the star-gazing fetus') at the onset of labour is important so that caesarean section can be planned.

The prevention of spinal cord obstetric injuries is clearly more important than their treatment, which is unfortunately mostly supportive. If a fracture-dislocation of the spine is suspected a myelogram should be performed in the hope of showing a surgically treatable lesion. The relief of cord compression by removing a bony fragment or evacuating an epidural haematoma offers theoretical hope of improving neurological function but in practice the results are often disappointing.

BRACHIAL PLEXUS BIRTH INJURY

The anatomy of the brachial plexus, with its contributions from the fifth, sixth, seventh and eighth cervical and the first thoracic nerve roots, renders it vulnerable to damage by stretching forces, particularly in its upper part. Such injuries are most often seen after difficult delivery but are relatively uncommon in communities with good obstetric services, their frequency in one New York hospital in 1962 being 0.4 per 1000 births (Adler & Patterson 1967). Traction on the baby's shoulders or arms, or extreme lateral flexion of the neck are the forces usually involved. Most often injury to nerve roots results from compression by haemorrhage and oedema within their sheaths. Less often a nerve is torn or a root avulsed from the spinal cord, sometimes with damage to the grey matter in the cord at the same level. Traction injuries of increasing severity affect first the fifth cervical root, then the sixth and successively the lower components of the plexus.

The condition may be unilateral or bilateral, and effects the right side more often than the left, perhaps because the common left occipito-anterior presentation leaves the right shoulder against the pubic arch for longer than other presentations. In one series of 25 infants with brachial plexus palsy (Eng 1971), the condition was right-sided in 15, left-sided in 7 and bilateral in 3.

The severity of the traumatic forces involved is shown by the frequency with which other evidence of trauma is seen in affected infants. Eng (1971) found that 17 of 25 babies had other signs of trauma; these included fractured clavicle or humerus in 4 cases, dislocations in 4, facial palsy in 4, and cephalhaematoma in one.

Three main clinical pictures are recognized, the commonest with involvement of the fifth and sixth cervical roots and the much rarer conditions affecting the lower roots or the entire plexus.

Erb's (upper brachial plexus) palsy

Muscles innervated by the fifth and sixth cervical segments are paralysed (deltoid, biceps, brachioradialis, supra-and infraspinatus). A typical posture of the arm results from unopposed action of antagonists, with extension of the elbow, adduction and internal rotation at the shoulder and pronation of the forearm, sometimes with flexion of the wrist. The term 'waiter's (or sometimes 'policeman's') tip position' describes the position graphically. The proximal paralysis is confirmed by the finding of an absent or greatly reduced Moro reflex on the affected side. It can be shown that distal power is preserved by eliciting the palmar grasp reflex (Ch. 1) which should be equal on both sides. The limb may be hypotonic and the biceps reflex is lost. Sensory loss is difficult to demonstrate in the newborn period, but may be shown over the areas of skin innervated by the fifth and sixth cervical segments. Phrenic nerve palsy may be associated when the fourth cervical root is also affected, and this can occasionally occur without brachial plexus injury. The features of respiratory distress will suggest the diagnosis. Fractures of the clavicle or humerus are commonly associated with Erb's palsy. A Horner's syndrome is often present on the side of the lesion.

Unilateral Erb's palsy has been reported coming on many hours after delivery in two infants treated for respiratory distress syndrome by constant positive pressure airways pressure (Turner et al 1975). Both had been treated in a head box and it was thought that ischaemic damage to the upper roots of the brachial plexus by the neck seal might have been responsible. The infants both recovered from their paresis.

Klumpke's (lower brachial plexus) palsy

This type of brachial plexus palsy is much rarer than Erb's palsy, constituting between 2 and 3% of cases. The lower roots, the eighth cervical and first thoracic, are affected with paralysis of the intrinsic hand muscles and wrist flexors producing a claw hand which cannot be closed to make a fist (such as the normal newborn infant shows). Testing the neonatal automatic responses shows a normal Moro reflex but no palmar grasp. An ipsilateral Horner's syndrome is often present due to interruption of cervical sympathetic fibres in the first thoracic root. Loss of sensation and sweating may be found in the hand, and trophic skin changes with ulceration may develop. When there is segmental damage to the spinal cord signs of an upper motor neurone lesion may develop in the legs to produce a confusing clinical picture.

Total brachial plexus palsy

It is very rare for all the elements of the plexus to be affected. A severe degree of injury is needed, often causing avulsion of many nerve roots from the spinal cord, and often with other signs of trauma. The arm is totally paralysed and hypotonic with absence of all tendon reflexes and of the Moro and grasp reflexes. At lumbar puncture the CSF may contain blood and myelography may show localised disruption of the dura. Muscle wasting develops and the growth of the arm is slowed down. Pyramidal features in one or both legs are more likely than with less extensive lesions.

The prognosis for the commoner C 5 and 6, and C 5, 6 and 7 injuries is much better than that of the rare C 8 and T 1 lesions. In Eng's (1971) series permanent weakness or deformity developed in two of the ten infants with C 5 and 6 injuries, in three of the ten with C 5, 6 and 7 lesions and in three of the five in whom all the roots of the plexus were damaged. Of 20 infants adequately followed up, six had recovered by six months of age with minimal deficit, 11 had recovered by one year with moderate deficits and 3 showed significant handicaps.

Treatment is aimed at correcting abnormal postures by appropriate splinting and preventing contractures by repeated passive movement of the arm.

With Erb's palsy the arm should be partially immobilized in a position of optimum function, achieved by placing a folded towel in the axilla and applying a sling to hold the arm in flexion.

In Klumpke's palsy attention is focussed on the hand with small pads of cotton wool placed in the palm and between the fingers loosely bandaged in place to hold the hand and fingers slightly flexed.

REFERENCES

Adler J, Patterson R L 1967 Erb's palsy. Long-term results of treatment in 88 cases. Journal of Bone and Joint Surgery 49: 1052a–1064

Batten F E 1903 Congenital cerebellar ataxia. Clinical Journal 22: 81

Black P D 1980 Ocular defects in children with cerebral palsy. British Medical Journal 281: 487a–488

Bobath B 1967 The very early treatment of cerebral palsy. Developmental Medicine and Child Neurology 9: 373

Bresnan M J, Abroms I F 1974 Neonatal spinal cord transection secondary to intra-uterine hyperextension of the neck in breech presentation. Journal of Pediatrics 84: 734a–737

Brown C 1970 Down all the days. Secker and Warburg, London Bundey S, Griffths M I 1977 Recurrence risks in families of children with symmetrical spasticity. Developmental Medicine and Child Neurology 19: 179a–191

Byers R K 1932 Transection of the spinal cord in the newborn. A case with autopsy and comparison with a normal cord at the same age. Archives of Neurology and Psychiatry 27: 585a–592

Byers R K 1941 Evolution of hemiplegia in infancy.American Journal of Diseases of Children 61: 915

Carpenter E B, Seitz D G 1980 Intramuscular alcohol as an aid in management of spastic cerebral palsy. Developmental Medicine and Child Neurology 22: 497a–501

Chapalain M-Th 1978 Perinatality: French Cost-benefit studies and decisions on handicap and prevention. 193–204

Christensen E, Melchior J 1967 Cerebral palsy — a clinical and neuropathological study. Clinics in Developmental Medicine No. 25, Spastics Society Medical Education and Information Unit and William Heinemann Medical Books, London

Crothers B 1923 Injuries of the spinal cord in breech extractions as an important cause of fetal death and paraplegia in childhood. American Journal of Medical Science 165: 94

Crothers B, Paine R S 1959 The natural history of cerebral palsy. Harvard University Press, Cambridge, Mass., Oxford University Press, London

Davies P A, Tizard J P M 1975 Very low birthweight and subsequent neurological defect (with special reference to spastic diplegia). Developmental Medicine and Child Neurology 17: 3a–17

Drillien C M 1964 The growth and development of the prematurely born infant. Livingstone, Edinburgh

Egan J M 1977 The physical management of cerebral palsy. In: Drillien C M, Drummond M B, (eds) Neurodevelopmental problems in early childhood, Assessment and management. Blackwell Scientific Publications, Oxford

Eng G D 1971 Brachial plexus palsy in newborn infants. Pediatrics 48: 18a–28

Evans P R, Polani P E 1950 The neurological sequelae of Rh sensitization. Quarterly Journal of Medicine 19: 129a–149

Finnie N R 1974 Handling the young cerebral palsied child at home, 2nd ed. Heinemann, London

Fixsen J A 1979 Surgical treatment of the lower limbs in cerebral palsy: a review. Journal of the Royal Society of Medicine 72: 761a–765

Freud S 1897 Die Infantile Cerebrallähmung (Nothnagel's Specielle Pathologie und Therapie). Hölder, Vienna div 2,pt 2, vol 9

Glenting P 1973 Cerebral parese — patienter i danska amter øst for storebaelt i årene 1940–1969. Meddelelser fra C. P. Registret, 1

Gordon N 1966 The electroencephalogram in cerebral palsy. Developmental Medicine and Child Neurology 8: 216–218

Gordon N 1976 Paediatric neurology for the clinician. Clinics in Developmental Medicine nos 59/60. Spastics International Medical Publications, William Heinemann Medical Books Ltd, London, J. B. Lipincott, Philadelphia

Gowers W R 1876 On athetosis and post-hemiplegic disorders of movements. Medical Clinical Transactions 59: 271

Hagberg B 1975 Pre-, peri- and postnatal prevention of major neuropediatric handicaps. Neuropädiatrie 6: 331a–338

Hagberg B, Hagberg O, Olow I 1975a The changing panorama of cerebral palsy in Sweden 1954–1970 I. Analysis of the general changes. Acta Paediatrica Scandinavica 64: 187a–192

Hagberg B, Hagberg O, Olow I 1975b The changing panorama of cerebral palsy in Sweden 1954–1970. II. Analysis of the various syndromes. Acta paediatrica Scandinavica 64: 193–200

Hagberg G, Hagberg B, Olow I 1976 The changing panorama of cerebral palsy. III. The importance of foetal deprivation of supply. Acta paediatrica Scandinavica 65: 403–408

Hagberg B, Sanner G, Steen M 1972 The dysequilibrium syndrome in cerebral palsy. Acta paediatrica Scandinavica, suppl 226

Hammond W A 1871 On athetosis, Medical Times (London) 2: 747

Holt K S 1965 Assessment of cerebral palsy. I. Motor function locomotion and hand function. Lloyd-Luke, London

Holt K S, Reynell J K 1967 Assessment of cerebral palsy. II. Vision, communication and psychological function. Lloyd-Luke, London

Holt K S, Jones R B, Wilson R 1974 Gait analysis by means of multiple sequential exposure camera. Developmental Medicine and Child Neurology 16: 742a–745

Ingram T T S 1955 The early manifestations and course of diplegia in childhood. Archives of Disease in Childhood 30: 244a–250

Ingram T T S 1964 Paediatric aspects of cerebral palsy. Livingstone, Edinburgh

Ingram T T S 1966 The neurology of cerebral palsy. Archives of Disease in Childhood 41: 337a–357

Jones R B 1975 The Vojta method of treating cerebral palsy. Physiotherapy 61: 112

Joynt R L, Leonard J A 1980 Dantrolene sodium suspension in treatment of spastic cerebral palsy. Developmental Medicine and Child Neurology 22: 755a–767

Little W J 1843 The deformities of the human frame. Lancet 1, 5, 38 et seq

Little W J 1862 On the influence of abnormal parturition, labour, premature birth and asphyxia neonatorum on the mental and physical condition of the child, especially in relation to deformities. Transactions of the Obstetrical Society of London 111: 293

Little Club 1959 Memorandum on terminology and classification of cerebral palsy. Cerebral Palsy Bulletin 1(5): 27

Lloyd-Roberts G C 1971 Orthopaedics in infancy and childhood. Butterworths, London

Loring J, Holland M 1978 The prevention of cerebral palsy. The basic facts. Spastics Society

Manning J 1972 Facilitation of movement. The BOBATH approach. Physiotheraphy 58: 403

Milla P J, Jackson A D M 1977 A controlled trial of baclofen (Lioresal®R) in children with cerebral palsy. Journal of International Medical Research 5(6): 398

Minear W L 1956 A classification of cerebral palsy. Pediatrics 18: 841–852

Nolan C 1981 Dam-burst of dreams. The writings of Christopher Nolan. Weidenfeld and Nicolson, London

O'Reilly D E 1971 The Future of the cerebral palsied child. Developmental Medicine and Child Neurology 13: 635a–640

O'Reilly D E 1974 The adult with cerebral palsy. Developmental Medicine and Child Neurology 16: 707

Perlstein M A 1952 Infantile cerebral palsy; classification and clinical correlations. Journal of the American Medical Association 149: 30a–34

Perlstein M A, Hood P N 1954 Infantile spastic hemiplegia. I. Incidence. Pediatrics 14: 436a–441

Phelps W M 1950 Etiology and diagnostic classification of cerebral palsy. Nervous Child 7: 10

Rapp D 1980 Drool control: long-term follow-up. Developmental Medicine and Child Neurology 22: 448a–453

Robson P 1970 Shuffling, hitching, scooting and sliding, some observations in 30 otherwise normal children. Developmental Medicine and Child Neurology 12: 608a–617

Robson P 1978 Essential hypotonia in infants and young children. In: Jukes A N (ed) Baclofen — spasticity and cerebral pathology. Cambridge Medical Publications, Northampton

Robson P, MacKeith R C 1971 Shufflers with spastic diplegic cerebral palsy: a confusing clinical picture. Developmental Medicine and Child Neurology 13: 651a–659

Sachs B 1891 Contributions to the pathology of infantile cerebral palsies. Quoted by Sachs & Hausman (1926)

Sachs B, Hausman L 1926 The proper classification of the cerebral palsies of early life. American Journal of Medical Science 171: 376

Samilson R L (ed) 1975 Orthopaedic aspects of cerebral palsy. SIMP Clinics in Developmental Medicine nos 52/53, William Heinemann, London, J B Lipincott, Philadelphia

Sanner G, Hagberg B 1974 188 cases of non-progressive ataxic syndromes in childhood. Neuropädiatrie 5: 224a–235

Sanner G, Sundequist U 1981 Acupuncture for the relief of painful muscle spasms in dystonic cerebral palsy. Developmental Medicine and Child Neurology 23: 544a–545

Scrutton D, Gilbertson M 1975 Physiotherapy in paediatric practice. Butterworth, London

Sheridan M D 1976a Manual for the STYCAR Vision Tests, 3rd edn. National Foundation for Educational Research, London

Sheridan M D 1976b Manual for the SYTCAR Hearing Tests, 3rd edn. National Foundation for Educational Research, London

Sheridan M D 1977 Development and assessment of vision and hearing in Drillien C M, Drummond M B, edn Neurodevelopmental problems in early childhood. Assessment and management. Blackwell Scientific Publications, Oxford

Tardieu C, Tardieu G, Hariga J, Gagnard L 1968 Treatment of spasticity by injection of dilute alcohol at the motor point or by epidural route. Clinical extension of an experiment on the decerebrate cat. Developmental Medicine and Child Neurology 10: 555a–568

Tizard J P M, Paine R S, Crothers, B 1954 Disturbances of sensation in children with hemiplegia. Journal of the American Medical Association 155: 628a–632

Towbin A 1969 Latent spinal cord and brain stem injury in newborn infants. Developmental Medicine and Child Neurology 11: 54–68

Turner T, Evans J, Brown J K 1975 Monoparesis. Complication of constant positive airways pressure. Archives of Disease in Childhood 50: 128

Volpe J J 1976 Perinatal hypoxic – ischaemic brain injury. Pediatric Clinics of North America 23: 383a–397

12

Epilepsy and convulsions

E. M. Brett

'Lastly we may observe, to the great comfort and satisfaction of the parents of those children subject to convulsions, or the epilepsia infantilis, that they need not be apprehensive of its changing into the true epilepsy, for it generally disappears by degrees, as they grow older and acquire more strength.'

von Rosenstein 1776 *Diseases of Children and their Remedies,*
British edition

The great Swedish proto-paediatrician, von Rosenstein, in his rather optimistic prognosis for early convulsions, showed remarkable insight, not only into the concerns of parents, but also into the tendency towards spontaneous improvement. He clearly recognized the distinction to be made between those young children who are subject to seizures for a limited period, and those who, showing a tendency to recurrent attacks somewhat later, justify the use of the word 'epilepsy'. There is still no unanimity about the precise application of this word, and an ideal definition of epilepsy is not easy to find. The classical definition of Hughlings Jackson, 'epilepsy is the expression of occasional, sudden, excessive, rapid, local discharge in the grey matter', is of little practical use to the paediatrician involved in the problems of childhood seizures. His approach to these problems must be largely empirical and pragmatic, since many questions of aetiology, natural history and epidemiology remain unanswered.

The paediatrician must draw a clear distinction between children who have one or more convulsions in certain specific situations only, such as transient biochemical disorders in the newborn period or febrile infections at a slightly later age, and others who show a definite tendency to repeated seizures in the absence of provoking factors and can therefore be regarded as 'epileptic', since the concept of *recurrence* of attacks is central to any definition of epilepsy. To apply the term to children who have had a single attack, especially when associated with clear provoking factors, is inadvisable and can be harmful in many ways. Time is a major factor in any history, and only the passage of time will show whether a clear pattern of unprovoked attacks will emerge or not. Great harm can be done to a child (or, indeed, an adult) by prematurely and incorrectly applying to him the emotive label 'epilepsy'. Prejudice and misunderstanding are still widespread so that the diagnosis of epilepsy carries overtones of terror and despair, and should be made only after very careful consideration.

CLASSIFICATION OF EPILEPSY

The problems of classifying epilepsy are rather similar to those of classifying cerebral palsy (Ch. 11) but more complex. Marsden (1976) pointed out the difficulty of devising a single code to cover three basically incompatible systems of classification, relating to the clinical features of the fit, to the anatomical and electrophysiological evidence of the source of the fit, and to its aetiology (when known). For those dealing with children a pragmatic approach is needed emphasizing the chronological aspect, since the stage of maturation of the nervous system is an important factor determining the occurrence and the type of seizures.

The International Classification of Epilepsy (Gastaut 1969, 1970) was developed at the behest of the International League against Epilepsy and has come to be widely accepted. Seizures are classified into the following categories:

1. 'Partial' seizures or those beginning locally. These are subdivided into those with 'elementary' symptomatology, (generally without impairment of consciousness) those with 'complex' symptomatology (generally with impaired consciousness) and partial attacks becoming secondarily generalized.

2. Generalized seizures or those which are bilaterally symmetrical and without local onset. These include petit mal absences, bilateral massive myoclonus, infantile spasms, clonic and/or tonic seizures, tonic-clonic seizures (grand mal) and atonic and akinetic seizures.

3. Unilateral seizures.

4. Unclassifiable seizures.

The advantages of this classification in facilitating communication about epilepsy have caused it to be increasingly adopted, but it has not entirely ousted the older classification with its terms (grand mal, petit mal, temporal lobe epilepsy, focal epilepsy etc.) derived from different sources. The International Classification has been slower to gain adherents in the field of childhood epilepsy, and in this chapter the older system will be used, with the newer terms given in parenthesis.

In assessing children with seizures and epilepsy the associated problems which may co-exist, in particular the two other common chronic neurological handicaps of childhood, mental retardation and cerebral palsy, must be considered since these may in themselves closely affect the prognosis. The EEG may show a variety of abnormal patterns, or may be normal and it may — rarely — give clues to the aetiology of the seizures. This aspect is discussed by Dr Harris in Chapter 24.

Classification may also be attempted according to aetiology, when known, based upon history, examination and investigation, but it must be stressed that in many cases of childhood epilepsy (as in mental retardation and, to a lesser extent, cerebral palsy) the cause remains unknown.

In analysing the clinical phenomena of seizures in children the paediatrician is usually denied the history of subjective symptoms which an older, more articulate patient can give, but this may be partly balanced by the greater likelihood of a detailed account of the attacks from an observer, usually the mother.

MATURATION AND THE CHRONOLOGY OF SEIZURES

The stages of maturation or development of the child is an important factor in determining both his liability to seizures and the type of seizure he may have. Thus, a range of seizures occurs in the newborn period some of which are seldom seen in older children. Febrile convulsions and infantile spasms are also closely related to age. Temporal lobe attacks are not often seen under the age of three years.

It is convenient and logical therefore to consider in chronological sequence the common problems of epilepsy and convulsions in childhood from neonatal (and prenatal) life onwards. This pragmatic approach is adopted with success by O'Donohoe (1979), whose monograph *Epilepsies of childhood* is perhaps the best available guide to the subject for the clinician.

NEONATAL SEIZURES

The incidence of seizures in the newborn period is variously assessed as between 0.2 and 1.2% of all live births. In the newborn the attacks can take many different forms. Many neonatal attacks resemble isolated aspects of generalized seizures in older infants. (Their fragmentary nature is probably related to the functionally incomplete state of the nervous system at this age before the final architecture of cortical neurons, elaboration of axonal and dendritic networks and establishment of synaptic connections have been attained.) Their features have been well reviewed by several authors (Brown 1973, Volpe 1973, Snodgrass 1974). In the commonest type of neonatal seizure the unwary observer may fail to recognize that the baby is having a fit so subtle are the features, with slight jerking or horizontal deviation of the eyes, fluttering of the eyelids, sucking or other movements of the mouth, and often a short apnoeic spell. Tonic, clonic and myoclonic seizures are more dramatic and easily recognized. Tonic fits usually result from brain damage, can occur in very immature infants, and often carry a bad prognosis with early death or chronic handicap in the survivors. Clonic fits are unusual before 37 weeks of gestation, occur without a preceding tonic phase and may be focal or multifocal. They often occur in metabolic disturbances. Clonic jerking may migrate from one part of the body to another in a random way. Sometimes the baby may appear unaffected by the attacks, even to the extent of continuing to feed during them.

Jitteriness in the newborn period is sometimes confused with seizures and should be clearly distinguished from them. This movement disorder of the newborn is rarely seen in older children. It occurs in babies with hypoxic-ischaemic brain disorder, hypocalcaemia, drug withdrawal and occasionally in otherwise normal infants. Volpe (1977) has stressed the main points of distinction — that jitteriness is unaccompanied by abnormalities of gaze or extra-ocular movements, but is exquisitely stimulus-sensitive unlike seizures, and that the dominant movement of jitteriness is tremor with rhythmic alternating movements of equal rate and amplitude, while in seizures the main movement is clonic jerking with a fast and slow component.

Causes

The causes of neonatal seizures are many and varied. Volpe (1973) lists them in descending order of frequency as perinatal hypoxic-ischaemic injury, subarachnoid haemorrhage, hypoglycaemia, CNS infection and congenital cerebral malformations.

The aetiology can be fairly well correlated with the day of onset of seizures and the prognosis. Rose & Lombroso (1970) in their detailed study of 137 full-term babies with neonatal fits followed up for an average of 4 years found that the peak incidence of seizures occurred on the second day of life, intracranial haemorrhage and cerebral contusions being the commonest cause. The second highest incidence was on the first day of life when perinatal anoxia was the single most common cause. With attacks starting between 4 and 7 days of age, hypocalcaemia accounted for one third: three-quarters of hypocalcaemic fits began after the fourth day. By contrast hypoglycaemia caused fits mainly in the first 3 days. The prognosis was found to be good in simple hypocalcaemia and primary subarachnoid haemorrhage, but less good in hypoglycaemia and very poor when cerebral anoxia was the cause.

Metabolic causes have come to account for an increasing proportion of neonatal convulsions in the past 15 years while anoxia and birth injury have decreased in importance as causes. In some seven of the 12 per 1000 infants with convulsions born in one Scottish centre the fits were due to primary uncomplicated hypocalcaemia/hypomagnesaemia (Brown 1973), while in 45 of the 112 infants studied by Keen and Lee (1973) the seizures were associated only with hypocalcaemia. The prognosis was good in these cases; of the 45 infants with hypocalcaemic fits, only two had an intelligence assessment under 85 and only one had a further convulsion. By contrast hypoglycaemia, cerebral haemorrhage and anoxia carried a much worse prognosis. Hypocalcaemia occurs mainly in artificially fed infants and is a theoretically preventable cause of seizures, readily treated, if detected, when it occurs. Amino-acid disorders and those of the urea cycle and organic acidaemias may occasionally present with neonatal convulsions (Ch. 6 and 7).

Infection, particularly meningitis, is an important cause of neonatal seizures to be considered and excluded or treated as soon as possible.

Cerebral malformations are another cause, but account for only a small proportion of cases of neonatal fits. They may be suspected when there are abnormalities of the ears, palate or lip, but special X-rays are needed to confirm their presence. With the exception of the Sturge-Weber syndrome (Ch. 20) fits in the newborn period are not often due to the neurocutaneous syndromes.

Seizures may occur in the newborn baby as a withdrawal symptom in the case of mothers who have been taking phenobarbitone or other anticonvulsant drugs therapeutically, alcohol or certain drugs of addiction during pregnancy. Careful enquiry should be made for such a history, but it may be deliberately concealed by addicts. Withdrawal fits in infants may result when the mother is addicted to barbiturates (Desmond et al 1972) or to narcotic drugs. Herzlinger & Herbert (1977) found that 18 of the 302 babies born to narcotic-dependent women at the Bronx Memorial Center had seizures, coming on at a mean age of 10 days. These were usually generalized motor seizures or rhythmic myoclonic fits. Most responded quickly to treatment, paregoric (camphorated tincture of opium) being more effective than Diazepam.

A small proportion of neonatal seizures remain unexplained after detailed investigation. A few such cases may be examples of the rare 'benign familial neonatal convulsions' reported by Carton (1978) and Tibbles (1980). The fits are often frequent and intractable but recovery is usually complete if they can be brought under control and brain damage avoided. However, Tibbles (1980) found that 13% of the reported patients later developed epilepsy. He believes the condition may be less rare than it seems from the paucity of reports.

A recent Swedish study (Eriksson & Zetterström 1979) into the causes and short term prognosis of neonatal convulsions in infants under 4 weeks of age concerned 77 full term infants born in Stockholm between 1970 and 1976. In 48% hypoxia was considered the main aetiological factor, while infection (12%) and metabolic disease including hypoglycaemia and hypocalcaemia (12%) were the next commonest. The aetiology was unknown in 29%. The total mortality was 13%. At one year of age 19 of the surviving 64 children (30%) had severe psychomotor retardation. Of 11 with normal mental development at one year 6 had cerebral palsy and 5 had epileptic seizures. 34 children (53%) had no signs of any sequelae. The worst prognosis was in the group with hypoxia as the main probable aetiology. The incidence of neonatal convulsions over this period was 1.5 per 1000 full term deliveries. This was less than half that in a similar study made in Gothenburg 10 years earlier from 1960–1962 (Zetterström 1963) in which the incidence was 3.7 per 1000. The reduced incidence of neonatal seizures was rather similar to that for perinatal mortality in Gothenburg (23.8) and Stockholm (13.5) in the same period.

The EEG is of some prognostic help in neonatal convulsions (Harris & Tizard 1960, Tibbles & Prichard 1965, Rose & Lombroso 1970). This aspect is discussed by Dr Harris (Ch. 24).

DRUG TREATMENT OF NEONATAL SEIZURES

Phenobarbitone is the drug of choice for seizures in the newborn period. Apart from acting as an anticonvulsant it has the advantage of reducing the cerebral metabolic rate. This is particularly beneficial in cases of hypoxic-ischaemic encephalopathy (Ch. 1) in which seizures are often a major problem aggravating an already parlous situation by markedly accelerating the metabolic rate of the brain. Experimental data suggest that barbiturates in high doses also protect against cerebral hypoxic-ischaemic injury. They have also been shown to prevent or reduce cerebral oedema of ischaemic origin. Volpe (1981) believes that Phenobarbitone given before the onset of clinical seizures reduces the likelihood of later, uncontrolled fits in hypoxic-ischaemic encephalopathy and has treated seriously asphyxiated, full-term infants in the first hours after birth with the drug prophylactically in the absence of seizures. He does not recommend it use for this purpose in premature infants since its depressant effect may obscure the subtle signs of intraventricular haemorrhage and embarrass respiration.

There is a tendency to underestimate the loading dose and to overestimate the maintenance dose of phenobarbitone in treating neonatal seizures. Fischer et al (1981) have shown that loading doses of 15–20 mg/kg are needed for adequate plasma levels, whereas maintenance doses between 3.1 and 3.8 mg/kg per day will produce plasma concentrations of 20 to 25 μg/1. The plasma half-life of the drug is longer in the newborn than at older ages, so that a watch should be kept for signs of respiratory depression, and it is advisable to monitor blood levels.

Phenytoin is better avoided in the newborn period since the developing cerebellum may be vulnerable to permanent damage from toxic levels. Diazepam, useful in the treatment of status epilepticus and severe fits in older patients by the intravenous route, should not be used in the newborn since the complex of bilirubin and albumin may be unbound by the sodium benzoate present in its vehicle with an increased risk of kernicterus.

INTRA-UTERINE CONVULSIONS AND PYRIDOXINE-DEPENDENT EPILEPSY

Convulsions may rarely begin during intra-uterine life. The mother may experience fetal movements which are episodically and briefly abnormal and tumultuous and the infant may be born convulsing or be seen to convulse soon after birth. In these cases it is reasonable to regard the convulsions as having started in utero. This situation occurs most often with the rare recessively inherited disorder, pyridoxine (pyridoxol or vitamin B6) dependency (Hunt et al 1954, Bejšovec et al 1967) in which the infant has a grossly increased requirement for this vitamin.

The disease should always be considered in any convulsing newborn and a therapeutic test made with 100 mg of pyridoxine by intravenous injection. The effect is dramatic in definite cases and the drug should then be continued regularly by mouth, since the abnormal requirement persists for a variable period. The oral dose required varies from one case to another. In one personal case doses of up to 1 g per day were needed to prevent fits.

The prognosis is usually good when the condition is recognized and treated effectively, but unfortunately the possibility is often not considered until the child has been convulsing for some hours or days. After prolonged status epilepticus in the newborn period (and indeed at any age in childhood) the outlook is often poor since neuronal damage may have resulted from the seizures whatever their cause.

Heeley et al (1978) have studied certain aspects of pyridoxine metabolism in 3 patients believed to suffer from pyridoxine-dependency and compared the findings with those in healthy children and adults and in children with mental handicap. The size of the initial rise and subsequent fall in plasma pyridoxal phosphate (PALP) concentrations after a load of pyridoxal suggested that the B6-responsive patients were able to synthesise PALP normally but could not maintain the prolonged high levels normally found in the plasma. The urinary excretion of 4-pyridoxic acid was within normal limits, but the excretion of pyridoxal after the load was increased. The authors postulate an instability of the PALP-albumin complex in this condition.

INFANTILE SPASMS

This variety of generalized seizure is known by at least 21 synonyms in six languages (Jeavons & Bower 1964). The first description (which can

scarcely be bettered) appeared in a letter to the *Lancet* in 1841 by Dr W. J. West, a Kent practitioner who reported the onset of the attacks at 4 months of age in his own son, a previously normal infant, who was thereafter severely retarded (whence the name 'West's syndrome' sometimes used for the condition although West's own term 'salaam spasms' is more informative.)

The attacks figured rarely in the English literature over the next hundred years, although recognised in continental European publications. In 1883 Féré listed the many names attached to the seizures and commented both on the frequently associated mental defect and the fact that the children were 'epileptic apprentices', subject to epilepsy (i.e. recurrent convulsions) in later life. He also recognized two aetiological groups, the symptomatic and the idiopathic. The condition reappeared in the British literature in 1955 with Illingworth's report of 'Sudden mental deterioration with convulsions in infancy'. The clinical aspects were fully analysed by many writers and in the 1950s the EEG features of the syndrome were also studied and the grossly abnormal pattern usually associated with it was described (Vazquez & Turner 1951, Gibbs & Gibbs 1952).

The onset of the attacks is in the first year of life in 90% of cases, and in the first six months in nearly 70%, with a peak at about 5 months. Onset under three months is uncommon. A preponderance of males over females of up to two to one has been reported by some authors, but others have found no sex difference.

The word 'salaam' or 'jack-knife' provides a useful shorthand description for the typical attack of the more common flexion variety. The events are dramatic, with sudden, brief flexion of neck and trunk, raising of both arms forwards or sideways sometimes with flexion at the elbows, and flexion of legs at the hips. Less often the legs extend at the hips. In some cases flexion of the neck may be the only or main feature: this may occur at an early stage of the history and be followed by more complex and dramatic attacks later on. A cry is often associated with the attacks: this may form part of the attack or occur afterwards as an expression of disquiet (the episodes are clearly distressing for the infant just as they are for the onlooker). Sometimes it is difficult to be certain as to its relationship. The spasms are usually symmetrical but may occasionally show lateralising features with the head turned to one side or one limb moving more vigorously. It is understandable that many different terms should be used for these attacks. 'Spasmes en flexion' enjoys wide currency in France. In Germany 'Grusskrampf' shows analogies with 'Salaam attacks', but the term 'Blitz-Nick and Salaamkrämpfe' (BNS), (lightning, nodding and salaam attacks) is more descriptive. 'Massive myoclonic jerks' seems to have certain disadvantages, since this term can be applied to attacks in older children which differ from infantile spasms, and the duration of the episodes is slightly longer than that of a myoclonic jerk in an older patient. In many ways the term 'infantile spasms' seems the most suitable.

Although the experienced observer will have no difficulty in recognising the attacks they are often misinterpreted. It is not easy for an anxious mother to note carefully or to give an accurate description of the events, and it is helpful to persuade her to *imitate* an attack rather than merely to describe it. Sometimes, with less observant parents, it is helpful to demonstrate a typical attack oneself (the child neurologist must have a repertoire of such ictal mimes), but this should not be done until the mother has made at least an attempt at a demonstration.

Confusion often occurs with more benign phenomena, such as a Moro reflex, attacks of colic or even attempts to sit up. This can be avoided if, in addition to obtaining a detailed account of the individual events, the doctor studies the pattern of occurrence of the attacks. Infantile spasms are unique among seizures in coming 'not as single spies, but in battalions'. It is rare for a single attack to occur. In the earlier stages of the history they will often occur two or three times in succession, but quite soon they come in series of between 5 and 50, or even more, the attacks being separated by a few seconds. Towards the end of a series, the interval between spasms lengthens and their severity decreases until they gradually cease, often leaving the child exhausted. The twilight state, just before sleep or just after waking, often acts as a precipitating factor, and feeding may also provoke the spasms.

The findings on examination vary according to the aetiology, which is very variable. The findings, and the previous history, are more likely to be normal in the idiopathic or cryptogenic group than in the symptomatic. In many cases the spasms occur in children who have given clear evidence of an abnormal nervous system in delayed developmental milestones related to mental retardation sometimes accompanied by microcephaly or hydrocephalus or by the early signs of cerebral palsy (spasticity, dystonia, and abnormal asymmetric tonic neck reflex, exaggerated tendon reflexes). When this occurs with a history of severe perinatal difficulties, it is very likely that the onset of the spasms is merely the latest evidence of abnormal brain function. Spasms symptomatic of previous brain pathology may occur in children damaged by intrauterine infections, such as toxoplasmosis, cytomegalic inclusion disease or rubella. In these cases there are often pointers to the cerebral abnormality or its cause, in retardation, microcephaly, hydrocephalus, choroidoretinopathy or intracranial calcification. In 50% or more of cases there is no evidence of previous abnormality, and these children must be examined very carefully for underlying disorders which might have prognostic or genetic implications. Infantile spasms are now recognised to be a common presenting symptom of tuberose sclerosis; sometimes the infants have shown delayed development from birth, though this may have been unrecognized, but in some cases their previous developmental history cannot be faulted. Some 30% of infants referred in recent years to the Hospital for Sick Children, Great Ormond Street, with infantile spasms have been found to show cutaneous evidence of tuberose sclerosis most often in the form of pale, leaf-shaped amelanotic naevi (see Ch. 20) which should be searched for meticulously with the naked eye and ultraviolet light. The genetic implications of this diagnosis are so important that it must not be missed. Phenylketonuria and other inborn errors of metabolism must be excluded. Occasionally a cerebral malformation or other anomaly may be found on special X-rays. Hydrocephalus or porencephalic cysts may be found. Hydranencephaly was present in one child (Neville 1972). Agenesis of the corpus callosum (Ch. 17) may be shown on X-rays, either alone in either sex or in girls in association with a peculiar form of choroido-retinopathy constituting the

Aicardi syndrome (Aicardi et al 1969, Dennis & Bower 1972).

A possible relationship between infantile spasms and immunization, particularly against diphtheria, pertussis and tetanus (DPT), has been discussed for many years. Baird & Borofsky (1957) found that 9 out of 24 children who had been normal until the onset of their spasms had a history of DPT immunisation just before the onset. This temporal association has been observed in many cases and some paediatricians are convinced of a causal relationship, although it is obviously very difficult to be certain in the individual case. Such factors as the previous normality of the children and the interval between immunisation and onset of spasms are critical, but details of these may be missing.

Studies from Japan (Fukuyama et al 1977) and from Denmark (Melchior 1977) did not lend support to an aetiological role of DPT in infantile spasms. The Danish immunization programme was changed from a régime of triple immunization at 5, 6 and 15 months to one of monovalent vaccine at 5 and 9 weeks and 10 months. Comparison of the cases of spasms reported with these different régimes showed no change in their age of onset.

The whole problem of serious neurological reactions to DPT is at present very topical, with questions of compensation and litigation tending to cloud the issue. The pertussis element (Kulenkampff et al 1974) has been most often blamed for such adverse reactions and it is advisable to omit it in all children who have shown any signs of previous neurological abnormality or who have had seizures, or have first-degree relatives who have had seizures, since there is an impression that adverse reactions are more likely in these. It is particularly important to avoid immunisation in children with a history of a recent infection, especially of the respiratory tract.

Progressive degenerative brain disease and neoplasms are rare as causes of infantile spasms.

The major importance of the syndrome lies in the close association with mental retardation. Whether his development has previously been normal, suspect or clearly abnormal, it is usual for the onset of the spasms to be followed quickly by slowing down in the infant's development and often by dramatic regression with loss of his acquired skills and of social responsiveness. This is sometimes so dramatic that the parents believe the child has suddenly become deaf or blind, since he ceases to react to visual and auditory stimuli. Regression in motor skills is usually less striking, but often the ability to sit up, if already acquired, is lost. In untreated (and in many treated) cases persisting severe mental retardation is very common, even though the spasms usually cease by the age of two years, often being followed later by major convulsions. Treatment with conventional anticonvulsants was early noted to give very disappointing results, in terms of the attacks, the grossly abnormal EEG and the outlook for future development. More recently the benzodiazepine drugs, diazepam, nitrazepam and clonazepam, have been found to abolish or reduce the attacks in many cases, and sometimes to improve the EEG, but the ultimate prognosis for intelligence seldom seems to be improved thereby. Sodium valproate has given good results in some cases.

ACTH and adrenal cortical steroids were introduced in the treatment of infantile spasms in 1958 (Sorel & Dusaucy-Bauloye) in the belief that there might be an underlying neuro-allergic encephalitis which could be controlled by these drugs. This is unlikely in most cases, but nonetheless good results were obtained, and this approach is the most hopeful one at present available. The response to steroids and ACTH is often dramatic, the spasms ceasing within a few days, the EEG becoming less abnormal and the children often becoming socially responsive again. The best results seem to follow when treatment is started soon after the onset of the spasms. ACTH is usually given in large doses of the order of 40 units daily, similar to the dose found effective in many adult patients with disseminated sclerosis, and prednisolone in a dose of 2 mg/kg per day. Smaller doses may be ineffective, and I believe that one should not accept that ACTH has failed when the dose used has been less than 40 units daily; occasionally 60 units are found to be effective when 40 units have produced no benefit. 80 units are recommended by Lerman and Kivity (1982). Similar flexibility is needed in the length of treatment; it is usual to treat for two weeks and in most cases improvement has occurred during that time, but occasionally improvement is delayed until after 3 or 4 weeks of treatment and too early acceptance of defeat may prevent the child from benefitting. The side-effects of treatment, with almost invariable weight gain and a Cushingoid appearance, occasional hypertension and gastro-intestinal upset with frequent irritability, must be accepted as a small price to pay for the hope of a satisfactory outcome. In some cases longer-acting preparations of ACTH are effective, and the use of alternate day injections or prednisolone, sometimes in a higher dose, may help to reduce side-effects. Gratifying and encouraging though the response may be, for parents and doctor alike, relapses in the spasms are unfortunately common when the treatment is stopped or reduced. In many cases the attacks remain in abeyance when the conventional two week course is discontinued, but in other cases they recur, and it may then be justified to resume treatment and to continue with the smallest dose which seems effective for a period of further weeks or even months. Some doctors prefer not to use ACTH or steroids in cases in which the spasms are symptomatic of obvious brain damage or of tuberose sclerosis, but I personally feel that most children should be given the chance of the most effective treatment, since the results are unpredictable in the individual case, and occasional patients with perinatal brain damage or tuberose sclerosis respond very well.

It is advisable to start treatment with conventional drugs such as nitrazepam or clonazepam while the child is still on ACTH or steroids, and to continue these when the latter are withdrawn.

Mental retardation is very common in children who have had infantile spasms, occurring in from 70 to 96% of patients according to various authors. In most cases the degree of subnormality is severe, so that formal education at school age is of limited value. Delay is most marked in the field of social and personal abilities, while motor skills may develop more normally. A common and tragic outcome is a severely subnormal child, without speech, who is hyperactive, needs constant supervision and shows many autistic traits and mannerisms. Harris (personal communication) has noted that there may be a significant increase in intellectual functioning in some children at school age.

The prognosis for developing severe epilepsy in later childhood years is also poor. In most children spasms have ceased by three years of age, but many later develop intractable seizures of myoclonic and akinetic type and present some of the most difficult problems of epilepsy in paediatric practice. Such cases form an important contribution to the so-called Lennox-Gastaut syndrome, which overlaps many others (Aicardi 1973).

The prognosis depends to some extent on the aetiology, being better in the cryptogenic than the symptomatic group. Jeavons and Bower (1964) found that their symptomatic group had the highest incidence of mental subnormality (78%) and of neurological abnormalities. The crytogenic group contained the majority (13) of the 16 patients who were normal or only mildly abnormal on follow-up. Jeavons et al (1970) reported later on a longer term follow-up study of 98 of their original 112 cases. The patients were aged 5 years or more. Fifty-eight had been treated with steroids. Eighteen had died, mostly under the age of 4 years. Only nine of the 80 survivors still had spasms, but nearly two-thirds had other types of fit at some time, and only a third were free from all types of epilepsy at follow-up. Half of the children showed neurological abnormality; this was commonest in those with a history of perinatal insult. Only 13 appeared to have made a complete recovery. A good prognosis seemed to depend more upon the cause than upon treatment, the best mental outcome occurring in the cryptogenic and immunization groups, in which a third attended normal schools. The prognosis in the other aetiological groups was uniformly bad. This study confirmed the authors' view that steroids and other drugs had no significant effect on intelligence.

Nonetheless it is hard to deny a child with infantile spasms the possible benefits of treatment with ACTH or steroids, even if these benefits prove only transient. The spasms themselves are distressing for the infants, parents and onlookers, and enough individual cases are seen with a good eventual outcome after treatment to make it difficult to withold it. It is reasonable to make certain exceptions, such as babies who are initially severely retarded with other evidence of neurological abnormality, e.g. microcephaly and cerebral palsy, before the onset of spasms, in whom the attacks are a relatively trivial problem among many more severe ones. Such patients may be treated with nitrazepam or clonazepam alone. It is a very personal decision whether to treat or not, but the difficulty of making an accurate prognosis for the future development of any handicapped infant should encourage the doctor to err on the side of over- rather than under-treating.

FEBRILE CONVULSIONS

Introduction

One of the commonest situations in which seizures occur in childhood is with pyrexia. Convulsions have been known for centuries to occur with fever due to non-cerebral infections in certain otherwise normal children between the ages of six months and six years (with occasional cases at younger and older ages). Such attacks are described as febrile convulsions and are particularly associated with viral upper respiratory infections including roseola (exanthem subitum). Their mean incidence in six large populations studied was 29 per 1000 children under 5 years (Lennox-Buchthal 1973). This may well be an underestimate since surveys in Newcastle (Miller et 1960) and Israel (Costeff 1965) have shown that many childhood seizures never come to medical attention despite good medical facilities. The true figure may well be 5 or 6% of children under 5 years of age. Boys outnumber girls and convulsions with fever often occur in close relatives, especially siblings and often a parent or grandparent. In some families the attacks are accepted as a family trait and, being mild and brief, excite little comment or concern. This genetically determined tendency to convulse with fever usually ceases by the age of five or six years.

Most children who have one febrile convulsion and are not given prophylactic treatment will not have a second attack, but 30 to 40% will do so. Few affected children have more than three febrile seizures but those who have frequent attacks arouse great concern. Most of the second convulsions occur within one year of the first.

Factors determining the risk of recurrence after a first attack have been examined with conflicting results, but the age at the time of the first seizure is important. If it occurred in the first year of life, the recurrence rate within 3 years was 45% in van den Berg's prospective study of 368 children

(1974); if in the second year 42%, and if in the third or fourth year only 25%. Similar findings have emerged from the work of Nelson & Ellenberg (1978), the recurrence rate being about 40 to 50% for those under 18 months of age at the time of their first convulsion, and 20 to 30% for those over 18 months.

Discussion of this common problem has been confused by varying criteria and definitions of febrile convulsions and of epilepsy (good reviews are provided by Nelson & Ellenberg (1976), O'Donohoe (1979) and Wallace (1979) (whose contributions over many years have illuminated the subject). Clearly it is important, and not usually difficult, to distinguish between classical febrile convulsions and the less common situation in which *some* seizures in early life are provoked by fever whereas others are not. Some writers (e.g. *British Medical Journal* 1972) have applied rigid criteria and have excluded convulsions which occur under 6 months or over 6 years of age, cases without an obvious rapid rise in temperature or clinically obvious illness before the fit, cases in which a second seizure occurs during the same infection, and also cases in which a fit lasts more than 10 minutes, is focal or is followed by post-ictal weakness. These exclusive criteria seem unjustified in view of the many exceptions seen in practice both within a sibship, and also in the same child from one time to another when a careful history is taken. For example 23% of 142 children with febrile convulsions admitted to one British hospital in 1972 had two convulsions in the same febrile episode, and seven per cent had three or more (Brett 1975). The four last criteria (multiple fits, duration over 10 minutes, focality and post-ictal weakness) are often taken to define 'complicated' seizures for the purpose of epidemiological analysis.

Stephenson (1978b) had found that ocular compression produced an abnormally long period of cardiac asystole in a substantial proportion of children with presumed 'febrile convulsions' and believes that some of these attacks are 'reflex anoxic seizures' due to cerebral ischaemia mediated by a vagal inhibitory effect. The contribution of this mechanism to seizures with fever is still debatable.

The duration of febrile convulsions is very variable. Most are brief and last 15 or 30 seconds, but many attacks exceed 10 minutes in duration and some last 30 minutes or more and so fulfil the criteria of status epilepticus. Febrile convulsions may be described as the commonest 'cause' of status in young children and this consideration alone means that they should be treated with respect, since status from *any* cause is potentially harmful. Rare complications of febrile seizures have long been recognized, and occasional children may die in the attack or show neurological deterioration following it. Longer delayed problems may also arise. Recurrent, unprovoked non-febrile convulsions have been known for many years to follow in a small minority of children, who then become, by definition, epileptic. A link has been shown between febrile convulsions and the later development of temporal lobe epilepsy (TLE) by the work of Ounsted et al (1966) at the Park Hospital, Oxford. Falconer and others (Falconer & Taylor 1968, Falconer 1971) have shown mesial temporal sclerosis (a term preferred to Ammon's horn sclerosis) to be the lesion responsible for the evolution of TLE in such cases, and have also shown that selected patients in this group are helped by temporal lobectomy to a degree not found in cases of different aetiology. These collaborative studies have confirmed that febrile convulsions are potentially harmful and must be stopped as soon as possible (Taylor & Bower 1971).

An analysis of 438 children with febrile convulsions (Ounsted, 1971) gave some striking and sobering results. The male-female ratio was 1.5:1, similar to that in most series. Thirty-three of these children convulsed to death, of whom twice as many were boys (22) as girls (11). 120 of the survivors had further fits and 71 of these had mild, remittent attacks, the male-female ratio being preserved in this group. Severe subsequent fits occurred in 49 children, of whom 28 were girls and 21 boys. The reversed sex ratio in this group may be due to the fact that girls are more resistant to death in convulsion than boys, so that more girls survived. Taylor (1969) has studied sex differences in this connexion by correlating the age of onset of febrile convulsions with the side of the brain affected in a series of patients who had undergone temporal lobectomy for the relief of TLE which began under 10 years of age combined with 100 unoperated children from the series of Ounsted et al (1966). The risk to the *left* hemisphere of damage

by febrile convulsions was highest under 12 months of age and fell steeply and exponentially, while the risk to the right had its peak at the age of two years. In boys the decline in risk was smooth over the first 4 years, but in girls it fell much more sharply, mainly in the second year of life. The longer vulnerability of the left hemisphere to damage from seizures in boys compared with girls may be due to the less functionally active hemisphere being at risk; the acquisition of verbal skills, which usually occurs earlier in girls compared with boys, is associated with the left hemisphere becoming the more active in those whose right hand is the eventually preferred one.

The prevention of morbidity and death from febrile convulsions is clearly related to the control and prevention of the attacks. The problem is a very common one, and many febrile convulsions do not come to the attention of a doctor; if they do this is more often the family doctor than a hospital physician. The hierarchy involved is therefore usually mother–family physician–hospital doctor. Much can and should be done by parents or other 'caretakers' of young children to prevent the attacks. This involves the doctor in his rôle as teacher. There is much ignorance in the general public about febrile convulsions (and all seizures) and most uninstructed parents when faced with the first convulsion in their child make the mistake of covering him with blankets, closing the windows and trying to raise the already rocketting temperature, the worst thing to do. Rutter & Metcalfe (1978) in a Nottingham survey of 89 children admitted to hospital with a first febrile convulsion found that parental management of the fit was often wildly inappropriate. Half of them had taken no steps to lower the temperature and 30% volunteered that they thought their child was dying or dead. Fear and panic were often the predominant reaction and it is understandable that appropriate action was often not taken. Education of the public is needed. Parents should be taught, with simple written instructions, the importance of reducing the body temperature by stripping the child, tepid sponging, fanning, opening windows and the use of aspirin. These measures, taken at the first sign of fever, will often prevent a seizure, or prevent a second attack when one has already occurred in a particular infection. If aspirin cannot be taken by mouth because of vomiting or lack of co-operation, it can be given rectally in suppositories.

Specific treatment for the causal infection may be needed and this falls to the medical adviser who needs to satisfy himself that the child does not have meningitis and decide whether a viral or bacterial infection is responsible. In many cases no definite cause is found, and examination may show, to the eye of faith, slight reddening of the pharynx or of an ear-drum.

THE MANAGEMENT OF STATUS EPILEPTICUS WITH FEBRILE CONVULSIONS

Specific treatment

Since febrile convulsions are the commonest 'cause' of status epilepticus in young children, it is appropriate to discuss the management of status at this point.

The acute problem of how to stop the convulsion associated with fever when its duration exceeds ten or fifteen minutes and parental anxiety prompts appeals for medical help usually falls to the family doctor. He must understand the potential seriousness of prolonged seizures and must be able to provide emergency treatment. Advice to send the child to hospital without attempting to stop the attack is dangerous and indefensible, since half an hour or more has often passed between the start of the seizure and the arrival of the doctor in the home. Various injectable agents are available, and the choice depends on the situation and the doctor's experience.

In the ideal situation, i.e. in hospital or a well equipped and staffed doctor's office or surgery, diazepam (Valium) given intravenously is the drug of choice. It is much less effective by the intramuscular route. To inject it into a vein in a convulsing infant calls for skill which not all doctors possess. Given as a single intravenous bolus the dose is between 0.2 and 0.3 mg/kg body weight. An alternative formula, for use in an emergency when the exact weight is unknown, is 1 mg per year of age plus 1 additional mg (so that a 2-year old child would require $2 + 1 = 3$ mg). Respiratory depression and respiratory and cardiac arrest may

occur, and it is important to realize that resuscitation may be needed. The risks are higher when the child has already received barbiturates or paraldehyde (Bell 1969) and when convulsing children are despatched to hospital full details of their regular medication and of all emergency treatment should accompany them, just as patients evacuated from the battlefield had details of the morphine given attached to their clothing. Experience in one Boston hospital (Lombroso 1966) showed that 25% of the deaths with status epilepticus were due to overdosage with hypnotic agents while trying to control the convulsions. Often diazepam exerts only a transient effect on fits, and so further doses may be needed. Herein lies a danger, since it is easy to give repeated injections until the cumulative effect puts respiration at risk. The use of a continuous intravenous infusion by which the drug can be given in larger doses over some hours is safer. Doses of 50 to 100 mg may be given in this way in 500 ml of $\frac{1}{5}$ normal saline spread over six hours, and the rate of infusion can be altered as needed.

The rectal administration of diazepam is being used increasingly for the control of status in childhood. Suppositories have not usually been found helpful but direct instillation of diazepam as the intravenous preparation into the rectum can produce adequate absorption of the drug and blood levels which are clinically effective (Agurell et al 1974). This is consistent with the recent experience of many paediatricians. Encouraging results have been obtained in Denmark by Knudsen (1979) with rectal diazepam solution in the acute treatment of convulsions in infants and children. In a prospective study of 44 children, aged 6 months to 5 years, admitted to hospital with febrile convulsions or epilepsy, the drug was used in 59 generalized attacks. It was effective in 80% of cases. In 10% of cases the rectal approach failed, whereas intravenous diazepam gave immediate results. Another 10% of cases were resistant to diazepam, whether given rectally or intravenously. The therapeutic effect was correlated with the duration of convulsions before treatment began. Early treatment (duration 15 minutes or less) was effective in 96% of cases and late treatment (duration over 15 minutes) in only 57%. A total of 317 children admitted with febrile convulsions were also treated prophylactically with rectal diazepam whenever their rectal temperature reached 38.5°C or above. The same dose was used for both therapeutic and prophylactic purposes, children of 3 years or less receiving 5–7.5 mg of diazepam (0.5–0.9 mg/kg), while those over 3 were given 7.5–10 mg (0.6–0.8 mg/kg). No significant respiratory depression or other serious side-effect was seen in the 317 children treated prophylactically, although sedation was common. In 2 patients who developed purulent meningitis stiffness of the neck and back were not obscured by the drug and the diagnosis was easily made. In a third patient with meningitis the diagnosis may have been delayed by a few hours as a result of diazepam.

Prepacked sets were used containing ampoules of 2 ml, a disposable plastic syringe and a 6 cm long plastic tube with a blunt tip through which the drug was injected into the rectum. Knudsen believed that this method of treatment is an effective and simple alternative to intravenous diazepam and found that most parents were able to use it to treat their children at home prophylactically or in cases of recurrences. It is advisable that the child's reaction to the treatment should be studied in hospital before home treatment is given, especially if he is receiving phenobarbitone, and the parents should be carefully instructed, verbally, in writing, and by demonstration, in the technique of injection.

The newer benzodiazepine clonazepam (Rivotril®) is often very effective intravenously, either in a single bolus injection (0.05 mg/kg) or by continuous infusion (1–3 mg in 250 ml of $\frac{1}{5}$ normal saline over 6–12 hours). The drug may depress respiration and blood pressure and may also, like nitrazepam, lead to excessive bronchial secretion which can also endanger respiration.

Paraldehyde is an old-fashioned but useful and generally safe drug for the treatment of status epilepticus. It is traditionally given intramuscularly (into the lateral aspect of the thigh or upper and outer quadrant of the buttock) in a dose of 0.3 ml/kg of body weight, but the injection is painful and large volumes should not be given into one site. When more than 3 ml are needed the dose should be divided between two sites. The drug can also be given rectally in a dose of 0.3 ml/kg dissolved in an equal volume of olive or arachis oil, and this route deserves wider use. Paraldehyde

should not be given intravenously unless much diluted. There were problems with the drug when the older type of disposable plastic syringe was used since it tended to dissolve with paraldehyde and an abscess could result. The newer type of plastic syringe or a glass instrument are safe and preferable. It is important that the paraldehyde should be fresh and be kept in the dark, since it may otherwise be ineffective

Intravenous phenytoin and phenobarbitone are sometimes used to treat status in an initial dose of 5 mg/kg of body weight. Phenobarbitone carries a risk of depressing respiration and blood pressure. Intramuscular injection of these drugs is considered ineffective through slow absorption, but there is some evidence that phenytoin may be effective by this route, at least in adults.

Resistant cases of status may yield to intravenous treatment with Chlormethiazole (Heminevrin®) using continuous infusion of an aqueous solution containing 8 g/l in 4% dextrose and a dose of 5–10 mg/kg per hour (Lingam et al 1980). Complications of treatment reported by these workers include reaction of the drug with the plastic giving sets, thrombophlebitis, fever and headache. Certain giving sets are more resistant to Chlormethiazole than others, but these problems make it necessary to use the drug carefully and preferably for short periods only. Respiratory depression and hypotension do not seem serious hazards with this drug.

Lignocaine is another drug for which good results have been claimed when given intravenously in a dose of about 4 mg/kg per hour. Intravenous thiopentone has also proved successful in some cases. Respiratory depression is a risk with both these drugs.

The emergency treatment of febrile convulsions may sometimes be given by a parent if she (or he) is emotionally and intellectually capable of the task, by the use of rectal diazepam, as described, or of rectal or intramuscular paraldehyde. This is not within the capacity of all parents and should not be demanded of them when there is any doubt as to their coping, but in many cases it can save precious time and benefit the child greatly (Brown & Sills 1977, Knudsen 1979). Brown and Sills in a useful account of status epilepticus in childhood described how they provide some mothers of children at risk with ampoules of diazepam or paraldehyde and the necessary equipment, so that the family doctor when summoned can be sure of finding what he needs at hand. This is valuable in cases in which parents are unable to treat the child themselves.

Supportive measures

Attention to general supportive measures in prolonged febrile seizures and status is essential, above all the maintenance of a clear airway and adequate respiration. The child is safest in the semi-prone position. The airway should be kept clear with suction of secretions and vomit, and an anaesthetic airway inserted when possible. Oxygen should be available and given freely. Respiratory failure will require artificial respiration. If there is known or suspected cerebral oedema (which can develop rapidly in status) dexamethasone or mannitol may be helpful in reducing it, and the fluid intake should be restricted. Hypoglycaemia may occur as a result of the excessive workload of neurons, and should be corrected when present.

THE PREVENTION OF FEBRILE CONVULSIONS

The number of children in the United Kingdom who had had one or more febrile convulsion in 1973 was estimated as between 114 000 and 190 000. The figures are probably similar in most of the 'developed' nations. It is clearly neither practicable nor justified to treat such large numbers of children; as Costeff (1965) pointed out, neither physicians nor parents are likely to have the moral fervour to ensure continuous, well-supervised drug treatment in all cases; the more serious side-effects of long-term anticonvulsants must also be considered.

The problem then is to select from all who have had one febrile convulsion those children who are likely to have further attacks and, in particular, severe attacks. Studies from Denmark (Lennox-Buchthal 1973), the United States (van den Berg 1974) and the United Kingdom (Wallace 1974, 1975a) have given some pointers towards identifying these vulnerable patients, but the results have

not shown full agreement. The age at the time of the first seizure was important, the recurrence rate being highest in those with onset under 14 and 12 months of age in the Danish and American studies. Van den Berg did not find any other characteristics of the initial seizure related to recurrence of febrile convulsions or late occurrence of non-febrile seizures, but Wallace (1974) found three features of the first fit to be positively correlated with recurrence. The features were a prolonged attack (lasting at least 30 minutes), a repeated initial seizure during the febrile illness, and a persisting neurological deficit (most often a hemiparesis), even if minimal, after the initial illness had subsided. These features (which some authors would claim place the attacks outside the category of febrile convulsions) seemed to be dependable warning signs that the children were at greater risk of recurrence. Other risk factors were, for males, a positive family history in parents and/or siblings, and in females age of onset under 19 months.

The prospective American study by Nelson & Ellenberg (1976), based on the Collaborative Perinatal Project of the National Institute of Neurological and Communicative Disorder and Stroke, has greatly illuminated the problem. 1706 children from a total sample of 54 000 had had febrile convulsions between the ages of one month and seven years. These children were followed to the age of seven. Epilepsy (defined as afebrile seizures not symptomatic of an acute neurological condition at least one of which occurred after the age of 48 months) developed by the age of 7 in 20 per 1000. It was much commoner in children whose neurological or developmental status was suspect or abnormal before any seizure and whose first seizure was 'complex' (i.e. longer than 15 minutes, multiple or focal). In this group the rate of epilepsy was 18 times higher than in those with no febrile seizures. In the largest group with febrile seizures, those previously normal with non-complex first attacks, epilepsy developed in 11 per 1000. This rate, though moderate, was greater than that for children with *no* febrile seizures (5 per 1000).

Although rectal diazepam has (Knudsen & Vesterman 1978, Knudsen 1979) proved helpful in preventing febrile convulsions in the acute situation of a febrile illness, in most cases anticonvulsant drugs must be given regularly to be effective. The natural history of the condition means that treatment must be prolonged for several years.

In the past the drugs most often used have been phenytoin and phenobarbitone. The results with pheytoin have been disappointing. Melchior and his colleagues (1971) found it was more effective in children whose attacks began over 3 years of age, a group less at risk from the attacks than younger children. Phenobarbitone has until recently seemed to be, at least in theory, the drug of first choice. A collaborative Danish study (Faerø et al 1972) showed that it was effective if the serum level were kept above 16 mg/ml. Wolf et al (1977) in California obtained similar results. Wallace (1975b) found an impressive reduction in the recurrence rate of febrile convulsions in 108 children in her high risk group treated with continuous phenobarbitone or primidone for at least 18 months compared with untreated patients, the rate falling from 59 to 17%. Thorn (1975) in her controlled study of long-term phenobarbitone for febrile convulsions found that serum levels were often low at the time of recurrence. By contrast Heckmatt et al (1976) found that pheobarbitone failed to prevent further febrile convulsions in children who had had their first attack between the ages of 6 months and 3 years when followed over a period of 6 months. Although compliance was not good, the plasma levels were in the so-called therapeutic range in the four children with recurrent attacks from the 49 who took the drug regularly.

In practice the poor tolerance of many young children for phenobarbitone (Wolf & Forsythe 1978) with severe problems of irritability, aggressiveness and overactive behaviour (especially if a tendency to this is already present), makes its use unacceptable to many parents, who prefer to run the risk of further fits in their children. Parents will often stop the drug themselves; in other cases the doctor is forced to discontinue it on the principle of primum non nocere. Wolf & Forsythe (1978) found that of 109 children treated with phenobarbitone after their first febrile convulsion 42% developed a behaviour disorder, most often overactivity. These symptoms did not depend on the blood level of the drug. They enforced cessation of treatment in many cases and improved after this.

At present interest is growing in the use of sodium valproate for the prevention of febrile convulsions. The results of the reported studies have been rather conflicting, and the structure of the trials has varied. Cavazzuti (1975) treated 47 children after their first simple (i.e. without complex factors) febrile convulsion with sodium valproate in the rather moderate dose of 20 mg/kg per day and an equal number with phenobarbitone or primidone. The recurrence rate was 4% in both groups followed over one year compared with 55% in untreated patients. No side-effects were seen. Wallace & Aldridge-Smith (1980) compared sodium valproate and phenobarbitone treatment in children aged 6 to 42 months after their first febrile convulsion. Both drugs were significantly better than no treatment, their efficacy being comparable. Ngwane & Bower (1980) compared the same two drugs in a double-blind trial in children aged 6 to 18 months who had had a single simple febrile convulsion. Sodium valproate was found to be more effective than phenobabitone, though the difference was not significant. Severe side-effects enforced stopping treatment in two children on each drug. By contrast with these encouraging results Williams et al (1979) in treating 30 children with simple febrile convulsions after their *second* attack with sodium valproate for one year, found that it was not effective despite good compliance and infrequent side-effects.

Good results, however, seem to exceed poor ones, and since sodium valproate is generally better tolerated than phenobarbitone, it seems reasonable to regard it as the drug of first choice for the prevention of febrile convulsions, though it would be naive to believe that *any* drug is the ideal treatment for *all* children with convulsions, whether febrile or non-febrile, and undesirable side-effects can certainly occur with valproate.

A 'consensus development conference' on febrile seizures was held at the National Institutes of Health in May 1980 to consider the subject in detail. The factors separating children at high risk of developing non-febrile seizures from those at low risk were regarded as a family history of non-febrile seizures, abnormal neurological or developmental status before the attack, and an atypical febrile seizure, such as a prolonged or focal episode. Only 2 to 3% of children with none or only one of these risk factors later develop non-febrile seizures. Two or more factors put a patient in the high risk group. Prophylaxis is believed to reduce the risk of subsequent febrile seizures but not that of non-febrile attacks or of significant neurological defects. The consensus statement recommends that anticonvulsant prophylaxis be considered under the following conditions: previous neurological abnormality (e.g. cerebral palsy, mental retardation or microcephaly), when a febrile seizure lasts longer than 15 minutes, is focal or followed by transient or persistent neurological abnormalities, or if there is a history of non-febrile seizures in a parent or sibling. Further indications included multiple febrile seizures or occurrence of seizures in an infant under 12 months of age.

Addy (1981) in a helpful recent review has discussed the potential advantages and disadvantages of prophylactic treatment in children who have had a febrile convulsion. The possible advantages are the prevention of further febrile convulsions and the prevention of neurological damage resulting from such further convulsions and manifested as later epilepsy, mental retardation or other neurological defect. The two aims are quite separate. The risk of neurological sequelae to prolonged febrile convulsions is of developing mesial temporal sclerosis and later TLE, and other neurological deficits. This risk seems to be more often recognized in Britain, where the work of Ounsted and his colleagues on the relationship between febrile fits and TLE is well known, than in the United States, where the epidemiological study by the National Institutes of Health of 1706 children with febrile convulsions showed no cases of death or permanent motor deficit. The disparity is interesting and raises the possibility that the risk may have been over-estimated in Britain and under-estimated in the United States. Addy's own view is that prophylactic treatment should be given (1) if the diagnosis seems to be epilepsy (recurrent afebrile convulsions) or in the presence a clear pre-existing neurological abnormality, such as microcephaly, hydrocephalus or cerebral palsy, which makes epilepsy more probable; (2) for frequent convulsions (arbitrarily two in 6 months or three in 18 months) and (3) when parental anxiety is very great, especially in children aged under 18 months.

Investigations in febrile convulsions

These have usually given normal results, apart from abnormalities resulting from the infection responsible for the pyrexial illness (Gerber & Berliner 1981).

Viral studies may indicate infection with a particular virus and recent investigations have given interesting results. In a Newcastle study (Stokes et al 1977) of 276 children admitted to hospital with febrile convulsions the overall virus identification rate was 49%, but there were no striking clinical differences between the virus-positive and virus-negative children. More intensive investigation is likely to yield more evidence of virus infection. A disseminated viral illness was demonstrated by isolating a virus from the CSF, blood or urine in only 27% of 73 children admitted to hospital after a first febrile convulsion (Lewis et al 1979). However, a viral aetiology could be implicated in 86% of children after combining the results of tissue culture, electron microscopy, mouse inoculation, complement fixation tests and interferon assay. Parallel bacterial cultures showed a possible pathogen in 29% of children but in only 4% was this isolated from CSF, blood or urine. No correlation was found between the nature of the pathogen, or evidence of its dissemination, and the severity of the convulsion, degree of fever, CSF protein level or white cells, or white cell count in the blood. These results suggests that a febrile convulsion may be a response to invasion of the blood stream or CNS by a micro-organism, usually a virus. The short duration of the invasion may explain why successful isolation of the virus is relatively rare with routine investigation methods.

Seizures in a febrile setting may occur with bacterial or viral meningitis and this possibility must be kept in mind and lumbar puncture performed whenever there is doubt. Some authorities consider that examination of the CSF is mandatory in a first febrile convulsion; while this may be a good rule for beginners, the more experienced will exercise their clinical judgement.

A possible immunological factor predisposing to febrile convulsion has been suggested by the findings of Seager and his colleagues (1975). These workers studied 32 children with seizures treated with phenytoin (diphenylhydantoin). Five of these had low levels of serum-IgA before treatment, and all of these 5 were among the 15 who had had febrile convulsions in infancy. The immunological aspects of epilepsy have been well reviewed recently by Aarli & Fontana (1980).

Skull X-rays are usually normal in children with febrile convulsions and more detailed radiological tests such as air encephalography and CT scans are not indicated in the average case.

The EEG is not usually helpful since it may be normal or show slow wave activity related in a non-specific way to infection or to medication. Discharges are rarely seen, and when present may raise the question whether non-febrile seizures may occur later, though this can never be assumed. Doctors and parents may derive comfort from a normal EEG, but the investigation is not essential in managing most cases of febrile convulsions.

TEMPORAL LOBE EPILEPSY ('PARTIAL SEIZURES OF COMPLEX SYMPTOMATOLOGY' OR 'PARTIAL COMPLEX SEIZURES')

Clinical features

Discharges arising in the limbic system of the temporal lobes give rise to a chronic form of epilepsy, temporal lobe epilepsy (TLE), which is perhaps the commonest form of focal seizure in childhood. The word 'psychomotor' is sometimes used as an alternative, but the terms are not synonymous, since similar psychic and motor activity may be seen in seizures arising in other parts of the brain, such as the frontal lobes.

The frequency of TLE in childhood is often underestimated since understandably the psychic elements of the attacks may be overlooked in a child who is too young to describe his symptoms, and only the more dramatic motor features may be noticed. Careful enquiry should be made of the parents or other observers as to what they have seen in the child during an attack. Failure to question closely is one reason for the common confusion of TLE with petit mal attacks, since rather similar 'blank spells' may occur in both. The parents should be asked not only to describe in detail what

they observe (and questioned directly about specific features) but also to imitate the attacks. Occasionally provocation by over-breathing in a coöperative child will indicate the nature of the seizures.

The extensive connexions of the temporal lobes explain the rich repertoire of psychic, motor and autonomic disorders that may occur in temporal lobe seizures. Hallucinations of sight, sound, smell or taste, often of an unpleasant or frightening kind, may be experienced. Threatening phrases may be heard in the auditory hallucinations, sometimes incorporating comments or criticisms related to the child's everyday experience, or sometimes commonplace phrases imbued with a sinister character An example of the first was the phrase, 'It's not your turn. Mary', habitually heard in her attacks by one girl, and of the second the words 'We make smarties' spoken in a terrifying voice. Visual hallucinations may be complex and resemble dreams; younger children, as with all these symptoms, cannot describe them, but older ones may describe them vividly or may be persuaded to try to draw or paint them. Vertigo may be a feature of the attacks. Disorders of thought or of perception of the self or surroundings may occur, with feelings of depersonalization or 'derealization', or states of high emotion, joy, fear or anxiety, for which there is no appropriate cause. The child may utter jumbled phrases, or indicate distress, saying 'No, no, take it away' or 'Go away' and may appear visibly frightened, often running and clinging to his mother, though occasionally fighting her off during the attack but seeking close contact and consolation afterwards. The disorders of **déjà vu** and **jamais vu** are occasionally described by articulate children as features of their attacks. Sometimes amnesia for the attack itself or even for events just before it may occur and this disorder of memory will destroy all recollection of it. The understandable unwillingness of some older children to describe their bizarre experiences, due to fear that they are 'going mad', is another possible obstacle to obtaining a full account of the symptoms. With encouragement and reassurance that such feelings are well recognised and harmless the child may talk freely, and share and shed his anxieties in a very therapeutic way.

The motor phenomena of the attacks are more

readily seen and analysed. Their variety is endless, but whether simple or complex they have in common the fact they are actions which appear purposive but are inappropriate at the time, though in a different context they could be entirely apt. Their tempo is that of normal willed actions and quite unlike the jerking and twitching movements of convulsive seizures. Sometimes they are influenced by the day-to-day activities of the patient. The mildest type of movements include repetitive fumbling with buttons or clothing, which may go on to a partial undressing, or rubbing of the face or other part of the body with one hand. Cursive attacks in which the patient runs are sometimes seen. The classical 'Hippocratic dash' was described by the father of medicine. Complex movements as of rowing a boat while sitting on the floor or the motions of carrying out domestic tasks such as sweeping or cleaning may be seen. Often the child will wander around the room in an abstracted fashion, perhaps picking up and dropping objects on the way. Throughout such activities he is clearly out of touch and 'not with it', usually being inaccessible to verbal contacts, but occasionally seeming to respond to a limited degree. One mother described how when she put out her hand to touch her daughter during an attack the latter took her hand and shook it, and was very embarassed afterwards to be told of this. Oral movements of lip smacking, chewing or swallowing are common, and probably occur with hallucinations of taste or smell. Frequently the automatic type actions are regarded by teachers and others as day-dreams or as naughty or antisocial behaviour and may lead to conflict with authority and to undeserved sanctions.

Autonomic phenomena are very frequent but are often overlooked by parents, and should be specifically inquired for. Pallor and flushing are the commonest, but sweating, erection of skin hair, pupillary changes, tachycardia and borborygmi also occur. Urinary incontinence is fortunately uncommon but passage of wind, upwards or downwards, may occur (embarrassment may prevent parents from mentioning this).

Examination of the patient is unlikely to show any features specific for this type of seizure, but the usual evidence of CNS abnormality should be sought, such as hemiplegia, asymmetry of limbs, chorioretinopathy or stigmata of neurocutaneous syndromes. Signs of new neurological deficit which might indicate progressive pathology should be looked for.

A subtle but important sign in many patients with TLE is facial asymmetry. Remillard et al (1977) found this to be a useful clinical sign in the lateralization of temporal epileptogenic foci. Mild unilateral weakness of the lower face was noted which was rarely apparent at rest, but more obvious on voluntary movement and greatly enhanced on emotional movement. 23 of the 37 patients with a unilateral temporal focus showed contralateral facial weakness. Another sign noted occasionally was a slightly wider palpebral fissure.

Aetiology

As with most forms of seizure in childhood, there is nothing specific about the aetiology of temporal lobe attacks, and they may occur in patients with clear evidence of previous neurological abnormality, such as mental retardation, cerebral palsy or other forms of seizure, or in children who have been entirely normal. The causes of TLE in childhood differ from those in adult life, and the work of Ounsted and his colleagues (1966), already referred to, has shown the importance of previous febrile convulsions as a causal factor. In their study of 100 children with TLE these workers found three roughly equal groups, one being idiopathic with no obvious aetiological factors discernible in the history, one related to previous brain insults such as birth injury or meningitis and one in which the only previous abnormality was a history of one or more febrile convulsions in infancy. The risk of seizures in the siblings of the last group was high (30%), compared with 9 or 10% in the organic insult group, and 2% in the idiopathic group. The seizures in these siblings were often simple febrile convulsions which differed from those of the probands only in their shorter duration. Thus there seems to be a strong genetic factor in the aetiology of TLE following febrile convulsions, operating through the dominantly inherited tendency to the latter. The mean age of onset of TLE was lower in the children with previous febrile convulsions (mean 4 years 2 months with a mean interval of 2 years 7 months) than in the 'insulted' group (5 years 7 months) or the idiopathic (7 years 6 months).

The surgical treatment of TLE by the late Murray Falconer by a generous anterior temporal lobectomy including the hippocampus, amygdala and uncus (structures often left in situ by other surgeons) has led to fruitful neuropathological studies and correlation with clinical features (Falconer & Taylor 1968, Falconer 1971). In two published series of surgically treated patients mesial temporal sclerosis (MTS) was found in half the cases (this term was proposed by Falconer as preferable to 'Ammon's horn sclerosis' since the lesion often involves other mesial temporal structures such as the amygdala, uncus and hippocampal gyrus). This group was not only the largest in the surgical material but also the only one in which most patients had the onset of habitual seizures in the first decade, very often with a past history of febrile convulsions in infancy. Falconer argued convincingly that the lesions shown in these cases, with neuronal loss in the H1 or Sommer zone with sparing of the H2 or resistant sector, are not explicable by the theory of incisural sclerosis related to birth injury put forward by Penfield and the Montreal school. The practical preventive implications of these clinicopathological correlations for the management of febrile convulsions have already been mentioned, but can hardly be over-emphasised, since we cannot afford to overlook any method of preventing epilepsy (Taylor & Bower 1971). A further practical implication is that the results of surgery in this group were very gratifying, 92% of patients being benefited.

In 20 to 25% of the removed temporal lobes hamartomas or small cryptic tumours, mostly of glial origin, were found which were thought to be developmental abnormalities. No patients in this group had a positive family history of seizures, but the results of surgery were as successful as in the MTS group. In 10% scars and infarcts were found, but it was not clear whether these had caused the epilepsy or resulted from it. A non-specific group of about 20% of cases showed no definite structural abnormality.

Neoplasms are rare as a cause of TLE in childhood, but low grade gliomas or ependymomas may occasionally cause such seizures over many years before they are detected with the onset of neurological deficits. The rarity of neoplasms as a cause of TLE and of focal seizures in general in childhood means that investigation is often not pushed to the limits so that the tumours may be missed for some years. The advent of the CT scan has made easier their detection at any earlier stage. The contrast with the situation in adults is well shown by the survey of 666 patients with TLE from the London Hospital (Currie et al 1971) in which 64 patients had brain tumours, only one of whom had the onset of his attacks under the age of 10 years.

These aetiological considerations affect the selection and intensity of investigation of children with TLE. The history may give clear pointers to birth injury or to previous febrile status as the cause. Skull X-rays may suggest mesial temporal sclerosis when the middle cranial fossa appears smaller on one side than the other and the EEG shows appropriate discharges or other changes. An expanded fossa on the other hand or calcification might suggest a neoplasm. The EEG may be helpful in showing abnormalities in the temporal region on one or both sides, and a slow wave focus, especially if increasing, will suggest a tumour. Lumbar airencephalography or carotid arteriography were previously needed to demonstrate a space-occupying lesion such as a tumour or an angioma, but the CT scan will usually show such lesions and is preferable when available.

Associated problems in childhood TLE

The two other chronic neurological handicaps of childhood, mental retardation and cerebral palsy, which so often accompany epilepsy, may be present in TLE. Two troublesome chronic behaviour problems often also co-exist. The hyperkinetic syndrome is often seen, as with any organic brain disorder of childhood, and episodes of catastrophic rage and aggressive behaviour may occur, which have a profound effect on the schooling and management of the child in the family and community.

Management

The frequency of the attacks and the associated problems mentioned above may necessitate special educational arrangements for a few children. In most cases, however, as in all forms of epilepsy, the child can and should remain in his normal home and school environment, though some modifications of this may be needed. Anxious teachers may need reassurance, and their tolerance is often the critical factor which will allow or prevent retention in the normal school.

The drug treatment of TLE is empirical, but often very successful. No one drug (despite advertising claims to the contrary) proves effective in *all* cases but good results are often obtained with carbamazepine. One drug to be avoided is phenobarbitone which is likely to aggravate the hyperkinetic and aggressive behaviour so often present. Primidone is better tolerated and may be helpful. Phenytoin may also help, but the benzodiazepines are usually ineffective. The results obtained with sodium valproate in TLE are less striking than in some others forms of epilepsy.

The use of anticonvulsant level estimation in the blood allows all drugs to be more fully and logically exploited.

The surgical treatment of TLE has been mentioned. It has proved very effective in carefully selected cases, particularly in patients with mesial temporal sclerosis resulting from previous febrile status and some patients with hamartomas. Falconer (1971) insisted on three criteria in choosing patients for temporal lobectomy: the attacks must be frequent and have resisted adequate medical treatment, neuroradiological studies must have excluded a gross space-occupying lesion, and preoperative EEG recordings, including the use of sphenoidal electrodes with activation by natural or drug-induced sleep, have shown a consistent spike-discharging focus which was either unilateral or, if bilateral, strongly predominant in the temporal lobe to be removed.

Improvement is often noted post-operatively, not only in relief of seizures, but also in behaviour, particularly in cases with mesial temporal sclerosis, as shown by a review of the outcome in the first 40 patients, aged 15 years and under, operated on by Falconer (Davidson & Falconer 1975).

COMPLEX PARTIAL STATUS EPILEPTICUS (CPSE)

Under this title have been reported (Engel et al 1978, Mayeux & Lueders 1978, McBride et al 1981) a number of children with episodes of impaired consciousness, reduced speech and social reactions, intermittent staring, and wandering eye movements or eye deviation. The four girls reported by McBride et al were aged between 1 and 4 years. The children would pick intermittently at their clothing or nearby objects during the attacks and three of them showed smacking of the lips. Three of them developed focal clonic activity during their seizures and one progressed to a generalized motor seizure after four hours in CPSE. In two patients the EEG during the episodes showed polyspikes and slow waves in the temporo-occipital regions. Two other patients had EEGs only after the episodes had ended and these showed focal slowing in one posterior quadrant. In three patients the episodes of CPSE seem to have been the first recognized manifestation of epilepsy. The child reported by Mayeux and Lueders developed CPSE after resection of a craniopharyngioma. The condition may be commoner than the relatively few reports would suggest.

The prognosis of temporal lobe epilepsy in childhood

It is desirable to know the long-term outlook for children with TLE and the factors which influence it for many reasons, including the problem of when to consider surgical treatment.

Light has been thrown on this subject by work done at the Park Hospital, Oxford, reported in a series of recent papers by Lindsay et al (1979a, b, c), and summarized in the *British Medical Journal* 1980. The Oxford study was based on 100 consecutive children who met the clinical and EEG criteria of TLE. Neuropathological confirmation was later obtained in some of the patients who were treated surgically.

Of the 100 children, five died under the age of 15. About one third of the survivors became adults free of seizures and leading independent lives. Another third were socially independent but receiving anticonvulsants and the remainder were dependent, living as adults with their parents or confined to institutions. The social prognosis could be predicted from factors ascertainable in childhood. Eight adverse factors were seen (Lindsay et

al 1979a). These were an IQ below 90, onset of seizures before the age of 2 years 4 months, five or
more grand mal attacks (in addition to TLE), a seizure frequency of once daily or more, a left-sided
EEG focus, the hyperkinetic syndrome, episodes
of catastrophic rage, and a need for special schooling. All but one of those who became fit-free and
independent had attended normal schools.

An important positive genetic factor for prognosis was a history of febrile convulsions in a first
degree relative. This favourable factor seemed to
cancel out the bad effects of the eight adverse factors. When this family history was absent, the adult
social prognosis was related to the number of
adverse factors. When more than three of these
were present in childhood the patient was likely to
be dependent and to have continuing epilepsy in
adult life.

The prognosis for marriage and parenthood was
related to gender (Lindsay et al 1979b). In boys
TLE persisting after the age of 12 years was
associated with lack of development of a sexual
appetite.

The psychiatric prognosis was more encouraging
(Lindsay et al 1979c). Though 85% of the children
had psychiatric problems, most of those who were
not mentally retarded became psychiatrically
healthy adults. Ten per cent developed schizo-
phrenia-like psychoses and all these had left-sided
temporal foci on the EEG. Antisocial conduct in
adult life was related to several factors — male sex,
a focus opposite to the preferred hand, unremittent
epilepsy, low intelligence, and childhood rages
were prominent correlates.

These findings suggest that much clearer guide-
lines are now available to us for selecting patients
for consideration of temporal lobectomy. Persisting
seizures, male sex, more than 3 of the adverse factors, and absence of a first degree relative with
febrile convulsions would suggest a poor chance of
spontaneous remission of fits and a bad outlook for
social and sexual normality in adult life. Surgery,
to be most effective in such cases, should be carried
out before adolescence has begun.

MYOCLONIC EPILEPSY

This term is used for a form of generalized epilepsy
in which a sudden, involuntary and momentary
contraction occurs in a single muscle or group of
muscles, often without loss of consciousness. In
adults these attacks may occur in isolation or in
association with grand mal and other types of epilepsy. In children they may occur as symptoms of
various progressive degenerative diseases previously described (Ch. 5) e.g. in progressive
myoclonic epilepsy, Batten's disease in its various
forms and Gaucher's disease, but much more commonly they represent a more benign condition. The
syndrome of infantile spasms is sometimes designated 'massive myoclonic seizures' but these
attacks are so different from true myoclonic epilepsy in childhood (Harper 1968), in their clinical
features, age of onset and prognosis, that the term
has grave disadvantages.

In true myoclonic epilepsy of childhood the
average age of onset is $3\frac{1}{2}$ years (Harper 1968) and
the attacks are often preceded by other forms of
seizure, usually grand mal, for a period between 3
months and 2 years. The attacks are typically violent and sudden in onset without any warning or
aura, so that the child is caught unawares and cannot protect himself, as he may often do in other
seizures. They are very brief and without loss of
consciousness. A sudden violent contraction of the
muscles of the neck and trunk, often with a jerk
of the arms, occurs and often causes the child to
fall forwards or backwards and to hurt himself. He
makes no attempt to save himself by putting out
his hands, and so often injures his head or face,
with cuts, bruises and fractures of the teeth or chin.
If standing he will often fall as if pole-axed or
thrown to the ground. If sitting at table, his face
is often plunged into his dinner plate. Objects held
in the hands may be thrown some distance during
an attack. Recovery is usually immediate, provided
no serious head injury is sustained, and the child
can quickly resume the activities in which he was
previously engaged, though often upset and crying.
Some children are remarkably stoical about their
attacks and may even deny they have had a seizure
and attempt to rationalize it by claiming that they
tripped over an obstacle. The attacks are often
more frequent in the morning in the hour or so
after waking or when tired towards evening. Sometimes they occur when the child is woken from
sleep, but not when he wakes up spontaneously.

Attacks may be precipitated by flashing lights, and television and discotheques are frequent offenders. Loud or unexpected noises, such as the telephone, may be provoking factors in some cases and cutaneous stimuli in others.

Examination shows no abnormality in most cases, but there may be signs indicating long-standing neurological abnormality related to perinatal problems (microcephaly, retardation, cerebral palsy, etc.). Skull X-rays usually show no specific features but may give further evidence of brain abnormality. The EEG is almost always abnormal, usually with atypical bilateral spike and wave discharges and often with polyspikes. Typical 3 per second spike and wave discharges are not seen. Photic stimulation during the EEG recording may provoke myoclonic jerks and sometimes an associated increase in dicharges.

There is usually little difficulty in recognizing the rare cases in which myoclonic attacks are due to degenerative brain disease, since these are usually assocaited with other indications of progressive neurological deficit, particularly ataxia, dementia, visual impairment and pyramidal signs. Occasionally myoclonic attacks due to non-progressive pathology may be very frequent and intractable, amounting to status myoclonicus. The term 'minor epileptic status' (Brett 1966) has been used to describe some cases of this kind, in which the frequency and severity of the attacks is so disabling as to produce at times a 'pseudodementia' and 'pseudo-ataxia', in which the child's mental and willed physical activities are grossly impaired. This alarming clinical picture may arouse suspicion of a degenerative brain disease, a cerebellar tumour or drug intoxication, but an essential point of distinction from these is the striking fluctuation seen in 'minor epileptic status', so that a child may be grossly disabled for a time, yet by contrast be alert, seizure-free and functioning normally at other times. The EEG abnormality, which may fluctuate greatly, not always correlating closely with the clinical state, is also diagnostically helpful. The aetiology of this condition is variable; in some cases it is unknown, and in others related to brain damage of perinatal origin. The prognosis is also variable, but in some cases the outcome is good with complete cessation of seizures and reasonable educational progress.

This condition should be distinguished from the rarer petit mal status, in which petit mal absences are continuous or succeed one another with scarcely any interval so that the child is rendered confused and incompetent. The clinical and EEG features here differ markedly from 'minor epileptic status' and the response to ethosuximide and sodium valproate is usually dramatic.

'The Lennox syndrome', a term suggested by Gastaut and co-workers (1966) for 'childhood epileptic encephalopathy with diffuse slow spike waves' or 'petit mal variant', is a somewhat controversial concept, as the term is apparently used with different meanings, sometimes primarily referring to an EEG pattern and sometimes to a clinical picture. This problem has been well discussed by Aicardi (1973) who has stressed the electrical features of diffuse slow spike-waves (petit mal variant) and the commonly, but not invariably, associated clinical features of the seizure pattern. Most paediatricians are primarily concerned with the clinical seizures which are of three types, head-dropping or head-nodding spells, atypical absences and brief tonic fits, especially during sleep. The attacks are very frequent, but may fluctuate widely, bad periods with many seizures, sometimes amounting to status, alternating with good phases of freedom from fits and normal or near-normal functioning. The aetiology is very variable, some cases arising de novo in previously normal children, and others in neurologically or mentally handicapped patients. It is common for children with infantile spasms which persist after the first year of life to evolve into the 'Lennox syndrome'. There is probably some overlap between this syndrome and 'minor epileptic status', and in both conditions conventional anticonvulsant treatment is often disappointing. Benzodiazepines, such as nitrazepam and clonazepam, and sodium valproate are helpful in some cases, and corticosteroids or ACTH may have a dramatic effect, though relapses commonly follow withdrawal of treatment. A ketogenic diet may be beneficial when drug treatment fails.

STATUS EPILEPTICUS

Major status epilepticus has already been mentioned under the heading of febrile convulsions, which are probably the commonest 'cause' of status in childhood. Other causes have been analysed in a review by Aicardi & Chevrie (1970) who studied the aetiology and prognosis in a group of 239 children with status. In 77% of cases the status was the first sign of epilepsy, and it was common for seizures to follow this episode. When seizures had occurred previously there was often a change in the type of epilepsy, and the subsequent fits tended to be of the kind associated with organic brain disease, focal fits, psychomotor attacks, infantile spasms, tonic fits classified as the Lennox syndrome and generalized tonic-clonic convulsions. The causes of the status were divided into three groups, acute brain injuries (meningitis, encephalitis, anoxia, dehydration and subdural haematoma), chronic encephalopathies often of obscure origin but sometimes related to birth-injury or cerebral malformation and a cryptogenic group, the largest contribution, which included convulsions with fever. The prognosis in this series was bad. 11% of the children died either during the status or later. 37% showed neurological abnormalities and in over half the affected children the disability, usually a hemiplegia, followed the status. Mental handicap was found in nearly half the children, most of whom had previously developed normally. The risks of permanent disability after status seemed to be highest under the age of 40 months. Another common cause of status is the sudden stopping of anticonvulsant drugs: this is not always the fault of parents (who must always be firmly instructed about its risks), but is sometimes done at the behest of misguided doctors. When little success attends the use of drugs there is sometimes a tendency to stop the drugs suddenly and 'see what happens'. It is not difficult to guess what will happen and the experiment is dangerous.

Aicardi & Baraton (1971) have produced dramatic radiological evidence of brain atrophy following status in 15 children who had air encephalograms performed immediately after the event and again a few weeks or months later. In 13 cases gross ventricular enlargement was seen on the second study, whereas the first was normal or showed only slight enlargement. The ventricular dilatation was unilateral or bilateral and related to the predominant localization of the convulsions. The CT scan allows similar observations to be made more easily and has sometimes shown evidence of cerebral infarction, previously unsuspected, indicating a vascular mechanism. In some cases of acute hemiplegia in childhood (Ch. 19) with the neurological deficit appearing in a setting of unilateral convulsions (the hemiconvulsions-hemiplegia-epilepsy (HHE) syndrome of Gastaut et al 1957) arteriography has shown occlusion of the anterior or middle cerebral arteries. Cerebral oedema, bilateral or unilateral, may be shown on arteriograms or CT scan, and this is often followed by atrophy in the same distribution.

Whatever the cause of status in childhood (and sometimes the cause may remain uncertain) the most urgent need is to stop the convulsions, maintain adequate oxygenation and lower the temperature. These problems are discussed earlier.

OTHER FORMS OF FOCAL EPILEPSY IN CHILDHOOD ('PARTIAL SEIZURES OF ELEMENTARY SYMPTOMATOLOGY')

Jacksonian and adversive attacks

Seizures with focal motor and sensory features are common in childhood and include Jacksonian attacks with a motor and sensory march. Focal convulsions are very frequent in patients with congenital hemiplegia and are probably due to cerebral scars, with porencephalic cysts or developmental cerebral anomalies accounting for a minority. A transient post-ictal increase in weakness is often seen in such cases. Another common form of focal seizure is the adversive attack in which the head and eyes are turned to one side (away from the focal lesion) and often the arm is extended on the side to which the head turns. Focal fits are seen with many types of cerebral pathology including vascular lesions, such as angioma, arteriovenous malformation, the Sturge-Weber syndrome and hydrocephalus treated by ventriculoatrial shunt (Hosking 1974). Progressive diseases of the brain may present with focal seizures. Degenerative disorders rarely cause attacks which are persistently focal and tend to produce generalised convulsions or myoclonic attacks. Neoplasms, by contrast, often cause focal seizures, but account for only a small proportion of such attacks in children. Progressive neurological deficits, such as hemiplegia, sensory loss and dysphasia, often accompany the focal attacks caused by neoplasms and signs of raided intracranial pressure usually develop fairly early. Among 114 cases of Jacksonian epilepsy in infancy and childhood (Holowach et al 1958) only one patient had an expanding intracranial lesion. In nearly half the cases the Jacksonian seizures began under 3 years of age, reflecting the substantial contribution of birth injury and congenital cerebral defect to the aetiology. In many cases no definite cause can be found, and in others there is only suspicion that perinatal difficulties may be responsible.

The benign nature of the pathology in many cases of focal childhood epilepsy is associated with a commonly good prognosis for the cessation of attacks, although a relapse rate of 53% was noted by Holowach and her colleagues (1972) in children with Jacksonian and focal epilepsy.

Benign focal epilepsy of childhood

One form of benign focal epilepsy apparently limited to childhood and with an excellent prognosis is a type with 'Sylvian seizures' and midtemporal spike foci. The onset is usually between 7 and 10 years. The characteristics of these attacks are sensory involvement, usually of the tongue but sometimes of the inner cheek, lips, gums or teeth, dysarthria, pooling of saliva, tonic or tonic-clonic involvement of the facial muscles, and occasionally spread of sensory disturbance to the ipsilateral arm. Rarely a motor Jacksonian march occurs and convulsions may affect one side of the body or spread to become generalised. This is more likely to occur during sleep so that nocturnal attacks may rapidly propagate and their initial focal nature may be hidden. In most cases consciousness is preserved. An older child may try to indicate what is happening to him by pointing and grunting or by writing a message for his mother. Though distressing for the child and observers, the attacks are not usually accompanied by psychic or perceptual disorders, or by chewing and swallowing movements, nor followed by amnesia or postictal confusional states.

Mental retardation and learning and behaviour disorders, so common in children with classical temporal lobe epilepsy, are fortunately very rare in this form of focal seizure. Neurological examination is normal in most cases, though mild facial asymmetry is often seen. The prognosis for cessation is excellent. Lombroso (1967) in a prospective study of 58 consecutive cases found that almost half were seizure-free within three years of onset and the EEG had become normal in over 30%. After 5 years over 75% were fit-free and about 60% had normal EEGs. The commonest EEG correlate of these seizures is the finding, between attacks, of mid-temporal spike foci, often with spread to the central or Rolandic region, usually with normal or nearly normal background activity. Gibbs & Gibbs (1960), who first recognised this EEG pattern, noted that children with mid-temporal lobe spike foci had a far better prognosis than those with anterior temporal spike foci. A similar excellent outcome was found by Lerman & Kivity (1975) in a study of 100 patients in all of whom the attacks ceased and the EEG became normal before adult life was reached. Treatment with Carbamazepine gives excellent results in many cases (Lerman & Kivity-Ephraim 1974, O'Donohoe 1977).

A strong genetic component in these attacks has been suggested with variable dominant inheritance from a study of 19 probands and their families (Heijbel et al 1975).

Epilepsia partialis continua (Koshewnikow's syndrome)

Partial continuous epilepsy affecting a limb, part of a limb, the face or tongue, or the limbs and face on one side of the body, may occur in childhood. In adult life epilepsia partialis continua has a rather poor prognosis and is caused by neoplasms or by infarcts or cerebral haemorrhage in a high proportion of cases (Thomas et al 1977). In childhood the aetiology remains unknown in many cases after full investigation, and in some children the condition is associated with progressive hemiplegia and radiological atrophy of the opposite hemisphere. In some of these cases the seizures have proved intractable to all forms of medical treatment and relief has sometimes followed subtotal hemispherectomy. Neuropathological examination in such cases has sometimes failed to show an identifiable pathological process.

OTHER FORMS OF MINOR SEIZURE

Various forms of minor seizure were previously grouped together despite having more differences than similarities. At one time petit mal absences, myoclonic attacks and some forms of akinetic attacks were classified together under the heading 'the petit mal triad'. This classification is no longer appropriate on clinical, therapeutic and neurophysiological grounds, and it has the disadvantage of encouraging the grouping of all non-major convulsions under the misleading umbrella of 'petit mal'. This confusion is seen in the fact that temporal lobe attacks and other forms of focal seizure are often referred to hospital with the diagnosis of 'petit mal'. Careful study of the clinical features of the various minor attacks and of their EEG correlates will usually allow them to be distinguished from one another.

PETIT MAL ATTACKS ('PRIMARY GENERALIZED EPILEPSY')

The main clinical feature of the true petit mal attack, a benign and relatively uncommon form of seizure, is a sudden, brief blank stare accompanied by unawareness and amnesia and sometimes by flickering of the eyelids and upward deviation of the eyes. The words 'absence attack' describe these features very well, but absence attacks and the motor and autonomic phenomena that may accompany them can occur in other types of seizure, particularly those of temporal lobe origin. The brevity of the attacks may make it difficult to analyse their clinical features and to distinguish their differences. The frequency of associated phenomena is probably underestimated since even the trained observer witnessing an attack may find it difficult, in the few seconds involved, to notice everything that happens.

Although the blank spell and cessation of speech and other activities are the features noticed by the careful observer, it is unusual (contrary to earlier teaching (Lennox & Lennox 1960)) for these to be the only phenomena in petit mal absences. One of the most instructive studies is that of Penry and his colleagues (1975) who followed 48 patients, aged 4 to 24 years, with recurring absence seizures.

They recorded the patients and their EEGs simultaneously by a multicamera videotape technique. From the 48 patients 374 clinical absence seizures were recorded and classified according to the International Classification of Epileptic Seizures. Simple absences with no other features constituted only 9.4% of the seizures. The other attacks most often contained, in order of frequency, either automatisms (seen in 88% of patients), mild clonic components (seen in 71%) or decreased postural tone (seen in 41%) or a combination of two or more of these features. The attacks in individual patients were not always stereotyped and 40% of patients, showed on occasions seizures with only blank staring, unawareness and amnesia, although they had more complex attacks at other times. 88% of patients had seizures lasting 10 seconds or less and very few seizures lasted longer than 45 seconds, an important point of distinction from temporal lobe attacks (complex partial seizures) most of which exceed 10 and often 30 seconds in duration. Automatisms were seen in 236 seizures, containing 655 complex movements. These most often involved the face or head (67%) and less often the limbs. The commonest events were lip-smacking (24%), chewing (18%), and fumbling with the fingers (15%), but many other complex and quasi-purposive movements were seen.

Two main categories of automatisms were seen. In the perseverative type the patient continues an activity engaged in before the onset of the attack, such as walking or handling an object, but does so in an aimless and distorted fashion, so that he may wander off the path. In the de novo automatisms movements begin after the onset of the seizure and are usually of oral, scratching or fiddling type. It was rare for automatisms to occur as the initial event in the seizures, and the probability of their occurring was closely related to the length of the attacks, being 95% for those lasting at least 18 seconds, over 50% with duration longer than 7 seconds, and only 22.6% with attacks lasting 3 seconds or less. This correlation between automatisms and duration of seizure supports the suggestion of Penry & Dreifuss (1969) that automatisms are reactive in mechanism and represent a released form of behaviour when the cortex is impaired by spike-wave discharges.

Mild clonic movements, occurring in 71% of

patients, affected the eyelids in 87% of cases. In contrast to automatisms, these movements tended to occur early in the attacks and showed a negative correlation with seizure duration. Decreased postural tone in trunk or limb muscles, seen in 41% of patients, resulted in drooping of the head, slumping of the trunk, dropping of the arms and relaxation of the grip, so that knife and fork, pen or other object in the hand was dropped. Only rarely did the patient fall, though he might buckle at the knees, a helpful point of distinction from myoclonic attacks. Increased postural tone was much rarer, occurring in only 4.5% of seizures. It caused some patients to show extension of the neck and trunk, sometimes taking a few steps backwards, and in others the head or trunk were pulled to one side.

The effects of the seizures on responsiveness and recall were tested in over 200 attacks by speaking a standard test phrase (a nursery rhyme) to the patients who were asked to repeat it afterwards. There was no recall after 188 seizures, and recall was imperfect after the other attacks. The implications of such gaps in recall for a child's education if attacks are frequent are obvious.

The EEG showed typical 3 per second regular spike and wave discharges in 323 of the 374 seizures, and in most of the others showed variations on the theme of spike and wave. There was no difference in the incidence of automatisms with 3 per second spike-wave and those with other spike-wave abnormalities.

The clinical analysis of absence seizures is particularly helpful in indicating the differences from temporal lobe attacks. Important points are that in absence attacks the onset is abrupt and is not preceded by an aura, that the end of the episode is also abrupt with mental clarity returning at once, and that the seizures usually last less than ten seconds.

A careful history is essential in order to obtain as full a picture as possible, and an attack can often be provoked in a co-operative child by persuading him to hyperventilate. Similar techniques during EEG recording often allow clinical and electrical features to be studied simultaneously. It is possible in most cases to be fairly certain about the diagnosis of petit mal absences from the history and usually the EEG confirms this, although in rare cases doubt may remain. In such cases a therapeutic trial with

ethosuximide is reasonable, since in most cases of true petit mal this drug produces dramatic improvement. Sodium valproate may be used in the same way.

It is very rare for true petit mal attacks to be due to serious brain lesions, and this form of 'centrencephalic' epilepsy is thought to arise in the diencephalon often with a genetic basis. Metrakos & Metrakos (1966) found that the incidence of seizures among the parents and siblings of children with petit mal of centrencephalic origin was 12%, while 45% of siblings had an abnormal EEG. Intensive investigation is therefore seldom justified in this form of epilepsy, and is likely to be harmful by causing unnecessary anxiety to parents and children.

The prognosis is usually excellent in these seizures, the tendency to attacks often ceasing spontaneously after a few years. It is unusual to find adults still suffering from seizures of this type.

Drug treatment is usually very effective. Until recently ethosuximide (Zarontin) was the drug of choice, and its effect is often immediate. Being well tolerated, with few serious side-effects, it can be given for several years, and the dose can be 'titrated' according to need: parents usually discover what is the minimum effective dose. Sodium valproate (Epilim), a newer drug, is also very effective in most cases. Although well tolerated generally, it is not entirely free from side-effects.

ACQUIRED APHASIA IN CHILDREN ASSOCIATED WITH SEIZURES AND EEG ABNORMALITY (LANDAU'S SYNDROME)

'A syndrome of acquired aphasia with convulsive disorder in children' was first described by Landau & Kleffner (1957) and later reported by other writers (Worster-Drought 1971, Deonna et al 1977, Rapin et al 1977). The clinical picture in this rare condition is dramatic and puzzling. A child, who has usually developed speech and language normally, suffers the abrupt or gradual loss of speech. At about the same time or soon afterwards he develops seizures of generalized or focal motor type. The two problems persist, often fluctuating markedly, the dysphasia sometimes becoming worse when the fits are more severe, and improving when they are in abeyance. There is a severe receptive aphasia with loss of comprehension of spoken language followed by loss or reduction of executive speech. Intelligence is usually intact. The child appears bewildered and looks blank or may repeatedly say 'Pardon?' or 'What?' when spoken to, so that often deafness is wrongly suspected. Acute anxiety about his sudden predicament often causes him to develop behaviour disorders which may lead to psychiatric referral. When seizures occur, as they commonly do, these point to the organic nature of the disorder, but may understandably raise concern about progressive brain pathology, neoplastic or degenerative. The EEG shows paroxysmal abnormalities with spike foci mainly in the parietal and posterior temporal regions (Deonna et al 1977). The discharges are almost always bilateral and asynchronous, usually with a left-sided predominance.

The age of onset of the disorder is between 3 and 9 years and its course is variable. There may be prompt initial recovery and later relapses or the condition may persist with little variation. In a few cases seizures are absent or rare. Worster-Drought's (1971) experience with 14 cases was that recovery was more or less complete in 6, partial in 3 and slight or very limited in 5 children whose comprehension and production of spoken language remained very defective. The recent review of 9 cases (Mantovani Landau 1980) [6 of them from the original report by Landau & Kleffner (1957)] showed a rather better outcome 10 to 28 years after onset. Four patients had recovered fully and 5 had mild or moderate language dysfunction. In severe cases speech is laboured and telegraphic with a poor vocabulary and many periphrases. Understanding of the written word may be preserved but writing spontaneously or to dictation may be severely affected (Rapin et al 1977) so that education in a normal school is impossible. The term 'verbal auditory agnosia' has been used by Rapin and her colleagues to emphasize the problems which these children have in encoding and decoding using the acoustic channel, and the implications for their remedial education. Their patients were somewhat atypical since two of them had evidence of structural brain disease (presumed megalencephaly and a left parietal angiomatous anomaly) whereas most have shown no evidence for this clinically or radiologically. The aetiology of the syndrome remains mysterious. Speculation about a very localized encephalitic or inflammatory process is unsupported by any evidence. A consistent feature is the EEG evidence of bilateral brain dysfunction which may in some way be responsible.

Recognition of this rare syndrome and its differentiation from deafness, psychiatric illness and progressive brain dissease is essential so that remedial help can be given. Education requires abundant and skilled help from therapists and teachers familiar with these problems. Schools for the mentally handicapped are not suitable for most of the victims of this disorder, for whom adequate help can usually only be provided in a specialized residential school.

PROVOKING FACTORS IN CHILDHOOD EPILEPSY: REFLEX OR SENSORY-EVOKED SEIZURES

We do not know why most seizures occur when they do rather than at some other time, and this is true even of the many children whose attacks show a regular periodicity, occurring at intervals of days, weeks or months.
Certain conditions, however, do predispose to fits and many children suffer some or all of their seizures in particular situations. These include certain physiological, psychological and metabolic states, which appear to lower the seizure threshold, and various sensory stimuli. Reflex epilepsy, the term formerly used for attacks provoked by these latter factors, is misleading, since the mechanism is not as simple or automatic as a reflex, and sensory-precipitated or sensory-evoked seizures seems preferable.

Sleep

Sleep and the twilight state before and after sleeping are associated with infantile spasms and myoclonic seizures. Temporal lobe attacks often occur at night, so that their true nature, or even their very existence, may be overlooked. The benign focal 'sylvian seizures' with mid-temporal spike foci are more likely to become generalized when they occur in sleep. Many children may have unrecognised nocturnal attacks since there is often a history of unexplained wet beds, disturbed nights and sore tongues preceding the first recognized seizures.

Boredom and emotional factors

Boredom is a potent precipitant of seizures in children with epilepsy and attacks are relatively rare while the child is engaged in interesting activities. Emotional factors, of both pleasurable and unpleasant type, may provoke fits and the excitement of Christmas, birthdays or bonfire nights is a common trigger. Worry and anxiety over problems at school and at home, such as the prospect of a move to a new school or new class, or parental illness often act in the same way.

Fever

Fever is the specific trigger in the many children subject to febrile convulsions, but there are also many cases of seizures with a later age of onset in which some but not all attacks occur in a setting of febrile infections such as tonsillitis. The premenstrual state is often associated with an increase in fits in girls as in older women.

Sensory stimuli

Sensory stimuli which may provoke fits include sight, sound and touch but very rarely smell or taste, despite the frequency with which olfactory or gustatory hallucinations occur in temporal lobe attacks.

Photosensitive and television epilepsy

Stroboscopic stimulation is an effective activating procedure during the EEG (Ch. 24) and precipitation of seizures by photic stimuli has been recognized for many centuries, sunlight being the usual trigger until recently. The incidence of photosensitive epilepsy probably exceeds 1 in 10 000. A rare but difficult problem is that of the child, often retarded or disturbed, who induces attacks by staring at the sun or other source of bright light, waving one hand in front of his eyes with fingers outspread. It has been suggested (Ames 1971) that

the hand waving is part of the ictus itself rather than a voluntary action provoking it, but this is probably not true of all cases. Some children are known to stare at a bright light and blink rapidly apparently to induce attacks. Others seem able to provoke fits by staring at particular patterns of black and white or lines set at certain angles, as in wire netting.

Television is now the commonest photic precipitant of seizures in the developed nations. Television-induced epilepsy usually starts under the age of 20 years, most often between 6 and 12, and is commoner in girls than boys. There is evidence of a genetic factor with photic sensitivity among many asymptomatic relatives of affected children. The commonest type of fit provoked by light is a tonic-clonic convulsion, sometimes preceded by myoclonic jerking. The relationship of these seizures to television is a specific one, and not merely a reflexion of the many hours spent by children in front of the television set. Television epilepsy is rarer in the United States than in Europe, due perhaps to the difference in the mains AC frequency, 50 Hz in Europe and 60 Hz in the USA (Bower 1963). The result is that the two half scans produce flicker at the dangerous rate of 25 cycles per second in Europe and at 30 in the United States.

Although it has been suggested that a malfunctioning television set is an important factor in provoking these attacks, Jeavons & Harding (1975) believe the major factor to be the nearness of the patient to the set. Attacks often occur on approaching the set to change channels, switch off or correct a fault. They found that 7% of their patients were impulsively attracted to the television screen, and males predominated among these in contrast to all other photosensitive patients.

Discotheques and home movies are other possible triggers of photically induced seizures. The risks of the former were lessened by the ban placed by the Greater London Council in 1971 on the use of flicker rates faster than 8 per second in discotheques, but 42% of the patients reported by Jeavons & Harding were still sensitive to this rate of flicker.

Jeavons & Harding found spike and wave discharges in the basic EEGs of 54% of their patients. This finding was relevant to treatment, since those without spontaneous discharges did not usually need anticonvulsant therapy. Photoconvulsive responses of various kinds were seen, the commonest being a spike and wave discharge with a 3 per second slow wave component. It proved helpful to establish the lowest and highest flash rate which consistently induced a photoconvulsive response since this allowed improvement or deterioration to be detected and showed the dangerous flicker rates.

The most effective treatment for all photosensitive patients is avoidance of the provoking stimulus. This may be difficult in the case of children who deliberately seek to provoke attacks by hand waving or other techniques or by approaching close to the television set. Anticonvulsants are often ineffective in such cases. The parents of children with television-induced seizures should ensure that they do not view closer than six feet (2 meters) from the set, nor approach it to switch or adjust the controls. If they must approach it, they should cover one eye. The set should always be viewed in well-lit surroundings, with another light source in addition to the set, preferably a lamp placed on top of it.

Patients who develop fits with sunlight may be helped by wearing polarized glasses in sunny weather.

Most photosensitive patients do not need anticonvulsant therapy, but those with spike and wave discharges in their basic EEG should probably be treated, and also those whose EEGs show an abnormal response to photic stimulation although their fits have not been associated with this. Sodium valproate has been found helpful clinically and electrically.

The prognosis for improvement in most photosensitive children is probably good, although recovery is unlikely before the age of twenty. The EEGs of the parents of photosensitive children rarely show abnormal responses, even when their past history suggests that they may have been photosensitive.

Reading epilepsy

This much rarer form of visually provoked epilepsy was first described by Bickford (1954). Reading in these cases leads to increasing twitching of the jaw associated with epileptic activity in the EEG in the temporo-parietal region. The twitching ceases when the child stops reading, but if he continues a generalized convulsion may occur. The EEG does not usually show an abnormal response to flicker in these children. Subclinical reading epilepsy has been suggested as a cause in some cases of unexplained reading difficulty (Oettinger et al 1967). Excellent therapeutic results have been reported with clonazepam (Hall & Marshall 1980).

Auditory provocation of fits

The commonest example of auditory precipitation of seizures is the acousticomotor attack induced by a sudden noise, usually with an element of startle. The attacks are often myoclonic. They may be the only form of seizure in a patient or be accompanied by other attacks occurring spontaneously. Usually a loud noise is needed as an effective trigger, but in some cases a sound as quiet as that caused by switching a light on or off is adequate. Clinically it is often possible to show habituation; a hand clap may provoke an attack three or four times in succession but later fail to do so.

More complex forms of auditory provocation of seizures are seen in musicogenic epilepsy (Critchley 1937) and voice-induced epilepsy (Forster et al 1969), both induced by very specific patterns of sound. Language-induced epilepsy has also been described (Geschwind & Sherwin 1967) in an adult in whom seizures could be triggered by attempts to use three modalities of language, reading, writing and speaking.

Tactile stimuli

Tactile stimuli act as provoking factors for seizures in some patients. Seizures induced by movement have been described by several authors (Lishman et al 1962). These have often been provoked by the initiation of movement and the sensory stimuli involved may arise from receptors in tendons and muscles. In some cases paroxysmal choreoathetosis may be responsible for the involuntary movements, and the absence of EEG changes during the attacks in some patients throws some doubt on their epileptic nature (Ch. 10).

Drug withdrawal

Injudicious reduction or withdrawal of drug treatment is a common precipitant of seizures, and of status epilepticus. The parents of children with epilepsy, and their doctors, must be aware of these risks, and no patient with epilepsy should ever be told to stop all drugs before an EEG examination, as sometimes happens.

Menstruation and epilepsy

Many women with epilepsy have an increase in attacks in association with their menstrual periods, often at a time of premenstrual tension. This may be a problem in adolescent girls in whom behaviour and mood may deteriorate with increased fits at these times. Sometimes this occurs only for the first few periods, especially if these are initially irregular and heavy. In some cases relief is obtained by taking acetazolamide for some days before the onset of the periods.

TRAUMA AS A CAUSE OF CHILDHOOD EPILEPSY

Although trauma is included in most lists of the causes of epilepsy, *postnatal* injury, as Jennett (1973) has pointed out, has received scant attention in many paediatric texts in contrast to perinatal brain injury. With improvements in obstetrics the latter has become rarer, but postnatal trauma has achieved prominence with the hazards of accidents on the roads and at home and the emergence, or recognition, of non-accidental injury as an important contribution to childhood trauma in the bosom of the family (Ch. 18). Jennett (1973) calculates, on the basis of 100 000 patients admitted each year to British hospitals with head injuries, with 25 000 of these under 16 years of age, that between 1000 and 1500 children leaving hospital after a head injury each year are likely to develop late traumatic epilepsy. A series of head injuries admitted to hospitals in Oxford, Glasgow and Rotterdam included 1000 patients with depressed skull fractures, of whom one half were under 16 at the time of injury. Road accidents remain an important cause of head trauma in children. Cynthia Illingworth (1979) in a recent review of 227 road accidents to children seen at the Children's Hospital, Sheffield, in a 9 month period, found that 169 of these involved pedestrians, 31 cyclists and 27 passengers. 29.6% of the 227 children had severe head injuries (concussion with or without skull fracture). Comparison with 225 previously described skateboard injuries and 200 playground equipment injuries showed that the injuries sustained in road accidents were serious in a much higher proportion, 37%. It was of interest that 55 of the 227 children had had previous accidents, many of them two or more. 5 of these 55 children came from known 'problem families', in which accident-proneness is recognized.

Jennett has analyzed the occurrence and significance of early epilepsy after head injury in children and adults, and has stressed the differences between seizures starting within a week of injury and those starting in the subsequent seven weeks. Epilepsy occurs 30 times more often in the first week after injury than the average in any of the next seven weeks. Focal motor attacks account for 40% of fits in the first week but only 17% in the next seven weeks and 3% after three months. Less than a third of patients with one or more fits in the first week after injury have any further fits in the next 4 years, but the recurrence risk rises to 71% if the first fit occurs within the next 7 weeks. Fits in the first week in the whole series were fairly evenly divided in time of onset between the first hour after injury, the next 23 hours and the remaining 6 days, but children under 16 were far more likely to have their first fit in the first 24 hours than adults.

Status epilepticus was much commoner in children, especially those under 5, during the first week after injury. Children whose early fits were *focal* were significantly less liable to recurrence than those with non-focal attacks, or than adults with either type of attack. Whether early epilepsy followed a trivial injury (with no post-traumatic amnesia, depressed fracture or intracranial haematoma) or a more serious one, the risk of subsequent late epilepsy was as high.

The EEG prediction of post-traumatic epilepsy was considered by Jennett & Van de Sande (1975).

The EEGs from 722 patients with injuries associated with a high risk of late traumatic epilepsy were analyzed. Although abnormal records were commoner in patients who developed epilepsy, they reflected the more severe brain damage in these patients, which was already evident on clinical grounds. In individual patients the EEG did not improve the accuracy of the prediction calculated from clinical data.

In the prophylaxis of post-traumatic epilepsy Young and his colleagues (1979) have obtained good results from a regime of Phenytoin specifically tailored for the patient with acute head injury and designed to provide immediate and sustained plasma concentrations of the drug between 10 and 20 μg/ml. This involves an immediate intravenous dose of 13 mg/kg of body weight, followed by an immediate intramuscular dose of 13 mg/kg, and daily i.m. doses of 8.8 mg/kg until oral medication is tolerated. Of 84 patients so treated only 6% had seizures in the first year (excluding fits in the first week), a considerably lower rate than reported in previous series. Since only one third of patients were known to have continued to take Phenytoin after the first month, and only half of these had plasma levels in the desired range, it seems possible that the drug had a prophylactic rather than merely a suppressive effect.

THE DIFFERENTIAL DIAGNOSIS BETWEEN CERTAIN NON-EPILEPTIC EVENTS AND EPILEPTIC SEIZURES

The misdiagnosis of epilepsy and its causes

Epilepsy is often over-diagnosed and many children, and some adults, have the label wrongly applied to them. The consequences of this can be disastrous: not only is the label 'epilepsy' well known as a 'passport to prejudice', but the side-effects of inappropriate medication may compound the problem.

Jeavons (1975) found that 20% of 470 patients (children and adults) seen at two epilepsy clinics in Birmingham did not have epilepsy. Of these 93 patients, 35 had syncope and 39 had attacks of psychological origin. Others had migraine, breath-holding attacks, night terrors, day dreams or narcolepsy. The misdiagnosis of epilepsy in these cases arose from four main causes:

1. inadequate history, or jumping to conclusions
2. the occurrence of clonic movements or incontinence in attacks
3. a family history of epilepsy, a past history of febrile convulsions, or the finding of an 'abnormal' EEG
4. insufficient knowledge of the nature of epilepsy.

The first cause is probably the most important. A detailed history will usually distinguish true seizures from other types of disorders of consciousness, but once the label 'epilepsy' has been wrongly applied it is seldom critically examined and the patient all too often suffers the associated stigma indefinitely. It is common to see the words 'known epileptic' written in case notes by junior doctors who have not taken the trouble to question the parents about the history. The diagnosis of epilepsy is so important that it is better to err on the side of under rather than overdiagnosing it, and often the data available are so limited that the physician must keep an open mind. If the final diagnosis of epilepsy is made after some months of observation and reserving judgement, little is lost, whereas the harm done by diagnosing it wrongly is incalculable. Some of the conditions misdiagnosed as epilepsy are described below.

Syncopal attacks (faints)

Fainting attacks are common in older children, occurring more frequently in girls than boys. They illustrate well Jeavon's dictum that the differential diagnosis of epilepsy depends much more on what precedes or follows an attack than on what occurs during it. Syncopal attacks often occur while standing in a tense or emotionally fraught situation such as school assembly or church, with emotional upsets such as the prospect of an injection or the sight of blood, or a sudden change in posture, particularly standing up from the lying or sitting position. The onset of symptoms is slower than in a fit, and the patient experiences 'faintness', giddiness, and visual blurring. Sometimes he is able to sit or lie down and prevent himself from falling, but often he will fall or slump and can sometimes afterwards remember falling and even hitting the floor. If he sustains a head injury he may lose consciousness as a result and may even convulse so that the interpretation of events is made more difficult. After an ordinary syncopal attack, however, the child usually recovers quickly, without confusion or a period of sleep, whereas recovery is slower and sleep common after a fit. If the pulse rate is recorded during the attack, bradycardia is usually noted in syncope and tachycardia during a seizure. Older children should always be asked what they remember of the onset of attacks since only they can describe their sensations, and parents are often amazed at what they can recall. If a child describes the feelings of giddiness and visual blurring, remembers falling and recalls the agitation of his teachers as he lay on the floor, he has probably not had a fit, but a faint.

Breath-holding attacks

One of the more satisfying experiences of a paediatric neurologist's life is to obtain a clear history of breath-holding spells in a child who has been referred with the diagnosis of epilepsy.

These attacks are self-limited and usually outgrown by school age, but their dramatic onset with cyanosis or skin pallor may cause intense anxiety to parents and doctors alike until the situation is 'defused' by explanation and reassurance.

Two major types of breath-holding spells occur; the classical cyanotic type, and the pallid syncopal attack (Lombroso & Lerman 1967). In a review of 184 children at the Mayo Clinic in whom the diagnosis had been made (Laxdal et al 1969) 87% of the children had their first attack before the age of 18 months and none later than $3\frac{1}{2}$ years. In 5% of cases the spells began in the newborn period. The usual pattern was for the attacks initially to occur at intervals of weeks or months, to reach a peak in the second year of life and to decrease in frequency thereafter. Most lasted less than one minute, though few were accurately timed.

The commonest precipitating factors were a painful stimulus (such as a fall in a toddler, a cut or a venipuncture) or anger or frustration. Fear provoked some attacks and excitement or fatigue caused a small number. Following such a stimulus the child cries, stop breathing in expiration, becomes cyanosed, limp and unconscious. In the

shorter attacks he regains consciousness within a few seconds and may resume crying. If apnoea lasts longer, the limp phase is followed by an opisthotonic phase sometimes with sporadic clonic movements of the limbs and sometimes incontinence of urine or faeces. This convulsive phase may be followed by another brief limp phase before consciousness is regained and the child may then sleep for several hours. The cyanotic attacks were most often provoked by anger or frustration in the Mayo Clinic series whereas pallid syncopal attacks usually followed a painful stimulus, often a slight blow to the head, the child gasping and becoming apnoeic and unresponsive usually without significant crying.

Most children in the series had either cyanotic (54%) or pallid (27%) spells, but 12% had either type at different times, and 5% had mixed attacks in which both cyanosis and pallor occurred. Clonic limb movements were noted in 43 children and incontinence in 21, always related to attacks with opisthotonos (usually cyanotic) but never to those with limpness. Most of the children were neurologically and intellectually normal but abnormal behaviour was recorded in 45, frequent temper tantrums, overactivity, irritability and stubbornness being the main features. EEGs were obtained in 116 children and were normal or showed non-specific abnormalities.

48 of the 127 children in whom the family history was known had a relative who had breath-holding attacks at the time or in the past.

The prognosis for the attacks was excellent in the 123 children followed up, since none had attacks after the age of 7 years 7 months and 90% had stopped having them before their sixth birthday. Four patients aged between $16\frac{1}{2}$ and 21 years had had recurrent syncopal attacks. The literature contains at least one report (Paulson 1963) of a child dying during a breath-holding attack, but this is exceptional and parents can and should be reassured.

Stephenson (1978b) has studied 58 children with 'white' or pallid breath-holding attacks which he has called reflex anoxic seizures due to vagal cardiac inhibition with asystole. Ocular compression was performed under EEG and ECG control and the length of induced systole was noted. In 55% of cases it was 4 seconds or longer, which is an abnormal response, and in 78% 2 seconds or more. He finds that atropine is helpful in preventing this vagal-mediated reflex cardiac arrest and has also suggested (1978a) from similar studies that a proportion of febrile convulsions are due to the same mechanism.

In most cases explanation and reassurance that the attacks will cease is enough and this is often followed by a marked decrease in their frequency. Great concern may have been felt because a label of epilepsy has already been applied (in 34 children in the Mayo Clinic series a diagnosis of some form of epilepsy had been made) and the removal of this label may be very therapeutic. The children concerned are often difficult and easily frustrated, differing in temperament from their siblings. Parents can often be advised on how to avoid the battles of the will which often provoke the attacks in a determined toddler by diverting his attention to something else before flash-point is reached. Occasionally skilled psychiatric help may be needed when the parent-child relationship seems particularly unhappy. In general anticonvulsant treatment is not recommended and phenobarbitone often exacerbates the problem, being badly tolerated by an already rather irritable child. Some of the 30 children in the series of Laxdal et al treated with phenobarbitone, however, did seem to derive benefit.

Benign paroxysmal vertigo

Sudden brief attacks of vertigo in small children may be mistaken for epilepsy or even attributed to a brain tumour. Benign paroxysmal vertigo (Basser 1964) is a condition affecting boys and girls equally, usually starting between one and three years of age, with attacks coming on suddenly without warning or provocation. The child appears distressed and calls for help, sometimes indicating that he feels a sense of rotation of his surroundings or self or a sense of falling. He may say 'fall down.' He often appears unsteady, and may cling to his parents or to furniture for support. He may stagger or fall in the attacks. Sometimes he will lie down on the floor and refuse to move. Consciousness is fully preserved and there are no convulsive movements. Pallor, sweating and vomiting are common. Nystagmus may be noted during attacks. Torticol-

lis is seen in some attacks and it has been suggested (Dunn & Synder 1976) that paroxysmal torticollis may occur in the children when younger and evolve into benign paroxysmal vertigo. A relationship to migraine has also been suggested (Fenichel 1967).

The frequency of attacks varies but is commonly between one and four per month. Most episodes last less than five minutes and some only a few seconds, but occasionally the duration is over ten minutes. The outlook for cessation of attacks is good, many of them ceasing after four years.
Between attacks the children are well with no abnormal neurological signs, but some may show signs of ear infection. Caloric testing, with iced water instilled into the auditory canal, is often abnormal, failing to provoke the usual nystagmus. The EEG is usually normal.

It is not difficult to distinguish these attacks from epilepsy if a good history is taken. Vertigo is not uncommon as a feature of epilepsy, especially of temporal lobe type, but in these cases there are usually other indications of its epileptic nature.

Medication is often unhelpful. Dimenhydrinate (Dramamine) may be of some benefit, as may Stemetil. Anticonvulsants should not be used.

Narcolepsy and the narcoleptic syndrome

Narcolepsy has been defined (Parkes & Fenton 1973, modified from Yoss & Daly 1957) as a condition with periodic and frequently irresistible sleep in the day-time which may occur at inappropriate times and is often produced by monotony. The narcoleptic syndrome includes three other symptoms with which narcolepsy is often associated, although all four symptoms are present in only a third of patients.

The other symptoms are:

Cataplexy

Loss of voluntary movement produced by emotion or sudden startle which results in head nodding, immobility, collapse or double vision.

Sleep paralysis

Paralysis of voluntary movements on waking from sleep.

Hypnagogic hallucinations

Vivid and commonly visual sensory impressions, often frightening, which occur during half-sleep.

These symptoms will occasionally come into the differential diagnosis of epilepsy in childhood.

The subject has been usefully reviewed by Zarcone (1973).

The rapid eye movement (REM) phase of sleep is abnormal in patients with the narcoleptic syndrome in whom night sleep begins with a REM phase. Narcolepsy has been described as a regression to the sleep pattern of infancy, in which REM predominates and in which there are sleep-onset REM periods. These phenomena and the effect of medication upon them can be studied polygraphically, by the combined use of EEG, EMG and electro-oculography.

The prevalence of the syndrome is uncertain and is probably underestimated. In about 50% of cases the age of onset is between 10 and 20 years, and in about 5% under 10, (Zarcone 1973) but the diagnosis is often delayed until adult life, when the disruption of daily activities, and the complications of driving and other accidents and of amphetamine abuse or habituation motivate a deeper medical analysis of the problem.

The history of the narcoleptic sleep attack is characteristic and should not be confused with epilepsy. It is of sudden onset, usually lasting about 15 minutes, but sometimes longer if the patient is lying down, and may be accompanied by dreams. It occurs most often in a boring situation. It can be put off by an effort usually for minutes and sometimes for some hours. The patient usually wakes refreshed from the attack and has a refractory period of one to five hours before the next. Some patients are drowsy between attacks. Of great importance in distinguishing narcoleptic sleep attacks, cataplexy and sleep paralysis from epilepsy is the fact that the patient can be easily awoken by calling or shaking him.

In investigating patients suspected of having narcolepsy the routine EEG is of value in lacking 'epileptic features', but most help is gained by polygraphic studies which show a direct transition from wakefulness into REM sleep which is pathognomonic.

The syndrome is usually idiopathic, having a genetic basis in some families. In rare cases narcolepsy is secondary to encephalitis or trauma.

Management

Recognition of the diagnosis is essential for correct management. A punitive or moralistic attitude is misplaced, and anti-convulsant drug therapy is even worse, carrying with it the dreaded label 'epilepsy'. Once narcolepsy has been recognized, minor adjustments to a child's daily time-table may help to avoid awkward sleep attacks by allowing regular breaks for sleep.

Drug treatment (reviewed by Zarcone 1973 and by Parkes & Fenton 1973) has been mainly with the amphetamines or methylphenidate (Ritalin®). Parkes & Fenton (1973) found that both laevo- and dextroamphetamine abolished narcolepsy in adult patients, but did not affect cataplexy. Good results were also obtained in adult patients with Clomipramine Hydrochloride (Guilleminault et al 1976).

Two other phenomena related to sleep are sometimes mistaken for epilepsy but should be clearly distinguished from it.

Pavor nocturnus or night terrors

These occur in many, if not most children and in some adults. The episodes come on in the earlier hours of sleep during the deep non-REM sleep associated with high-voltage slow waves in the EEG. Polygraphic recording of night terrors by Gastaut & Broughton (1965) showed them to occur during intense and sudden arousal from deep slow wave sleep. The affected child may mutter or cry, and then screams and often sits up in bed staring and apparently terrified, not recognising his parents and sometimes getting out of bed. He soon settles down again into a sound sleep and usually has no memory of the event next morning. Incontinence and tongue-biting are rare, in contrast to nocturnal convulsions. Emotional disturbance does not seem to be commoner in those subject to these episodes than in those who are not. Severe and frequent attakcs may respond to a small dose of Diazepam at bedtime which has the effect of reducing the amount of non-REM sleep. The disorder is basically one of arousal rather than of sleep. The

EEG is normal during the episodes and it is essential not to confuse them with attacks of temporal lobe (complex partial seizures) or other forms of epilepsy. Hypoglycaemia or hypocalcaemia can occasionally result in similar symptoms.

Nightmares

These are familiar to most parents, who are usually wise enough to recognise them for what they are and to avoid consulting a doctor when they occur in their children and so running the risk of their being mistaken for epilepsy.

Masturbation and 'gratification phenomena'

Two daytime physical activities which may be misdiagnosed on occasion as 'epileptic' in younger children are the movements of masturbation (commoner in girls in this age group) and the so-called 'gratification phenomena'. In the latter the child engages in, and derives great pleasure from, stereotyped movements while appearing withdrawn. A common pattern is rapid flapping movements of both hands carried out when he is excited. The movements may have a ritualistic quality and be performed when the child is bored. His face may appear blank so that he seems out of touch, but he will respond at once when called and the movements will stop.

Hysterical or simulated seizures

The older literature contains many references to hysterical fits or seizures as a manifestation of conversion hysteria (e.g. Gowers 1881). Frankly hysterical fits in childhood are probably rare nowadays and are not usually difficult to recognise, though confusion may occur with psychomotor seizures. The child often indicates his awareness of his audience and his surroundings by a graded performance, more dramatic and varied when observed, and by a contrast between his often frenzied motor activities and the lack of any injury to himself. I have seen a child roll along the floor in such an attack until he came to an obstacle in his path, when he stood up, walked around it, lay down again and pursued his previous course. Such extreme instances are rare. In some cases there is a history of seizures in a close relative or friend and familiarity with the phenomena of fits may allow a more convincing performance. Teachers and other staff in schools for children with epilepsy are often well aware of the histrionic abilities of certain of their charges and can distinguish without much difficulty between the genuine and the simulated episodes.

The difficulties that may be posed by pseudo-epileptic seizures in children and adolescents are discussed by Finlayson & Lucas (1979) who reviewed 18 patients aged from 4 to 20 years seen at the Mayo Clinic over a 6-year period. Seventeen of these had previously been treated with anticonvulsants and most had been subjected to many diagnostic procedures.

THE DIAGNOSIS AND INVESTIGATION OF EPILEPSY

The problems and importance of distinguishing other episodes from epileptic events and of avoiding the misdiagnosis of epilepsy have been referred to. Erroneous application of the label 'epilepsy' can be as crippling psychologically as the misinterpretation of an innocent cardiac murmur which can cause cardiac invalidism.

The first essential is to decide whether the episodes complained of are epileptic or not. Having concluded that they are, the second is to decide what type of epilepsy is involved. The third is to try to determine the cause of the epilepsy, recognising that this is often not possible and ensuring that serious causes, which are rare, are excluded. The approach to those questions is basically clinical with the history of major importance. The clinician must be prepared to make liberal use of the 'test of time', to show whether attacks recur, what form they take, in what situations they occur, and whether symptoms develop which indicate a possible progressive pathology.

The investigation of epilepsy should be determined by the clinical features. Investigations, in general, should not be used to try to decide whether episodic events are epileptic or not, and it is unwise to invoke an abnormal EEG as evidence for epilepsy or a normal one as evidence against it. EEG abnormalities are so common in childhood and the record is so readily altered by physiological and metabolic factors that undue reliance on the EEG can be misleading.

The diagnostic probabilities will determine the investigation programme. It will clearly be different for a newborn baby with fits, for an infant with infantile spasms, for a child of one year with febrile convulsions, for a child with a congenital hemiplegia who develops unilateral convulsions at the age of five years, for a child with classical petit mal absences or television-induced seizures and for another with temporal lobe attacks starting at the age of ten.

In each of these examples the clinical features may indicate certain possible diagnoses, and hence the choice of tests. The past history may show that the child was clearly abnormal developmentally and neurologically before seizures began. This is most common in children with infantile spasms, and those with previously recognised cerebral palsy and/or mental retardation who develop seizures. In such cases the seizures, like the previous handicaps, are likely to be symptoms of long-standing abnormality of the brain. Perinatal difficulties may be relevant, or prenatal factors such as intrauterine infections or cerebral malformation may be suspected and evidence will be sought for them. Evidence for tuberose sclerosis must be sought in all children with fits and especially with infantile spasms, since the cutaneous and other stigmata of this (and other neurocutaneous syndromes) (Ch. 20) are diagnostic.

Certain forms of seizure are rarely due to serious organic brain disease, for example, the classical petit mal absence and benign focal epilepsy with midtemporal spike foci. Focal seizures in general must indicate focal pathology, but this is seldom neoplastic in childhood. Temporal lobe attacks are more likely to be due to atrophic than to expanding lesions. When progressive pathology, either neoplastic or degenerative, *is* responsible for focal fits in childhood, evidence of this usually appears with neurological deficits, such as hemiplegia, dysphasia, dementia or visual problems.

The value of the EEG in childhood epilepsy is discussed by Dr Harris in Chapter 24. This investigation is rarely diagnostic of precise diseases, although in some progressive disorders such as subacute sclerosing panencephalitis and some forms of

Batten's disease, it shows pathognomonic features. Serial EEGs are of value in suggesting progressive pathology be showing, for example, increasing focal abnormality in cerebral neoplasms, and to some extent indicating a good prognosis when the record shows improvement.

Plain skull X-rays may be helpful in investigating childhood epilepsy. Some of the diagnostic features are discussed in other chapters. Intracranial calcification may be seen in tuberose sclerosis, the Sturge-Weber syndrome, some neoplasms, and intrauterine infections such as toxoplasmosis and cytomegalic inclusion disease. They may also indicate the likelihood of an expanding or atrophic cerebral lesion by showing enlargement or relative smallness of the skull or cranial fossae on one side. Contrast radiography, such as air encephalography and carotid arteriography, are not necessary in most children with epilepsy. They are unjustified unless there is suspicion of a neoplasm, angioma, vascular malformation, subdural haematoma or other surgical lesion, of a porencephalic cyst or of a cerebral malformation such as agenesis of the corpus callosum. The value of air-encephalography in the investigation of focal epilepsy when neoplasms are not suspected is limited. Cerebral atrophy was found in only 45% of children with focal epilepsy compared with 73% of those without focal features to their fits in one series (Brett & Hoare 1969). Atrophy was slightly commoner when focal fits were associated with hemiplegia, but the proportion with unilateral or markedly asymmetrical atrophy was the same among hemiplegic and non-hemiplegic patients. Comparison of hemiplegic patients with focal and non-focal epilepsy also showed no difference in the frequency of unilateral atrophy.

The advent of the CT scan has helped greatly in the investigation of epilepsy, as well as that of mental retardation and other neurological handicaps of chilhood, and this non-invasive technique is much easier to justify than the older radiological investigations. Although the CT scan occasionally shows surprising results, disclosing a neoplasm which had not been suspected in a child with epilepsy, calcification which was not shown on plain skull X-rays, a porencephalic cyst, or localised cerebral atrophy, it is certainly not essential for the management of most cases of epilepsy. Sometimes its use is specifically to exclude a tumour when parents are anxious about this possibility, perhaps because of a family history of a neoplasm or because of ill-founded comments of relatives — or even doctors. In this situation the demonstration of normal brain structure on the scan can be tactically helpful, and facilitate future management.

Biochemical and metabolic disorders should be excluded. Hypoglycaemia and hypocalcaemia, though rare as causes of epilepsy, are easily treatable and deserve exclusion. Disorders of amino-acid metabolism are often associated with epilepsy. Though clinical features may suggest a particular disease (phenylketonuria or homocystinuria) there may not be evidence of this, and so chromatographic examination of blood and urine are advisable.

THE MANAGEMENT OF CHILDHOOD EPILEPSY

'She's much better, doctor, but of course I'm not satisfied'
— The father of a young girl with epilepsy

To treat or not to treat?

When it has been decided that the child is subject to epileptic attacks of one kind or other, and when appropriate investigations have excluded a serious cause, the next question is whether to treat him with regular anticonvulsants or not. In most cases the decision is easy, as there is a clear pattern of regular seizures which may have caused great concern to parents, teachers and the child himself and created difficulties in his daily activities. If, however, the child has had only a few attacks it is often reasonable to defer treatment while waiting to see if further episodes occur. Many children have one, two or three seizures and no more. To treat all children who have had one attack only would result in the unnecessary treatment of many, and it seems preferable not to treat in this situation but to adopt a policy of 'wait and see'. Little is lost by this, and much may be gained. After two or three attacks it is reasonable to start regular medication, but the decision may be affected by the type, severity and timing of the seizures, and by parental attitudes towards the idea of long-term treatment.

Education and support of parents

Parents must be fully informed of the aims and implications of treatment. Without this they cannot be expected to be faithful in the giving of drugs, nor to know how the need for regular dosage will affect the life of the family. Often parents gain the impression that medication will be for a short time only, perhaps for one or two weeks as with antibiotic treatment for infections, and sometimes they believe it will have the same curative effect as the latter. It must be explained that treatment is only suppressive and symptomatic and that one cannot speak of cure in epilepsy, although there is room for optimism about the attacks ceasing spontaneously. Parents must be taken into the doctor's confidence about the nature and side-effects of the drugs prescribed. It is indefensible to leave them in ignorance of what their children are taking, as was common in years past when doctors were more authoritarian than today. They may need to be reassured that the drugs prescribed are not drugs of addiction, and that treatment will not need to continue permanently, although the length of treatment cannot be predicted in advance. This uncertainty, and the many others inherent in epilepsy, are hard for parents to understand and accept, and time spent early on in educating them in frank discussion pays dividends in their greater acceptance of the problem (few parents ever *completely* accept the fact of their child's epilepsy) and in their informed co-operation in treatment.

The mythology of epilepsy

Parental acceptance and understanding of the problem are often marred by myths and misunderstandings about epilepsy which make the idea of it worse than the substance and which encourage prejudice and unhealthy attitudes to the child, who is looked on as different. The extent of these feelings is often shown by the question posed by many parents, 'It isn't epilepsy, is it, doctor?' The doctor who is asked this question will be wise to devote much time to his reply, which can usefully begin by asking what the questioner understands by the word 'epilepsy'. The answer will often disclose depths of ignorance and old wives' tales in which epilepsy is equated with insanity and is said to continue throughout life, 'once an epileptic, always an epileptic'. Most parents, seeing their child's first convulsion, believe he will die in it. Many fear that a brain tumour is the cause but are usually too frightened to voice this fear. Strong reassurance can be given on both these scores. It is helpful to elicit these concerns and deal with them one by one: if they are not mentioned it may nonetheless be helpful for the doctor to comment that such fears are often present in the minds of parents and are of course unfounded.

It is also helpful for him to give a simple operational definition of epilepsy as a condition in which there is a tendency to recurrent seizures, and to draw an analogy with other symptoms such as cough, to illustrate the fact that it is a common problem with very varied causes, few of which are serious. If the idea of epilepsy as a *disease* in its own right can be destroyed, much of the anxiety with which it is invested can be dispelled and a more relaxed attitude be promoted, increasing the chances that the life of the child and his family will remain relatively normal. Many of these factors have been usefully explored by Ward & Bower (1978) in a study of certain social aspects of epilepsy in childhood.

Sometimes the lot of the parents has been made harder by well-meaning relatives prophesying doom. Doctors are not guiltless and parents are often needlessly disturbed by being told that with each attack more damage results to the child's brain and that it is therefore essential to prevent attacks at all costs. Since there are many children whose attacks *cannot* be completely controlled even by massive doses of anti-convulsants, this unfounded statement ensures the maximum of misery for their parents.

'Overprotectiveness' and the problem of restrictions

Parental anxiety about the child's seizures is understandable, but it can aggravate his problems. Sometimes his parents develop an extreme degree of protectiveness, fearing that he will come to harm in an attack, and they may so restrict his activities that he cannot become independent and is denied much of what makes life enjoyable. He may never be let out of his mother's sight nor allowed to play with other children. Sometimes he is not even allowed to feed or dress himself. Such extreme overprotectiveness (called 'hyperpaedophilia' by Ounsted) constitutes a gross handicap for the child, hindering his normal emotional and educational maturation. The same phenomenon is seen with other chronic handicaps, but it tends to be most severe with epilepsy because of the greater anxiety engendered by this disorder.

How far the activities of the child with epilepsy should be restricted depends on the frequency and severity of his attacks, on their timing and provoking factors, on associated problems such as mental retardation and overactive behaviour, and — not least — on the attitudes of his parents. The risks are clearly far less in the case of a child with nocturnal seizures or attacks occurring at regular intervals of weeks or months than in that of another who has frequent and severe convulsions without warning. The aim should be to impose as few restrictions as seems consistent with reasonable safety. Some risks must be accepted: no child can be guarded from *all* conceivable hazards. Games and sports seldom present problems since seizures are rare when a child is pleasantly occupied in such pastimes and more often occur when he is tense or bored. However, competitive athletic effort pushed to the stage of exhaustion should be avoided. Swimming is possible with adequate supervision. Often teachers feel unable to accept responsibility for an epileptic child when supervising a large group of children. A white swimming cap may help by making him instantly recognizable to the instructor, but may be unacceptable as it emphasises his difference from his fellows, in the same way as a crash-helmet worn for protection. If swimming at school is inadvisable the child can still swim with his parents or other adults in attendance. Though some children with epilepsy have drowned while swimming in the sea or in swimming-baths, the problem may be put in perspective by the finding (Pearn 1977) that only two out of 76 consecutive chilhood drownings in Southern Queensland were caused by epileptiform seizures, both occurring in the family bath-tub.

Many of the problems of children with epilepsy stem from society's attitudes towards them and from a stereotyped image of 'the epileptic child', which is as false and misleading as the concept of the 'epileptic personality' in adults, now happily extinct. The late Ronald MacKeith insisted that his colleagues, junior and senior, should never refer to 'the epileptic child,' but rather to the child with epilepsy, lest they should forget that they were dealing with a child first and a symptom second. The rule is sound one.

EDUCATIONAL ASPECTS, LEARNING AND BEHAVIOUR PROBLEMS

Certain problems nonetheless occur more often in children with epilepsy than in normal children. Some of these problems are common to children with other evidence of organic brain disease in the form of mental retardation and cerebral palsy, and these common chronic neurological handicaps of childhood often occur together or in combinations of two. Mental retardation occurs in about one third of children with epilepsy and when present affects management and prognosis. Apart from retardation, various behavioural and educational difficulties are seen in many children with epilepsy which may constitute a greater handicap than the seizures themselves. There has been disagreement about the prevalence, specificity and mode of production of psychiatric disorder in children with epilepsy, and these questions were investigated in an epidemiological study of school children in the Isle of Wight (Rutter et al 1970). In the 5 to 14 year old child population of 11 865 there were 86 children with epilepsy, a prevalence of 7.2 per 1000. 64 of the children were classed as having 'uncomplicated epilepsy', showing no evidence of any other brain disease, disorder or injury, and 22 children had cerebral palsy or other evidence of structural brain disorder. 52 of the 86 children had had a fit in the previous 12 months and 34 had had a fit since the age of 5 years and had taken regular anti-convulsants during the previous year. The prevalence of psychiatric disorder in the children with epilepsy was found to be several times higher than in the general population and over twice that in children with chronic physical handicaps not involving the brain. Assessment of clinical, social and other factors suggested that this difference was not explained by differences in age or sex, by the presence of a chronic physical handicap per se, nor

by the severity and visibility of the handicap. Social prejudice was not apparently a major factor, and low intelligence was only partially significant. The presence of dysfunction specifically of the brain seemed to be the most important factor. The characteristics of the seizures themselves did not seem relevant to the presence of psychiatric disorder with the important exception of pyschomotor attacks. The reason for this association is not clear, but it is possible that states of partial consciousness, such as occur in these seizures, are more threatening to the child than total loss, and the rejecting attitudes of adults who fail to recognise that he is unaware of his actions may also be a factor.

Stores and his colleagues at the Park Hospital, Oxford, (Stores 1973, Stores & Hart 1976, Stores & Piran 1978, Stores et al 1978) have studied children with epilepsy from the point of view of their EEG abnormalities in a search for factors carrying a high risk of educational and other behavioural problems. Measurement of reading retardation, inattentiveness, dependency and other aspects of disturbed behaviour at school, especially overactivity, has suggested that male sex and the presence of a persistent left temporal lobe spike discharge are consistently associated with these problem.

The prevalence of epilepsy in children of school age (5 to 16 years) in the United Kingdom is of the order of 8 per thousand, with about 60 000 school children affected and an inception rate of between 2 and 4 per thousand per annum.

Most children with epilepsy and normal intelligence can and should be educated in normal schools. The seizures themselves seldom constitute a bar to this, provided teachers are aware of the problems of epilepsy, are emotionally able to cope and are not frightened by the thought or the fact of a fit. Other children are usually tolerant of seizures and will take their cue from the reaction of their teacher. If this is matter-of-fact and unruffled, they will not be upset. The complaint of parents that their children may be disturbed by seeing a fit usually reflects their own ignorance and anxiety. The lot of the child with epilepsy is easier if his teacher has already met the problem in other pupils or in his own family. Unfortunately communication between teachers and school doctors about pupils with epilepsy is often far from ideal.

(Holdsworth & Whitmore 1974b) and sometimes teachers have not been told of a child's epilepsy by either school doctor or parents. Although parental reticence is understandable, it is not advisable, except perhaps in the case of a child whose seizures have all occurred at night.

There is a need for more education of teachers, and the public at large, in the facts of epilepsy and good work is done in this field by voluntary bodies such as the British Epilepsy Association. It is seldom necessary for a child who has had a seizure to be sent home from school, yet unfortunately many children are sent home after a mild attack to vegetate for the rest of the day and in this way can lose much time and have their confidence sapped.

Learning problems in the child with epilepsy need careful assessment and often remedial help. Failure to provide this help can exacerbate behaviour problems and render the child more unacceptable and 'different'. Teachers may need to be warned against an 'over-protective' attitude to the child with epilepsy, which can lead to failure to exploit his potential and to under-achievement. Children are more likely to have fits when bored than when engaged in interesting and stimulating work. Sometimes the occurrence of very frequent minor attacks, unrecognised by the teacher, may cause educational problems: the child may be 'peppered with unconsciousness' as Brown (1977) has put it. In some cases lack of concentration may prevent a child of normal or superior intelligence from applying himself in the ordinary class-room setting, and he may need to be taught, at least for part of the time, individually. The educational problems of the child with epilepsy require careful thought and close co-operation between social, educational, psychological and medical services. Holdsworth & Whitmore (1974a) in a survey of 85 school-children with epilepsy found that 53.1% were holding their own at a below-average level and 15.6% were falling seriously behind. Behaviour problems were prominent in 21.1% and were closely related to the frequency of seizures.

Rarely the frequency and severity of seizures, the adverse reactions of teachers towards them, the presence of specific learning difficulties and of behaviour problems may make it impossible for a child to progress in a normal school. A school for children with epilepsy may then be indicated, where medical and teaching expertise are available and where fits will cause minimum disruption of his education. Such schools are usually residential, and are therefore undesirable for younger children, but older children often show impressive gains in education and fit control. The children also benefit by being able to enjoy a social life and to take part in games and sports to a degree impossible in their normal schools where they may have been virtual outcasts standing on the side-lines. It is often possible, if fits cease or decrease, for children to transfer to a normal school and the situation should be kept under review. In some cases a school for physically handicapped or educationally subnormal children may be appropriate for the child with epilepsy because of the presence of one or both of these handicaps. Such schools will allow provision for his educational and physical needs while avoiding the trauma of separation from home, though the staff will seldom be as familiar with the problems of epilepsy as those in more specialized schools. For the child with epilepsy who happens in addition to be severely handicapped mentally and/or physically it is unfortunately very difficult to arrange suitable schooling.

An unusual and creditable attempt has recently been made to portray the problems of the child with epilepsy in a work of fiction written for children, which could however be read with benefit by all adults, especially teachers. 'What difference does it make, Danny?' be Helen Young (1980) is a moral tale. The attitudes of the hero's teachers are, with one exception, exemplary and enlightened to a degree not often matched in real life.

The problems and concerns of the adolescent with epilepsy require much investment of patience, tact and general support by his medical adviser. 'When the brisk minor pants for twenty-one', and the adolescent boy or girl is struggling for independence from parental control and desperate, perhaps, to obtain a driving licence for a car or motorcycle, the restrictions necessitated by his epilepsy are hard to bear. He may feel at odds with society and see all authority as enemies, including his doctor, with an exaggeration of the normal emotional turmoil of adolescence. Psychiatric help may be needed for some patients. Contact with others who have faced and surmounted the same problems may be very beneficial. O'Donohoe (1979) has discussed this subject helpfully. Ideally, at this age, the patient should come to have a deeper knowledge of his disorder and to take more responsibility for its management. An excellent simple guide, *Epilepsy explained* has been prepared by Laidlaw & Laidlaw (1980) for the use of patients and their friends, teachers and others with whom they come in contact. It discusses the common anxieties of those with epilepsy, including marriage, inheritance, employment and driving licences, and gives information about helpful organizations, such as the British Epilepsy Association, which itself publishes a series of useful leaflets on various aspects of epilepsy.

DRUG TREATMENT OF EPILEPSY

The principles of drug treatment are that it should be regular, as simple as possible, and cause the minimum of side-effects and disturbance to the life of the child and his family.

Whenever possible one drug should be used rather than two, and 'polypharmacy' with three or more drugs should be avoided, though it may unfortunately sometimes be necessary. Combined tablets such as those uniting phenytoin with phenobarbitone, and primidone with phenobarbitone are dangerous and should be avoided in children. They allow no flexibility of dosage and often contain too high a dose of phenobarbitone (e.g. 50 mg of phenobarbitone plus 100 mg of phenytoin). They are also very expensive.

Changes in treatment, whether starting, reducing, withdrawing or substituting a drug, should be gradual and never made rapidly. To start a child on high doses of anticonvulsants increases the chances of side-effects which make the drug less acceptable to the child and his parents. Rapid withdrawal carries the risk of provoking status epilepticus.

The dose of any anticonvulsant should be carefully calculated for the child concerned, based on his weight or surface area: his weight should be recorded at each clinic visit so that weight gain (or loss) can be noted and appropriate changes made in dosage. This is especially important with sodium valproate, which may cause excessive weight gain (Egger & Brett 1981). The introduc-

tion of methods of measuring the blood levels of many drugs has made anticonvulsant treatment more scientific and less empirical than in the past.

It is seldom possible to predict in advance which drug will be most effective for a child's seizures, and some of the glowing reports of drug trials in epilepsy which have appeared in the literature cannot fail to provoke scepticism in those who treat many epileptic children. It is also impossible to predict the side-effects. The term 'drug of choice' is often misleading when considering certain forms of epilepsy because of the variability of response, and the situation is different from that in, for example, the treatment of bacterial infection with antibiotics. Nonetheless it is possible to speak in broad terms of the drug or drugs most likely to help with particular types of seizure, and these are considered below.

Grand mal and focal seizures

The drugs most often used for these attacks until recently have been phenobarbitone, diphenylhydantoin (phenytoin: Epanutin) and primidone (Mysoline).

Phenobarbitone, in use since 1912, is often an effective and well tolerated anticonvulsant in adults. Some children benefit from it and tolerate it well, but many, 30% or more, develop irritability, aggressive behaviour, overactivity or depression and are so disturbed that its use is unacceptable to their parents (Wolf & Forsythe 1978). The peace of the whole family may be so disrupted that parents regard the treatment as far worse than the disease and often discontinue the drug themselves. Children who are already overactive with behaviour disorders, including many with temporal lobe epilepsy are particularly likely to tolerate phenobarbitone badly. It is advisable, as always, to start with small doses and increase gradually. When tolerated the usual daily dose is 3–4 mg/kg.

Primidone (Mysoline), although partly metabolized to phenobarbitone, is better tolerated, causing behaviour and psychological problems in only 5 or 10% of children. It often produces side-effects, such as nausea, vomiting, abdominal pain or sedation, in the first week of treatment, especially if large doses are given initially. Small doses of about one quarter of the calculated final dose (20 mg/kg daily) should be given first and increased gradually. Parents should be warned of these possible side-effects and can be told that they usually pass off after two or three weeks, so that the drug should not be prematurely condemned as not tolerated.

Phenytoin, in use since 1938, is often very effective but in normal doses (5–7 mg/kg) often causes unsightly side-effects. Gingival hypertrophy is common and sometimes severe. This can to some extent be limited by good oral hygiene and the importance of regular tooth cleaning should be stressed to parents when the drug is started. Gross gum swelling may necessitate a change of drug but if, for any reason, it seems essential to continue phenytoin, gingivectomy can be performed with excellent cosmetic results (Fig. 12.1).

Children who take phenytoin for many years may develop thickening of the soft tissues of the

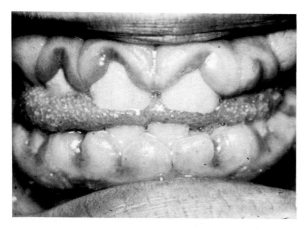

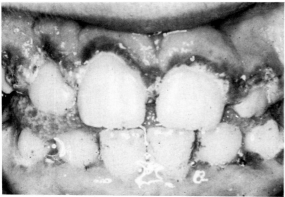

Fig. 12.1 Gum hypertrophy caused by phenytoin — before and after gingivectomy.

nose, lips and face, which produces a coarsening of their features. This, together with its tendency to cause hirsutism, may make it unacceptable for long term use in girls (though it is not altogether logical to accept these drawbacks in boys either.)

Ataxia is usually only seen with excessive doses and nystagmus is rarer in children than in adults taking phenytoin. The non-linear relationship between dose and blood level, with small increases in dose causing steep rises in blood level when the dose exceeds 7 mg/kg, means that the therapeutic range for the drug is rather narrow and the level quickly passes from it into the toxic range. (Eadie et al 1973.) Great care is therefore needed in adjusting the dose, and measurement of anticonvulsant blood levels is particularly helpful with this drug, especially in view of the many interactions known to occur between phenytoin, and other anti-epileptic drugs.

A progressive encephalopathy due to chronic phenytoin intoxication has been reported in ten children on long term treatment (Vallarta et al 1974). The patients showed the usual cerebellar signs of hydantoin toxicity together with progressive neurological deterioration similar to that seen in degenerative CNS disease. After stopping the drug the deterioration abated in all cases and six patients recovered to their premorbid level of functioning.

Carbamazepine (Tegretol) is regarded by many as the drug of choice for temporal lobe epilepsy, although others (Dam et al 1975) found it more effective when combined with phenytoin or phenobarbitone than when used alone. Good results are often obtained in benign focal epilepsy of childhood. The effective dose is usually between 10 and 20 mg/kg per day.

Sulthiame (Ospolot) has also been claimed to reduce temporal lobe attacks, but this has not been the general experience. When given with phenytoin, sulthiame greatly increases the level of the latter, and this may be of some indirect therapeutic value but can also be hazardous. (Houghton & Richens 1974)

Acetazolamide (diamox) may be helpful in generalized and focal seizures, when added to other drugs, especially Carbamazepine. It is also effective in preventing fits related to menstruation when used before the periods.

Sodium valproate (Epilim), one of the newer anticonvulsants, may be helpful in focal epilepsy and grand mal seizures though less effective in temporal lobe attacks. There have been enthusiastic reports about its success rate and freedom from side-effects, but although its effects are often gratifying it is not a panacea and it is not entirely free from side-effects. It is far less likely to have a sedative effect when given alone, and in some cases seems to make patients more alert. A study in adult males, however suggested that the drug does have a sedative effect (Boxer et al 1976). When added to phenobarbitone it may cause a significant increase in the serum level of this drug: similar effects have been found with phenytoin in some studies but not in others. These interactions make it important to monitor the blood drug levels when sodium valproate is added to other drug régimes. Hair loss is a fairly common side-effect, but fortunately is usually transient. The hair may also become curly. Occasionally a catastrophic worsening of behaviour ensues as soon as the drug is started, similar to that seen more commonly with phenobarbitone, and some children seem unable to tolerate it. Rarely thrombocytopenia may develop. A particularly troublesome side-effect is increased appetite and weight gain. (Egger & Brett 1981) In some cases the latter can be precipitous, so that the weight crosses several centile lines in a few months. As a result the dose becomes inadequate for the excessive body weight and seizures may become more frequent so that the unhappy patient has the worst of both worlds. The weight should be carefully charted when sodium valproate is used. Sometimes dietary control can restrict weight gain to acceptable limits, but in some cases excessive gain necessitates stopping the drug, after which the weight may fall dramatically with a consequent rise in the blood levels of other drugs. Severe hepatic side-effects and pancreatitis have been reported, but are very rare.

The effective dose usually lies between 30 and 60 mg/kg daily, but is sometimes as low as 20. In some cases the response is very dramatic with attacks ceasing after only a few doses. The drug should be started in small doses, preferably of about 10 mg/kg, and increased gradually in order to avoid the gastro-intestinal side-effects. These are less likely to occur with the enteric-coated tablets (now available in the UK in both 500 and 200 mg strengths) than with the original plain 200 mg tablets.

It was previously thought necessary to give the doses three times a day for best effect, since the half-life of sodium valproate is only about 10 hours, but once-daily dosage has been found effective in recent studies (Covanis & Jeavons 1980).

Myoclonic epilepsy

The benzodiazepine drugs, originally diazepam (Valium) and more recently nitrazepam (Mogadon) and clonazepam (Rivotril) are often very effective in myoclonic attacks. Their sedative effect makes it advisable to start with a small dose and increase it gradually. In this way they are more likely to be tolerated. Nitrazepam and clonazepam are often used in the treatment of infantile spasms with benefit. ACTH and cortical steroids usually give the best results but cannot be continued for more than a few months and can usefully be combined with or followed by one or other of the benzodiazepines. There is an impression that diazepam may exert only a transient anticonvulsant effect, and there are advantages in keeping it in reserve for the control of status epilepticus. The tolerated and effective doses of nitrazepam and clonazepam vary widely. Many children seem to tolerate daily doses of 10 or 15 mg of nitrazepam and 6 mg or more of clonazepam which would heavily sedate most adults. Salivation and bronchial secretion may be increased by nitrazepam with risks to retarded infants and to those with chest infections.

Petit mal absences

Ethosuximide (Zarontin) is usually very effective in reducing or abolishing petit mal absences with 3 c/s spike and wave discharges on the EEG. The drug is well tolerated, with hiccups one of the few side-effects. The dose varies between 250 and 1000 mg per day. Troxidone and Paradione are rarely used since the introduction of Ethosuximide. Excellent results have also been found with sodium valproate, which many now consider the drug of choice, since it may control absences in the rare cases when ethosuximide has failed.

Television-induced seizures

Sodium valproate is probably the drug of choice in those cases in which drug treatment is indicated.

Febrile convulsions

In theory phenobarbitone is the 'drug of choice', but in practice it is often not tolerated, and the choice then lies between phenytoin and sodium valproate. The results of studies referred to earlier suggest that the latter is often effective.

SIDE-EFFECTS OF ANTICONVULSANT DRUGS

Many of these have been mentioned above for individual drugs but there are numerous other side-effects, some specific to one drug and others common to several. There is now a vast literature on the subject: a useful review is that of Reynolds (1975) on chronic antiepileptic toxicity, which contains over 300 references, and classifies the toxic effects according to the system affected.

The nervous system

Mental changes

These are probably much commoner than is realised. Teachers often express concern that anticonvulsant drugs are dulling the child and impairing his scholastic performance and, although it is difficult to assess the contribution of the seizures themselves, the short attention span and lack of concentration so common in children with epilepsy and the attitudes of adults towards the child, such a dulling effect is probably present in many cases. It is most likely to occur in children treated with the more sedative drugs (phenobarbitone, primidone, nitrazepam and clonazepam) and in those on multiple therapy. The effects of phenobarbitone in four adult volunteers in doses used for grand mal seizures were studied by Hutt et al (1968). Perceptual motor performance was found to be affected in 6 tasks to an extent depending on the blood level of the drug, the difficulty and duration of the task and the degree of external constraints being exercised over the performance. The well-known effect of phenobarbitone and, to a less extent, primidone in provoking or aggravating overactivity and behaviour disorders has already been mentioned, and many paediatricians in cynical mood have concluded that their single most helpful therapeutic intervention has been the withdrawal of phenobarbitone. It is a common experience also for teachers and parents to notice a marked improvement in mood and performance when a child is finally weaned off his anticonvulsant therapy.

Ataxia

Cerebellar ataxia is a common effect of acute anticonvulsant toxicity, especially with phenytoin (Ch. 9). Although it has been claimed that chronic cerebellar dysfunction can result from this drug, the relationship is still uncertain. Reduced Purkinje cell counts have been found in the brains of epileptic patients treated with high doses of phenytoin, but these changes may have resulted from frequent seizures.

Involuntary movements

Unwanted movements of choreo-athetoid and dystonic type have been seen in some children and adults receiving phenytoin. These are often, but not always, related to high dosage and blood levels of the drug, are independent of cerebellar ataxia and usually disappear when the dose is reduced. However, Chalhub et al (1976) have reported two retarded boys who developed involuntary movements while serum phenytoin concentrations were in the therapeutic range. The movement disorder may be mediated by changes in serotonin. It is important to be aware of this effect since the dramatic movements may otherwise suggest an underlying progressive disease of the basal ganglia.

Peripheral neuropathy, with loss or reduction in tendon reflexes, slowing in nerve conduction velocity and reduction in nerve action potentials, has been reported in adult patients on prolonged phenytoin therapy. The mechanism is uncertain.

The haemopoietic system

A relationship between anticonvulsant therapy and megaloblastic anaemia due to folic acid deficiency has been recognised for many years. This probably occurs in less than one per cent of drug-treated epileptics. It is usually associated with phenytoin, alone or combined with phenobarbitone, but has occasionally been reported with either phenobarbitone or primidone alone. It may occur at any age and after as little as one month of treatment. Serum and red cell folate levels are low, macrocytosis is common in the peripheral blood and megaloblastic changes are often seen in the bone marrow. The mechanism of this drug-induced folate depletion is not clear: the rival hypotheses have been reviewed by Reynolds (1972). It has been suggested that the anticonvulsant action of the drugs may be due, at least in part, to their antifolate effect, and some authors have reported worsening of seizures with administration of folic acid. Many studies however, including that of Bowe et al (1971) on children, have failed to confirm this, and my own experience of treating folate-deficient epileptic children with folic acid supplements has shown no increase in their seizure frequency. Psychiatric illness has been described in adult patients with anticonvulsant-associated megaloblastic anaemia, with improvement after folic acid treatment.

Folic acid depletion in children on anticonvulsants is not common, but it seems wise to measure the level in serum and red cells at least once a year.

The skeletal system

Metabolic bone disease and vitamin D deficiency have been reported in the last ten years in up to one third of drug-treated epileptic patients in all age groups. Overt rickets and osteomalacia are rare, but subclinical abnormalities of calcium metabolism are common, with low serum calcium levels, elevated alkaline phosphatase and radiological changes of rickets and osteomalacia. Many of the studies have been based on mentally subnormal epileptic patients in institutions. Richens & Rowe (1970) showed that hypocalcaemia was correlated with a high dosage of drugs and multiple therapy and with the use of pheneturide, primidone, phenytoin and phenobarbitone in descending order of frequency.

The metabolic bone changes are thought to be due to vitamin D deficiency caused by drug induction of liver enzymes involved in the metabolism,

especially hydroxylation, of the vitamin. (Dent et al 1970). Its metabolism is thereby diverted along pathways producing more inactive compounds.

Those particularly at risk of these anticonvulsant side-effects are children, dark-skinned people, pregnant women and patients on long-term treatment with many drugs. It seems logical to carry out biochemical screening tests of serum calcium and alkaline phosphatase from time to time to avoid the more serious effects which may possibly include aggravation of seizures by hypocalcaemia. If prophylactic vitamin D is given to these patients at risk the dose needs to be at least 4000 international units per week (Hann et al 1972).

Connective tissue

Gum hypertrophy and facial skin changes with coarsened facial features occur in many patients on prolonged phenytoin treatment. *The skin* is also affected by hirsutism in some 5% of patients on phenytoin. This may make it unsuitable for use in girls.

The liver

Phenobarbitone and phenytoin cause induction of hepatic microsomal enzymes involved with the metabolism of drugs, steroids, bilirubin and lipids. These effects have many implications for the drug treatment of epilepsy apart from the production of folate deficiency and metabolic bone changes already mentioned. When two anticonvulsant drugs are given together, interactions may occur, through induction of hepatic enzymes which alter the level of one of them in the blood. One of the best known interactions is the reduction of phenytoin levels by phenobarbitone. It is equally important to realise that withdrawal of phenobarbitone in a patient who has been taking both drugs can cause a rise in phenytoin level which could be dangerous.

Periodic measurement of the blood levels of drugs can be particularly helpful in adjusting the dose when two or more drugs are used. (See below)

Immunological disorders

Several unusual idiosyncratic reactions to anticonvulsant drugs are recognised. (Booker 1975)

Lymphadenopathy is seen as a rare complication of phenytoin treatment, usually within four months of starting and associated with fever, rash or other signs of hypersensitivity, but sometimes later than this and without other clinical features.

Systemic lupus erythematosus (SLE) may occasionally occur in patients taking anticonvulsant drugs, including phenytoin, phenobarbitone, primidone and ethosuximide. Antinuclear antibodies have been found in many symptomless epileptic children and adults on drug treatment.

ANTICONVULSANT BLOOD LEVELS

Indications

The indications for measuring anticonvulsant blood levels in epilepsy and its implications have been reviewed by Gardner-Medwin (1973) and Brett (1977). Gardner-Medwin listed five kinds of patient in whom serum levels are of immediate practical help — the patient with refractory seizures, the intoxicated patient on many drugs, the patient whose intoxication may be confused with symptoms of underlying disease, the patient with hepatic or renal disease in whom drug metabolism may be impaired and the patient in whom, for any reason, it is thought undesirable that *any* further seizures should occur. A further very important indication (Livingston et al 1975) is the need to discover whether a patient is taking his drugs or not. All paediatricians are aware that parental 'compliance' in ensuring that their child takes his medication regularly is often imperfect. Another major indication is the need for precise adjustment of dose in patients who show signs of intoxication on small or conventional doses of a drug. With phenytoin this may occur in the rare congenital deficiency of the hepatic parahydroxylation enzyme system, intercurrent infection, impaired elimination mechanisms and numerous drug interactions (17 drugs are known or suspected to impair phenytoin metabolism). The non-linear relation between dose of phenytoin and blood level, with small increments in dose producing rapid rises in blood level to the toxic range, is another reason for careful monitoring of the level. The value of blood

levels in avoiding polypharmacy was well shown by a recent report (Reynolds et al 1976) on the use of one drug (phenytoin) in the treatment of epilepsy. Though based on 31 adult patients, previously untreated, its lesson applies a fortiori to children, who are more often the victims of polypharmacy. With careful monitoring of the serum phenytoin levels and adjustment of the dose to keep them in the therapeutic range, only three patients needed a second drug. An unexpected finding in this study was a slow fall in the serum phenytoin level in 14 patients, despite a constant or increasing dose, perhaps because of increased hydroxylation through enzyme induction. This downward drift of the blood level further underlines the value of monitoring the level, since the drug could well be considered inadequate and another drug be added if the fall were not detected. It may possibly explain the common observation that the results of an anticonvulsant may be initially gratifying but shortlived. The prophylaxis of febrile convulsions is another field where the chances of success can be improved by regular monitoring of the blood level.

It seems probable that further drug interactions as yet unknown may occur, and these will be detected only by careful monitoring, especially with the newer drugs. These interactions may possibly differ from one person to another, and even from one time to another.

Variable binding of phenytoin to plasma proteins and advantages of estimation in saliva

The variable binding of phenytoin to plasma proteins needs consideration, since it is the 'free' unbound phenytoin rather than the total plasma level which reflects the CSF level and thus probably the concentration of phenytoin in the brain. Variations in the degree of phenytoin binding account for the poor correlation sometimes seen between its total plasma level and toxic effects. The degree of protein binding is decreased by various drugs, including acetylsalicylic acid. Ideally the level of *unbound* phenytoin should be measured as well as the total concentration, but at present this requires larger volumes of blood than are desirable in paediatric practice in which micromethods are preferable.

Since the concentration of phenytoin in saliva is

similar to that of the free unbound fraction, measurement of the salivary level of the drug may possibly replace blood level estimation in time. Rylance & Moreland (1980) regard salivary estimation as useful for phenytoin, carbamazepine and ethosuximide, possibly useful for phenobarbitone and primidone and not useful for sodium valproate and diazepam.

THE KETOGENIC DIET

The beneficial effect on epilepsy of ketonuria induced by a ketogenic diet was noted by Wilder (1921) and this dietary treatment has since been widely used for intractable seizures, especially of the minor motor type — myoclonic, akinetic and atypical petit mal attacks. Children suffering from these seizures usually show an EEG with an atypical spike and wave pattern and the prognosis is often very poor for control of attacks and intellectual development. The diet is more likely to be effective in younger children between two and five years of age than in older patients in whom adequate ketosis is more difficult to maintain.

The cost, difficulty and unpalatable nature of the diet, which restricts protein and carbohydrate and supplies 80% or more of the daily calories in the form of fats, has limited its use in the past. The use of the triglycerides of octanoic and decanoic acids (medium-chain triglycerides or MCT) is an important advance since these tasteless and water-miscible compounds are rapidly absorbed from the gut and have a high calorie value. Good results have been obtained in many children with intractable fits especially of minor motor type (Huttenlocher et al 1971, Huttenlocher 1976, Gordon 1977). Side-effects are usually few. They include diarrhoea, and abdominal cramps; a mild, symptomless hypoglycaemia may also occur. Huttenlocher (1976) compared the metabolic and anticonvulsant effects of a standard high-fat diet and MCT in children with epilepsy. Long-term MCT treatment did not cause hyperlipidaemia or significant change in the pH of venous blood.

The blood glucose fell below 50 mg per 100 ml in a third of the children, the lowest levels occurring 2 to 3 weeks from the start of the diet. Plasma levels of β-hydroxybutyrate (BHB) and acetoacetate rose gradually after starting diet, the highest figures being achieved after about one month. These levels were similar on the two diets. The plasma BHB levels showed a significant correlation with the anticonvulsant effect of the diet. This effect and the ketonaemia were both rapidly reversed by intravenous infusion of glucose. Stephenson et al (1977) recommend fasting the child for 48 hours before starting MCT since the rapid development of ketosis may cause seizures to cease with a beneficial effect on morale. They start with only 10 ml of the MCT oil and increase gradually. It may be taken in a milk shake made with skimmed milk. The diet is cheap since the oil provides 60% of the daily calories, but vitamin and calcium supplements are needed. The urine should be monitored for ketones with ketostix which must be kept in a cool, dark place but not in a refrigerator.

THE PLACE OF SURGERY IN CHILDHOOD EPILEPSY

In a small number of carefully selected children with epilepsy surgery may be indicated and may give good results when medical treatment has clearly failed.

Two main groups of children with epilepsy have been subjected to surgical treatment.

In the past children and young adults with hemiplegia of early onset, intractable epilepsy and severe behaviour disorder have undergone hemispherectomy. This approach was introduced by Krynauw (1950) and good results were reported by McKissock (1953) and others. The early results were often gratifying, not only in terms of cessation or reduction of seizures, but also in improvement in behaviour problems which had sometimes made the management of the child very difficult for his family and teachers. The hemiplegia was seldom made worse, and there was an impression that intelligence might improve after surgery, or at least cease to deteriorate. Unfortunately delayed complications of hemispherectomy have come to be recognized more recently and have made it necessary to be much more critical about its results. After a trouble-free period of between 4 and 12 years deterioration is seen with evidence of bleeding into the CSF pathways and later of obstructive hydrocephalus. Autopsy has shown a superficial haemosiderosis of the CNS with chronic granular ependymitis, associated with obstruction of CSF pathways and evidence of multiple bleeding points in the membrane which has replaced the missing hemisphere and its extension on to the lining of the ventricular system. This delayed complication is undoubtedly commoner than was realized: Wilson (1970) believes that it develops in 30 to 40% of patients after hemispherectomy. Its management is difficult, requiring shunt procedures for the hydrocephalus. Fortunately with improvements in anticonvulsant treatment in the past 20 years a surgical approach to the hemiplegic child with epilepsy is much less necessary and less justified than previously.

A more fruitful field for the surgical treatment of childhood epilepsy has been that of temporal lobe epilepsy, already referred to. The more radical approach of a generous anterior temporal lobectomy, including the hippocampus, amygdala and uncus, by Falconer (1971) has given good results particularly in those children in whom the aetiology of the seizures seemed related to a past history of febrile convulsions in infancy and in whom mesial temporal sclerosis was the pathological substrate. Good results were also obtained in patients in whom harmartomas were found in the removed temporal lobe (some 20 to 25% of surgically treated cases).

The selection of patients with intractable epilepsy for resective surgery has recently been reviewed by Polkey (1980).

Further surgical approaches to epilepsy in adults are being developed, but the paediatrician is likely to feel somewhat conservative about these until more experience has been gained of their advantages and risks.

THE PROGNOSIS OF EPILEPSY IN CHILDHOOD

This complex problem is well discussed by O'Donohoe (1979). The wide variety of clinical situations in children with seizures reviewed in this chapter makes it obvious that generalizations are misleading and that much depends on the type of epilepsy and its cause. Although the prognosis is so varied, it is appropriate for the physician involved to present, if he does not always feel, an attitude of guarded optimism rather than to project an aura of helpless gloom. Parents need much support and should never be denied all hope. The prognosis for spontaneous improvement and cessation of seizures is good in many cases. In other cases it is unpredictable and may appear poor, but dogmatic forecasts of a life-time of seizures are seldom if ever justified. The question is often linked with the prognosis for mental development which in some conditions, e.g. certain neonatal convulsions and infantile spasms, is far from promising, but here again some rays of hope should be permitted to lighten the darkness and a presumed poor prognosis should not be allowed to lead to an attitude of therapeutic nihilism.

The prognosis of neonatal convulsions and of infantile spasms has already been discussed.

With regard to other types of seizure, two studies from the United States have given helpful results. Holowach and her colleagues (1972) followed up 148 children with epilepsy who had been seizure-free for 4 years on treatment for a further 5 to 12 years after cessation of medication in order to determine the frequency of relapse and to discern any prognostic criteria. Seizures recurred in 36 cases (24%). Relapse showed no relation to sex, race, heredity, puberty or seizure frequency. The recurrence rate was lowest (13%) with an early age of onset of epilepsy and prompt seizure control. It was at least twice as high in cases with late onset and prolonged duration of seizures and with neurological, psychological or EEG abnormalities. As regards types of seizure, the relapse rate was lowest in grand mal (8%) and highest in Jacksonian seizures (53%) and in 'multiple seizure types' (40%). It was 12% in febrile seizures and 25% in psychomotor attacks (TLE).

Higher remission rates than previously reported were found by Annegers et al (1979) in a longitudinal study of patients with epilepsy in Rochester, Minnesota. The probability of being in remission (at least 5 consecutive years seizure free) at 20 years after the diagnosis of epilepsy was 70%. The prognosis was poor in those with associated neurological dysfunction recognized from birth. It was better for patients with idiopathic epilepsy and for the survivors of postnatally acquired epilepsy. It was probably highest in patients with generalized onset fits diagnosed under 10 years of age, and was less favourable in those with partial complex seizures and adult type epilepsy. The probability of remission was 85% for those with generalized tonic-clonic seizures, 80% for absence seizures with or without tonic-clinic seizures, and only 65% for partial complex seizures.

The age of onset was important. The probability of remission was 75% for those with epilepsy diagnosed under 10 years of age, 68% with diagnosis between 10 and 19, and 63% with diagnosis between 20 and 59.

When discontinuation of medication was considered as well, the differences in remission according to age at diagnosis were even greater. At 10 years after diagnosis the probability of no seizures and no medication for at least 5 years was 51% for those diagnosed under 10, 40% with diagnosis between 10 and 19, 28% with diagnosis between 20 and 59, and only 6% with diagnosis at 60 or later. Among patients diagnosed at the youngest age, those with focal onset seizures had higher remission rates in the first few years after diagnosis but had fewer late remissions.

Encouraging results were also found by Emerson et al (1981) in their study of 68 children with epilepsy who had had no seizures for four years. The probability of their remaining free of seizures for four years after stopping medication was 69%. Recurrence of fits was more likely if children were mentally retarded, if their seizures had started before two years of age (unlike the findings of Holowach et al), if they had had many generalized seizures before control, or if they had had a definitely abnormal EEG before medication was stopped. The best predictors of outcome were found to be the EEG taken at cessation of treatment and the number of seizures before control.

The very good prognosis for benign focal epilepsy of childhood and its excellent response to treatment have been mentioned.

REFERENCES

Aarli J A, Fontana A 1980 Immunological aspects of epilepsy. Epilepsia 21: 451–457

Addy D P 1981 Prophylaxis and febrile convulsions. Archives of Disease in Childhood 56: 81–83

Agurell S, Berlin A, Ferngren H, Hellstrom B 1975 Plasma levels of diazepam after parenteral and rectal administration in children. Epilepsia 16: 277–283

Aicardi J 1973 The problem of the Lennox syndrome. Developmental Medicine and Child Neurology 15: 77–81

Aicardi J, Baraton J 1971 A pneumoencephalographic demonstration of brain atrophy following status epilepticus. Developmental Medicine and Child Neurology 13: 660–667

Aicardi J, Chevrie J J, Rouselle F 1969 Le syndrome spasmes en flexion, agènèsie calleuse, anomalies chorio-retiniennes. Archives Françaises de Pèdiatrie 26: 1103–1120

Aicardi J, Chevrie J J 1970 Convulsive status epilepticus in infants and children. A study of 239 cases. Epilepsia 11: 187–197

Ames F R 1971 'Self-induction' in photosensitive epilepsy. Brain 94: 781–798

Annegers J F, Hauser W A, Elveback L R 1979 Remission of seizures and relapse in patients with epilepsy. Epilepsia 20: 729–737

Baird H W, Borofsky L G 1957 Infantile myoclonic seizures. Journal of Pediatrics 50: 332–339

Basser L S 1964 Benign paroxysmal vertigo of childhood. A variety of vestigular neuronitis. Brain 87: 141–152

Bejšovec M, Kulenda Z, Ponča E 1967 Familial intrauterine convulsions in pyridoxine dependency. Archives of Disease in Childhood 42: 201–207

Bell D S 1969 Dangers of treatment of status epilepticus with diazepam. British Medical Journal 1: 159–161

Bickford R G 1954 Sensory precipitation of seizures. Journal of the Michigan Medical Society 53: 1018

Booker H E 1975 Idiosyncratic reactions to the antiepileptic drugs. Epilepsia 16: 171–181

Bowe J C, Cornish E J, Dawson M 1971 Evaluation of folic acid supplements in children taking phenytoin. Developmental Medicine and Child Neurology 13: 343–354

Bower B D 1963 Television flicker and fits. Clinical Pediatrics 2: 134–138

Boxer C M, Herzberg J L, Scott D F 1976 Has sodium valproate hypnotic effects? Epilepsia 17: 367–370

Brett E M 1966 Minor epileptic status in children. Journal of the Neurological Sciences 3: 52–75

Brett E M 1975 The prognosis of seizures in the first three years of life. In: Williams D (ed) Modern trends in neurology, 6th edn, Butterworths, London

Brett E M 1977 Implications of measuring anticonvulsant blood levels in epilepsy. Developmental Medicine and Child Neurology 19: 245–251

Brett E M, Hoare R D 1969 An assessment of the value and limitations of air encephalography in children with mental retardation and epilepsy. Brain 92: 731–742

British Medical Journal 1980 Prognosis of temporal lobe epilepsy in childhood. 280: 812–813

Brown J K 1973 Convulsions in the newborn period. Developmental Medicine and Child Neurology 15: 823–846

Brown J K, Sills J A 1977 Status epilepticus. Journal of Maternal and Child Health 2: 383–389

Carton D 1979 Benign familial neonatal convulsions. Neuropädiatrie 9: 167–171

Cavazzuti G B 1975 Prevention of febrile convulsions with dipropylacetate (depakine). Epilepsia 16: 647–648

Chalhub E G, Devivo D C, Volpe J J 1976 Phenytoin-induced dystonia and choreoathetosis in two retarded epileptic children. Neurology 26: 494–498

Costeff H 1965 Convulsions in childhood. Their natural history and indications for treatment. New England Journal of Medicine 273: 1410–1413

Covanis A, Jeavons P M 1980 Once-daily sodium valproate in the treatment of epilepsy. Developmental Medicine and Child Neurology 22: 202–204

Critchley M 1937 Musicogenic epilepsy. Brain 60: 13–27

Currie S, Heathfield K W G, Henson R A, Scott D F 1971 Clinical course and prognosis of temporal lobe epilepsy. A survey of 666 patients. Brain 94: 173–190

Dam M, Jensen A, Christiansen J 1975 Plasma level and effect of carbamazepine in grand mal and psychomotor epilepsy. Acta paediatrica scandinavica suppl. 60: 33–37

Davidson S, Falconer M A 1975 Outcome of surgery in 40 children with temporal-lobe epilepsy. Lancet 1: 1260–1263

Dennis J, Bower B D 1972 The Aicardi syndrome. Developmental Medicine and Child Neurology 14: 382–390

Dent C E, Richens A, Rowe D J F, Stamp T C B 1970 Osteomalacia with long-term anticonvulsant drugs. British Medical Journal 4: 69–72

Deonna Th, Beaumanoir A, Gaillard F, Assal G 1972 Acquired aphasia in childhood with seizure disorder: a heterogeneous syndrome. Neuropädiatrie 8: 263–273

Desmond M M, Schwanecke R P, Wilson G S, Yatsunaga S, Burgdorff I 1972 Maternal barbiturate utilisation and neonatal withdrawal symptomatology. Journal of Pediatrics 80: 190–197

Dunn D W, Snyder H 1976 Benign paroxysmal vertigo of childhood. American Journal of Diseases of Childhood 130: 1099–1100

Eadie M J, Tyrer J H, Hooper W D 1973 Diphenylhydantoin dosage. Proceedings of the Australian Association of Neurologists 10: 53

Egger J, Brett E M 1981 Effects of sodium valproate in 100 children with special reference to weight. British Medical Journal 283: 577–581

Emerson R, D'souza B, Vining E P, Holden K R, Mellits E D, Freeman J M 1981 Stopping medication in children with epilepsy. New England Journal of Medicine 304: 1125–1129

Engel J, Ludwig B I, Fetell M 1978 Prolonged partial complex status epilepticus: EEG and behavioral observations. Neurology (Minneapolis) 28: 863–869

Faërø O, Kastrup K W, Lykkegaard-Nielsen E, Melchior J C, Thorn I 1972 Successful prophylaxis of febrile convulsions. Epilepsia 13: 279–289

Falconer M A 1971 Genetic and related aetiological factors in temporal lobe epilepsy. Epilepsia 12: 13–31

Falconer M A 1972 Place of surgery for temporal lobe epilepsy during childhood. British Medical Journal 2: 631–635

Falconer M A, Serafetinides E A, Corsellis J A N 1964 Etiology and pathogenesis of temporal lobe epilepsy.

Falconer M A, Serafetinides E A, Corsellis J A N 1964 Etiology and pathogenesis of temporal lobe epilepsy. Archives of Neurology (Chicago) 10: 233–248

Falconer M A, Taylor D C 1968 Surgical treatment of drug-resistant epilepsy due to mesial temporal sclerosis Archives of Neurology (Chicago) 18: 353–361

Fenichel G M 1967 Migraine as a cause of benign paroxysmal vertigo of childhood. Journal of Pediatrics 71: 114–115

Fèrè C 1883 Le tic de Salaam. Les salutations neuropathiques. Progrès Médical 11: 970

Finlayson R E, Lucas A R 1979 Pseudoepileptic seizures in children and adolescents. Mayo Clinic Proceedings 54: 83–87

Fisher J H, Lockman L A, Zaske D, Kriel R 1981 Phenobarbital maintenance requirements in neonatal seizures. Neurology 31: 1042–1044

Forster F M, Hansotia P, Cleeland C S, Ludwig A 1969 A case of voice-induced epilepsy treated by conditioning. Neurology (Minneapolis) 19: 325–331

Fukuyama Y, Tomori N, Sugitate M 1977 Critical evaluation of the role of immunization as an etiological factor of infantile spasms. Neuropädiatrie 8: 224–237

Gardner-Medwin D 1973 Why should we measure serum levels of anticonvulsant drugs in epilepsy? Developmental Medicine and Child Neurology 15: 87–90

Gastaut H, Broughton R 1965 A clinical and polygraphic study of episodic phenomena during sleep. In: J. Wortis (ed) Recent advances in biological psychiatry. Plenum, New York, vol 7

Gastaut H 1969 Clinical and electroencephalographical classification of epileptic seizures. Epilepsia 10 suppl: 2–21

Gastaut H 1970 Clinical and electroencephalographical classification of epileptic seizures. Epilepsia 11: 102–113

Gastaut H, Roger J, Soulayrol R, Tassinari C A, Règis H, Dravet C et al 1966 Childhood epileptic encephalopathy with diffuse slow spike-waves (otherwise known as petit mal variant or Lennox syndrome). Epilepsia 1: 139–179

Gastaut H, Vigouroux M, Trevisan C, Règis H 1957 Le syndrome 'hémiconvulsion-hémiplègie-epilepsie' (syndrome HHE). Revue neurologique 97: 37–52

Geschwind N, Sherwin I 1967 Language-induced epilepsy. Archives of Neurology 16: 25–31

Gibbs F A, Gibbs E L 1952 Atlas of electroencephalography. In: Epilepsy, 2nd edn, Addison-Wesley, Cambridge, Mass, vol 2

Gibbs F A, Gibbs E L 1960 Good prognosis of mid-temporal epilepsy. Epilepsia 1: 448–453

Gordon N S 1977 Medium-chain triglycerides in a ketogenic diet. Developmental Medicine and Child Neurology 19: 535–537

Guilleminault C, Raynal D, Takahashi S, Carskadon M, Dement W 1976 Evaluation of short-term and long-term treatment of the narcolepsy syndrome with clomipramine hydrochloride. Acta neurologica scandinavica 54: 71–87

Hall J H, Marshall P C 1980 Clonazepam therapy in reading epilepsy. Neurology 30: 550–551

Hann T J, Hendin B D A, Scharp C R, Haddad J G 1972 Effect of chronic anticonvulsant therapy on serum 25-hydroxycholecalciferol levels in adults. New England Journal of Medicine 287: 900–904

Harper J R 1968 True myoclonic epilepsy in childhood. Archives of Disease in Childhood 43: 28–35

Harris R 1978 Personal communication

Harris R, Tizard J P M 1960 The electroencephalogram in neonatal convulsions. Journal of Pediatrics 57: 501–520

Heckmatt J Z, Houston A B, Clow D J, Stephenson J B P,

Dodd K L, Lealman G T, Logan R W 1976 Failure of phenobarbitone to prevent febrile convulsions. British Medical Journal 1: 559–561

Heeley A, Pugh R J P, Clayton B E, Shepherd J, Wilson J 1978 Pyridoxal metabolism in vitamin B6-responsive convulsions of early infancy. Archives of Disease in Childhood 53: 794–802

Heijbel J, Blom S, Rasmuson M 1975 Benign epilepsy of childhood with centrotemporal EEG foci: a genetic study. Epilepsia 16: 285–293

Herzlinger R A, Kandall S R, Vaughan H G 1977 Neonatal seizures associated with narcotic withdrawal. Journal of Pediatrics 91: 638–641

Holdsworth L, Whitmore K 1974a A study of children with epilepsy attending ordinary schools. I Their seizure patterns, progress and behaviour in school. Developmental Medicine and Child Neurology 16: 746–758

Holdsworth L, Whitmore K 1974b A study of children with epilepsy attending ordinary schools. II Information and attitudes held by their teachers. Developmental Medicine and Child Neurology 16: 759–765

Holowach J, Thurston D L, O'Leary J 1958 Jacksonian seizures in infancy and childhood. Journal of Pediatrics 52: 670–686

Holowach J, Thurston D L, O'Leary J 1972 Prognosis in childhood epilepsy. Follow-up study of 148 cases in which therapy had been suspended after prolonged anti-convulsant control. New England Journal of Medicine 286: 169–174

Hosking G P 1974 Fits in hydrocephalic children. Archives of Disease in Childhood 49: 633–635

Houghton G W, Richens A 1974 Phenytoin intoxication induced by sulthiame in epileptic patients. Journal of Neurology, Neurosurgery and Psychiatry 37: 275–281

Hutt S J, Jackson P M, Belsham A, Higgins G 1968 Perceptual-motor behaviour in relation to blood phenobarbitone level: a preliminary report. Developmental Medicine and Child Neurology 10: 626–632

Huttenlocher P R 1976 Ketonemia and seizures: metabolic and anticonvulsant effects of two ketogenic diets in childhood epilepsy. Pediatric Research 10: 536–540

Huttenlocher P R, Wilbourn A J, Signore J M 1971 Medium-chain triglycerides as a therapy for intractable childhood epilepsy. Neurology 21: 1097

Iilingworth Cynthia M 1979 227 road accidents to children. Acta Paediatrica Scandinavica 68: 869–873

Illingworth R S 1955 Sudden mental deterioration with convulsions in infancy. Archives of Disease in Childhood 30: 529–537

Jalling B 1974 Plasma and cerebrospinal fluid concentrations of phenobarbitone in infants given single doses. Developmental Medicine and Child Neurology 16: 781–793

Jeavons P M 1975 The practical management of epilepsy. Update 1: 11

Jeavons P M, Bower B D 1964 Infantile spasms. Clinics in Developmental Medicine No. 15, SIMP and Heinemann Medical Books, London, J B Lippincott, Philadelphia

Jeavons P M, Bower B D, Dimitrakoudi M 1973 Long-term prognosis of 150 cases of 'West syndrome'. Epilepsia 14: 153–164

Jeavons P M, Clark J E, Maheshwari M C 1977 Treatment of generalised epilepsies of childhood and adolescence with sodium valproate (Epilim). Developmental Medicine and Child Neurology 19: 9–25

Jeavons P M, Harding G F A 1975 Photosensitive epilepsy. Clinics in Developmental Medicine no. 56, SIMP, Heinemann Medical Books, London

Jeavons P M, Harper J R, Bower B D 1970 Long-term prognosis in infantile spasms: a follow-up report on 112 cases. Developmental Medicine and Child Neurology 12: 413–421

Jennett B 1973 Trauma as a cause of epilepsy in childhood. Developmental Medicine and Child Neurology 15: 56–62

Jennett B 1977 Traumatic epilepsy — the scale of the problem. In: Jennett B, Whitty C W M (eds) Epilepsy, trauma and the family doctor. Hull, Reckitt and Colman Pharmaceutical Division 4–5

Jennett B, Van de Sande J 1975 EEG prediction of post-traumatic epilepsy. Epilepsia 16: 251–256

Jennett W B 1975 Epilepsy after non-missile head injuries. Heinemann, London

Keen J H, Lee D 1973 Sequelae of neonatal convulsions. Study of 112 infants. Archives of Disease in Childhood 48: 542–546

Knudsen F U, Vestermark S 1978 Prophylactic diazepam or phenobarbitone in febrile convulsions: a prospective controlled study. Archives of Disease in Childhood 53: 660–663

Knudsen F U 1979 Rectal administration of diazepam in solution in the acute treatment of convulsions in infants and children: anticonvulsant effect and side effects. Archives of Disease in Childhood 54: 855–857

Krynauw R A 1950 Infantile hemiplegia treated by removing one cerebral hemisphere. Journal of Neurology, Neurosurgery and Psychiatry 13: 243–267

Kulenkampff M, Schwartzman J S, Wilson J 1974 Neurological complications of pertussis inoculation. Archives of Disease in Childhood 49: 46–49

Laidlaw M V, Laidlaw J 1980 Epilepsy explained. A Churchill-Livingstone Patient Handbook. Churchill Livingstone, Edinburgh

Landau W M, Kleffner F R 1957 Syndrome of acquired aphasia with convulsive disorder in children. Neurology 7: 523–530

Laxdal T, Gomez T L, Reiher J 1969 Cyanotic and pallid syncopal attacks in children (breath-holding spells). Developmental Medicine and Child Neurology 11: 755–763

Lennox W G, Lennox M A 1960 Epilepsy and related disorders. Little, Brown, Boston, Mass.

Lennox-Buchthal M A 1973 Febrile convulsions: a reappraisal. Electroencephalography and Clinical Neurophysiology Suppl 32

Lepintre J, Schweisguth O, Labrune M, Lemerle J 1969 Les neuroblastomes en sablier. Archives françaises de Pèdiatrie 26: 829–847

Lerman P, Kivity-Ephraim S 1974 Carbamazepine sole anticonvulsant for focal epilepsy of childhood. Epilepsia 15: 229–234

Lerman P, Kivity S 1975 Benign focal epilepsy of childhood. A follow-up study of 100 recovered patients. Archives of Neurology 32: 261–268

Lerman P, Kivity S 1982 The efficacy of corticotropin in primary infantile spasms. Journal of Pediatrics 101: 294–296

Lewis H M, Parry J V, Parry R P Davies H A, Sanderson P J, Tyrell D A J, Valman H B 1979 Role of viruses in febrile convulsions. Archives of Disease in Childhood 54: 869–876

Lindsay J, Ounsted C, Richards P 1979 Long-term outcome in children with temporal lobe seizures. I. Social outcome and childhood factors. Developmental Medicine and Child Neurology 21: 285–298

Lindsay J, Ounsted C, Richards P 1979 Long-term outcome in children with temporal lobe seizures. II. Marriage, parenthood and sexual indifference. Developmental Medicine and Child Neurology 21: 433–440

Lindsay J, Ounsted C, Richards P 1979 Long-term outcome in children with temporal lobe seizures. III. Psychiatric aspects in childhood and adult life. Developmental Medicine and Child Neurology 21: 630–636

Lindsay J, Ounsted C, Richards P 1980 Long-term outcome in children with temporal lobe seizures IV. Genetic factors, febrile convulsions, and the remission of seizures. Developmental Medicine and Child Neurology 22: 429–439

Lingam S, Bertwhistle H, Elliston H M, Wilson J 1980 Problems with intravenous chlormethiazole (heminevrin) in status epilepticus. British Medical Journal 280: 155–156

Lishman W A, Symonds C P, Whitty C W, Willison R G 1962 Seizures induced by movement. Brain 85: 93–108

Livingston S, Berman W, Pauli L 1975 Anticonvulsant drug blood levels. Practical applications based on 12 years' experience. Journal of the American Medical Association 232: 60–62

Lombroso C 1966 Treatment of status epilepticus with diazepam. Neurology (Minneapolis) 16: 629–634

Lombroso C T 1967 Sylvian seizures and mid-temporal spike foci in children. Archives of Neurology 17: 52–59

Lombroso C T, Lerman P 1967 Breath-holding spells (cyanotic and pallid infantile syncope). Pediatrics 39: 563–581

Mantovani J F, Landau W M 1980 Acquired aphasia with convulsive disorder: course and prognosis. Neurology 30: 524–529

McBride M C, Dooling E C, Oppenheimer E Y 1981 Complex partial status epilepticus in young children. Annals of Neurology 9: 526–530

McKissock W 1953 Infantile hemiplegia. Proceedings of the Royal Society of Medicine 46: 431–434

Marsden C D 1976 Neurology. In: Laidlaw J, Richens A (eds) A textbook of epilepsy. Churchill Livingstone, Edinburgh

Mayeux R, Lueders H 1978 Complex partial status epilepticus: case report and proposal for diagnostic criteria. Neurology (Minneapolis) 28: 957–961

Melchior J C 1977 Infantile spasms and early immunization against whooping cough: Danish survey from 1970–1975. Archives of Disease in Childhood 52: 134–137

Melchior J C, Buchthal F, Lennox-Buchthal M 1971 The ineffectiveness of diphenylhydantoin in preventing febrile convulsions in the age of greatest risk, under three years. Epilepsia 12: 55–62

Metrakos K, Metrakos J D 1966 Genetics of convulsive disorders, Part 2: Genetic and electroencephalographic studies in centrencephalic epilepsy. Neurology (Minneapolis) 11: 464–483

Miller F J W, Court S D M, Walton W S, Knox E G 1960 Growing up in Newcastle-upon-Tyne: a continuing study of health and illness in young children within their families. Nuffield Foundation, Oxford University Press, London, p 164–173

National Institutes of Health Consensus Development Panel. Febrile seizures: long-term management of children with fever-associated seizures 1980. British Medical Journal 281: 277–279

Nelson K B, Ellenberg J H 1976 Predictors of epilepsy in children who have experienced febrile seizures. New England Journal of Medicine 295: 1029–1033

Nelson K B, Ellenberg J H 1978 Prognosis in children with febrile seizures. Pediatrics 61: 720–727

Neville B G R 1972 The origin of infantile spasms: evidence from a case of hydranencephaly. Developmental Medicine and Child Neurology 14: 644–647

Ngwane E, Bower B 1980 Continuous sodium valproate or phenobarbitone in the prevention of 'simple' febrile convulsions. Comparison by a double-blind trial. Archives of Disease in Childhood 55: 171–174

O'Donohoe N V 1979 Epilepsies of childhood. Butterworths, London

Oettinger L, Nekonishi H, Gill I G 1967 Cerebral dysrhythmia induced by reading (subclinical reading epilepsy). Developmental Medicine and Child Neurology 9: 191–201

Ounsted C 1971 Some aspects of seizure disorders. In: Gairdner D, Hull D (eds) Recent advances in paediatrics, 4th edn, Churchill Livingstone, Edinburgh, p 363–400

Ounsted C, Lindsay J, Norman R M 1966 Biological factors in temporal lobe epilepsy. Clinics in Developmental Medicine no. 22, Heinemann Medical Books, London

Parkes J D, Fenton G W 1973 Levo (−) amphetamine and dextro (+) amphetamine in the treatment of narcolepsy. Journal of Neurology, Neurosurgery and Psychiatry 36: 1076–1081

Paulson G 1963 Breathholding spells: a fatal case. Developmental Medicine and Child Neurology 5: 246–251

Pearn J H 1977 Epilepsy and drowning in childhood. British Medical Journal 1: 1510–1511

Penry J K, Porter R J, Dreifuss F E 1975 Simultaneous recording of absence seizures with video tape and electro-encephalography. Brain 98: 427–440

Penry J K, Dreifuss F E 1969 Automatisms associated with the absence of petit mal epilepsy. Archives of Neurology (Chicago) 21: 121–149

Pilgaard S, Hansen F J, Paerregaard P 1981 Prophylaxis against febrile convulsions with phenobarbital. Acta paediatrica scandinavica 70: 67–71 (Copenhagen)

Price D J E 1977 Prophylaxis of post-neurosurgical epilepsy including the use of sodium valproate (Epilim). Epilepsy, trauma and the family doctor. Medicine Meeting 2, Glasgow, Reckitt and Colman Pharmaceutical Division

Rapin I, Mattis S, Rowan A J, Golden G G 1977 Verbal auditory agnosia in children. Developmental Medicine and Child Neurology 19: 192–207

Remillard G M, Andermann F, Rhi-Sausi A Robbins N M 1977 Facial asymmetry in patients with temporal lobe epilepsy: a clinical sign useful in the lateralization of temporal epileptogenic foci. Neurology 27: 109–114

Reynolds E H 1972 Anticonvulsant drugs, folate deficiency and metabolic bone disease. British Medical Journal 2: 656–657

Reynolds E H 1975 Chronic antiepileptic toxicity: a review. Epilepsia 16: 319–352

Reynolds E H, Chadwick D, Galbraith A W 1976 One drug (phenytoin) in the treatment of epilepsy. Lancet 1: 923–926

Richens A, Rowe D J 1970 Disturbances of calcium metabolism by anticonvulsant drugs. British Medical Journal 4: 73–76

Riikonen R, Donner M 1979 Incidence and aetiology of infantile spasma from 1960–1976: a population study in Finland. Developmental Medicine and Child Neurology 21: 333–343

Rose A L, Lombroso C T 1970 Neonatal seizure states. Pediatrics 45: 404–425

Rosenstein Von 1776 Diseases of children and their remedies, British edn.

Rutter M, Graham P, Yule W 1970 A neuropsychiatric study in childhood. Clinics in Developmental Medicine nos. 35/36, SIMP and Heinemann Medical Books, London

Rutter N, Metcalfe D H 1978 Febrile convulsions — what do parents do? British Medical Journal 2: 1345–1346

Rylance G W, Moreland T A 1980 Drug level monitoring in paediatric practice. Archives of Disease in Childhood 55: 89–98

Seager J, Jamison D L, Wilson J, Hayward A R, Soothill J F 1975 IgA deficiency, epilepsy and phenytoin treatment. Lancet 2: 632–635

Snodgrass G J A I 1974 Seizures in newborn infants. Developmental Medicine and Child Neurology 16: 92–94

Sorel L, Dusaucy-Bauloye A 1958 A propos de 21 cas d'hypsarhythmia de Gibbs: son traitement spectaculaire par l'ACTH. Acta neurologica psychiatrica belgica 58: 130–141

Stephenson J B P 1978a Two types of febrile seizure: anoxic (syncopal) and epileptic mechanisms differentiated by oculocardiac reflex. British Medical Journal 2: 726–728

Stephenson J B P 1978b Reflex anoxic seizures ('white breath-holding'): non-epileptic vagal attacks. Archives of Disease in Childhood 53: 193–200

Stephenson J B P, House F M, Stromberg P 1977 Medium-chain triglycerides in a ketogenic diet. Developmental Medicine and Child Neurology 19: 693–694

Stokes M J, Downham M A P S, Webb J K G, McQuillin J, Gardner P S 1977 Viruses and febrile convulsions. Archives of Disease in Childhood 52: 129–133

Stores G 1973 Studies of attention and seizure disorders. Developmental Medicine and Child Neurology 15: 376–382

Stores G 1978 School-children with epilepsy at risk for learning and behaviour problems. Developmental Medicine and Child Neurology 20: 502–508

Stores G, Hart J A 1976 Reading skills in children with generalised or focal epilepsy attending ordinary school. Developmental Medicine and Child Neurology 18: 705–716

Stores G, Hart J A, Piran N 1978 Inattentiveness in children with epilepsy. Epilepsia 19: 169–175

Stores G, Piran N 1978 Dependency of different types in schoolchildren with epilepsy. Psychological Medicine 8: 441–445

Taylor D C 1969 Differential rates of cerebral maturation between sexes and between hemispheres. Lancet 2: 140–142

Taylor D C, Bower B D 1971 Prevention of epileptic disorders. Lancet 2: 1136–1138

Thomas J E, Reagan T J, Klass D W 1977 Epilepsia partialis continua. Archives of Neurology 34: 266–275

Thorn I 1975 A controlled study of prophylactic long-term treatment of febrile convulsions with phenobarbital. Acta neurologica scandinavica suppl. 60: 67–73

Tibbles J A R, Prichard J S 1965 The prognostic value of the electroencephalogram in neonatal convulsions. Pediatrics 35: 778–786

Tibbles J A R 1980 Dominant benign neonatal seizures. Developmental Medicine and Child Neurology 22: 664–667

Van den Berg B J 1974 Studies on convulsive disorders in young children. III. Recurrence of febrile convulsions. Epilepsia 15: 177–190

Vazquez H J, Turner M 1951 Epilepsia en flexion generalizada. Archivos Argentinos de Pediatria 35: 111

Volpe J J 1973 Neonatal seizures. New England Journal of Medicine 289: 413–416

Volpe J J 1977 Neonatal seizures. Clinics in Perinatology 4 (1): 43–63

Wallace S J 1974 Recurrence of febrile convulsions. Archives of Disease in Childhood 49: 763–765

Wallace S 1975a Factors predisposing to a complicated initial febrile convulsion. Archives of Disease in Childhood 50: 943–947

Wallace S J 1975b Continuous prophylactic anticonvulsants in selected children with febrile convulsions. Acta neurologica scandinavica suppl. 60: 62

Wallace S J, Aldridge Smith J 1980 Successful prophylaxis against febrile convulsions with valproic acid or phenobarbitone. British Medical Journal 280: 353–354

West W J 1841 On a peculiar form of infantile convulsions. Lancet 1: 724–725

Wilder R M 1921 Effects of ketonuria on the course of epilepsy. Mayo Clinic Proceedings 2: 307

Williams A J, Evans-Jones L G, Kindley A D, Groom P J 1979 Sodium Valproate in the prophylaxis of simple febrile convulsions. Clinical Pediatrics 18: 426–430

Wilson P J E 1970 Cerebral hemispherectomy for infantile hemiplegia: a report of 50 cases. Brain 93: 147–180

Wolf S M, Carr A, Davis D, Davidson S, Dale E P, Forsythe A et al 1977 The value of phenobarbital in a child who has had a simple febrile seizure: a controlled prospective study. Pediatrics 59: 378–385

Wolf S M, Forsythe A 1978 Behavior disturbance, phenobarbital and febrile seizures. Pediatrics 61: 728–731

Worster-Drought C 1971 An unusual form of acquired aphasia in children. Developmental Medicine and Child Neurology 13: 563–571

Young B, Rapp R, Brooks W H, Madauss W, Norton J A 1979 Post-traumatic epilepsy prophylaxis. Epilepsia 20: 671–681

Young, H 1980 What difference does it make, Danny? Andrè Deutsch, London

Zarcone V 1973 Narcolepsy. New England Journal of Medicine 288: 1156–1166

13

Mental retardation

E. M. Brett

What a piece of work is a man! How noble in reason!
How infinite in faculties! In form and moving, how
express and admirable! In action how like an angel! In
apprehension, how like a God!

Hamlet, Act ii, scene 2

Mental retardation is one of the three common
chronic neurological handicaps of childhood, the
others being cerebral palsy and epilepsy, with one
or both of which it is often associated. Whether it
occurs alone or in combination with other handicaps, it is one of the commonest problems confronting the paediatrician and paediatric neurologist,
causing great anxiety to parents and making
immense demands of the physician and his professional colleagues in terms of time, support and
sympathy.

TERMINOLOGY, CLASSIFICATION AND PREVALENCE

Definitions of mental retardation, subnormality or
deficiency are difficult and the terminology and
classification still far from ideal. Tredgold in the
early years of this century defined mental deficiency as a state of arrested or incomplete development of the mind, while the World Health
Organisation has defined mental retardation as an
'incomplete or insufficient general development of
mental capacities'. The *social* dimension of mental
defect, as Penrose (1954) has pointed out, was early
recognised as an important factor and is included
in recent attempts at definition and classification,
and in legislation. In the United Kingdom under
the 1927 Mental Deficiency Act, three classes of

mentally subnormal persons were recognised, the
idiot (low-grade defective), imbecile (middle-grade
or trainable) and feeble-minded or moron (high-
grade or educable). These were defined in terms of
the individual's capabilities for self-care, avoidance
of common physical dangers and management of
his own affairs. In terms of formal psychometric
assessment these three groups corresponded to
Intelligence Quotients (IQ) of 0–20, 21–50 and
51–75 respectively. Their relative proportions in
the general defective population are of the order of
5, 20 and 75%. There is no doubt that the words
'idiot', 'imbecile' and 'moron', often used by the
general public as terms of abuse, were distressing
for the parents of the children so described (as are
the terms 'mongol' and 'gargoyle', now largely
replaced by 'Down's syndrome' and other eponyms
or biochemical terms). They were happily
superseded with the reclassification of mental deficiency under the 1959 Mental Health Act into
'severe subnormality' and 'subnormality'. *Severe
subnormality* is defined as a state of arrested or
incomplete development of mind which includes
subnormality of intelligence and is of such a nature
or degree that the patient is incapable of living an
independent life or of guarding against serious
exploitation or will be so incapable when of an age
to do so. *Subnormality* is used to mean a state of
arrested or incomplete development of mind (not
amounting to severe subnormality) which includes
subnormality of intelligence and is of such a nature
or degree which requires or is susceptible to medical treatment or other special care or training of
the patient. In the United States the American
Academy of Mental Retardation (1973) has defined
mental retardation as 'significantly sub-average intellectual functioning, existing concurrently with de-

ficits in adaptive behaviour and manifested during the developmental period'. (Adaptive behaviour is defined as 'the effectiveness with which the individual meets the standards of personal independence and social responsibility expected of his age and cultural group'.) These definitions are of necessity based largely on sociological rather than clinical criteria.

Statistics on the prevalence of mental handicap in the childhood population vary from one community to another. In the United Kingdom in the age group 7 to 14 years, the age by which most cases have been identified, about 20 per 1000 children are mentally handicapped, having an IQ of 70 or lower. Of these less than 5 per 1000 are severely mentally handicapped, with IQs below 50, and the remainder moderately handicapped with scores between 50 and 70. Alberman (1978) has compared the prevalence rates of IQ under 50 in children in age groups in which all subjects are likely to be known in nine series (seven from the United Kingdom and two from North America) and has found remarkably little variation between these, the rates ranging from 3.3 to 4.9.

The terms 'Educationally Subnormal (Moderate)' and 'Educationally Subnormal (Severe)' [ESN(M) and ESN(S)] have been introduced in the United Kingdom in recent years to refer to those with IQs between 50 and 69, and below 50 respectively. This reflects the increased emphasis on education for all handicapped children which has been an encouraging development in this period. The expressions 'severe' and 'profound retardation' have been applied to children in the ESN(S) category to designate those with IQs above and below 30.

From a clinical point of view the mentally subnormal can be divided into two further categories. The first comprises patients with undifferentiated mental deficiency, who do not show signs of gross cerebral involvement in terms of obvious neurological deficits such as cerebral palsy and in whom metabolic or infectious causes and malformations or other structural anomalies of the brain are excluded by appropriate investigation. These contrast with the second group of patients showing gross neurological deficits resulting from identifiable insults or diseases in the prenatal, natal or postnatal periods. It seems likely that the first, undifferentiated group includes many individuals whose subnormality may be 'physiological' or 'subcultural' rather than pathological, in the sense that they represent the lower end of the distribution curve of intelligence. This curve seems to show a Gaussian pattern which is skewed towards the lower end, so that there are more children whose scores are under 70 than over 130. The cases of 'physiological' subnormality are probably of complex aetiology, due to a combination of adverse genetic and environmental factors each of little effect alone, but summating to produce a condition of low mental development. These children tend to have parents whose average intelligence is below that of the general population, which is not the case with the 'pathological' group. Social differences can be seen between the two groups, the 'physiological', but not the 'pathological', defectives tending to occur in larger families of below-average economic status. (In a survey of mental handicap in Aberdeen, Birch et al (1970) found a recorded prevalence among the children of unskilled urban manual workers roughly nine times greater than among the children of those in non-manual occupations.) Though sociologically important, members of the 'physiological' group of subnormal children are less likely to be brought for medical advice than the 'pathologically' subnormal, since their parents are also likely to be of below average intelligence and to have lower expectations and aspirations for their children.

The point must be made that mental subnormality, like any other neurological deficit, may be present from birth or acquired after an interval of normality. The degree of mental subnormality may be fixed or may increase. It is essential to distinguish between *amentia*, in which mental defect is present from birth and is not progressive, and *dementia*, in which the defect develops in a child of previously normal intelligence. In the second case the dementia may be catastrophically acute in onset and maximal at the start of the illness (as with meningitis, encephalitis, head injury or status epilepticus) or insidious and subacute in onset as in progressive degenerative disease of the nervous system such as the neurometabolic disorders or subacute sclerosing panencephalitis. The implications for prognosis and genetic counselling of these two situations are so different that they must be clearly distinguished by a detailed developmental history, examination, investigation and, when indicated, repeated psychometry. This distinction between progressive and non-progressive disorder, in which time is an essential test, is one of the most important decisions which the child neurologist is required to make. The difficulties encountered, especially in the younger child, are referred to in Chapter 5 in relation to dementing diseases.

AETIOLOGY

In general, mental subnormality may be caused by hereditary and environmental factors. It may be determined by a single abnormal gene or combination of genes, or by various harmful external factors affecting the brain early or late in embryonic, fetal or postnatal life. As mentioned above, a combination of genetic and environmental factors may conspire to produce the 'physiological' or 'subcultural' form of subnormality. In many cases of subnormality the aetiology cannot be determined, even after detailed investigation directed towards excluding genetic disorders and environmental insults.

It is convenient to consider the causes under the headings of prenatal, perinatal and postnatal factors. Prenatal factors have come in recent years to account for an increasing proportion of subnormality (Sabel et al 1976, Laxova et al 1977, Drillien 1978, Alberman 1978, Hagberg 1978) and are responsible for about three quarters of the cases in most series. Prenatal causes may be genetic or nongenetic, with a large contribution from chromosomal disorders, particularly Down's syndrome.

PRENATAL CAUSES

GENETIC CONDITIONS

Chromosomal disorders

Chromosomal anomalies are known to be associated with many congenital conditions with mental retardation and dysmorphic features. Down's syndrome, or mongolism (Trisomy 21), with an incidence of 1 in 600 newborns, is the commonest identifiable cause of subnormality, accounting for

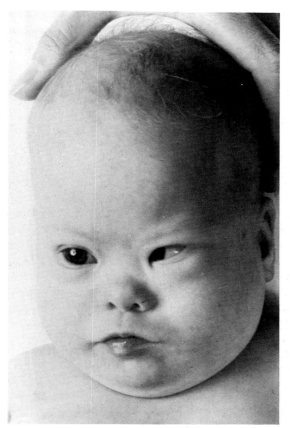

Fig. 13.1 Seven-week-old girl with Down's syndrome

about one third of all published series (Fig. 13.1 and 13.2). Other chromosomal aberrations involve other forms of trisomy, various patterns of deletion and abnormalities of the X-chromosome. These are associated with various anomalies of the eyes, nose, mouth, neck, genitalia, skeleton, heart, lungs and renal tract. With more intensive investigation of subnormal and 'dysmorphic' children increasing numbers of such syndromes are defined each year. A good guide is given by Smith (1976), the second edition of whose monograph lists 21 chromosomal anomalies compared with 12 in the first edition (1970). Chromosomal syndromes were present in 36% of a Swedish series of severely retarded children (Gustavson et al 1977): Down's syndrome accounted for most of these cases.

Genetic conditions — non-chromosomal

A large number of genetically-determined condi-

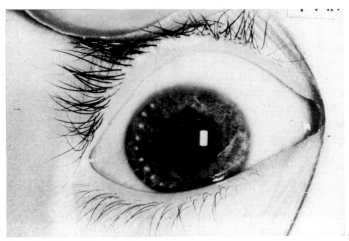

Fig. 13.2 Brushfield spots in Down's syndrome

tions are known to be associated with mental subnormality of non-progressive type: many of these show epilepsy as an added symptom while a few may also show various forms of cerebral palsy. They are usually inherited as autosomal recessive characters, but some are autosomal deominant or X-linked.

The neuro-ectodermal disorders (see Ch. 20) such as tuberose sclerosis and neurofibromatosis, which may be associated with mental subnormality, are usually inherited as dominants, though some cases are sporadic. Others in this group, such as Feuerstein's syndrome and the Sjögren-Larsson syndrome, are recessively inherited. Incontinentia pigmenti (the Bloch-Sulzberger syndrome) may be due to a single mutant gene lethal in the male. (The Sturge-Weber syndrome, in which encephalofacial angiomatosis may be associated with subnormality in addition to epilepsy and hemiplegia, is usually not genetically determined.)

Many inborn errors of metabolism are associated with subnormality and sometimes with epilepsy. These account for only a small proportion of the retarded population, but it is particularly important to recognize them because of their genetic implications (most have an autosomal recessive mode of inheritance) and because some of them with early dietary treatment may be compatible with normal or almost normal development. These disorders include phenylketonuria, galactosaemia, maple-syrup urine disease, the mucopolysaccharidoses, homocystinuria and a large number of other amino-acidurias and organic acidurias, new examples of which are recognized each year. In some of these metabolic disorders the child's development is clearly retarded from the beginning and in others it starts to lag after a period of relative normality in relation to dietary factors. For example, developmental retardation is obvious early in life in children with untreated maple-syrup urine disease, which is more often lethal than most inborn metabolic disorders, but it may not be evident until 2 or 3 years of age in homosystinuria (which is compatible with normal intelligence) while untreated phenylketonuria is intermediate between the two diseases in this respect. In most of the disorders of mucopolysaccharide metabolism associated with subnormality there are striking skeletal and facial abnormalities which may increase with age; the mental retardation may also be progressive.

Some of these metabolic disorders are considered in more detail in other chapters. For a fuller description the reader is referred to Smith (1976) and Stanbury et al (1978).

Microcephaly, which is usually non-specific and a descriptive rather than a diagnostic term, occurs very rarely as an autosomal recessive inherited condition. Hydrocephalus, which is also multi-factorial in origin, can occur rarely on an inherited basis as an X-linked recessive character when it may be associated with retarded development. X-linked inheritance is also seen in the syndrome of moderate retardation *without* specific facial or other abnormalities sometimes associated with the name of Renpenning in which the pattern of inheritance when more than one boy is affected in a sibship provides the clue (see below).

Many cerebral malformations, which may be gross and obvious, such as the various forms of cranium bifidum and hydranencephaly, or mild and detected only radiologically, such as agenesis of the corpus callosum, are associated with mental subnormality and sometimes with congenital anomalies affecting other structures. There may be a genetic element in cranium bifidum, but hydranencephaly and callosal agenesis are usually not genetically determined.

An increasing number of genetic syndromes of mental retardation without chromosomal anomalies is recognized, in which a great variety of congenital defects of different organs and systems occur in various combinations. Some of these have been referred to in other chapters (e.g. dystrophia myotonica, ataxia-telangiectasia, Menkes' syndrome.) Various oral, facial and digital defects seem to group themselves together into specific syndromes, some of which are associated with mental retardation. Genital anomalies occur as a striking feature of some syndromes of retardation, such as the Smith-Lemli-Opitz syndrome, (Fig. 13.3) in association with a variety of other commoner abnormalities such as microcephaly, simian crease, polydactyly, and dislocated hips; the identification of these cases in the male is facilitated by the ease with which cryptorchidism and hypospadias are recognized, so that female cases may be underdiagnosed. The number of 'recognisable patterns of human malformation' in the second edition of Smith's (1976) monograph is 345 compared with 135 in the previous edition, and there are probably many more syndromes as yet unreported, since many experienced paediatricians have observed striking patterns of defects in retarded children which have not yet been described. (There is perhaps a Procrustean tendency to try to make the features fit the described syndrome, and the problem is made more difficult by the fact that minor anomalies of eyes, ears, nose, hands and feet are common in the normal population, so that undue weight can sometimes be given to such features in a retarded child.)

The increased incidence of minor congenital anomalies of other organs in idiopathic mental

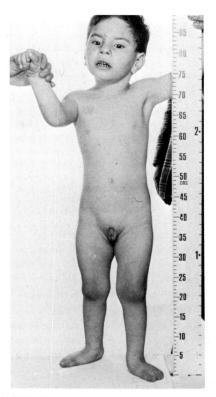

Fig. 13.3 Smith-Lemli-Opitz syndrome in a 4-year-old boy

retardation was shown by the study of Smith & Bostian (1964) who determined the frequency of associated congenital structural anomalies in 50 children with idiopathic mental retardation, 50 with ventricular septal defect, 50 with cleft lip and palate and 100 control children. The highest frequency of anomalies (42%) was found in the retarded group compared with none in the control group, 18% in the ventricular septal defect and 10% in the cleft lip and palate group. 71% of the anomalies detected involved the hand, eye, face, mouth or ear. The finding of three or more associated congenital anomalies in a patient seems to indicate a significant abnormality in prenatal development, and the discovery of multiple associated congenital anomalies in a child with idiopathic mental retardation can reasonably be taken to suggest, if not to prove, that the defect of brain function also has its basis in a congenital anomaly. This group of sporadic, unexplained, but presumably prenatally determined cases of mental retardation forms the multiple congenital anomaly-mental retardation ('MCA/MR') category in the classification of Kaveggia et al (1973). (The term 'provisional private syndrome' has been proposed by Opitz et al (1978) for cases of this kind with similarly affected close relatives.) In the Swedish series of 122 severely retarded children of Gustavson et al (1973) 24 showed major or minor anomalies of prenatal onset, but only two of these could be fitted into recognized syndromes, the Cornelia de Lange and Prader-Willi syndromes.

Renpenning's syndrome or X-linked mental retardation and its wider genetic implications

An excess of males over females among mentally retarded patients in institutions was noted by Penrose (1938) in a survey of 1280 cases of mental defect. Certain X-linked syndromes with mental retardation and progressive neurological deterioration are well recognized (e.g. Menkes', Lowe's, Lesch-Nyhan syndromes and adrenal-leucodystrophy) but these dramatic diseases are too rare to account for the male preponderance and are, in most cases, lethal.

Priest et al (1961) in family studies of mentally retarded people in a state institution noted more families with two affected brothers than with a brother and sister or two sisters affected. Martin and Bell (1943) reported 'a pedigree of mental defect showing sex-linkage' with eleven affected males in two generations, and Renpenning et al (1962) described a large Canadian family with 21 affected males. Similar pedigrees were reported from Australia by Turner et al (1971) who found five such families over two years in a clinic for the mentally retarded and suggested the term 'Renpenning's syndrome' for the condition. In some families males in four generations were affected. The retarded males were remarkably free from physical abnormalities on examination. All had head circumferences in the normal range and none had more than two minor congenital anomalies. Some patients had had a few fits, but in none was epilepsy an important feature. Most had IQs in the *moderately* retarded range (IQ 36–51). No biochemical abnormality was detected. Further studies of patients with X-linked mental retardation have confirmed their physical normality apart from macro-orchidism which has been noted in many (Turner et al 1980a). The patients are often described as well-built and physically strong, sometimes with rather prominent ears (Renpenning et al 1962).

A chromosomal anomaly has now been noted in many patients with X-linked mental retardation (Lubs 1969, Sutherland 1977) with a constriction near the end of the long arm of the X-chromosome resulting in a small knob separated from the body of the chromosome by a thin and fragile stalk. Sutherland has referred to this as a 'fragile site'.

The importance of the recognition of X-linked mental retardation of this kind is shown by the fact that it may account for about ten per cent of cases of moderate retardation in males. Its genetic implications have recently been extended even further by the work of Turner et al (1980b). These workers found that males affected by one form of X-linked mental retardation possessed the X-chromosomal marker fra (X) (q27) and were physically normal apart from macro-orchidism. In a group of physically normal, mildly retarded Sydney schoolgirls (with IQs 55–75) they found five who carried the same marker X. They then investigated the relatives of these girls and found retarded males in 4 of the 5 families and identified a further 18 heterozygotes of whom six were intellectually or educationally retarded. They conclude that expression of the X-linked mutation in female carriers contributes to *mild* mental retardation of girls, that those who are physically normal should be screened for the marker X and the their relatives should be investigated in order to identify additional females with a high risk of conceiving affected males.

Recent re-examination of the Renpenning family has shown that affected men do not have the fragile site on the X chromosome. They are characterised by short stature and rather low skull circumference (Fox et al 1980) and do not have the macro-orchidism, large ears and prominent forehead and mandible seen in most of those with the fragile site on the X chromosome. The latter condition is then perhaps best called the 'Fragile X-mental retardation syndrome'.

Leber's amaurosis

In this autosomal recessive disorder with blindness mental retardation may also be present, though not invariable. Sometimes known as congenital tapetoretinal degeneration (and not to be confused with Leber's optic actrophy), it affects both sexes and presents with visual loss from birth. The absence of the electroretinogram (ERG) helps to distinguish it from most other causes of early blindness.

In a series of 30 patients with Leber's amaurosis seen at the Hospital for Sick Children, Great Ormond Street, moderate or severe mental subnormality was present in eleven of the twenty one who were assessed psychometrically (Vaizey et al 1977). Lumbar air encephalography gave abnormal results in eight of nine patients, with cerebral atrophy in eight and cerebellar atrophy in three. Microcephaly was present in some cases.

In 24 children the visual loss was very severe while another six were later shown to be less severely affected.

In the patients with severe amaurosis no useful vision could be detected. They showed roving eye movements and a poor pupillary response to light. Enophthalmos was common and many children manipulated their eyes, pressing on them probably in an attempt to provoke an impulse in the optic nerve which may produce a crude visual perception. (There is a risk of corneal scarring from repeated manual stimulation of the eyes.) In young infants in the series slight increase in pigmentation with an equatorial distribution and attenuation of retinal arteries was sometimes noted. In patients over one year of age retinal artery attenuation was invariable with increased granular pigmentation which might be equatorial or diffuse in distribution or concentrated at the macula. Macular pigmentation, when present, helps to distinguish Leber's amaurosis from tapetoretinal degeneration of later onset in which it is rare. Optic atrophy was noted in only 5 patients.

The combination of visual defect and mental subnormality in this disorder, as in others in which they co-exist, produces a severe degree of handicap. Some of these children may be regarded merely as mentally retarded with the visual defect and genetic implications overlooked. The condition should be considered in any retarded and visually handicapped child and investigation by ERG arranged.

Non-genetic prenatal causes

Many environmental factors may affect the central nervous system in fetal life causing later mental subnormality as well as other neurological handicaps and sometimes deficits in the structure and function of other organs.

Maternal infections, particularly rubella, toxoplasmosis, cytomegalovirus (CMV), herpes simplex, syphilis, the Epstein-Barr virus and possibly influenza, can cause severe brain damage in the fetus with resultant microcephaly, retardation, epilepsy and sometimes hydrocephalus and cerebral calcification. The contribution of these intrauterine infections has been underestimated in the past, especially that of CMV infection. The clinical features of these fetal infections may be diagnostic, as with a typical rubella syndrome, or highly suggestive with intracranial calcification and choroidoretinopathy pointing to CMV or toxoplasma infection. On occasion they may be less striking and the diagnosis may only be made by serological investigation or culture. CMV infection in particular may be easily overlooked. These infections and the diagnostic approach are considered in Chapter 22.

Antepartum haemorrhage, toxaemia of pregnancy and intrauterine growth retardation producing a 'light for dates' infant are often incriminated as causes of mental subnormality, alone or in association with other neurological handicaps. There was disagreement about the importance of these factors in earlier series probably reflecting differences in the populations studied and changing patterns of care. In a review of birth records of subnormal children in Baltimore, Pasamanick & Lilienfeld (1955) found significantly more complications of pregnancy and delivery, prematurity and abnormal neonatal condition than in a series of matched controls. Non-mechanical abnormalities such as bleeding in pregnancy and toxaemia seemed to be important factors in this association. By contrast, Barker (1966a) in a British survey of

607 subnormal children found no evidence for a contribution from toxaemia or ante-partum haemorrhage. In the same survey Barker (1966b) studied the relationship between low intelligence and length of gestation and rate of fetal growth. He found the former to be associated with both a slower rate of intrauterine growth and a higher incidence of birth below 38 weeks gestation than are found in the general population.

More recent studies agree on the importance of acquired prenatal factors, particularly intra-uterine growth retardation, in the aetiology of severe mental retardation and cerebral palsy. Sabel et al (1976) in Sweden found that babies with intra-uterine malnutrition were the major remaining group at risk of these handicaps, two thirds of the children affected being recruited from the 16% of children with birth weights more than one standard deviation below the mean for their gestation. Similar findings have emerged from retrospective Swedish (Hagberg 1978) and Scottish (Drillien 1978) studies. Babies with a low birth weight appropriate for gestational age and an uncomplicated history do not seem to run a special risk of severe mental retardation (Gustavson et al 1977a) and there has been a striking reduction in the incidence of spastic diplegia in this group (Ch. 11.)

Many drugs taken in pregnancy can have teratogenic effects and give rise to microcephaly and retardation in addition to abnormalities in many other systems. Anticonvulsants, Warfarin, aminopterin (Smith 1976) and alcohol (Robinson 1980, Little & Streissguth 1981) are implicated in specific syndromes of fetal malformation when taken in the early weeks of pregnancy. Anticonvulsant effects are particularly important. In the case of phenytoin, which has been incriminated more often than other drugs, the effect may be mediated by folic acid deficiency; the teratogenic effect of folic acid antagonists such as aminopterin and methotrexate in man is well known, and in rats folate deficiency can cause cleft lip and palate. Unfortunately the critical period occurs very early in pregnancy so that the damage has probably been done before it is realised that the epileptic woman is pregnant. A dysmorphic syndrome with retardation and a typical facial appearance has been described in children exposed to tridione (Troxidone) in pregnancy.

Alcohol fetopathy is being recognised increasingly as an important cause of mental retardation and chronic neurological handicap. Its incidence probably varies from one community to another. In a recent survey from Sweden (Hagberg et al 1981) of 91 children with mild mental retardation (with IQs between 50 and 70) alcohol fetopathy was considered to account for 8% of cases. This horrifying statistic is likely to be matched in some other communities and must prompt educational measures aimed at prevention. Bacchus is no friend to the unborn. Smoking and drinking commonly go together, so the fetus is often exposed to two adverse influences.

PERINATAL CAUSES

Obstetric problems such as prolonged and difficult delivery with fetal distress and neonatal asphyxia have figured prominently in the past histories of many children with mental subnormality and other chronic neurological handicaps. In some cases the causal relationship seems certain but in others it is speculative. Often the handicaps are of multifactorial origin, with maternal factors, such as malnutrition, short stature, infections and smoking contributing to varying and imponderable degrees. Improvements in such maternal factors and in standards of obstetric and neonatal care have led to a marked reduction in handicaps related to perinatal brain damage. This has particularly affected cerebral palsy with reduction in total numbers per 1000 live births most marked in the 'spastic-ataxic diplegic' syndromes (Hagberg 1975). The perinatal contribution to a severely retarded series of 122 Swedish children was 10% (Gustavson et al 1977b). Ten of these children had suffered asphyxia and/or intracranial haemorrhage in the perinatal period. Two children were retarded as a sequel to neonatal infections of the CNS. Low birth weight was not a factor unless associated with additional adverse circumstances. Other recent studies have agreed in showing only a small contribution from perinatal problems (Drillien 1978).

The prevention of handicap caused by perinatal problems is clearly linked with improved obstetric techniques, resulting in less hypoxia and trauma, and improved neonatal care with reduction in hypoxia, acidosis, hypothermia, hypoglycaemia, hyperbilirubinaemia and other biochemical abnormalities. Early feeding has also been an important factor in the improved outlook for babies of very low birth weight.

POST-NATAL CAUSES

The contribution of post-natal factors to the causation of mental subnormality and other neurological handicaps has decreased in the developed countries with improvements in nutrition, housing, hygiene and paediatric care. Post-natal factors accounted for between 1 and 12% in 5 recent epidemiological studies of severe mental retardation (Laxova et al 1976, Hagberg 1978). The list of postnatal factors capable of damaging the brain in infancy and childhood and causing intellectual impairment is similar to the list of serious diseases occurring in this epoch. Infective, traumatic and toxic conditions all contribute. Bacterial meningitis and its complications, (subdural effusion and hydrocephalus), encephalitis, cerebral abscess and dehydrating illness are important infective causes. Some of the infections which can damage the brain in fetal life may also do so after birth (see Ch. 22). Subdural haematoma and intracranial bleeding due to trauma including non-accidental injury may be followed by severe retardation and microcephaly or hydrocephalus. Repeated trauma, which may be associated with anaemia, fractures of the skull and other bones, malnutrition and emotional deprivation, carries a particularly poor prognosis for mental development. This is a special hazard for the children of parents with Huntington's chorea (Ch. 8) and infants who are in some way already abnormal, with slow development and posing management problems for their parents, are also at risk. Craniostenosis when severe enough to restrict growth of the brain may result in mental retardation if untreated or unsuccessfully treated. Progressive hydrocephalus from any cause may be followed by mental deterioration, quite apart from the developmental effects of the causal condition (intra-uterine infection, subarachnoid bleeding). Recurrent hypoglycaemia and status epilepticus from any cause may be followed by mental impairment. The syndrome of infantile spasms is an example of mental impairment associated with fits

in infancy (Ch. 12): though many cases are cryptogenic, the mental handicap is probably related to the causal disease rather than to the seizures themselves. Chronic lead poisoning may be a cause of mental retardation, (apart from causing acute encephalopathy) but the relationship is obscured by the fact that many retarded children have pica and so eat lead-containing material which may aggravate the retardation.

THE DIAGNOSIS OF MENTAL SUBNORMALITY

There are two problems in the process of diagnosis The first is the recognition that mental subnormality is, or may be present. The second, having decided that it is present, is to define the cause when possible.

THE RECOGNITION OF MENTAL SUBNORMALITY

In a few syndromes associated with mental retardation the diagnosis of the syndrome may be made or suspected by the recognition of clinical features in the infant at birth, and the doctor is thereby alerted to the strong possibility of subsequent subnormality. Examples are Down's syndrome and other chromosomal anomalies, cretinism (Fig. 13.4) microcephaly, hydrocephalus, obvious forms of cerebral maldevelopment, certain intra-uterine infections and tuberose sclerosis, (if the typical amelanotic naevi are detected early, which is unusual). In other cases the history shows severe abnormalities in the prenatal, perinatal or postnatal period and early examination shows evidence of dysfunction of the CNS in the form of irritability, tremulousness, seizures, apathy, overactivity, breathing difficulties, an abnormal cry, hypo-or hypertonia, or weakness of one or more limbs. Apart from these gross neurological abnormalities the pattern of neonatal postural automatisms may be aberrant, responses such as the Moro, palmar and plantar grasp, positive supporting, automatic walking, crossed extension (see Ch. 1) being absent or depressed to a level appropriate for an earlier stage of gestation. Some workers have

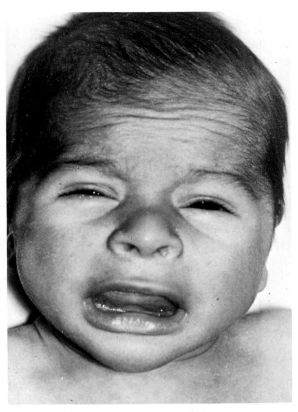

Fig. 13.4 Cretinism. Congenital hypothyroidism (untreated) in 4-month-old boy

claimed that a high correlation exists between the finding of neurological abnormalities in the newborn period and later abnormality but other studies have suggested that these physical signs have a poor predictive value for abnormality detected at one year of age (Donovan et al 1962). It is certainly wise to be guarded in giving a prognosis with a history of prenatal or perinatal problems and in the presence of abnormal neurological signs of conventional type or abnormal neonatal postural responses, but it is seldom justified to be dogmatic. Indeed the premature assumption of subnormality, even though it may prove later to be justified by events, is tactically unwise, since to deny hope to parents in this way may seriously affect the delicate 'bonding' process between mother (and father) and child, jeopardising his development in another way, and may even lead to outright parental rejection.

The 'test of time' is an essential ingredient in resolving the inevitable doubts: time is needed before one can see whether or not the child's development is progressing normally and sometimes a long period of observation is needed. As Illingworth (1960) has emphasised, the essential principle in the early diagnosis of mental retardation is the fact that the mentally retarded child is backward in *all* fields of development, except occasionally in gross motor development and rarely in sphincter control. He is relatively less retarded in gross motor development than in other fields, unless there is an associated mechanical difficulty such as cerebral palsy. He is relatively more retarded in speech, and in the interest he shows in his surroundings, in concentration, alertness and promptness of response.

Conventional neurological signs, such as disorders of tone, power, tendon reflexes, cerebellar ataxia and involuntary movements are lacking in many mentally subnormal children and, when present, are evidence of additional neurological dysfunction usually constituting cerebral palsy in its various forms. In the subnormal child without such dysfunction, examination generally shows a pattern of neurological performance appropriate for a younger child and consistent with the history of delayed developmental milestones. At the severest level and earliest stage, a full term newborn baby may be totally lacking in the expected repertoire of neonatal postural responses or an older infant may behave like a neonate. In later months persistence of certain automatic responses such as the Moro may provide additional evidence of abnormality to complement the obvious failure to achieve motor milestones such as head control, independent sitting, reaching and grasping, rolling over, crawling etc. and to develop social and speech skills. Persistence of hand regard, the child gazing for long periods at his own hand, beyond the age of one year is often a sign of subnormality. The late development and undue persistence of a normal pattern such as the 'index approach' to an object with prodding forefinger, normally present at ten months of age, indicates that the child is functioning at this lower level.

The patterns of sleeping and feeding of the mentally retarded child are often grossly abnormal, the infant sleeping far more than usual and never crying. The description 'a very good baby' for this situation often occurs in the early histories of subnormal children: silence in this case is not golden. Illingworth (1960) quotes the comments of mothers of severely defective children in their early weeks: 'he never cried', 'we didn't know we had him', 'she seemed to live in a world of her own'. The child may not demand his feeds in the usual way and may have difficulty in sucking and trouble with regurgitation. His lack of social responsiveness may sometimes give a false impression of deafness or blindness in the first year of life, although it later becomes clear that the child can hear and see but has earlier simply failed to react in the usual way to the stimuli. This social unresponsiveness may also sometimes give rise to a wrong diagnosis of infantile autism.

In the older retarded child a pattern of motor immaturity is often seen with a persistence of synkinetic movements, choreiform movements of the outstretched hands and difficulty with discrete finger movements and rapidly alternating movements appropriate for a much younger child. The performance of these children in gross motor tasks such as jumping, hopping, standing on one foot, tapping the feet on the floor, walking on toes and heels and in manipulative tests may resemble that of a child of half their age, though there is no defect detectable on more 'formal' neurological examination. An easily elicited age-dependent sign of motor immaturity is given by the Fog test. Here the child is asked to stand on the outer sides of his feet and the movements of his arms and hands are noted. Most normal children show marked supination of the forearms under 10 years of age but rarely above this age. Such signs of motor immaturity are not confined to the mentally retarded but may be seen also in children whose normal intelligence contrasts with their poor motor performance, so that they are sometimes classed as clumsy children and regarded as having 'minimal cerebral dysfunction' or 'minimal brain damage' (Ch. 15).

Observation of the spontaneous play activity of mentally handicapped children can give valuable insights into their level of functioning. The late Mary Sheridan defined play as 'the eager engagement in pleasurable physical or mental effort to obtain emotional satisfaction'. Her graphic illustra-tions of spontaneous play in normal and handicapped children (Sheridan 1977) with their detailed captions provide a delightful guide to this important aspect of development.

Clinical pitfalls in mental retardation

Pitfalls abound in the diagnosis of mental retardation, both in the direction of not recognising it and of suspecting it incorrectly.

A common source of error is failure to appreciate the variation in normal developmental milestones. In many families the children tend to walk, to talk, or to become dry and clean at later ages than are regarded as normal, but nonetheless master all these skills perfectly in time. Undue reliance on gross motor milestones such as walking may prevent retardation from being recognised, since this may be within normal limits in a child whose delay in social and speech skills betokens severe subnormality.

'Pseudo-retardation' may result from lack of opportunity and stimulation in a normal child living in deprived circumstances, perhaps cared for by a baby-minder who is responsible for several children who spend all day in one room with minimal attention. The children of sick, depressed and otherwise mentally disturbed parents may give a false impression of dullness and lack of interest which is rapidly corrected when they are exposed to the interest and affection of and stimulation by an involved adult. This picture was previously seen, unhappily, in children in long stay hospitals and institutions. Clues are usually found in watching the interaction between child and parents: more visible clues may be seen in the scars or bruises of trauma in the child victim of 'non-accidental injury'. A similar pseudo-retardation may be seen in children with severe medical illness, such as heart disease or syndromes with malabsorption and malnutrition, in which prolonged stay in hospital may also be a factor. (When a child's development seems to blossom in the artificial setting of a hospital ward when he is admitted for investigation of developmental delay it is wise to consider whether his home environment may fall short of the ideal, in lack of love and stimulation or even calories.)

The child who is deaf or has poor vision may be

wrongly thought to be mentally subnormal because he fails to respond normally to stimuli. These sensory defects may also co-exist with subnormality but be unrecognised. They should always be positively considered and excluded so that help may be given. The child with a severe physical handicap such as gross dyskinetic or athetoid cerebral palsy with deafness and difficulty with speech may be wrongly regarded as dull, and particular care should be taken in assessing his intellectual status and checking for auditory and visual defects. The dull-looking, expressionless face of many children with myopathies, such as congenital dystrophia myotonica, may wrongly suggest mental subnormality; careful psychometry must form part the comprehensive assessment in such cases.

Childhood autism may be confused with mental subnormality and the reverse may occur. This psychosis is much rarer than mental subnormality. Most autistic children show some degree of mental retardation, and conversely autistic traits and mannerisms are very common in retarded children. There is a tendency among parents of subnormal children, and perhaps their doctors also, to prefer a diagnosis of autism, as if it were a lesser and more respectable evil. In many children so labelled the justification for this is minimal and the strength with which the label is grasped indicates the difficulty the parents have in accepting the true situation.

Finally developmental assessment itself and the assignment of a developmental or intelligence quotient may be misleading if this figure is regarded as fixed and immutable. The difficulties in accurate assessment of young children are immense. IQs may be underestimated or overestimated. Many factors, such as the state of health of the child at the time, the occurrence of unrecognized seizures, the effect of drugs, physiological factors such as state of tiredness or alertness, powers of concentration and distractibility, rapport with the psychologist, anxiety or tension in the child, his parents or the psychologist, may conspire to cause his potential to be underestimated. There is often doubt about the results of an assessment and it may need to be repeated at a later date. Parents are rightly concerned if they feel that an assessment, on the results of which important decisions

depend, may have been unreliable. These problems are discussed more fully in Chapter 14.

INVESTIGATION INTO THE CAUSE OF MENTAL RETARDATION

Investigation should be directed particularly towards excluding recognizable genetic disorders. Though these account for only a small fraction of cases in most series, the implications for parents are so important that this priority is very high. Careful examination for cutaneous or other stigmata of tuberose sclerosis or other neurocutaneous syndromes is needed. Biochemical tests for the aminoacidurias, organic acidurias and mucopolysaccharidoses allow detection of these metabolic, genetic disorders in some of which (phenylketonuria, homocystinuria and some organic acidurias) dietary treatment may be helpful. It is essential to exclude hypothyroidism since it is one of the few treatable diseases causing retardation: neonatal population screening for congenital hypothyroidism is the ideal preventive measure. Serological tests and culture of urine for CMV are needed in the younger child to exclude intrauterine infections, whether or not there are clinical pointers to these.

The EEG in general is not of great help in the investigation of mental retardation. Commonly it shows a pattern of rhythms appropriate for a younger age. More specific features may be seen in patients with epilepsy, hemiplegia and other forms of cerebral palsy, but these are not diagnostic.

Plain skull X-rays should be taken and may be helpful in showing calcification suggestive of tuberose sclerosis, the Sturge-Weber syndrome or intra-uterine infections. Special X-rays are not usually indicated in the investigation of mental retardation. In the past many retarded children were subjected to pneumo-encephalography but the diagnostic yield was low, cerebral atrophy being the commonest finding with neither aetiological, genetic nor clear prognostic implications (Brett & Hoare 1969). A major malformation of the brain such as agenesis of the corpus callosum or septo-optic dysplasia, or a porencephalic cyst may be shown. The CT scan allows these to be recognized easily with less risk to the patient, and may also show calcification, not visible on plain X-rays, which may be of diagnostic value.

Chromosome analysis is indicated in subnormal children in whom dysmorphic features suggest a chromosomal anomaly.

COUNSELLING THE FAMILY OF THE MENTALLY SUBNORMAL CHILD

Helping the parents of the mentally handicapped child calls for patience and tact. The idea of *any* handicap in their child is tragic and painful for parents, but the limitations on development implied by mental retardation make this handicap particularly distressing. The situation is sometimes all too clear at birth or at an early age, as with easily recognizable disorders such as Down's syndrome, and the parents will then have to cope early with the emotions of guilt, anger, resentment and sometimes rejection, and with the process of mourning for the normal child they have wanted and have lost. Most parents manage in a remarkable way to adjust to the situation and to accept it in large measure, (though perhaps never completely) so that the child becomes part of the family and as precious as, or perhaps even more so than his normal siblings.

More often the possibility of mental retardation is not recognized until some months or even years have passed when concern is felt because the child is clearly not making the expected progress. In the case of a first child, parents may not become anxious until later since they have no yardstick with which to measure his progress. It is then sometimes a grandparent, a doctor in an infant welfare clinic, a health visitor or a nurse who first feels and voices concern, which leads to referral to hospital for specialist advice. Often it is possible at first referral to see that the child's development is indeed far from normal, but sometimes there is uncertainty and he may appear possibly to be 'within normal limits', recognising how wide these limits may be. Even when the doctor feels confident that the child is mentally subnormal at first attendance, it is probably wise to avoid being dogmatic at this stage, but to acknowledge that there is cause for some concern and that careful observation will be needed. When

there is room for doubt, unqualified reassurance should *not* be given, and can militate against acceptance of the true situation as this becomes clearer. As a significant lag develops between the actual and expected performance it becomes easier for the parents to recognise and accept the situation than if they are suddenly presented with a categorical and, to them brutal, statement that their child is abnormal.

The concept of mental age can often be usefully introduced at his stage and can help towards an acceptance of the facts. Many parents, especially those with normal children for comparison, will assess the mental age of the retarded child fairly accurately. Even if they overestimate it, the recognition of a lag and its possible significance is a step in the right direction.

The personality and attitudes of the parents must be considered in the approach to be adopted. Some parents will be well aware of the truth and would resent anything but complete frankness, while others may need months or years before they seem able to accept the truth and its full implications. Others will seek frantically and pathetically for alternative explanations and will embrace the diagnosis of 'infantile autism', which is often misapplied to the subnormal child as it were a talisman. In their desire for a physical explanation some parents will be distressed to be told that their child does *not* have cerebral palsy or a neuromuscular disorder (and this reaction may strike the inexperienced doctor as bizarre and contrary, making it more difficult for him to communicate with them in a helpful way). Second opinions may be sought repeatedly in the hope that a more favourable and acceptable opinion will be given. No paediatrician should feel aggrieved that parents should want to have another opinion, but the hazards of multiple opinions are well known: even though the opinion given will usually be the same, it will often be expressed differently and will all too often be interpreted as different. Lack of time for discussion is undoubtedly a factor of importance. Repeated discussions are often needed and experience has shown that parents often take in little of what is said at an initial interview and that it must be reinforced by repetition. The help of an experienced medical social worker can be invaluable in such situations, and it is essential that all those involved, both medical and para-medical, should be fully aware of the medical facts and should speak with one voice. Well-meaning but ill-informed grandparents may be a factor making parental acceptance more difficult. As with epilepsy, many myths and misunderstandings surround the subject of mental subnormality in the lay mind. Mental handicap may be equated by parents or others with insanity and with the inevitable later development of problems of delinquency and of physical and sexual aggression. As with epilepsy also, parents should be encouraged to voice these fears so that they may allayed.

Every effort must be made to discuss the problems with both parents together: it is rarely justified to place the burden of knowledge or doubt on one parent alone, and when a father seems, as often happens, to be opting out of the situation, tactful efforts are needed to share the discussion with him. His absence from home for long periods may make it difficult for him to appreciate the reality, but may also be an escape mechanism to avoid painful confrontation with the facts.

At an early stage it is important to exclude the presence of any other defect such as cerebral palsy or sensory deficits such as blindness and deafness which might simulate mental retardation or — more commonly — coexist with it. Even a minor hearing defect may be enough to prevent a mentally retarded child from developing normal speech. If poor vision from myopia can be helped by suitable glasses, this aid should not be overlooked or witheld, no matter how difficult if may be to ensure the glasses are worn. An uncorrected squint may add to a child's problems by increasing the risks of social rejection, and treatment in some cases may be justified on cosmetic grounds.

With mental handicap, as with all neurological deficits in childhood, parents feel a great need to know, not only 'Why has this happened to us?' (an unanswerable question), but also what is the cause, scientifically speaking, for their child's condition. In most cases an aetiology is not found: this uncertainty is unsettling and hard to accept and in part explains the search for further opinions. Parents may feel that if only a cause *could* be found some specific treatment could be applied. The doctor knows that this is rarely the case and must explain

that few of the possible causes are treatable, but that he will ensure that these are not overlooked. A more important reason for a thorough search for the cause is to exclude genetic disorders so that accurate advice can be given as to whether there is a risk of recurrence of the problem in further children. Most parents will voice this fear early on and, even if they do not, the question must be raised and answered as far as possible. Identification of a clear genetic disorder, such as phenylketonuria or tuberose sclerosis with stigmata in a parent, allows a precise risk to be given. Similarly the diagnosis of a non-genetic cause, such as intra-uterine CMV infection or toxoplasmosis or of tuberose sclerosis with *no* stigmata in either parent allows reassurance to be given on the genetic risks. Cerebral malformations generally suggest a slightly increased risk of recurrence of the order of 3 or 4% (Ch. 21).

PRACTICAL HELP FOR THE FAMILY

The problems posed by the mentally handicapped child must be seen in the context of his family as a whole and much time and support must be given to his parents. Sometimes they need to be dissuaded from altering their entire way of life in a vain attempt at cure, either by concentrating on treating him at home according to an intensive scheme which prevents any family life or by uprooting themselves to move to an area where they believe effective treatment is available. Sometimes both parents or the mother will focus on the abnormal child to the neglect and detriment of his normal siblings, and even of the marriage.

The material and financial implications of mental handicap for the family may be profound. A mother who would otherwise be able to earn money by working outside the home is unable to do so, with resultant reduction in living standards. The employment of the father may even be affected. Additional, unexpected expenses, such as provision of extra clothing and napkins (diapers), laundry costs and payment of a 'baby minder' to look after the child while his mother goes out shopping or takes his siblings to school, may affect the family budget. The recent introduction of the attendance allowance and mobility allowance to help with the financial and transport problems of handicapped children in the United Kingdom is a welcome recognition of these needs, but in some cases further financial support must be sought from charitable agencies. The doctor should be prepared to fight for such help for his patients, who usually have few other champions.

The maternal instinct, though adequate in most cases for the successful rearing of normal offspring, is often not enough for the management of mentally handicapped child. It is not surprising that parents need help and advice and that opinions vary among the 'experts'.

Apart from the essential emotional adjustment to the slowness of their child's development, parents need to adjust to it also intellectually, so that they can recognise its implications for management. Instead of seeing a child develop a new skill, such as partially dressing himself, over a short period with only limited instruction and example, they must accept that this milestone will only be reached slowly with repeated efforts and assistance. Perseverance and patient repetition are the keynotes of learning for the mentally handicapped. Dressing and undressing need to be broken down into steps which are mastered one by one on the way to full acquisition of these skills. Conditioning is used to promote this process, the child being regularly rewarded by a kiss, a cuddle, a word of praise or a sweet soon after he has achieved the desired goal. He cannot usually cope with prolonged activity of any one kind, becoming tired and losing interest in it after the fourth or fifth reprise, and the recipe must be 'little and often' to be effective. A structured pattern of activities usually lends itself better to this than an entirely free and easy regime in which it is less easy consciously to exploit the opportunities for learning. Concrete rather than conceptual learning is an important principle in teaching the handicapped. Abstractions are to be avoided, and rote learning, for example the meaningless counting which some parents encourage in their child and quote as evidence of intelligence, is undesirable. To count to 20 while not appreciating the meaning of 'twoness' is an empty skill. Time is better spent in exploiting the opportunities provided by his own body and those of his parents for learning the ideas of two and of 'my' and 'Johnny's' attributes: two hands, two feet, two eyes, two ears, my nose, my mouth, Johnny's teeth etc.

Toys should be simple and strong, safe and cheap. An expensive teddy bear with detachable eyes which may be swallowed by a child is unsuitable: a ball, a box or cup from which he can take objects and replace them and wooden blocks are more valuable. A simple form-board or jig-saw puzzle is more suitable than a complex one, but progressively more complex models can be supplied as skills increase so that the child is challenged and 'stretched'.

Thought must be given to the position of the child who cannot yet walk, or perhaps even sit alone, because of mental subnormality or an additional motor handicap such as cerebral palsy. Special chairs with a firm support for head and back and a tray where toys can be manipulated may be very helpful and this posture is obviously preferable to lying prone or supine or crumpled up with chin on chest in a chair without support. Many parents show great ingenuity in designing equipment for their children, given a little guidance.

Difficult, destructive and antisocial behaviour in the retarded child may pose great problems for his parents or the other attendants. Temper tantrums, a normal feature in the younger child, may persist in the older retarded child who is backward emotionally as well as intellectually. These may be a potent weapon used to manipulate his parents to do his will and satisfy his every whim — for constant attention, food, drink, other consumer goods or access to the parental bed. Life for the entire family may be disrupted by the tyranny of temper tantrums when the undesirable behaviour pattern is reinforced by regular rewards. This state should be avoided or rectified when it has been reached, by a firmer approach in which the child's outburst does not lead automatically to gratification but may instead cause withdrawal of the desired privileges and temporary removal, for instance, from the living room.

Self-injury may be a serious problem in the mentally subnormal. Repetitive head-banging at night against the cotside or wall may result, even with padding, in disturbed nights for other members of the family and bruising of the scalp; fortunately it very rarely causes serious harm and parents can be reassured that brain damage does not result. Pulling out and swallowing of hair by a child may alarm his parents: though a trichobezoar may result in the stomach, serious complications are rare. Their fingers and lips may be bitten by retarded children, sometimes to an extent which raises suspicion of the Lesch-Nyhan syndrome (Ch. 8) or a sensory neuropathy (Ch. 4). Masturbation is also common in the retarded child, and care is needed lest it provoke a scandalized uproar and the child learn to use it as a most effective device to gain attention. Physical restraint to prevent such behaviour patterns, though often used, is seldom helpful, and techniques of distraction and conditioning are more effective. Drug treatment is most unlikely to help with these problems.

PICA

Pica, or perverted appetite (the Latin word 'pica', meaning a magpie, refers to a voracious appetite for unsuitable material), with the ingestion of substances usually regarded as inedible, is a common problem in subnormal children, though it may also affect those of normal intelligence who are bored, deprived or disturbed. Apart from the risk of mechanical injury to the stomach or intestines from objects swallowed, its main danger is that of lead poisoning from the ingestion of lead-containing material, such as old paint on window-sills and cots, or plastic toys. (The sources of lead are discussed in Chapter 18.) Lead poisoning has been well reviewed by Chisholm (1970) and Rutter (1980). Chronic ill-health can result with anorexia and anaemia. Acute encephalopathy, with raised intracranial pressure, brain damage and convulsions, is a less common but serious effect. (Ch. 18) Acute deterioration in a retarded child may result in this way from pica, and it is probable that some normal children may become retarded from the same cause.

Bicknell (1973), in her series of 15 children with severe pica, found that it did not develop after the age of 4, but could persist for up to 11 years. She found that parents and professional workers consulted, including doctors, seemed remarkably ignorant of the dangers of the habit. Barltrop (1975) found that the hazards of lead poisoning in general were less appreciated in Britain than in the United States. Bicknell points out that the retarded child who has not learned to communicate

but is mobile enough to explore his environment persists in using his mouth far beyond the age at which oral exploration is normal, partly to relieve his frustration and boredom. The cessation of pica often coincides with an improvement in the ability to communicate and the development of sophisticated play. Lead poisoning must always be considered in any retarded child with coma, convulsions or acute encephalopathy.

Poisoning from ingestion of drugs, (aspirin, tranquillisers, anti-convulsants, iron tablets) is also commoner in the retarded child than the normal, and the same is true of accidents generally (Williams 1973).

Stereotyped and repetitive behaviour patterns are common in severely subnormal children (Mitchell & Etches 1977). They include rocking, tapping the teeth, twiddling or braiding the fingers, playing incessantly with a piece of string or paper, and moving rapidly round in circles. These patterns are also seen as part of a more complex disorder in children with the syndrome of infantile autism and are often described as 'autistic features'. They are sometimes so prominent that the diagnosis of autism is incorrectly applied to retarded children. Parents may regard this label as more acceptable than one of mental retardation, feeling that it carries less stigma and a more hopeful prognosis. Hyperkinetic behaviour is seen in many retarded children and may make their management more difficult for all concerned.

In the severely subnormal child who is immobile, these troublesome physical behaviour difficulties do not arise, but problems of bed sores and infections, particularly of the chest and renal tract, may be prominent.

EDUCATION

The schooling of the subnormal child often causes grave concern to his parents. At an early stage the idea of his attending any but a normal school is unacceptable to them. This is often a reflexion of their inability to acknowledge the extent of his limitations. They will sometimes express concern that he will pick up bad habits from other retarded children or be upset by the idea of his mixing with children who are obviously different in appearance from normal. 'Mongol' children, who are the most easily identifiable group in schools for the subnormal, tend to be singled out for disapproving mention. In time most parents will recognise that a normal school is not suitable for their child, who would be out of his depth there, and that he will only receive the extra help he needs in a special school. In helping them to accept the situation it is useful to stress the importance of his receiving this extra help and the frustration and unhappiness he will suffer if expected to conform to a standard of work and behaviour of which he is incapable, and to sit quietly in class attending to formal lessons when this is beyond him. Sometimes it is helpful to parents to see how a child's self-esteem and happiness can benefit from being among the *better* performers in a group rather than being invariably a failure. The large size of the classes in many normal schools is a factor which parents can appreciate as harmful for the child who needs more individual attention. Nonetheless some parents are unable to accept the situation and may insist on normal schooling. Usually a trial of this will help them to see that it is not a success and to accept the alternative offered where the better adjustment and progress generally confirm its greater suitability. Often a retarded child has started in a normal school because his limitations have not been recognised and the problems resulting from his inability to conform and to meet the demands made usually prompt referral for assessment and advice on alternative placement.

In the United Kingdom since 1971 all children including the severely subnormal, who were previously regarded as unsuitable for education, have come into the compass of the national educational system and there is a statutory obligation to provide appropriate education for them. For most subnormal children education starts at the age of 5 years or soon after, but there is evidence that attendance at a suitable nursery school from an earlier age is beneficial for them, as it is for normal children. At or near school age decisions are taken as to the most appropriate school based on assessment of intellectual and physical status. Sometimes the presence of physical handicaps such as severe cerebral palsy or spina bifida, or defects of vision or hearing make it impossible to provide for all the needs of a handicapped child in one centre and difficult decisions

on priorities must be made. The needs of the severely subnormal child with severe cerebral palsy are among those least well catered for.

It is sometimes desirable for subnormal children attending special schools to remain after the usual age of leaving, which in the United Kingdom is 16, since their potential for learning may improve at this age (Brand et al 1969). On leaving school formal education usually ceases for the mentally handicapped. Their placement will vary according to the degree of their handicap. Most ESN (M) children are capable of employment in simple, gainful occupations, although high unemployment rates will often prevent them from finding jobs. For the severely subnormal, especially those with an additional handicap, the outlook is bleaker. In the United Kingdom places are usually available in Sheltered Workshops or Adult Training Centres, in which supervised work, necessarily simple and repetitive, gives opportunities for social contacts, regular routine, a small wage and — perhaps most important — a sense of self-esteem and of having a place in the community.

In the past provision for the severely subnormal adolescent or adult who cannot remain at home has usually been in mental subnormality hospitals, with a small number of beds available in hostels. More recently a trend has developed towards smaller units, such as those run by the Wessex Regional Hospital Board, for 20 to 25 individuals where it is hoped staff may be used more economically with closer relationships between staff, patients and their families, and avoidance of the worst effects of 'institutionalization'. The ideal solution has not yet been found, but more flexible and imaginative plans of this kind seem promising.

PREVENTION OF MENTAL RETARDATION

It is widely agreed that about 75% of cases of severe mental retardation, with or without neurological deficit, have their origin prenatally (Laxova et al 1977, Alberman 1978, Drillien 1978, Hagberg 1978) and that the contribution of perinatal factors is less important than in the case of cerebral palsy. Nonetheless there is room for improvement in obstetric and neonatal care in many regions. The impressive reduction in infant mortality and morbidity which can result from centralization of services, improvement of standards and encouragement of full use of obstetric and paediatric facilities indicate the need to ensure a more uniform spread of excellence in these fields.

The main scope for prevention is in the disorders of prenatal origin. For the purely genetically determined conditions the only form of prevention may be for women known to be at high risk to avoid conception, or for termination of pregnancy when an affected fetus is diagnosed. Cases of maternal infection may be prevented by immunization of girls before child-bearing age and termination if immunization fails. This approach is adopted with rubella and may be possible with cytomegalovirus.

For Down's syndrome, which accounts for about one third of all cases of severe subnormality, a reduction in incidence could be achieved by a lowering of the age at delivery since high maternal age is the most important risk factor. In Sweden Gustavson et al (1977c) have shown that this has occurred. In the northern county of Västerbotten there was a marked fall in the incidence of severe mental retardation due mainly to a reduction in cases of Down's syndrome, correlated with a decrease in mean maternal age at delivery. This approach is clearly far more 'cost-effective' than a programme of prenatal diagnosis with termination when the fetus is affected.

Some idea of the potential for prevention can be obtained from Alberman's (1978) analysis of the figures in a study of 146 severely retarded children born in Hertfordshire between 1965 and 1967 by Laxova et al (1977) (Table 13.1). She calculated that had these children been born today (or next year) the numbers of this group *might* have been reduced by 30 (20.5%). Children with Down's syndrome made up about one third of the total and offered the best field for prevention, with 9 theoretically preventable cases, based on an estimated 20% of mothers aged 40 years and over. Genetic conditions with a family history contributed 5 cases and cerebral palsy with birth complications 6. Five cases each of postnatal conditions and neural tube defects completed the list. Only one of the cases was due to phenylketonuria, a disease in the prevention of which much effort and expense has been invested.

Table 13.1 (From Alberman 1978) Possibly preventable conditions as estimated from the Hertfordshire study (Laxova et al. 1977)

'Preventable cases'	No. of cases
20% of Down's syndrome (estimated proportion in mothers aged 40+)	9
Genetic conditions with family history	5
Cerebral palsy with birth complications	6
Post-vaccination encephalitis Meningitis Rubella syndrome Cardiac arrest during exchange transfusion	5
Neural tube defects (excluding sibs after 1 affected case)	5
Total 'preventable' cases	30 (20.5%)
Remaining cases	116 (79.5%)

Congenital hypothyroidism offers scope for the prevention of mental retardation since the prognosis for intellectual development appears best in children treated from very early in life (Fig. 13.4). National screening programmes have been introduced in several countries. A pilot screening programme of 87 444 babies over a period of one year in the UK detected 26 cases of primary congenital hypothyroidism, giving an incidence of 1 in 3363. Only two of these had already been diagnosed on clinical grounds (Hulse et al 1980). Single dried blood spots, already available for Guthrie tests, were used for thyroid-stimulating hormone (TSH) assay. In the area screened the diagnosis by clinical methods has often been delayed, only 40% of cases being recognized before three months of age, and a similar pattern is seen in other European countries. The recently published report of the New England Congenital Hypothyroidism Collaborative (1981) on the prevention of mental retardation by treatment before clinical signs appear is most encouraging. Sixty-three infants with hypothyroidism diagnosed by neonatal screening and treated at the age of 25 ± 15 days had a mean score on the Stanford-Binet of 106 ± 16, compared with a figure of 106 ± 15 for 18 normal siblings and 39 euthyroid children. It seems clear that screening for congenital hypothyroidism linked to Guthrie screening for PKU on a national basis would greatly improve the prognosis for the affected children.

Alcohol

The dangers of alcohol during pregnancy have been stressed. Education of the public is essential in view of the Swedish experience (Hagberg et al 1981) of the substantial contribution of alcohol fetopathy to mild mental retardation. Smoking should also be discouraged in pregnancy.

ABNORMALITIES OF GROWTH IN CHILDREN WITH MENTAL RETARDATION

Many mentally retarded children are shorter and lighter than their peers of normal intelligence. Low birth weight and very short stature are constant features of certain rare mental retardation syndromes in which various dysmorphic features occur in diagnostic constellations. Microcephaly is common. These syndromes are well described and classified by Smith (1976). Some show autosomal recessive inheritance (e.g. Seckel syndrome of 'bird-headed dwarfism', and Smith-Lemli-Opitz syndrome) but many are sporadic (de Lange and Rubinstein-Taybi syndromes).

By contrast a few retarded children show 'gigantism' with early overgrowth and various associated defects.

Sotos syndrome or 'cerebral gigantism' is the best known of these syndromes. Affected children already show excessive weight and length at birth with a mean birth weight of 3.9 kg. Their growth is especially rapid in the first few years with a height age at 10 years of age corresponding to 14 or 15 years. There is often macrocephaly with a prominent forehead, downward-slanting palpebral fissures and hypertelorism (an increased distance between the inner canthi of the eyes). Most affected children have been moderately or severely retarded. X-rays of the limbs show advanced bone age. The patients' ultimate height is usually below normal.

The facial appearance is unusual, the children with Sotos syndrome resembling one another more closely than their normal siblings.

The diagnosis is a clinical one since there are no diagnostic features on investigation. Air encephalography or the CT scan may show some cerebral atrophy or may be normal. The EEG may be abnormal, especially in the considerable proportion of patients who have seizures.

Most cases have been sporadic and the diagnosis is of some value in genetic counselling in suggesting that there are no implications for recurrence of the condition in further children.

REFERENCES

Alberman E 1978 Main causes of major mental handicap: prevalence and epidemiology: 3–12. In: Major mental handicap: methods and costs of prevention. Ciba Foundation Symposium 59 (New Series), Elsevier, Excerpta Medica, North Holland

American Academy of Mental Retardation 1973

Barker D J P 1966a Low intelligence and obstetric complications. British Journal of Preventive and Social Medicine 20: 15–21

Barker D J P 1966b Low intelligence. Its relation to length of gestation and rate of foetal growth. British Journal of Preventive and Social Medicine 20: 58–66

Barltrop D 1975 Chemical and physical environmental hazards for children. In: Barltrop D (ed) Paediatrics and the environment. Fellowship of Postgraduate Medicine

Bicknell D J 1973 An investigation into the aetiology and ill-effects of pica in childhood. Symposia 9, 10 and 11. In: Clayton B E (ed) Mental retardation: environmental hazards. Butterworths, London

Birch H G, Richardson S A, Baird D, Horobin G, Illsley R 1970 Mental subnormality in the community. Williams and Wilkins, Baltimore

Brand J, Shakespeare R, Woods G E 1969 Psychological development of the severely subnormal after 16 years of age. Developmental Medicine and Child Neurology 11: 783–785

Chisholm J J 1968 The use of chelating agents in the treatment of acute and chronic lead intoxication in childhood. Journal of Pediatrics 73: 1–38

Chisholm J J 1970 Poisoning due to heavy metals. In: Coleman A B, Alpert J J (eds), Pediatric clinics of North America. Poisoning in children. W B Saunders Company, Philadelphia vol 17, no 3

Chisholm J J 1973 Management of increased lead absorption and lead poisoning in children. New England Journal of Medicine 289: 1016–1018

Donovan D E, Coues P, Paine R S 1962 Diagnostic implications of neurologic abnormalities in the neonatal period. Neurology (Minneapolis) 12: 910–914

Drillien C M 1978 Aetiology of severe handicapping

conditions in early childhood (Dundee), 17–27. In: Major mental handicap: methods and costs of prevention. Ciba Foundation Symposium 59 (New Series) 1978, Elsevier, Excerpta Medica, North Holland, Amsterdam

Fox P, Fox D, Gerrard J W 1980 X-linked mental retardation: Renpenning revisited. American Journal of Medical Genetics 7: 491–496

Gerald P S 1980 (Editorial) X-linked mental retardation and an X-chromosome marker. New England Journal of Medicine 303: 696–697

Gustavson K-H, Hagberg B, Hagberg G, Sars K 1977a Severe mental retardation in a Swedish county. I. Epidemiology, gestational age, birth weight and associated CNS handicaps in children born 1959–1970. Acta paediatrica scandinavica 66: 373–379

Gustavson K-H, Hagberg B, Hagberg G, Sars K 1977b Severe mental retardation in a Swedish county. II. Etiologic and pathogenetic aspects of children born 1959–1970. Neuropädiatrie 8(3): 293–304

Gustavson K-H, Holmgren G, Jonsell R, Son Blomqvist H K 1977c Severe mental retardation in children in a northern Swedish county. Journal of Mental Deficiency Research 21: 161–180

Hagberg B 1975 Pre-, peri-, and postnatal prevention of major neuropediatric handicaps. Neuropädiatrie 6: 331–338

Hagberg G 1978 Severe mental retardation in Swedish children born 1959–70: epidemiological panorama and causative factors (Göteborg), 29–41

Hagberg B, Hagberg G, Lewerth A, Lindberg U 1981 Mild mental retardation in Swedish school children. II. Etiologic and pathogenic aspects. Acta paediatrica scandinavica 70: 445–452

Harvey J, Judge C, Wiener S 1977 Familial X-linked mental retardation with an X-chromosome abnormality. Journal of Medical Genetics 14: 46–50

Hulse J A, Grant D B, Clayton B E, Lilly P, Jackson D, Sprachlan A, et al 1980 Population screening for congenital hypothyroidism. British Medical Journal 280: 675–678

Illingworth R S 1960 The development of the infant and young child. Normal and abnormal. E & S Livingstone, Edinburgh

Ilvanainen M 1974 A study on the origins of mental retardation. Spastics International Medical Publications and Clinics in Developmental Medicine no 51 Heinemann, London

Kaveggia E G, Durkin M V, Pendleton E, Opitz J M 1973 Diagnostic/genetic studies on 1244 patients with severe mental retardation. Proceedings of the Third Congress of the International Association for the Scientific Study of Mental Deficiency. The Hague, Netherlands, 4th–12th Sept.

Laxova R, Ridler M A C, Bowen-Bravery M 1977 An aetiology survey of the severely retarded Hertfordshire children, who were born between 1 January 1965 and 31 January 1967. American Journal of Medical Genetics 1: 75–86

Little R E, Streissguth A P 1981 Effects of alcohol on the fetus: impact and prevention. Canadian Medical Association Journal 125: 159–164

Lubs H A 1969 A marker X-chromosome. American Journal of Human Genetics 21: 231–244

Martin J P, Bell J 1943 A pedigree of mental defect showing sex linkage. Journal of Neurology, Neurosurgery and Psychiatry 6: 154–157

Mitchell R, Etches P 1977 Rhythmic habit patterns (stereotypies). Developmental Medicine and Child Neurology 19: 545–550

New England Congenital Hypothyroidism Collaborative 1981. Effects of neonatal screening for hypothyroidism: prevention of mental retardation by treatment before clinical manifestations. Lancet 2: 1095–1098

Opitz J M, Kaveggia E G, Durkin-Stamm M V, Pendleton E 1978 Birth defects: Original Article Series. vol XIV, no 6B, 1–38

Pasamanick B, Lilienfeld A M 1955 Association of maternal and fetal factors with development of mental deficiency. 1. Abnormalities in the perinatal and paranatal periods. Journal of the American Medical Association 159: 155–160

Penrose L S 1938 A clinical and genetic study of 1280 cases of mental defect (special report series no 299). Medical Research Council, London

Priest J H, Thuline H C, Laveck G D, Jarvis D B 1961 An approach to genetic factors in mental retardation. Studies of families containing at least two siblings admitted to a state institution for the retarded. American Journal of Mental Deficiency 66: 42–50

Renpenning H, Gerrard J W, Zaleski W A, Tabata T 1962 Familial sex-linked mental retardation. Canadian Medical Association Journal 87: 954–956

Robinson R 1980 Fetal alcohol syndrome. Journal of Maternal and Child Health 5: 466–468

Rutter M 1980 Raised lead levels and impaired cognitive/behavioural functioning: a review of the evidence. Spastics International Medical Publications in association with William Heinemann Medical Books Ltd, J B Lippincott, Philadelphia (suppl No 42 to Developmental Medicine and Child Neurology, vol 22, No 1)

Sabel K-G, Olegard R, Victorin L 1976 Remaining sequelae with modern perinatal care. Pediatrics 57: 652–658

Sheridan Mary D 1977 Spontaneous play in early childhood, from birth to six years. National Foundation for Educational Research

Smith D 1976 Recognizable patterns of human malformation. In: Major problems in clinical pediatrics. W B Saunders Company, Philadelphia, vol VII

Smith D W, Bostian K E 1964 Congenital anomalies associated with idiopathic mental retardation. Frequency in contrast to frequency in controls, in children with cleft lip and palate, and in those with VSD. Journal of Pediatrics 65: 189–196

Stanbury J B, Wyngaarden J B, Fredrickson D S 1978 (eds) The metabolic basis of inherited disease, 4th edn. McGraw-Hill, New York

Sutherland G R 1977 Fragile sites on human chromosomes: demonstration of their dependence on the type of tissue culture medium. Science 197: 265–266

Sutherland G R 1979a Heritable fragile sites on human chromosomes. I. Factors affecting expression in lymphocyte culture. American Journal of Human Genetics 31: 125–135

Sutherland G R 1979b Heritable fragile sites of human chromosomes. II. Distribution, phenotypic effects, and cytogenetics. American Journal of Human Genetics 31: 136–148

Tredgold A F 1908 A textbook of mental deficiency. Bailliere, Tindall and Cox, London

Turner G, Daniel A, Frost M 1980a X-linked mental retardation, macro-orchidism and the Xq27 fragile site. Journal of Pediatrics 96: 837–841

Turner G, Brookwell R, Daniel A, Selikowitz M, Zilibowitz M 1980b Heterozygous expression of X-linked mental retardation and X-chromosome marker fra (X) (q27). New England Journal of Medicine 303: 662–664

Turner G, Turner B 1974 X-linked mental retardation. Journal of Medical Genetics 11: 109–113

Turner G, Turner B, Collins E 1971 X-linked mental retardation without physical abnormality: Renpenning's syndrome. Developmental Medicine and Child Neurology 13: 71–78

Vaizey M J, Sanders M D, Wybar K C, Wilson J 1977 Neurological abnormalities in congenital amaurosis of Leber: a review of 30 cases. Archives of Disease in Childhood 52: 399–402

Williams C E 1973 Accidents in mentally retarded children. Developmental Medicine and Child Neurology 15: 660–662

14

Psychological assessment or What's in an IQ?

M. E. Lobascher

Orandum est ut sit mens sana in corpore sano.

Juvenal, *Satires*

INTRODUCTION: HISTORICAL BACKGROUND

The evolution of the mental testing movement must be seen within the context of the philosophical, religious, scientific and political movements of the day, for it was these which forged and determined social attitudes to the rejects of society, the lunatic and the idiot.

Abandoned and exposed in Ancient Greece and Rome; cared for in asylums and seen as 'les enfants du bon Dieu' in mediaeval times; whipped and chained 'Children of Satan' in the 16th century, sold by Parish authorities (Payne 1916) to mill owners in the 18th century, the lunatics and the idiots were finally rescued by the great educational reformers of the 19th century.

Although the 17th and 18th centuries had seen a great flowering of scientific, medical research and thought following the work of Galileo, Newton, Boyle and Kepler which laid the foundations for the experimental method, little of this interest was reflected in organising measures for safeguarding public health, or in the care or protection of the retarded and the insane.

Until the 19th century it was an implicit assumption of governments that the burden of health and social problems must be borne by the individual and not by the state.

The cholera epidemic of 1832 in England prompted the appointment of medical officers to report on the progress of the epidemic, and the first Public Health Act passed in 1848 created a General Board of Health which laid the foundations for legislation relating to public health (Davies 1963).

FRANCE'S GREAT CONTRIBUTION

Reformers at the Bicêtre

However it must be to France's lasting credit that serious interest, concern and compassion for the insane and retarded began with the work of Pinel, Esquirol and Seguin in the late 18th and early 19th century. Pinel had been appointed Superintendent of the asylum at Bicêtre in 1792 and he was so affected by the conditions and treatment of his patients who were kept in chains, treated as wild animals, and even exhibited to the public for money, that he made a personal plea before the Revolutionary Committee. He was allowed to dispense with the chains and to appoint competent physicians to look after his patients. Pinel was convinced that brain dysfunction must be related to their condition and in his book on mental diseases he pleaded for more humane and compassionate treatment of the insane and retarded (Pinel 1801).

There have always been men whose humanity and vision have radically changed the environment, and Pinel's work at the Bicêtre was not only enormously influential in establishing 'properly run mental hospitals', but also attracted after his death a number of illustrious physicians who were to continue and change the treatment of the insane and retarded throughout the world.

Esquirol, who succeeded Pinel as Superintendent, was the first writer, in a book published in 1838, explicitly to state the need to distinguish between the insane and the retarded (Esquirol 1838). He also pointed out the continuum from normality to low grade idiocy and attempted several procedures to differentiate grades of defectiveness, but concluded that 'the individual's linguistic skill was probably the most significant indication of intellectual level' (Anastasi 1968).

Seguin, Director of the first school for the feeble-minded

Seguin, a pupil of Itard, who was a contemporary of Pinel and Esquirol and the Physician and Superintendent of the Institute for Deaf Mutes, had watched Itard's attempt to teach the Wild Boy of Aveyron, and had been impressed and convinced of the importance of social training. Itard was to abandon in despair the teaching of the Wild Boy, considering that little had been achieved and failing to see that the training had been of great benefit to the boy in making him less of a burden to society.

Seguin's influence and work as an educator were of immense importance. In 1842 he convinced the French authorities of the need to educate the 'idiots' and 'imbeciles' at the Bicêtre and from this dates the foundation of the first state school for the retarded child and the recognition that in addition to housing and feeding him, the state must also train and educate (Seguin 1846, Pintner 1924).

Seguin's life was devoted to work with the retarded and the United States, England, Germany and Switzerland were to recognise that provisions must be made for the mentally defective (Mitchell 1916).

In 1846 and 1847 the Magdalen Hospital School in Bath, and Earlswood, the first 'idiot asylum', were established in England.

Seguin's Formboard, the first performance test

Seguin used a number of measures to determine the child's degree of feeblemindedness and his Seguin Formboard, in which the child is required to insert variously shaped blocks into corresponding recesses, is still in current use. In teaching the child Seguin pioneered sense and muscle training techniques which form the basis of physical therapy and are still used in institutions for the retarded in the United States.

Influence of eugenics — the Eugenics movement

Parallel with an awakening social conscience for the psychotic and the retarded in the 19th century was the development of scientific methods and concepts of physics and chemistry which were applied (more systematically than in previous centuries) to the understanding of the nature of plant and animal life. Klein (1970) notes: 'In terms of perspective, man's scientific interest in himself is relatively late', but 'brooding over the meaning of the diversity of plant and animal forms', Darwin's *Origin of the Species*, published in 1859, spurred psychologists to apply the experimental method in the investigation of human psychological phenomena.

Darwin's cousin, Sir Francis Galton, has often been seen as one of the pioneer figures responsible for launching the testing movement. His great interest in heredity led him to measure the physical traits of related and unrelated persons. Galton visited educational institutions and kept careful records of students. At the International Exposition of 1884 visitors paid 3 pence to be measured for keenness of vision and hearing (Galton's bar for discrimination of lengths, whistle for determining pitch), muscular strength, reactions and other sensori-motor functions. His laboratory at South Kensington Museum amassed enormous data on individual differences. Galton theorised that sensory discrimination might be a means of determining an individual's intelligence and he noticed that idiots were defective in discriminating heat, cold and pain.

Wundt's Laboratory

Whilst Galton pursued the study of individual differences in England, a quiet, shy man, Wilhelm Wundt, living the simple life of the old traditional southwest German family was appointed in 1875 as a Professor of Philosophy at Leipzig. In Wundt's laboratory the beginnings of modern experimental psychology were about to be born.

Little is known about Wundt's early life (Watson 1978) except that his childhood was solitary and his attachment to his tutor, a Lutheran pastor, was so great that when the vicar was transferred, Wilhelm was allowed to board with his family and continue his studies.

Like that of Itard and Seguin, Wundt's early training was in medicine, although it is probable that he used medicine as a means of entering a scientific career rather than as a means of practising medicine. His first appointment was as Dozent at Heidelberg in 1857 to lecture in physiology. In 1858 he published a study of muscular movement and elasticity during action. In the introduction of his work he stresses the primacy of method, careful observation by trained observers and the use of calibrated instruments.

The concept of psychology as a distinct science was emerging and Wundt knew that he was pioneering a new science. He wrote, 'Psychology is to take its place among the sciences and not as a branch of philosophy'.

In 1867 Wundt lectured at Heidelberg on 'Physiological Psychology' and these lectures, first published in 1873, were to go into 6 editions, the last in 1911. The first course in experimental psychology at Leipzig was attended by one student in 1879.

Wundt's laboratory attracted students from all over the world and experiments on sensation, perception, reaction times, attention and feeling were studied by psychophysical methods.

MENTAL TESTS

One of Wundt's students was the American James McKeen Cattell who had gone to Leipzig to complete his Doctorate, a dissertation on individual differences. Cattell lectured at Cambridge in 1888 and his interest in measurement was undoubtedly furthered by his association with Galton. On returning to America Cattell established laboratories for experimental psychology and in his article published in 1890 the term 'mental test' was used for the first time in psychological literature. The tests given to college students measured muscular strength, weight discrimination and memory but they yielded disappointing results which did not correlate with scholastic attainments.

The search for mental tests to differentiate intelligence which began with Seguin, Esquirol, Galton and Cattell had proved unsuccessful and one of the main critics was Alfred Binet. A lawyer and scientist who had studied hypnosis with Charcot, Binet criticised Cattell's 'tests' as being too sensory and as concentrating on simple, specialised abilities, rather than testing functions such as memory, imagination, attention, comprehension and aesthetic appreciation. 'How can one measure richness of inspiration, accuracy of judgment and the general ability of the mind?' he asked. Like Galton he attempted to answer these questions by 'sinking many shafts as it were at a few critical points. In order to ascertain the best points for the purpose the sets of measures should be compared with an independent estimate of man's powers' (Galton 1890). Binet was both original and ingenious and sank many shafts even to the extent of considering handwriting and palmistry in his search for better mental tests. He compared the child's performance with parental and teacher estimates and saw intelligence as a complex of different abilities.

Binet used his own daughters as subjects, asking them to solve problems and to report the steps they took to reach a solution. In general the results indicated that thinking processes could not be reduced to sensory or ideational elements. Although the girls were similar in their thinking, they were very different in personality and Binet's interest in individual differences was undoubtedly influenced by his study of his young daughters. From 1887 Binet, using his own battery of tests, assessed many schoolchildren in Paris and its environs. It was this wide experience which gained him an appointment on the commission set up in 1904 by the Minister of Public Instruction to consider recommendations for the administration of special classes in the public schools. His work on the commission led him to put his tests to practical use and the first 'Binet Scale' appeared in 1905.

Over the next 60 years the enormous success of the mental testing movement, accelerated by the Second World War and the use of tests to select officers in the armed forces, created a demand in commerce, industry, government schools and universities which unfortunately was not accompanied by technical improvements in the tests. Also great concern has been expressed that many tests are discriminating against children and adults from 'disadvantaged' socio-cultural backgrounds. These are valid concerns. However, despite the criticisms aroused by the indiscriminate use of mental tests, the process of psychological assessment must be seen as a holistic approach to the child and quite distinct from the mere administration of mental tests.

Although in good hands and in ideal conditions psychological assessment is believed to give accurate and usually reproducible results, the reservations about the validity of such tests expressed by Binet are to some extent shared by all who work with handicapping conditions and with education.

In the following section some of the difficulties involved are considered as a prelude to a review of the common tests.

DEFINITION

Developmental assessment should properly be seen as the assessment of the infant and young child under 30 months, whilst psychological assessment refers to the assessment of children over this age. The results of baby testing show only a modest correlation with future intellectual status because these early tests do not assess thinking processes such as reasoning and judgment but are based on the sensori-motor aspects of development. However, in a very retarded or very bright child the developmental quotient may provide a meaningful baseline of future potential.

Assessment should not only be seen as the measurement of intellectual abilities but also as the opportunity to collect and synthesise a number of impressions about a child's performance and behaviour within the context of the family, school and community so that useful decisions may be made in the light of this special information.

Assessment should always be linked to treatment and this is often based within a small specialist team either in a hospital, clinic or the school. The information derived from the assessment should form the 'blueprint of action' directed to providing for the child's social, educational and psychological needs.

The role of the psychologist in the past has tended to emphasise the diagnostic aspects of the assessment rather than the therapeutic and remedial possibilities available. Fortunately there are now wide-ranging therapeutic settings such as family, individual or group therapy and conselling, behaviour modification and 'crisis intervention' to offer families. Attempts at pharmacological control of hyper-active children with possible beneficial effects on learning motor and social skills allow the psychologist to assess the cognitive aspects of different drug régimes (Werry et al 1980). Remedial help with specific deficits of functioning such as reading retardation has been less successful and Yule (1976) has pointed out that this may be due to inadequate training of remedial teachers. However it is the pattern of strengths and weaknesses which assessment can reveal which will determine the best ways to help a particular child. Of special importance is the counselling offered to parents of handicapped or congenitally deformed children who may be shocked and bereaved at the birth of such a child.

Early intervention programmes for the high risk infant have shown that motor and cognitive skills can be improved by increased sensori-motor stimulation and by extra parental handling (Brown & Hepler 1976).

Parent-infant relationships differ depending on whether the infant is a high risk or normal full-term infant. The parents of premature infants persist more with feeding but are less responsive verbally and emotionally (Brown & Bakeman 1977) and there is extensive documentation to show that low birth weight infants are more often abused, battered and neglected than the normal infant (Schmidt & Kempe 1975).

Psychologists in the United Kingdom are now extending their expertise so that they can usefully become part of a team attached to hospital wards, day centres, cerebral palsy units and community health clinics working alongside paediatricians, general practitioners, physiotherapists, nurses, social workers and other ancillary workers. They have moved outside the narrow confines of the child guidance clinics, mental hospitals and school psychological services and now offer a wide ranging approach in terms of assessing a child's behaviour, social responsiveness and learning strategies by observing 'high risk' young children who may attend nurseries or observation units prior to eventual school placement.

Over the past two decades there have been concerted efforts, especially in America, to improve the intellectual status of children from socio-culturally impoverished communities. 'Head Start' has had its successes and failures and although there were children in these programmes who made important social and intellectual gains there were many whose performance deteriorated when they were returned to their own communities. More recent attempts to maintain the improvement of such children seem promising but the follow-up studies are still to be published (Heber & Garber 1974).

The formal aspects of educational placement, however, still depend on the psychological assessment, although most psychologists are very aware that there are social, cultural and psychological features of the child's personality and environment which cannot be assessed by tests but must be taken into consideration when placement is made. Also it should be stressed that special schooling for the child with moderate or severe subnormality should be continuously reviewed in order to re-evaluate behavioural and intellectual status.

DEVELOPMENTAL TESTING: SOME PROBLEMS AND PITFALLS

1. The effect of testing on the emotional state of the family and resultant difficulties

The developmental or psychological assessment begins when the psychologist first meets the child and his family. Often the child is secure and mature enough to separate from his mother or father for the testing session, but most small children and some older ones prefer to have their parent(s) with them. When parents bring a child for assessment it is often at the request of the family doctor, the paediatrician, or a teacher, but sometimes because they themselves are concerned. The possible rea-

sons for referral are many but the commonest relates to developmental 'lags', and since the results of testing may profoundly influence both the child's and his parents' futures, they are often very anxious about the procedure. Parental anxiety will sometimes communicate itself to the child. The mother or father or both may be tense and impatient with him, smack him and urge him not to be silly, while themselves giving the psychologist the answers to the test questions and so spoiling the results. Most psychologists are familiar with these problems and under such circumstances many prefer to establish a sympathetic relationship with the parents and create a setting in which the child can play under observation before any formal tests are given. Often the toys, games and the interest and encouragement shown in his spontaneous play will gain the child's confidence and attention so that formal psychometry can then be attempted. By the time he participates in testing much useful information will already have been gained about the level and complexity of language, the motor manipulative skills, the quality of social interaction with his family and the psychologist and in the case of the handicapped child the special signalling systems which the family employ. Experienced psychologists have their own norms and are so familiar with the interpretation of a wide range of language, motor and social tests that they may start to assess the child in an informal way on first meeting him. Nonetheless subjective observations can never replace careful measurement based on well-validated tests. Interpretation of the test results must always be interactional and take account of the opportunities which the environment has provided for the development of a skill. There are ethnic differences in the maturational rates of locomotor development; African children walk earlier than Caucasian children (Grantham-MacGregor & Back 1971). The child with sensory deficits such as the deaf child may not only be deprived of a 'talking' environment but also deprived of the verbal control which is necessary in the execution of certain performance tasks (Luria 1961).

Blind and physically handicapped children by virtue of their limited mobility become overly dependent on their parents and much learning and experience is withheld from them. Hence assessment of their practical social sense must be relevant and within the context of their limited life experience.

The first assessment of a young child should perhaps be seen as a useful baseline with which to compare future growth trends. It may help the psychologist to understand the parents' perception of their child if they are asked their views of his performance after the testing session. There is some evidence (Tew et al 1974) to suggest that parents of handicapped children overestimate their child's IQs and reject the results of testing if these do not coincide with their own preconceptions. Much can be learned by listening carefully to their answers, and an over-optimistic estimate of the child's performance should warn the psychologist that the parents may need time to accept his problem, whether this be mild retardation, average ability within an 'aspiring' family or specific sensory and physical handicap where handicap has been denied by the parents. In such cases an established contact and reassessment give opportunities to meet the family again and to chart the child's psychological growth. Ideally most children who are slow in some aspect of development should be reassessed yearly. Sometimes parents want more frequent reassessment, but this should be resisted as such requests reflect parental anxieties and it is these which should be explored and discussed rather than the passes and failures on a particular test item.

The assessment of the severely subnormal young child can cause the greatest distress, since many parents are unable to accept the school placements which are offered to such children. Despite the improvement in facilities recommended by successive committees, much still remains to be done, and most families shoulder heavy burdens in caring for severely handicapped children.

Despite the recommendations of Warnock (1978) most handicapped children are still placed in special schools, although the Heads of Normal Schools are becoming more willing to accept children with mild learning, physical and behaviour problems. Moreover it is probable that the average school has its fair share of children who are eligible for special schooling, and it will be the tolerance of the teachers and the temperament of the child which determine whether or not placement is

made. In 1977 12% of children eligible for special education were in normal schools in the United Kingdom.

Although most psychologists and paediatricians hope that children with mild learning and physical handicaps can be included within the normal school system, it is often the lack of speech therapy and physiotherapy services, the geography of the school, the size of the class and the under-supervised playground which make such placement problematic. In the case of children with mild or moderate learning problems neither teachers, time nor facilities will be sufficient to meet their particular needs and it will rarely be in the child's best interests to maintain him within a normal ability range. Inclusion in a special class or school will offer protection against a more competitive peer group and loss of self-esteem. Occasionally children whose parents find it difficult to accept ESN schooling will permit placement in a 'delicate' school which originally was designed for children rendered vulnerable by illness or circumstance. Rosenbloom (1980) has drawn attention to the 'stigma' of attending special schools and referred to the increasing practice of transferring the handicapped child to normal school at about 14 which allows him to relate better to a normal peer group before further training placement. However a recent OECD (1980) study which looks at the training provisions offered by nine local authorities has concluded that handicapped children leaving special schools are more likely to find and keep jobs than handicapped children leaving comprehensive schools. The main advantage of special schools and units, according to this study, is that they emphasise work potential skills under the Youth Opportunities Programme. Children in comprehensive schools may not have access to specialist careers officers. The research has also shown that mentally handicapped youngsters are more ready to adapt to boring and repetitive tasks than their peers in normal schools. The study further reveals that adult training centres are not making the separate provision for young people recommended by Warnock.

The maladjusted child may fare less well within the special schools sector. Often the background may be seriously detrimental to healthy development and the only solution will be 'maladjustment boarding placement' for a child already deprived and rejected. Over the last few years frequent changes and inadequate staffing of such schools have brought their own problems. Greater success has been achieved by short term placements in units specially designed to help with behaviour modification. Fostering can also be a helpful alternative to residential schooling.

By contrast the undetected bright child has been the victim of changing social and political attitudes which have discouraged academic excellence so that many such children fail to reach their potential and may present with a wide spectrum of functional and behavioural disorders (Lobascher & Cavanagh 1977).

2. Past medical, obstetric, social and cultural factors

Before accepting the results of a child's assessment it would be imprudent for the psychologist to ignore the early obstetric, developmental, social and family history. There may be factors such as prematurity or family patterns of slow maturing, which could prejudice the test results and perhaps suggest that the child may 'catch up'. Separations from the mother due to ill-health or hospital admission (of mother or child) may have interfered with 'bonding'. The quality of nurturing may be inferior both psychologically (O'Callaghan & Hull 1978) and nutritionally (Cravioto & de Licardie 1972) and there may be an interplay of both these factors. Cravioto and de Licardie's studies showed that the development of Mexican children was influenced both by their malnourishment and their family circumstances. Wolkind (1977) and Hall et al (1979) have also shown that the children of mothers who have themselves been at some time in local authority care are at serious developmental risk. These children are of lower birth weight, have more behavioural problems and perform less well on intelligence and language tests compared to other children.

Special problems arise in the case of immigrants who have lived in their native communities in the milieu of an 'extended family' with friendly interaction between children and adults across the generation gap. When the family is suddenly transported to an environment which is unsympathetic climatically, culturally and emotionally, the effects on all its members can be profound. A new language must be learned and exposure to two languages simultaneously may delay consolidation of the main language; schooling may be sporadic and indifferent and the mother often has to go out to work so that a succession of baby-minders or 'caretakers' is involved. Similar problems arise in one-parent families. The child may develop behaviour disturbance and depression, which affect his functioning and produce a misleading impression of retardation. The follow up study of 3-year-old pre-school children (Richman 1981) has emphasised the interaction between the difficult child and the depressed mother so that the child not only scores lower on neuro-developmental tests at 3 years but also continues to have problems at 8 years even if his mother is no longer depressed.

Sometimes the basic equipment of testing, such as paper, pencil, toys and picture books are strange to the child who has been reared in a home lacking these refinements. The lack of toys in homes of Asian immigrants to Britain has been noticed by many observers (Lobo 1978). In the Luton survey for lead toxicity in which many families of Pakistani immigrants were visited, the scarcity of toys, for example model cars and 'Dinky' toys, was very noticeable, especially in the poorest and illiterate families. The effects of overcrowding and large family size also constitute an adverse influence on a child's development and school achievement, although family size and social class have more effect than inadequate housing (Rutter & Madge 1976).

3. Effect of physiological and other factors on test results

Parents often ask how far such factors as fatigue, irritability and feeling 'out of sorts' affect the test results. There is some evidence that tests administered under very adverse conditions were surprisingly predictive when the same children were retested seven years later under more favourable conditions (Rutter et al 1967). A more important factor affecting test results may be the inexperience of the psychologist, and Gregory & Mohan (1977) cite this as one of the important sources of error and a major methodological weakness in the lead studies.

However, there are children, the depressed, the epileptic and the child with phenylketonuria, who may show marked fluctuations of test scores at different assessments. In the case of the depressed child, mood change or lack of motivation and interest may seriously interfere with rapport and affect the results of the tests. The child with epilepsy may have subclinical attacks during testing and if the psychologist is unfamiliar with the manifestations of milder attacks he may not appreciate that these are affecting the child's performance. Children with minor epileptic status (Ch. 12) may show marked variation in test results from one time to another. The sedative effect of some anti-convulsant drugs may also impair performance but not usually severely unless the dose is too high. Children with phenylketonuria can also show dramatic changes of intellectual function over a peiod of time associated with the control of the diet or when diet has ceased (Smith et al 1978).

1. Consistency and stability of IQ
2. Factors affecting the intellectual outcome of children

Studies of the consistency and stability of intellectual status from infancy to the age of 18 years (Jones et al 1971) suggest that children's test scores are labile during infancy but gradually become more stable. At school age the lability scores are about one third of a standard deviation or 5–6 IQ points. However, within any group of children there will always be a few children who make sweeping changes of function in the region of 20–40 IQ points. The younger the child the more difficult it is to make valid predictions for his future development, but at both ends of the distribution curve of intelligence, i.e. for the very retarded and for the child with superior intelligence, predictions are more valid.

Because important decisions are made as a result of the psychological assessment parents rightly question the validity and ethics of mental testing. Over the last decade the use of intelligence tests as a means of selecting the talented student both at school and at university, within industry and government has been challenged by those who con-

sider that such selection seriously interferes with and affects the education of black children. The more tests highlighted talents, the more they became associated with 'élitism' and 'meritocracy'. By 1975 the critics were so vociferous that the California Legislature attempted to prohibit mental testing in schools and in 1979 they were successful in doing so.

HERITABILITY OF INTELLIGENCE

Much of the concern expressed by critics of mental tests has arisen out of the controversy over the 'inheritability' of intelligence and the arguments are well summarised by a number of publications (Butcher 1968, Block & Dworkin 1977). Social scientists are still debating the extent of the inherited factor and it is probable that no study or research design can disentangle the infinitely complex interplay of genetic and environmental components of group differences. The potential written on the chromosomes is so variable, a polygenic situation in a huge sense, and the environmental variables are infinite.

However, there is good evidence to suggest that within families and across generations genetic factors play an important part in determining variations in intelligence.

There are studies which show that the IQs of adoptive children correlate poorly with their adoptive parents whilst the IQs of children brought up by their own biological parents bear a much closer correlation (Skodak & Skeels 1949). Twin studies also suggest that there is a genetic basis for intelligence. Dizygotic twins show a greater difference between their IQs than do monozygotic twins (Babson et al 1964, Willerman & Churchill 1967).

SOCIAL CLASS

The social class, quality of schooling and prolongation of education lead to gains in intellectual level in child- and adulthood whilst impoverished environments can lead to intellectual impairment.

ENVIRONMENT

Studies (Tizard 1970) of institutional children have shown that differences between institutions in patterns of child care are related to differences in children's understanding of language. Variations of up to 15 points on language tests were associated with the best and the worst institutions. The influence of social factors on intellectual development has been well documented in a large number of studies and from those specifically dealing with gypsy and canal-boat children. Verbal abilities appear to be more seriously impaired than visuo-spatial skills. Conversely, the level of language fluency within the home can have an incremental effect on verbal abilities so that a child of average abilities within a middle class family may show specific increase of verbal skills (Mittler 1970). Black children reared in white families show a mean IQ 15 points higher than black children reared in their own families (Scarr 1976).

CHANGED ENVIRONMENTS

Moving children to different environments may have a marked effect on intellectual development. The Koluchova twins with IQs in the 40s at the age of 7 were reported to have normal abilities when assessed at 14 (Koluchova 1976). However the younger the child is moved the greater the social and intellectual benefits (Tizard & Hodge 1978), but the enriching effects of early stimulation are quickly lost if family circumstances change, and children show a decrease in intelligence if there is a drift downwards in social class.

PARENTAL ATTITUDES

Parental attitudes are influential in determining educational progress. Two groups of children, the bright child (IQ > 115) and the dull child (IQ < 85) were investigated and the factors associated with the home and neighbourhood were found to be more important than those associated with the schools. Paternal interest was significantly associated with brightness, and lack of maternal care was associated with backwardness (Wiseman 1964)

High maternal criticism and low maternal warmth are associated with continuing behaviour problems at 8 years (Richman 1981).

PERSONALITY FACTORS

Personality factors also correlate with IQ shifts during school life. The aggressive child who has opportunities to show initiative and independence of judgment makes IQ gains whilst the passive dependent child may not show the same score increases. The active child evokes greater stimulus from his environment than the passive child and the child's own personality acts on and determines the quality of response from his parents, siblings and teachers. He exerts both action and reaction on his environment (Rutter 1977).

Work attitudes, drive level and task involvement, which are related to temperament, sex and psychosocial factors, are also associated with educational progress and behavioural adjustment.

BEHAVIOURAL DISTURBANCE

Children who suffer from lesions affecting the cortex (Rutter et al 1970) and children with phenylketonuria (Stevenson et al 1979) are now known to show a higher incidence of behavioural disturbance. Hence the problems confronting psychologists who work with such children are two-fold, not only the clarification of the intellectual deficits but also the investigation of possible environmental causes which might contribute to, provoke or reinforce an essentially vulnerable child.

INTELLIGENCE AND ACHIEVEMENT

Whilst a multifactorial approach has been adopted in considering the innate and extrinsic factors which may influence and prejudice the intellectual course of an individual from infancy to adulthood it is nevertheless essential to appreciate that intellectual level may bear little relationship to educational efficiency. There is only a modest correlation between academic achievement and intellectual status and this has been noted by many writers from

Binet to the present day (Binet 1908, Terman et al 1915, Wall et al 1962).

Frank (1976) notes that 'the closer the (mental) test material is to the "target" data of academic performance the better is the prediction that can be achieved'. Studies which have looked at the factors common to both success in intelligence tests and success in school and university have highlighted a verbal factor as being central to intellectual and scholastic achievement.

There may also be subtle deficits of function which may inhibit scholastic performance and require careful assessment. It is probable that many intellectually able children are penalised in both school and formal examinations by specific problems such as slow handwriting so that only half the work is completed or half the questions answered; memory deficits and hence problems with the retrieval of information; mild problems of expressive language so that the content of written work may be awkward and convoluted. The present policy of some schools, polytechnics and universities to accept continuous assessment of a student's work as an index of ability undoubtedly aids those individuals who may otherwise be quite handicapped in what has been called the cruel and silly examination system (Stone 1980).

In the foregoing the discussion has centred on the factors which may influence developmental and intellectual status and paediatricians and psychologists working in mental and physical handicap are sadly accustomed to the effects which adverse physical, social and psychological factors confer upon their patients but they are also often astonished by and grateful for the effective survival of many such children.

INVULNERABILITY AND SURVIVAL

What are the conditions, criteria and characteristics which enable some children to survive whilst others founder? Rutter (1977, 1979) refers to 'the study of the invulnerability of certain individuals' as being 'a growth area of the future'. He lists four factors which may be related to the adjustment of the individual. The multiplicity of stress and its transactional effects whereby if 2 stresses are present (biological or social) the risk of instability is not doubled but increased four fold. Second, the changed circumstances of the environment, so that if children are moved to improved environments there is less psychiatric risk. Third, the factors of sex, temperament and genetic background which are important in determining whether the child is at risk. Males are constitutionally more vulnerable and those children who are negative or have 'low malleability, low fastidiousness' are also more likely to be at risk, especially if the parental attitudes are critical. Fourth, whatever the discord in the home, one good relationship either between a grandparent or a parent with the child serves to confer 'positive protective effects'. Thomas et al (1968) in his social study of 141 New York middle class children from 3 months to adolescence showed that at 6 years of age those children who had been rated as being 'easy' with regular sleep and bowel patterns, cheerful mood and ready adaptability to changed environments were less likely to become behaviourally disturbed than those children who were negative, had irregular sleep and were resistant to new situations.

Amongst the aspects of personality which are rarely measured by tests but are often readily observed clinically, good sense, sensitivity to others and personal courage are qualities which make an individual a potential survivor and which are as important as intelligence and psychiatric stability.

THE ADMINISTRATION OF THE PSYCHOLOGICAL TESTS (Fig. 14.1)

There are no hard and fast rules for testing the child with handicaps; indeed flexibility and imagination on the part of the psychologist are essential. Some children require a brisk and structured administration of the tests and prefer to work in an organised way; others must be cajoled and enticed into communicating with the examiner and may prefer initially to settle into an impersonal relationship performing the easier motor tests. Not too much notice should be taken as to where the tests are performed. Woe betide the psychologist who insists it should be at a chair and table. The child may have his own ideas — in the sink, under the desk or on the floor. Sensitivity as to how to establish 'rapport' will be related to the training, per-

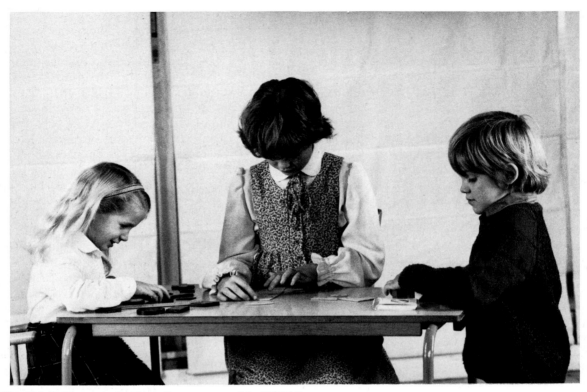

Fig. 14.1 Children enjoying the performance tests of the WISC R

sonality and experience of the psychologist who must in some way convince his companion that there is a good time coming, and interesting things to do. It is a rare child who shows lack of interest in everything.

The choice of tests must be relevant to the referring problems and take account of the child's problems. As important as the testing procedure is the proper evaluation and interpretation of the test results since there are many sources of error in the mere computation of IQs. If there is concern about the psychometric results, physicians and parents should not hesitate to request repeat assessments.

Children's attitudes to formal testing are infinitely variable and it is probable that these are as important for determining future potential as the test results themselves. 'Impulsive' children make more effort than 'reflective' children on a matching task and attentional problems relating to personality attributes are important predictors of future potential (Kagan 1965). The level of play a child indulges in during the tests is also a significant

pointer as to the developmental stage he may have reached; the early non-structured play (banging and casting) which occurs under 1 year, the arranging of blocks in rows or piles at a later age and the three-dimensional symbolic play emerging possibly at the same time as language. Lowe's work on play (Lowe 1975, Lowe & Costello 1976) shows that patterns of play follow a developmental and not an experiential sequence.

Most psychologists have their own personal preferences about which tests they find most useful and the following list (Table 14.1) is in no sense complete but merely documents a number of tests in common usage.

The United States has led the world in the development and standardisation of cognitive and specific tests and the United Kingdom is still using the American norms of the WISC R. A number of European countries, however, have established their own norms for the better known tests (Binet, WISC etc.).

Table 14.1 Tests used by educational and clinical psychologists in the assessment of intellectual and education status

Type	Name	Age range	Description and usage
1. Developmental Infant Test	Bayley Scales of Infant Development Psychological Corporation (1969)	0–2	Individually administered tests of mental and motor function which can be separately scored. Good for the non-speaking infant.
2. Pre-school cognitive tests	Merrill Palmer Scale of Mental Tests, Harcourt, Brace & World Inc. (1931, 48)	2.0–4.6	Individually administered test of language and performance function. Rather heavily loaded with motor items and predictively can be misleading.
3. Wechsler Pre-School and Primary Scale of Intelligence	Psychological Corporation (1967)	4.0–6.6	Individually administered test with 5 verbal and 5 performance tests giving 3 IQs (verbal, performance and full scale IQ). Children with attention problems may find the full battery stressful.
4. Pre-school and school	Stanford-Binet Intelligence Scale, Form LM. 3rd revision. Houghton Mifflin, 1960	2.0–18.0	Individually administered test using a mental age concept and testing at intervals of 6 months up to 5 years. Pre-school assessment gives good agreement with future WISC IQs. There are no separate motor or language scales but experience in interpreting the results of the tests often anticipates future problem areas of dysfunction. There is rarely any justification for using the Binet after 6 years of age.
5. School age cognitive tests	Wechsler Intelligence Scale for Children (WISC R) (Revised) Psychological Corporation 1974	6–15.11	This is a revision of the WISC. The individually administered tests of 5 verbal and 5 performance tests giving 3 IQs (verbal, performance and Full Scale). Probably the most important general intelligence test in present usage, translated and standardised in most countries and used extensively in longitudinal studies. The immense flexibility of the tests allows the deaf child to be tested on performance tests, the blind child to be tested on verbal tests; the dysphasic child with monosyllabic speech can respond and answer the arithmetic and information questions; the choreoathetoid child may be able to point to the picture completion cards.
6. Language tests	Reynell Developmental language scales a. Expressive language scale b. Comprehension language scale Reynell J. K. (1969) London NFER	0–5	Individually administered tests of executive language and comprehension of language. There is also a special scale for the handicapped child. The comprehension scale (B) allows assessment of a non-speaking child with limited motor skills.

Contd on p. 360

Type	Name	Age range	Description and usage
8.	Illinois Tests of Psycho-linguistic Abilities, University of Illinois Press	2.0–9.6	There are 9 subtests based on Osgood's (1957, 1963) theoretical communication model. They measure reception, expressive and associative language processes. The tests can be expressed in terms of a raw score, language age or standard score and a total score for the test. Use on children below 4 years is rather difficult.
9. Perceptual tests	Frostig Development Tests of Visual Perception Consulting Psychological Press 1961	3.0–10.0	These are tests of visual perception; there are 5 subtests, eye motor co-ordination, figure-ground discrimination; form constancy, position in space and spatial relations. The test measures perceptual ages. Frostig & Horne (1964) suggest a series of exercises which can be used to train poorly developed areas of perception.
10. Eye-pointing tests	a. Raven's Matrices b. The Peabody Picture Vocabulary c. Reynell Comprehension test	Wide age range	Problems of assessing the athetoid child whose eye hand movements may be uncontrolled or grossly inco-ordinated can be overcome by using a number of tests which can be scored by a child briefly fixating the named object or picture. Specific signalling systems can be conditioned; (yes–no for example) labelled on the arms of wheel chairs. These individually administered tests assess non-verbal reasoning and understanding of both language and abstract spatial problems.
11. Test for hearing impaired child	Hiskey-Nebraska Test of Learning Aptitude Univ. College Press 1966	3.0–16.0	Instructions can be given in mime. Test is more useful for very deaf child. Lengthy to administer, contents of tests lack some interest. Performance items of WISC R more suitable for partially hearing child.
12. Tests for children with defective vision	1. Reynell-Zinkin Scales: Developmental Scales for Young Visually Handicapped Children. N.F.E.R. Publishing Co. Ltd. November 1979. Ref: Child Care, Health and development, vol 1, p 61–69		Provides information on the stages pertinent to a blind child in the areas of sensori-motor development, sound production and speech, understanding of language, social adaptation. Separate norms for infants with or without visually directed reach.
	2. Williams (1957) University of Birmingham and RNIB		The Williams test is composed of items selected from material standardised on large groups of seeing children. Most items are verbal. At the younger age range a number of motor items have been included.

Type	Name	Age range	Description and usage
13. Test of social competence	Vineland Social Maturity Scale. Psychological Corporation (1965)	0–15	An excellent measure at the developmental level of the acquisition of self help skills. In the retarded child the resultant social age often correlates well with the mental age level derived from formal cognitive tests. The value of this test is that its administration and scoring can be carried out by non-psychologists.
14. Attainment: Reading	Neale Analysis of Reading Ability (Neale 1966)	6–13.0	This test explores the child's type of reading errors and his understanding of graded reading passages. 3 measures are derived: a reading accuracy age, a rate of reading age, and a comprehension age. There are 3 parallel forms which are useful clinically in making comparisons of reading ability over a period of time.

ILLUSTRATIVE CASES

Case No. 1

Andrew presented to the hospital at the age of 3 years with ataxia and tremor of the arms. He was the eldest adopted child of professional parents in their thirties. He had been born illegitimately. His father was an unstable married man and his mother had abandoned the baby soon after birth. At the time of referral there was uncertainty and anxiety about his intellectual status. On formal assessment he gained a Full Scale IQ of 80 and this was considered to be an underestimate of his potential. Executive speech was very limited but comprehension of language on the Reynell Language Scale suggested that his understanding was almost appropriate to his age. A hopeful sign was his concentrated imaginative play. At the assessment the parents discussed not only Andrew's slowness but also their concerns about the second child, a baby girl of 6 months whom they hoped to adopt. This child was born 6–8 weeks permaturely and was showing no reaching behaviour. The baby had been in a distressed state at the time of fostering and was said to be malnourished. Both prospective parents felt that they could not accept another handicapped child and were emphatic that her adoption must be conditional on the baby's normality. Neurological examination was normal although psychological assessment showed some

lag in development consistent with the degree of prematurity. Both parents, however, felt unable to continue fostering and the baby was eventually adopted by another family in which she settled well and eventually made good progress.

During this distressing period Andrew's behaviour had become disturbed. He was restless, slept little, rose early and became aggressive to both his parents and to the family pet. Over the next year there were many crises and Mrs. A. was in frequent telephone contact (they lived several hundred miles away from the hospital) to discuss various aspects of his management. Twelve months later she became pregnant and after the birth of her own child management became more relaxed. She commented: 'I can shout at Andrew and not feel guilty'. Reassessment of Andrew at 5 years showed marked increments of performance although his grasp and control of a pencil were immature. He still tended to fall down, bumping into objects and bruising himself. Over the next 2 years he continued to be an eruptive small boy, but motor control and skills gradually improved. At 7 years he was referred back because of a query as to school placement. He was head of his class and both his parents wondered whether this reflected a mediocre school or a boy who had improved intellectually. Assessment on the WISC supported the latter impression since Andrew gained an IQ of 128 with little discrepancy between verbal and performance skills.

The lowest score was related to a hand eye writing task (Coding). His behaviour had markedly improved although he still had outbursts of anger directed against his parents and his brother. The advent of another baby in the family and more confident experienced management resulted in an altogether calmer family.

A interesting postscript to this case was the remark of a remedial teacher who had been asked to help Andrew achieve a finer grasp of the pencil. 'Why, he's a perfectly normal boy. By the way the parents spoke I thought I was going to meet a very damaged child'.

Andrew's case emphasises 4 important factors which may be encountered in the assessment:

1. The problems which adoptive children may present.

2. The instability of the IQ — of particular significance in an ataxic child because early developmental tests assess motor and sensory aspects of development as opposed to cognitive development. In this child a normal comprehension age at the age of 3 years suggested normal intellectual potential.

3. The problems which may result from applying a diagnostic label, in this case ataxia, to a child. For the parents this label implied that the boy was damaged and it took many years for their attitudes to be modified.

4. The effect which such a diagnosis may have on bonding between the mother and a young child.

Case No. 2

Timothy was seen in a neurological clinic on account of delayed speech. He was the third child of healthy unrelated parents with no relevant family history. The pregnancy was uneventful and delivery was by forceps. He was slightly slow to suck and later feeding was prolonged and difficult. There was no concern about his progress in the first 2 years, his motor milestones being passed early. However, executive language was restricted to 6 words and he was therefore referred to the clinic at 4 years of age.

On neurological examination there were no significant findings apart from overactivity.

Psychological assessment suggested that his performance skills were advanced but executive language was markedly delayed although comprehension was within normal limits. There was some evidence of behaviour disturbance in that he was hyperactive, took a long time to settle at night and was loath to separate from his mother. Both his parents appeared tolerant and helpful. His mother worked part-time as a secretary and his father was a railway shunter. The parents belonged to a large extended family living in three separate but adjacent council houses. Few of the married children had moved away from their parents and there was limited social contact outside the family.

Timothy continued to be reviewed for the next 10 years. Speech therapy was offered weekly but the quality of executive language was so poor that his family and the school had great difficulty in understanding him as well as containing his physical restlessness.

At 7 years of age assessment on the WISC showed a marked discrepancy between verbal and performance skills. The Performance IQ was at the very superior level (IQ = 135) and the Verbal IQ within the dull normal range (IQ = 82).

Over the next 4 years Timothy attended the speech clinic, a reading class and general counselling sessions, although it was felt the parents might have benefited by family group work. He continued to be restless at night with occasional enuresis and had a limited linguistic repertoire. At 12 years Timothy developed school phobia and his parents requested home tuition which was refused. He was firmly told that the law required his daily attendance at school and over the next year he settled down. Now, at 14 years, he is 3½ years retarded in reading skills, still shows a verbal-performance discrepancy of 40 points, has rapid, explosive, poorly articulated speech which is not always understandable, and like his mother is overweight. He has no friends except his two cousins. His hyperactivity is no longer a problem, and indeed he has become hypo-active and is often depressed.

Timothy's case illustrates several problems not uncommonly seen by psychologists:

1. It shows how limited linguistic skills can create communication difficulties and later social problems which may well be lifelong.

2. It also highlights the effect of poor communication skills in childhood resulting in impoverished peer-relations and poor behavioural and school adjustment. The markedly reduced verbal

IQ may predict an increased risk of dyslexia, i.e. a reading age more than 2 years below the chronological age in a child of normal intelligence.

3. The hyperactivity of early childhood diminished and in this case was replaced in adolescence by hypo-activity and depression. The overeating could be seen as pleasure-substitute in a lonely child. This boy required both specific and general help with his language and behavioural adjustment and although this was offered to the family, the appointments were cancelled each time. The closed family system adopted by the family had not allowed Timothy to develop a rubust 'survival kit'. His problems beginning with a developmental dysphasia may have been reinforced by adverse family patterns and he illustrates well the complexity of the constitutional family factors which may be related to the original 'reason for referral'.

Case No. 3

Jane was born following a 31-week pregnancy to a 21-year-old mother. The birthweight was 3 lb 2 oz. There were cyanotic attacks during the first 2 days of life but later progress was satisfactory and no abnormality was found. She was referred at two years because of poor sleeping, difficult behaviour, hyperactivity and slowness in sitting up and in walking. She showed the signs of mild spastic diplegia but intellectually she seemed bright and normal walking was predicted. Chloral was prescribed for poor sleeping.

One year later Jane had a convulsion with an ear infection and her EEG was diffusely abnormal. Poor sleeping continued and tantrums were a problem. Psychometry on the Binet showed an IQ at the very superior level — 136+. Early school entrance was advised.

Three years later Jane had settled and her tantrums had lessened, although she showed specific problems with writing and arithmetic. Over the next 6 years she attended a normal school but at 13 she became increasingly sensitive about her diplegic gait and required a friend or teacher near her if she had to cross an open space or to walk down a corridor lined by children. At about this time her best friend had suffered from bullying and Jane developed school phobia, with complaints of dizziness and periods of misery. At her

own request boarding school placement was tried but was not successful. Over the years her relationship with her strict and religious parents had been ambivalent. She was their only child and had always been a disappointment to them; her father had wanted a boy and regretted her lack of athletic prowess. Because of her unhappiness Jane asked to be allowed to live with her mother's sister, a single middle-aged headmistress of a local grammar school, and she left home to do so at 14. Over the next 4 years she settled and did well at 'O' level and 'A' level examinations. A certificate of disability on account of slow handwriting was accepted by the Board of Examiners and she had the help of an amanuensis who wrote the answers to questions at her dictation. Jane gained University Entrance at 18 years and chose to read Law. She remains in close contact with her aunt but maintains a cool relationship with her parents. She enjoys the social life of her university and wears full skirts and loose slacks to disguise her diplegic gait. Her present boyfriend is a third-year medical student.

In discussing her handicap Jane is eloquent about the isolation and pain of being different physically. She asks 'Why did it happen to me?' She sees herself as being a physical girl who would have taken pleasure in sports and dancing. 'I watch the gymnasts and move with them in spirit. My intellectual life has been a substitute for all the other things I would have been and has given me a freedom I would never otherwise have achieved.'

This girl's story illustrates the needs of such children as Jane for help to foster their development and their talents. By her tantrums she won early school entrance, but despite her brightness and sensitivity she was unable to flourish either in her own family or in a normal comprehensive school. A supportive environment in the home of a relative and a challenging academic life brought her some measure of eventual fulfillment and freedom.

Case No. 4

David is now aged 14 years. His parents were concerned about his slow development when he was not yet sitting unsupported at 9 months of age. It was not until he was 13 months, when he presented with infantile spasms and retardation, that it was recognised that he was suffering from phenylketonuria (PKU). He was treated with a low phenylalanine (PA) diet and within a short time his fits stopped and his development speeded up to reach the low normal range by 4 years of age. He attended a normal school with remedial help. Because.of his overactive behaviour and persistently abnormal EEG, however, he was treated with a small dose of sulthiame from the age of 4 years.

At 8 years of age he wss assessed psychologically and all IQs were in the low 90s (VIQ = 90, PIQ = 96, FIQ = 92). He was then started on a normal diet. Four months later his school work deteriorated and he became lethargic and moody. His parents attributed these problems to his having moved to a large integrated class rather than a small streamed group of children, and they therefore moved him to a new school where he was placed at the bottom of a remedial class. During this time he was eating large amounts of protein. Psychometry at the age of 10 years showed a marked decrease in both verbal and performance IQs (VIQ = 71, PIQ = 79, FIQ = 72), and he developed a tremor of his hands and exaggerated knee reflexes.

A strict low PA diet was introduced and within a few weeks the tremor disappeared. Behaviour and school progress gradually improved along with his IQ results. At the age of 12 years 9 month his full scale IQ had risen to 82, with a verbal IQ of 81 and a performance IQ of 86. He attends a normal school and receives remedial tuition.

David's history emphasises the need for serial psychometry in children with phenylketonuria. The important but still uresolved question of when to stop diet must await the results of longitudinal follow-up studies such as that of the MRC DHSS PKU Register which now follows up over 1000 children with the disorder with respect to their behaviour and intelligence. David's improvement after a strict diet was reintroduced suggests that to some extent intellectual and behavioural regression may be reversible.

REFERENCES

Anastasi A 1968 Psychological testing. MacMillan, New York

Babson S G, Kangas J, Young N, Bramhall J L 1964 Growth and development of twins of dissimilar size at birth. Pediatrics 30: 327–333

Binet A, Simon T 1908 Le dévelopement de l'intelligence chez les enfants. L'année psychologique 14: 1–94

Block N, Dworkin G (eds) 1977 The IQ controversy. Anchor Press

Brown J V, Bakeman R 1977 Antecedents of emotional involvement in mothers of premature and full term infants. Presented at the Biennial Meeting of the Society for Research in Child Development, March, New Orleans.

Brown J, Hepler R 1976 Stimulation — a corollary to physical care. American Journal of Nursing 76: 578–581

Butcher J J 1968 Human intelligence: its nature and assessment. Methuen, London

Cravioto J, de Licardie E R 1972 Environmental correlates of severe clinical malnutrition and language development in survivors from Kwashiorkor and marasmus. In: Nutrition, the nervous system and behaviour. Pan American Health Organisation

Davies I G 1963 Modern public health. Edward Arnold, London

Esquirol J E 1838 Des maladies mentales. Boilliere, Paris

Frank G 1976 Measures of intelligence and conceptual thinking. In: Weiner I B (ed) Clinical methods in psychology. John Wiley & Sons, New York

Galton F 1890 Remarks on mental tests and measurements. Mind 15: 380

Grantham-Macgregor S M, Back E H 1971 Gross motor development in Jamaican infants. Developmental Medicine and Child Neurology 13: 79–87

Gregory R J, Mohan P J 1977 Effect of asymptomatic lead exposure on childhood intelligence: a critical review. Intelligence 1: 381–400

Hall F, Pawlby S J, Wokind S 1979 Early life experiences and later mothering behaviour: a study of mothers and their 20-week-old babies. In: Shaffer D, Dunn J (eds). The first year of life, Wiley, New York

Heber R, Garber H 1974 Progress Report III. An experiment in the prevention of cultural familial retardation. Proceedings of the Third International Congress, International Association of Scientific Study of Mental Deficiency

Jones H, Bayley N, McFarlane J W, Honzik M P (ed) 1971 The course of human development. Xerox College Publishing, Toronto

Kagan J 1965 Individual differences in the resolution of response uncertainty. Journal of Personality and Social Psychology 2: 154–160

Klein D B 1970 A history of scientific psychology: its origins and philosophic backgrounds. Routledge and Kegan Paul, London

Koluchova J 1976 The further development of twins after severe and prolonged deprivation: a second report. Journal of Child Psychology and Psychiatry 17: 181–188

Lobascher M E, Cavanagh N C 1977 The other handicap: brightness. British Medical Journal 2: 1269–1271

Lobo E de H 1978 Children of immigrants to Britain. Hodder and Stoughton, London

Lowe M 1975 Trends in the development of representational play. Journal of Child Psychology and Psychiatry 16: 33–47

Lowe M, Costello A J 1976 Manual for the symbolic play test. NFER Windsor

Luria A R 1961 The role of speech in the regulation of normal and abnormal behaviour patterns. Pergamon Press, London

Mitchell D 1916 Schools and classes for exceptional children. Cleveland Education Survey

Mittler P 1970 Biological and social aspects of language in twins. Developmental Medicine and Child Neurology 12: 741–757

O'Callaghan M J, Hall D 1978 Failure to thrive or failure to rear. Disorders in Childhood 53: 788–793

OECD 1980 Paper "What sort of life?" In: The handicapped adolescent. NFER Publishing, Windsor

Payne G H 1916 The child in human progress. Putnam, New York

Pinel P 1801 Traité médico-philosophique sur l'aliénation mentale. Caille & Revier, Paris

Pintner R 1924 Intelligence testing: methods and results. University of London Press, London

Richman N 1981 Follow-up study of pre-school children. Lecture given at the Spring Scientific meeting of the Royal College of Psychiatrists, London

Rosenbloom L 1980 Should handicapped children attend ordinary schools? Archives of Disease in Childhood 55: 581–582

Rutter M 1977 Individual differences. In: Rutter M, Hersov L (eds) Child psychiatry modern approaches. Blackwell, Oxford

Rutter M 1972–1978 Maternal deprivation. New concepts, new approaches. Child Development June 1979 50 (2): 283–305

Rutter M Greenfield D, Lockyer L 1967 A five to fifteen year follow-up study of infantile psychosis. British Journal of Psychiatry 113: 1183–1199

Rutter M, Graham P, Yule W 1970 A neuropsychiatric study in childhood. Clinics in Developmental Medicine Nos 39/40 Spastics International Medical Publications

Rutter M, Madge N 1976 Cycles of disadvantage. Heinemann, London

Rutter M, Quinlan D 1977 Psychiatric disorder — ecological factors and concepts of causation. In: McGurk H (ed) Ecological factors in human development. Amsterdam, North Holland

Scarr S, Wemberg R A 1976 IQ test performances of black children adopted by white families. American Psychologist 31: 726–739

Schmidt B D, Kempe H C 1975 Neglect and abuse of children In: Vaughan V C, McKay R J (eds) Nelson Textbook of Pediatrics, Philadelphia, p 107–111

Seguin E 1846 Traitement moral, hygiène et education des idiots. Reprinted 1906, Alcan, Paris

Skodak M, Skeels H M 1949 A final follow-up of one hundred adopted children. Journal of Genetic Psychology 75: 85–125

Smith I, Lobascher M E, Stevenson J E, Wolff O H, Schmidt H, Grubel-Kaiser S et al 1978 The effect of stopping the low phenylalanine diet on the intellectual progress of children with phenylketonuria. British Medical Journal 2: 723–726

Stevenson J E Hawcroft J, Lobascher M E, Smith I, Wolff O H, Graham P G 1979 Behavioural deviance in children with early treated phenylketonuria. Archives of Disease in Childhood 54: 14–18

Stone V 1980 University reform. British Psychological Bulletin 33: 15–16

Terman L M, Lyman G, Ordahl G, Ordahl L, Galbreath N, Talbert W 1915 The Stanford revision of the Binet-Simon Scale and some results from its application to 1000 non-selected children. Journal of Educational Psychology 6: 551–562

Tew B, Payne H, Laurence K, Rawnsley K 1974 Psychological testing: reaction of parents of physically handicapped and normal children. Developmental Medicine and Child Neurology 16: 501–506

Tew B, Laurence K, Samuel P 1974 Parental estimates of the intelligence of their physically handicapped child. Developmental Medicine and Child Neurology 16: 494–500

Thomas A, Birch H, Chess S, Hertzig M C, Korn S 1963 Behavior disorders in children. University Press, New York

Tizard J 1970 The role of social institutions in the causation, prevention and alleviation of mental retardation. In: Haywood H (ed) Social cultural aspects of mental retardation. Appleton Century Crofts, New York

Tizard B, Hodges J 1978 The effect of early institutional rearing on the development of eight-year-old children. Journal of Child Psychology and Psychiatry 19: 99–118

Wall W H, Marks E, Ford D H, Zeigler M L 1962 Estimates of the concurrent validity of the WAIS and normative distribution for college freshmen. Personnel and Guidance Journal 40: 717–722

Warnock M 1978 Chairman: Report of the Committee of Enquiry into the Education of Handicapped Children and Yound People: special educational needs. HMSO, London

Watson R I 1978 The great psychologists, 4th edn. J B Lippincott, Philadelphia

Werry J S, Amon N, Diamond E 1980 Imipramine and methylphenidate in hyperactive children. Journal of Child Psychology and Psychiatry 21: 27–35

Willerman L, Churchill J A 1967 Intelligence and birthweight in identical twins. Child Development 38: 623–629

Wiseman S 1964 Education and environment. Manchester University Press, Manchester

Wolkind S N 1977 Women who have been in care — psychological and social status during pregnancy. Journal of Child Psychology and Psychiatry 18: 179–182

Yule W 1976 Issues and problems in remedial education. Developmental Medicine and Child Neurology 18: 675–682

15

Specific disorders of learning: Motor skills and language

N. Gordon

INTRODUCTION

The number of neurones in the brain may well govern its potential and if they are reduced below a certain level the child's development will be restricted in all its aspects with resultant mental retardation however expertly the child is taught. Whatever the number of neurones in the brain, whether they are below average or well above, accomplishments must depend on the connections between the neurones, and therefore on the glial elements of the brain. Learning is dependent on the association of information derived from a variety of sensory inputs, linked to past memories and experiences, not to mention the emotional content. In the case of language function, for example, the human brain no doubt has the ability to extract the necessary data from the linguistic input to organise language into a consistent system, but this will not occur if there is an absence of the relevant information.

Not only do motor and language skills have to be learnt but so do patterns of behaviour. All these tasks are easier to accomplish in childhood than at a later age as the brain undoubtedly becomes less and less adaptable with increasing age. At birth there is a certain localisation of function, to the extent for example that the peripheral visual pathways terminate in the occipital areas, and the auditory impulses reach the temporal lobe. Meaning will only be given to these electrical impulses by their fate after they reach a cortical level; and it is this integration which is likely to involve the brain as a whole and, before well defined patterns are laid down, no particular pathways seem to be essential. As patterns of learning and behaviour do

become increasingly established, the adaptability of the brain decreases, and so does the potential for learning. Among the many factors which make it harder to learn with advancing age is the possibility of the long term suppression of sensory input which has for extended periods lacked meaning or been of no importance.

Most people, if honest with themselves, have to admit to learning disorders of some kind or another, although some are better than others at compensating for these. In the UK over 6% of 7 to 8-year-old children in normal schools have a significant degree of perceptual motor handicap (Brenner et al 1967) and 1.6% of boys and 0.8% of girls have almost unintelligible speech on starting school (Peckham 1973). The more a learning difficulty is confined to a particular skill the more specific it becomes, and the higher the level of general intelligence the more obvious the disability will be. However these disabilities are no respecter of the intelligence and may be significant at any level. For example although many mentally handicapped children are very agile, some are not. If they are particularly clumsy they may be in special need of help. Those of average or above average intelligence have a fair chance of working out ways of overcoming or circumventing their disability but if mentally handicapped, this is unlikely to happen unless skilled treatment and teaching are given.

In order to help children with learning disorders in their diagnosis, assessment, treatment and education a team of people from different disciplines is needed. To be really effective they must work together. The concept of the 'team approach' has produced many platitudes but the benefit to a particular child is likely to be lessened if those included hardly know each other and rarely meet. If the doctor is to act as the co-ordinator of such a team he must be aware of the ideas and opinions of the psychologists, therapists and others. If not, the parents are likely to be given contradictory advice and the end result will be increasing confusion and a deteriorating situation.

If these disorders are so common one of the main medical contributions must be to establish possible causes and then to try and provide more effective prevention.

CAUSATION

Genetic

The evidence that genetic factors play a major role in causing learning difficulties is relatively slight, although studies on twins do give some support to their role. The genetics of reading disabilities have been particularly studied and children showing specific reading retardation do seem to aggregate within families. However no single mode of genetic transmission is evident, suggesting genetic heterogeneity (Finucci 1976). Also it cannot be assumed that a reported familial incidence is necessarily evidence of a genetic origin when there can be so many causes for a particular disability (Naidoo 1972). There may, for example, be social reasons such as the size of the family. Complete concordance has been reported in uniovular twins but only in a third of binovular twins, which is certainly suggestive evidence (Hermann 1959), and as so often in conditions of this type there is likely to be an interaction of genetic and environmental factors. Those genetically vulnerable will succumb to adverse environmental factors while it is amazing how some children can surmount appalling circumstances. If there is occasional evidence of a dominant mode of inheritance of a learning disability it should not be a matter for surprise. If 'genius' seems to occur unusually often in some families there is no reason why the converse should not occur. In this context one cannot help speculating on the occurrence of such conditions as absence of the corpus callosum which may be genetically determined, and the possible absence of other association tracts on a genetic

basis. There have also been recent advances in the possible role of chromosome abnormalities in causing learning difficulties, for example among females who are heterozygous for the fragile X syndrome (Townes 1982).

Why boys should be more often affected with learning disabilities than girls is uncertain, but there are a number of possibilities. There could be a polygenic expression which has a lower threshold for males than females. It is also suggested that the expression of a mutant at a single locus is modified by sex. Sladen (1970) claimed that specific reading disability is dominant in males and recessive in females, but this can only account for some of the recorded pedigrees.

When learning disorders are due to acquired lesions, and this must often be the case, there is a possible reason for male predominance suggested by Ounsted and others (Ounsted & Taylor 1972). They argue that the message of the Y chromosome is translated through the regulation of the pace of development. The maturation of a number of functions is slower in the male and this has several consequences. It means that in males there is more time to elicit information from the genome; unfortunately both bad as well as good information. Also there is evidence that differential cerebral maturation is associated with particular risk to those brains and parts of the brain which are less functionally active (Taylor 1969). This means that boys are at greater risk for a longer time from various noxious agents if their brains develop at a slower rate than those of girls. Although this may be an explanation for the higher incidence of learning disorder from acquired lesions in boys it also has certain advantages in the long term as it gives the male a longer time to learn.

Acquired

Since learning disorders affecting the development of motor and language skills are so common it would be strange indeed if many of them were not due to acquired lesions.

The causes will be the same pre, peri and postnatal insults which will be found among children with cerebral palsy. This may well account for the boy whose siblings are all highly successful 'standing out like a sore thumb' because of his lack of skills. A careful review of the past history may show, for example, evidence of lack of oxygen during the pregnancy and birth or injury at birth, or some episode of cerebral infection in early life. Although difficult to prove this may mean that there is a spectrum of disabilities depending on the severity and location of the brain damage ranging from severe mental and physical handicap at one end to the more subtle disorders of higher cerebral function such as language at the other. Drillien (1972) showed that infants who had suffered from hypoxia and malnutrition in the third trimester, during which glial growth and myelination are establishing intraneural connections, are less likely to have major handicaps but may show an increase in mild degrees of mental retardation and minor neurological abnormalities. Insults to the developing fetus during the first trimester when the neurones are dividing are more often associated with severe mental handicap. Studies in Manchester, which have not been published, on children with perceptual-motor disorders appear to support this thesis. They were not able to involve any single factor in the past histories of clumsy children, except possibly for anoxia during pregnancy. Woods (1976) found in her Bristol and Leeds surveys of children with cerebral palsy that perinatal morbidity also caused delay in language development in a significant number of children. This perinatal damage caused both receptive and expressive disorders of language and defects of articulation. Also Brown (1976) followed up a group of infants with symptomatic neonatal asphyxia and found on comparison with normal controls, evidence of an association between the asphyxia and various handicaps, including motor inco-ordination, epilepsy, speech retardation and school problems.

However, the idea of a 'continuum of reproductive casualty' (Pasamanick & Knobloch 1960) is likely to be an over-simplification. It suggests that all infants exposed to such risks will have suffered brain damage even if this cannot be identified and this seems to be an unwarranted assumption. There are a number of other models: the additive model in which socio-economic variables are added to the medical events; the threshold model suggesting that there is a limit even to human adaptability and that if a series of medical and social risk factors

occur a point will come when evidence of a disability will be inevitable; the interaction model in which a 'continuum of caretaking casualty' is added to the 'continuum of reproductive casualty'; and perhaps the most favoured model, the transactional model, which recognises the continuing interplay of influences throughout development so that the child elicits responses from his environment according to his characteristics at the time, then the influence of the environment will produce a response from the child, which may in turn modify his environment, and so on. In particular this model emphasises the complexity of the problem (Stratton 1977).

Connections — possible pathogenesis

It is now well recognised that many of the acquired disorders of higher cerebral function, due for instance to cerebro-vascular accident, can be explained on the basis of the disconnection of one part of the brain from another (Geschwind 1965). Although they are often complex problems one of the factors underlying learning difficulties in children can be a failure to establish these connections; 'non-connection syndromes'. Such a failure must interfere with cerebral integration which underlies learning. For example a child who cannot develop adequate communication with spoken speech but is otherwise progressing normally may not be able to integrate information from the auditory cortex with patterns of movements subserving articulation, with the memory of past experiences, and with emotional factors.

What are the possible reasons for the failure to establish connections between neurones in the brain? They may never form due to an interference with the growth of the brain, for example when malnutrition occurs during the main spurt of brain growth. Since in humans this spurt takes place mainly in the later part of pregnancy and during the first two years of life and is due mainly to proliferation of the glial tissues of the brain, any interference at this time is bound to have a profound effect on the development of synaptic connections, and later, on learning. Such malnutrition before birth may well be one of the main reasons why dysmature babies are more likely to suffer from these disabilities as they grow older. The evidence (Dobbing 1970) suggests that if malnutrition does occur during the main spurt of brain growth complete recovery may be impossible.

The association fibres linking neurones can well be destroyed, and as has been stated anoxia during pregnancy or birth is a likely cause, although a combination of adverse factors rather than anoxia alone seems to be of importance. Finally if such connections are not used there is evidence that this may have a profound effect on functional organisation at a cortical level, and why not on structure? Experimental work on animals has been mainly on visual function by such procedures as occluding one eye or producing a squint, which interferes with the interaction of stimuli from the two eyes (Gaze 1970). When this occurs at a critical stage of development cells normally associated with afferent stimuli from one eye may be permanently linked to those from the other eye, even if normality is restored.

Another factor which may contribute to difficulties of learning, at least among older children, is inhibition. If a stimulus does not have any particular meaning or interferes with perception in some way or other, it may well be suppressed. A classical example is the double vision resulting from a paralytic squint which after a while will frequently resolve due to the suppression of one of the images.

'INTEGRATION' OF HIGHER CEREBRAL FUNCTIONS

When considering the role of 'connections' in subserving higher cerebral functions and the learning of skills it may help to discuss some of the possibilities on a framework suggested by Wedell (1968), although no doubt this is a gross over-simplification.

Sensory input and perception

The output of the brain is almost entirely dependent on input. Visual input is obviously very important in perceptual-motor functions and auditory input in the development of language. Perceptual disorders can occur in the squinting child, who is otherwise apparently normal (Abercrombie 1960),

and it is easy to illustrate the effect of impaired auditory information if one listens to speech from which the high tones have been extracted. It soon becomes unintelligible unless the meaning was previously known. Apart from peripheral hearing, auditory discrimination is obviously important and may sometimes be found to be defective when language development is delayed. Special tests (Markides 1978) will be needed to identify this defect such as the Wepman Auditory Discrimination Test (1973). This contrasts the classes of stops, fricatives and nasals as well as some of the vowels of English.

There is a prime responsibility to ensure that these input channels are intact, and if possible to rectify the fault. This is not always a simple procedure. For example 'deaf child plus hearing aid does not equal normal child' (Williams 1969). There are great technical difficulties in fitting a young child with a hearing aid, and as it amplifies background noise as well this must be particularly important at a time when auditory discrimination has not been developed. The parents will need constant guidance or else there is a risk that the child's language development may be delayed rather than improved. It is essential for the child to hear words in as meaningful a situation as possible. This must include not only the naming of objects but the use of language to describe the actions the child is performing and those of the caretakers.

Intelligence

The higher the intelligence level the easier it should be to give meaning to the sensory impulses reaching the brain to form perceptions and to integrate them into the various higher cerebral functions; and a certain degree of complexity in the structure of the brain will be necessary for their acquisition. Also mental and physical handicap by its nature adds secondary disabilities. People talk differently to children when they know they are severely retarded, and they often lack suitable toys, and the opportunity to acquire skills which are in fact within the scope of their abilities.

Physical disabilities

Physically handicapped children are deprived in so many ways. They cannot explore the environment and gain the experience upon which so much of early learning depends. The activities of a four year old child with spastic quadriplegia compared with a normal child of the same age are derisory. If a child has never poured water from a jug into a cup, the concept of this action will be harder to develop, and is true of all aspects of 'inner language' which must precede receptive and expressive language.

Psychoses

A child who is severely emotionally disturbed will find it difficult to learn, and this reaches a peak among children with psychoses, although this subject is more beset with confusion than most.

As far as the term 'infantile autism' is concerned it seems that some of the confusion has arisen from the tendency to regard this as a definitive diagnosis rather than the description of a behaviour pattern. If, as seems probable, these children suffer from severe disorders of language development and of perceptual functions (Rutter 1970), the world is bound to seem a frightening place to them and it is not surprising that some of them should withdraw and take refuge in stereotyped behaviour. Many of these children, but not all, will be mentally retarded to a severe degree, with an inevitably poor prognosis, but others can improve and learn if given a great deal of individual attention.

Hyperkinesis

Children who are distractible and unable to attend for long at a time and are grossly over-active for their age are bound to be at a disadvantage in the learning situation. The term 'hyperkinetic syndrome' is sometimes wrongly used to describe children who for example are emotionally disturbed, bored by inappropriate teaching, or over-sedated with barbiturates. When the 'hyperkinetic syndrome' occurs as a specific entity, which is rare, there may be various reasons for this pattern of behaviour. Some over-active children may be understimulated but probably only if they are also very anxious. Experimental evidence has shown a diminished response of the autonomic nervous system in these children compared with controls but it is possible that these findings are the result of the emotional

complications rather than being the primary cause of the overactivity (Conners 1976). A more attractive theory is the possible effect of overstimulation. Much of the sensory input to the brain is normally suppressed and never reaches a conscious level. Factors such as concentration, attention and interest are of obvious importance, and as has been suggested the selection of sensory input is a very active and complex function. If this system is disordered, with a primary defect in inhibition, or at a cognitive level with a defect in selective attention, due to injury or dysfunction of the diencephalon and brain stem in early life, too many stimuli may reach a conscious level (Conners 1976). The child then responds first to one stimulus and then to another in a seemingly endless series of disassociated actions (Laufer & Denhoff 1957). A hypothesis to account for such a disorder is a disturbance of catecholamine metabolism at a diencephalic level. The giving of a sedative would further depress a system already working inefficiently, and conversely stimulants such as amphetamines may improve its function by altering synaptic transmission. Also the child often seems to respond to a teaching situation in which stimulation is reduced to a minimum. This syndrome can affect children of varying intellectual levels and if it is due to a failure of normal development it can be considered as a specific learning disorder; in this instance of acceptable behaviour for the child's age. It is often found among children having learning disabilities of other kinds, such multiple handicaps resulting from a common aetiology.

Memory and imagery

Memory does not necessarily equate with intelligence, but it must play a fundamental role in the development of communication. When meaning has at last been associated by the child with the sounds we make and the receptive stage of language development is nearing an end, it is a vast step to using those same sounds to communicate; this skill will depend a great deal on memory and imagery. Those who have difficulty in acquiring foreign languages know that it is relatively easy to learn to understand them, but how much more difficult to speak them; and the same must surely apply to our mother tongue.

Sensory feedback

This must play an important part in the development and control of skills. There is no doubt about the obvious pleasure the baby takes in hearing the sounds he makes, and when words are used the child can monitor their correctness, as long as hearing is normal. Similarly at a later stage the eyes monitor what is written.

Motor organisation and the body image

Anyone acquiring a new motor skill is likely to be clumsy to begin with, but with practice this can usually be overcome. This is only accomplished when the movements become 'automatic' and are no longer at a conscious level. It will depend on the development of patterns and memory of movements which can be used as required. For example the concert pianist is obviously not thinking of his finger movements, but of factors such as timing, pitch and tone. The concert-goer is benefitting from the years of practice that the performer has devoted to his art. The concept of the body image is essential to this 'motor organisation' and many children with learning difficulties, especially in the field of movement take a long time to acquire this. If the skill necessitates the use of an instrument, or any extension of the body, for instance a tennis racquet or even a motor car, it is only when this has also become part of the body image, and its presence no longer a matter of awareness, that the person is likely to be any good at its use. Although involuntary movements must have certain effects on motor organisation and even on some aspects of perception, it is remarkable how the child of average intelligence can compensate for these disabilities.

LEARING DISABILITIES

A great deal of research is still needed into the mechanisms by which children acquire complicated skills in early life, as only then can such disabilities be understood, prevented and treated. It has been suggested that there is a fairly rigid hierarchy of learning; perceptual motor functions, followed by spoken language, and reading and writing. Higher cerebral functions can never be considered in isolation and defects in one are bound to have profound effects on others but no kind of rigid framework fits the facts.

PERCEPTUAL MOTOR DISABILITIES (THE CLUMSY CHILD)

Initially the development of perception will be paramount and there is no doubt that for the majority visual-perceptual function involves mainly the right side of the brain.

After the toddler stage children, by their very nature, have a grace of movement which is much to be admired. Hence the child who is clumsy may lead an unhappy life in many ways. There is likely to be a delay in motor development, the age at which sitting, standing and walking are accomplished. The clumsy child may not be able to do up buttons and tie shoe laces at the age when he should, and it is obviously easier for a busy mother to dress the child herself than allow him time for the practice which is so essential. Such children often drop things and trip over their feet, and can easily be regarded as fools and nuisances. When they start at school they will be in trouble in the class room particularly with their untidy writing. If the disability is not recognised for what it is and they are blamed for not trying when in fact they have been trying, sometimes harder than their peers, it is not surprising that they may opt out of learning and become lazy and badly behaved. The child's life in the playground may be no happier. Because of his clumsiness no one wants to play with him or have him in his team. All these troubles only too easily lead to lack of confidence and emotional complications of one kind or another.

Often these children show few abnormalities on 'routine neurological examination', although their movements are obviously awkward, and methods of detecting minor deviations of function are needed (Touwen 1979). Others have abnormal signs which suggest 'minimal cerebral palsy', such as a slight hemiplegia, diplegia or obvious choreiform movements. Even when these signs are present it may be better not to classify these children under the term 'cerebral palsy', but still refer to them as clumsy children with perceptual motor disabilities. If not, the label of cerebral palsy may have an adverse effect on the attitude of parents and teachers to the child, when the motor disability is likely to improve and there is no need for pessimism. The doctor may realise that a particular child has a form of cerebral palsy and this is not surprising if it is accepted that the main aetiological factors cause a spectrum of disabilities from severe physical handicaps to subtle disorders of perception.

Perceptual motor disabilities seem to be common. The Cambridgeshire survey in primary schools mentioned earlier (Brenner et al 1967) showed that 54 out of 810 seven-to eight-year-old children examined were affected with a significant disability of this type. It had been known for years that these children were awkward, clumsy, untidy, difficult and irritating, but little if anything had been done to help them. About the same figure of 6% has been found in the Isle of Wight after examination of all children of the same age (Rutter et al 1970). Early recognition is important if the child is to reach his full potential and avoid emotional and other complications. The more severely affected child is likely to be recognised by parents and is often identified in the good nursery school. However many are not, and a screening test of some kind may be needed. The development of percepts and concepts follows a recognisable pattern in early life. Piaget has shown that normal children under four show no conception of order when asked to copy a string of beads or a line of washing, and cannot make knots. They lack a mental representation of objects and the relationship of their parts. They are unaware of Euclidean properties such as the number of sides, verticals and parallels (Beard 1969). These finding must be taken into account in the examination of these children, and as most of them will not come under stress until they start formal schooling the best time to perform such an examination may well be at school entry or soon afterwards. The idea of such a screening test has been criticised because there is a danger of labelling a child as disabled and lowering everyone's expectations for his possible achievements. This seems unreasonable as it is only necessary to identify children who may be at risk of a learning disability of this type so that a watch can be kept on their progress and a further assessment organised if troubles do arise. Otherwise there will be unacceptable risks of the child's difficulties being unrecognised with all the problems that can follow.

Many workers in this field develop their own battery of screening tests, often using items from a number of standardised developmental and intelligence scales. As they have to be used on large numbers of children they must be able to be completed in about 15 minutes. After using a number of motor proficiency tests Gubbay (1978) has shown that four of them were the best guide to the severity of the disability: throwing a tennis ball into the air and clapping hands (up to four times) before catching it again; rolling a tennis ball underfoot in a zig-zag pattern between six matchboxes lined up 30 cm apart (timed); threading 10 beads of 3 cm diameter and 0.8 cm bore (timed); and inserting six differently shaped objects into appropriate slots (timed). He gives the 5th percentile values for the four tests between the ages of 6 to 12 years. Bax and Whitmore (1973) also showed that such screening tests do have predictive value as, using their protocol, over half the children with low scores were in difficulty three to four years later.

When it comes to the more detailed analysis of the more severely affected child's disability it can be accepted that the routine neurological examination is often not sensitive enough and is not orientated to the developmental changes in childhood. Some will work out standardised scales of their own (Peters et al 1975) and particularly for research purposes the examination must be structured in a way that allows for repetition to assess a child's progress (Touwen 1979). Tests such as the Frostig Developmental Test of Visual Perception and the Stott Test of Motor Performance can also be used in this way. The Extended Griffiths Mental Development Scale is particularly valuable for the assessment of the younger child, and in the school situation the Wechsler Intelligence Scale for Children with separate verbal and performance intelligence quotients is frequently applied to children with a mental age of 7 and over.

Once the nature of the child's disability has been identified teachers and psychologists are likely to plan a teaching programme suited to each child. If the main problem is lack of motor organisation presumably constant practice, suitably motivated, is the answer. On the other hand the child with severe perceptual disability cannot be told to carry out a certain task as the instructions will not be understood. The task will need to be broken down into simple parts and these demonstrated in detail. Also full use must be made of the child's verbal ability, and it is relatively common to find that the verbal IQ on the WISC is 10 to 20 points higher than the performance IQ.

As will be discussed later the physiotherapist and occupational therapist can do a great deal to help the clumsy child. If possible they should work in conjunction with the teacher, even if they are mainly involved in out-of-class activities. Apart from the treatment of the disability they can do so much to improve the child's confidence which is frequently sorely lacking, particularly among the less intelligent children. So often the child's response to a request to carry out a certain task is 'I can't' when the assessment has shown that it is well within his grasp. It is a situation where 'nothing succeeds like success'.

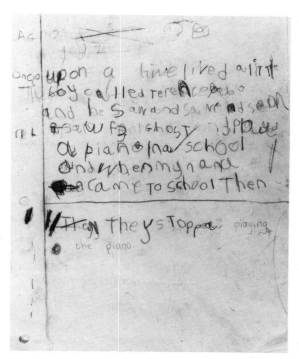

Fig. 15.1 Handwriting of a boy aged 9 (Case 1)

CASE REPORTS

In order to illustrate the kind of problems which affect these children the following two histories are given.

1. T. F., a boy aged 10. He first presented at the hospital following an accident in which he tripped over a dog and fractured his left leg. He was referred again at the age of five because of speech problems. According to his mother he talked 'like a baby' and this appeared to consist of an inability to pronounce some syllables clearly.

Birth had been normal with a birth weight of 3.5 kg. The child was said to have sat unsupported at the age of 6 months and to have walked at 11 months. On the Edinburgh Articulation Teest there was a low score with a number of difficulties with sounds. Speech improved and for a while he failed to attend the clinic.

When the boy was nine the School Medical Officer wrote to say that his teacher was worried about his progress. Very poor co-ordination was the main complaint, although reversal of numbers was also mentioned. To quote from a more detailed school report: 'He is unable to co-ordinate his arms and hands to catch a ball. He cannot run an obstacle course without knocking something over. He cannot colour within a confined space, and he tends to scribble across a shape, never up and down. Writing is very poor [Fig. 15.1]; it is as though his hand has a will of its own. The movements are very jerky and the end result is unreadable. He is so frustrated with his inability to produce written work that he is always wandering off, anywhere, as long as it is away from his books. If one looks at his work books the immediate reaction is — My God, he can't do anything — but he can. He once wrote a story in about six lines. I wrote it out for him and asked him to copy it in his best handwriting so that I could put it on the wall. He either couldn't or wouldn't. He lost his paper, lost his book, took an hour to write one line, tore his paper, dirtied his paper; and we both gave up. He can be witty and imaginative. He does not have any speech difficulties now, but has a spasmodic movement of his head when he is talking and sometimes stumbles over words'.

His reading is poor and spelling is very defective. He has difficulty in tying shoe laces, fastens buttons in the wrong hole, and cannot use a knife and fork properly. He does not mix with other children and has no friends at school. Routine neurological examination showed no abnormalities apart from jerky movements of the out-stretched arms, marked associated movements of the arms on performing Fog's tests and difficulty in balancing on one foot.

Vision on the Snellens Scale was 6/18 in both eyes and glasses have been prescribed. When assessed on the Stott Test of Motor Impairment and the Frosting Test of Visual Perception the child had a number of difficulties, particularly with balancing, with manual dexterity and with eye-motor co-ordination. On the Weschler Intelligence Scale for children the Verbal Scale IQ was 87 and the Performance Scale IQ was 76. The latter result showed areas of difficulty with visual perception. On object assembly he has no idea of what he was trying to do and his coding score was very poor. He was both slow and untidy.

This boy has reached a stage where he no longer wants to try and he is in urgent need of remedial help.

2. N.B., a boy referred to the hospital at the age of 7 because he was overactive, clumsy, distractible and attention-seeking. The mother had been given steriods to promote conception and the pregnancy was normal. The birth was normal with a birth weight of 3.25 kg, but the baby was jaundiced and there were considerable feeding difficulties in infancy.

The rest of the history will be left to the mother who provided a very detailed report. 'He was slow at sitting up, walking and talking. He never crawled. Feeding remained a problem and as a toddler he never attempted to feed himself. He never even put objects in his mouth as a means of exploring them. There have always been periods of waking in the night and even now sleep is very fitful and he travels all over the bed during the night.

'When the boy began to walk he was always falling and constantly stumbling. Outings were a nightmare as they always ended in tears, cuts and bruises; and he sometimes hurt himself quite badly when he fell. When tired he was much worse. At the age of 3 to 4 N. was very timid compared with other children and he could not use apparatus on the playground with the skill of other children of

his age. Drinking from a cup was difficult and it always meant half-filling the cup. No attempts were made to dress, do up buttons and so on. Learning to ride a bicycle was very difficult and there are still problems in turning circles for example.

'Attendance at a playgroup was started at the age of 3, and then he went to a nursery. He would not join in with the other children in anything they were doing, and would not play at one thing for even a short space of time. At his primary school the teacher soon said that she had washed her hands of him. It was hinted that the difficult behaviour was due to mismanagement at home. N. did not make or paint anything like the other children. It was considered that the boy would not do anything, rather than he could not, and he was labelled as lazy. A policy of not helping the child with anything was started but this was a complete failure. Transfer to a private school was arranged but the difficulties continued. The family doctor was seen on several occasions but it was a long time before a child phychiatrist was consulted.

'Recently at school N. has become very withdrawn and he will do nothing unless forced to do so on a one-to-one basis. The other boys tease him and ridicule him because he cannot do the work and cannot play games. He becomes very upset as he desperately wants to join in, but the other boys do not understand, in spite of the teacher's explanation, as they cannot see anything wrong. He irritates people and they usually jump to the conclusion he is lazy, spoilt and naughty. He still gets his right and left mixed up, and he has only just learnt to draw a square which previously had always ended up as a circle'.

A neurological opinion was requested because of the boy's obvious difficulties with co-ordination, for example he could not tie his shoe laces and his writing was very untidy (Fig. 15.2). There were marked associated movements on Fog's tests. On the WISC he was of low average ability with a marked scatter on the subtests with particularly low scores on the visual memory test. On two visual sequencing tasks from the Aston Index there were problems of retaining the correct sequences and with the orientation of individual pictures or symbols. On the Neale Reading Test the accuracy score was in keeping with the chronological age but comprehension was much higher. Copying was poor

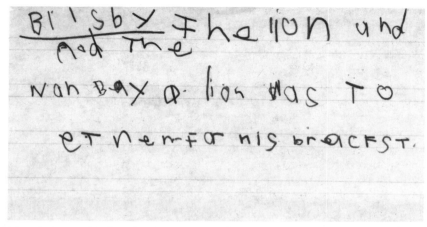

Fig. 15.2 Handwriting of a boy aged 7 (Case 2)

and there was no idea of spelling. The boy was disorganised in his approach to practical tasks and talked constantly while doing things. This chatter seemed to be aimed more at distracting the adult's attention from the inevitable failures than monitoring and controlling his actions. There was some difficulty with spatial awareness and to a less extent with knowledge of body position. He generally used his left hand for fine work.

In view of the child's learning difficulties and abnormal behaviour schooling is likely to remain a major problem and the main hope for the future lies in intensive help in the classroom, geared to his needs, and on as individual a basis as possible.

THE DEVELOPMENT OF SPOKEN LANGUAGE

In parallel with the development of perception and motor organisation, language will gradually take precedence and the left hemisphere will become increasingly active. Some (McNeil 1966) claim that children are born with a set of 'linguistic universals' as part of their innate endowment. They are neurologically so 'preprogrammed' with a language acquisition device that a minimum of stimulation is required for the realisation of this potential. More probably, children are born with certain propensities which enable them to extract from the linguistic input the relevant information to organise language into a consistent system (de Hirsch 1970). Also there is little doubt that language development goes through various stages; first of all the formation of an inner language with the use of concepts but initially without verbal symbols; then the stage of 'receptive language' when the child learn the meaning of the sounds we make; and finally 'expressive language' as he begins to use these verbal symbols to communicate.

Secondary speech disorders

There are a number of conditions which can interfere with the development of language. It is being increasingly realised that mentally handicapped children can be helped a great deal to acquire the ability to communicate, although not always by spoken speech. If the likelihood of the child making reasonable use of the spoken word seems remote then the use of signs and symbols must be considered. Such methods include the American Sign Language, the British Sign Language, the Paget-Gorman Sign System, Bliss Symbols, the Premark System and the Rebus system (Kiernan 1977). The diagnosis of mental retardation can of itself delay language development as it may lead to impoverishment of the child's environment in terms of reduced stimulation. This is obvious in institutions where the time which can be devoted to each child is limited, but may also affect the child at home. There is evidence that the way mothers talk to their normal children is related to social class but not when they have been diagnosed as mentally retarded. Presumably the mothers have been told to speak in very simple terms to their retarded children. This may well be important but can be overdone and deprive the child of adequate stimulation (Cashdan 1969).

As has been stressed, the lack of stimulation and opportunity is well seen among children who are physically handicapped. It may be necessary to give the child increasing experience of everyday life before any attempt is made to teach verbal symbols. For example, 'a boy was making no progress, and his vocabulary was so limited that it was impossible to converse with him. On visiting his home it was found that his world consisted of the view from the front door-step. No amount of reading, talking and explaining could help this child. He had to be taken out on many occasions to the shops to make his own purchases, to the park, on the bus and train, to the beach, to the zoo, to fish in the brook. Although of limited intelligence he absorbed the world like a sponge and was then able to begin a more formal type of education. After some months it was hard to convince people who had not seen him for a while that the alert happy child was the same boy they had met before'.

The importance of excluding any significant degree of peripheral hearing loss needs no emphasis, except to state again that even minor degrees of high tone deafness, sometimes difficult to identify in small children, can interfere with the acquisition of language, particularly if associated with other handicaps such as cerebral palsy. Intermittent deafness from middle ear disease, for example, may well interfere with language development if this occurs in the pre-school years; and can be difficult to diagnose unless tests of hearing are repeated on a number of occasions.

If speech, already acquired, is lost due to disease or injury, this is likely to have profound effects on the child's learning ability. Speech, particularly expressive speech, can often be permanently affected, but even a rudimentary beginning of language development before the brain damage occurs can significantly affect prognosis. The history of Laura Bridgman is a good example of this (Gordon 1969). It is taken from *American Notes*, an account by Charles Dickens of his visit to Boston in 1842. He graphically describes the story of Laura whom

he met at that time. There were a number of problems during the first 18 months of life including convulsions, but for the next six months she was said to have been perfectly well and 'to be displaying a considerable degree of intelligence'. Then the illness struck which left the child blind and deaf.

Admission to the Perkins Institution was arranged at the age of nearly eight and Laura was gradually taught to communicate by sign language. She even used her finger alphabet in her dreams. Intelligent as they must have been, it seems unlikely that Laura Bridgman or Helen Keller would have accomplished so much if at the onset of their illnesses language function had not reached the beginning of its expressive phase.

Adverse environmental conditions undoubtedly affect speech development; factors such as the place in the family, the social class of the parents, overprotection and deprivation. These will influence the richness and complexity of an individual's language, and the ability to express feelings and ideas. Severe emotional and behavioural disorders are also important; the overactive child, the depressed child, the frightened child will all be at a disadvantage if these disturbances occur in the early stages of language development. There is controversy over the role of delayed or deviant language development among children whose behaviour is classified as autistic, but there is no doubt that the language function of these children is profoundly affected. It is suggested that the basic defect may be a cognitive one and not one particularly affecting symbolisation (Boucher 1976).

SPECIFIC DISORDERS OF LANGUAGE DEVELOPMENT

Specific disorders of language development will often be of mild degree, and more of a delay than a deviation of development, and then will usually be overcome through advice to the parents and a sympathetic understanding of the child's difficulties without the need for special treatment. Those children who have developed a good comprehension of speech by the age of three almost always acquire adequate expressive speech without undue delay.

However if there is a significant impairment of both receptive and expressive speech, especially when reaching school age, special educational provision may be needed, if possible with the speech therapist and teacher working together in the class room.

Among the most severely affected children there are some who show not only a gross delay in language development but for a long time difficulties in understanding the meaning of other sounds as well. Some of these children with 'severe auditory agnosia' or 'central deafness' may not even react normally to sounds, as if they were peripherally deaf. This emphasises that we do not hear only with our ears; or see only with our eyes. They are excellent 'microphones' and 'cameras' to generate electrical currents in response to appropriate stimuli, but if the brain is unable to attach meaning to these electrical impulses the individual is just as deaf or blind as if he had no ears or eyes (Gordon 1966). Assessment of such children presents particular difficulties, and some of them may suffer from both central and peripheral deafness. Perhaps this is not surprising since causes such as anoxia at birth can so easily damage the cerebral cortex and the auditory nuclei in the brain stem, but it does have implications for teaching; and long term observation may be the only answer to the problem.

Among these severely affected children it may be important to keep alive an awareness of the meaning of sounds in early life, for instance by converting sounds the child makes into patterns on a television screen. Otherwise auditory sensations may be strongly inhibited if they remain meaningless for long periods. Griffiths (1979) in discussing language therapy for children makes the point that if children fail to learn language structure in the home environment, even under optimum conditions, there seems little justification for supposing that an attempt to duplicate this process in an educational setting is going to be any more successful. McNeil (1974) suggests that just as linguists and phoneticians have to become conscious of the language processes of syntax and phonology, so with children who have specific difficulties with language development.

For the majority of children the acquisition of the mother tongue may well be a question of hearing the auditory symbols in a meaningful situation with the brain at a stage of development capable of integrating the sensory input into the complex structure of a lexicon. If this method is not successful, as with any other skills it may be necessary to break down the language structure into its component parts so that these can be made conscious and practised. Skills are built up of 'sub-routines'. The more these are practised the more automatic they become; freed from the restraints of organisation, intention and feedback. Then these units, no longer having to be monitored, can be detached from the context in which they were learnt, discarded if proved inefficient, or used as the building blocks of more complex actions. The finite set of rules which constitute language function can be regarded as 'sub-routines' which can be presented to the child to practise until they become so habitual that the child can use them at will to generate an infinite set of sentences (Griffiths 1979).

A number of special teaching techniques have been advocated, stressing the importance of association but basically using a phonic approach. It seems more logical to use the unaffected visual pathways as much as possible, as in the method devised by Mr Lea (1965). In this scheme the parts of speech are differentiated by colour, nouns in red, verbs in yellow, adjectives in green, prepositions and conjunctions in blue and adverbs in brown. Words can be represented by lines of appropriate colour and the lines built into patterns to show what is required to describe pictures or events. Nouns are taught first, as whole words, in association with objects; first of all with an actual object and then with many different objects of the same type so that the full concept of what is represented by the particular symbol is demonstrated. Often the children can write and read to a greater extent than they can speak (Gordon 1966).

It is important to remember that language is not only a means of communication but is essential for learning, for categorisation to make sense of the environment, and is needed in the control of behaviour. There is no function more important to the development of the individual, and its growth in early life cannot be left to chance. Any suggestion that the child is failing to communicate as expected must be investigated as a matter of urgency (Gordon 1979).

Case report

This case history is an example of the very complex problems that can sometimes arise in the field of language development, particularly if there are defects of both auditory input and cerebral integration.

P. W., a boy aged 3 when he first attended hospital, had had a number of minor epileptic seizures. Pregnancy and birth had been normal and there was no other past history of note. The possibility of deafness had first been considered at the age of eight months although it was noted that his responses to sound varied. He did not sit up until a year old or walk till he was two.

On examination at the age of three there was little if any increase in muscle tone but the deep reflexes were brisk and the plantar responses extensor. The EEG showed a generalised dysrythmia but no epileptic activity. Treatment with phenobarbitone and then phenytoin was given but occasional seizures continued to occur.

An EEG audiogram was done at that time (1959) and apparent alerting responses were obtained to soft sounds during sleep. Doubts were also expressed about the results of clinical tests of hearing. His parents felt that he did sometimes respond to sounds of no great intensity and during some weeks there was a marked response to distracting techniques using stimuli of minimal loudness, and then for several weeks there seemed to be evidence of profound deafness. A number of detailed assessments were carried out and it was considered that the boy was suffering from a developmental dysphasia and peripheral deafness, and that his non-verbal IQ was around 80. The lack of progress in understanding of speech and the inability to communicate adequately was not the picture of uncomplicated peripheral deafness. At this time there was still generalised hypotonia and the plantar responses were extensor.

By the age of 6 years the boy was writing many words although he could not say them and he was using gestures. The results of pure tone audiometry were still uncertain. On clinical examination there was evidence of mild spasticity and his non-verbal IQ was again thought to be around 80. He continued to receive a great deal of special teaching in day and residential schools for children with disorders of hearing and language development. He had occasional epileptic seizures, in spite of treatment, and his impulsive and sometimes aggressive behaviour became more of a problem. EEGs during this time again showed a generalised dysrhythmia but no definite focal features or epileptic discharges.

When the patient was 13 years old it was impossible to condition him to any auditory signals and to get him to understand any association phenomenon. Lip reading ability was extremely limited; findings which suggested cerebral dysfunction. However there was also increasing evidence in support of a severe peripheral deafness. No response could be obtained to evoked response audiometry but on applying a vibrator to the finger tips there was a typical response showing that the cortex was capable of being reached by another route. A school report a year later said that progress had been made in reading, writing and communication by finger spelling and sign language. No spoken words were used.

After leaving school the patient began training in the bakery trade. Behaviour remained immature with a very low tolerance threshold, so that when employment began a number of jobs were lost in spite of very sympathetic handling. When 17 years old there did not appear to be any specific weaknesses on the non-verbal side and considerable progress had been made in manual communication. The epileptic seizures had stopped and the anti-epileptic treatment reduced to a very small dose. There were no longer any physical disabilities. By the time he was 20 he had had 9 different jobs but in spite of this showed considerable initiative in finding new ones. Various methods of controlling the aggressive behaviour were tried but with little if any benefit. The patient's present position in society is precarious but if the behaviour disorders improve there is no doubt that he is capable of supporting himself in full employment — at one time it had been thought that the only future was in a long-stay hospital for the mentally handicapped.

READING BACKWARDNESS, READING RETARDATION 'DYSLEXIA'

Once the development of perceptual-motor and language functions have reached a certain stage of complexity the child can acquire the skills of reading and writing. The age when a child starts to read will depend on such factors as intelligence, and the method of teaching. For example children can be taught to read at a very early age by the use of certain special techniques, but as this is likely to be without the understanding of what is read, it is of questionable merit.

Children may experience difficulty in learning to read and spell for many reasons. They may miss a great deal of time at school due to illness or truancy. They may be inappropriately taught. They may have defective vision, be emotionally disturbed or fail to acquire the abilito to read as part of a general retardation of development. All skills have to be learnt and reading is no exception. There must be opportunities to learn and there should be adequate motivation. In this context it should be remembered that a few hundred years ago there were not many people in the world who could read.

Reading backwardness has been defined as an attainment in reading accuracy or comprehension which on the Neale test is 28 months or more below the chronological age, but when this attainment is 28 months or more below the level predicted on the basis of the child's age and IQ on a modified WISC the term *'reading retardation'* was used with the implication of a specific disorder of learning (Yule & Rutter 1976). The rubric of 'dyslexia' no doubt has its uses in drawing attention to a group of children who are in great need of help but it should not obscure the fact that children with difficulties of reading present a complex problem of assessment, and that before anything else can be done the particular needs of the individual must be analysed in detail.

Among children of average intelligence with difficulties in learning to read, write and spell the largest number will have a basic defect of language development and in a smaller number the disability will be related to a disturbance of visual perceptual function. Boder (1973) found that among the chil-

dren she studied 67% had a deficit in symbol-sound integration (dysphonetic group). The child has difficulty in developing the phonetic word analysis-synthesis skills which affect the development of language. Children in this group recognise words globally and are unable to sound out and blend component letters and syllables of a word. Reading is easier in context when guesses at words can be made from minimal clues. Spelling is by sight, not by ear, and words are only spelt correctly when they can be visualised. 10% mostly among the younger age groups, were 'Gestalt-blind' with a deficit in the ability to perceive letters and whole words as configurations. These are the only children who are truly 'Word blind' and they may be, or may have been, clumsy in their movements with a more widespread perceptual motor dysfunction. They have a good auditory memory and can recite letters well. They are poor spellers but their errors are not bizarre. Those children with both types of disability which constitute the other 23% in Boder's series are obviously in most serious trouble as they have difficulties in reading by sight or by ear.

Studying children with 'dyslexia' Pavlidis (1979) has found that compared with a normal control group without reading difficulties and a group of slow readers the dyslectic children had obvious defects of eye movements. The normal readers moved their eyes in an orderly way from left to right and their eye movements had a consistent size, duration and pattern, while those with dyslexia showed erratic eye movements in a random scattered fashion. A particular difference between normals and dyslectics was in their regressive movements which were much more frequent in the latter group and were also irregular and often bigger than the preceding forward saccade. Unlike normal readers these children sometimes went far back to fixate on words in a manner that the normal and barkward readers did not. It was considered that the differences were sufficient to be the basis of a diagnostic test of specific developmental dyslexia. It seems unlikely that the findings are the cause of dyslexia but as the affected children also have other difficulties in sequential tracking, and in maintaining fixation, it is more probable that the malfunctioning of the eye movement control system and the dyslexia share a common cause; a central, non-modality specific, sequential disability. If so, there are obvious implications for remedial teaching.

Other children do not fit neatly into any of these groups. For example some seem to have a very specific defect of visual recognition. They have no difficulties with spoken language development and are not clumsy. They can spell words verbally without difficulty but not when they write them down as they cannot seem to recognise certain visual symbols correctly. Information on the exact nature of the disability is essential in order to plan the methods for helping these children. In the case of reading backwardness presumably any conventional methods of teaching can be tried as long as the teaching material is appropriate for the age of the child. When there is a specific learning disorder the teaching programme used should be geared to the defects shown by the particular child. If this is predominantly an audio-phonic one a 'look and say' approach may well be best, while if the child is truly 'word-blind' theoretically a phonic method should be easier. In fact each child is likely to respond in a different way and flexibility is essential, if possible a teaching programme being planned for the individual. Sometimes it may be necessary to borrow from a number of teaching methods.

THE ROLE OF THE DOCTOR

Diagnosis

The doctor, although not an educator, has a major role in helping children with learning disorders. Many aspects of this role are obvious. The importance of discovering causes from intra partum anoxia to epileptic status, and seeking to prevent them must be constantly stressed. Among children with handicaps, the disabilities are usually multiple, but even now high-tone deafness is sometimes missed among children with delayed language development and severe refractive errors among children with visual perceptual problems. Also there are dangers in allocating a child to a school catering for a particular disability and forgetting that he may have several significant handicaps. For

example, it is not uncommon for deaf children to have severe perceptual motor disorders which in their own right would seriously interfere with progress at school.

Assessment

The doctor has an important role to play in helping to analyse the child's difficulties so that a remedial programme can be planned. As Kinsbourne (1973) has said, if you ask a child to do something and he does not, you can ask again, and on the third occasion you can shout at the child; or you work out the components of the request, ask about them separately, and find out which one is not understood. This analysis will be much more effective if the doctor is a member of a team, with help from psychologist, teacher, speech therapist, and physiotherapist.

The fact that learning difficulties affect children with a wide range of intelligence makes it important to assess the child's strengths and weaknesses and not to pay undue attention to the formal IQ figure, and also underlines the need for those of below average intelligence to receive special help if indicated. Again it must be stressed that those of higher intelligence at least have a greater chance of working out their own solutions. As realistic an assessment as possible of the child's potential must be made and fully discussed with the parents. It may help to point out that one of the greatest disservices that one can do to a child is to put him into a school situation which is not meaningful to him. If he does not understand what is going on in the class he will become bored and this will almost inevitably lead to unhappiness and to emotional and behaviour disturbances. Then it is not only a matter of wasting precious time but negative attitudes to learning can easily develop which are hard to eradicate. It is surprising how often children come to the paediatric clinic with symptoms such as headache or abdominal pain and on investigation are found to be suffering from learning disorders of some kind or other.

Stress at home and at school

There are a number of adverse situations at home and at school which the doctor may be able to modify, especially with the help of the social worker and health visitor. If there is need of extra help, or a different type of help, at school the doctor can add his voice to those requesting this for a particular child. Apart from the teachniques of teaching, changes of attitude are often needed. If a child has already been given the label of 'lazy' or 'difficult', a change of school may be necessary. The child should be told that he has certain handicaps which have made life difficult and interfered with his ability to learn as fast as other children; that he can be helped both at home and at school by different methods from the ones he has already endured; and that constant practice will probably improve his performance but that some activities will need to be circumvented. The aims of testing must be explained to parents and the results discussed with them. The child's difficulties should be demonstrated and the fact that they do constitute a handicap; and above all it must be stressed that the child should be given the opportunity to succeed in some ways, however simple. Among other points to be discussed are the educational situation, and often a progress report from the school can be most informative. It is also helpful if the doctor talks to the teacher about the child's inherent difficulties, and the concept of the clumsy child, the child with a language disorder and the dyslexic child. Sometimes it must be stressed that the child *is* handicapped and not just dull and lazy, and that much can be done with fairly simple methods. The comments and advice of the teacher can be of great importance (Dare & Gordon 1970).

Treatment

Although for many learning disorders the school teacher will have a key role to play, there are others who have much to offer children with such disabilities (Gordon & McKinlay 1980). In the case of perceptual motor disabilities the physiotherapist has a major contribution to make in planning treatment and in developing a programme of exercises to improve co-ordination of both large and fine movements if this is indicated. The parents must be involved, if at all possible, so that these exercises can be carried out at home with periodic supervision by the physiotherapist. The more of a game that can be made of it the better and time must be given to the tasks that the child is good at as well as practising the difficult ones (Gordon & Grimley 1974).

The occupational therapist must also be involved, often in devising ways in which the child can cope with the disability, ranging from using a typewriter if his writing is illegible to aids in daily living such as garments with Velcro fastenings rather than buttons. The speech therapist must help in the assessment and treatment of children with speech and language disorders. Much more research is needed on the methods used and their effectiveness, but the individual approach of the speech therapist can undoubtedly complement the group role of the remedial teacher. If children with learning difficulties are under excessive pressure and spending most of their waking hours doing lessons, this is likely to be counterproductive, and the position should be reviewed at intervals. Also statements such as 'could do better if he tried' must be suspect, since often the child may be trying harder than average and the fault may lie in the method of teaching which is unsuitable for that particular individual. If the child is trying hard he must be given credit for this.

Emotional disorders

Emotional problems are a particular concern of the doctor. They often involve the whole family and can easily get out of proportion especially in families with learning high on their list of priorities. The doctor can often discuss these problems as someone outside the immediate situation. He can point out that there is rarely as ideal solution and that sometimes the school is doing all it can to help. If appropriate education is not given the parents, particularly the mother, can become so emotionally disturbed that realistic objectives are abandoned, and the correction of the child's disability becomes an obsession. When the situation reaches this stage it is very likely that more harm than good will result. If the child realises he is the centre of controversy, this is bound to cause tension unless he is exceptionally emotionally mature. Ensuring that the child succeeds in some task however simple is one of the ways in which the situation can be changed, increasing the child's confidence and possibly changing the atmosphere within the family from one of frustration and depression to one of optimism.

Behaviour disorders

Apart from emotional disturbances, behaviour disorders are common enough among children with learning difficulties, and the doctor must try to contribute to the treatment of these. Overactivity, truancy from school, destructive behaviour and aggression may well result from the same factors which cause depression and anxiety; abnormal stresses at home and at school. Drugs are likely to have a very limited role to play in treatment, except possibly in an emergency situation. The true hyperkinetic syndrome is rare but there is some evidence that it can be modified by treatment with drugs such as dexamphetamine sulphate, methylphenidate and pemoline. Dexamphetamine sulphate is given in a starting dose of 2.5 mg morning and mid-day, increasing to the limit of tolerance. Comparable doses for methylphenidate are 5 mg morning and mid-day, and pemoline can be started with a 20 mg tablet in the morning and increased as a single daily dose. If these drugs are given late in the day they may interfere with sleep, which anyhow tends to be disturbed in overactive children. Sometimes they aggravate the behaviour disorder, particularly if a wrong diagnosis has been made. If the dose is increased to too high a level, even after an initial improvement of behaviour, the child can become irritable and depressed, quite apart from sleep disturbances and lack of appetite sufficient to interfere with growth. It is not known how these drugs act but perhaps they enable systems controlling sensory input to work more efficiently. The converse is certainly true as sedatives such as phenobarbitone often aggravate overactivity and aggressive behaviour.

Reading retardation has been linked to delinquency (Critchley 1968); and other handicaps may lead surprisingly frequently to a life of crime. There may be a number of reasons for this and for the association with other types of behaviour disorder. One possibility is a failure of the cerebral integration that underlies maturation and learning, whether this is of skills such as language, or of behaviour patterns. Emotional factors must be of particular importance. A teenager or young adult who cannot read may be exposed to ridicule and scorn and he may be precluded from work that he is quite capable of doing with a little help and understanding. Anyone with a handicap has major adjustments to make and when this is added to the problems of any adolescent, it is hardly surprising that the situation can be too much to cope with.

THE DOCTOR AS CO-ORDINATOR

The doctor must be in the forefront of those pressing for more efficient services, and he is in an ideal position to act as a co-ordinator of all the different experts that may be needed. He must interpret and explain the various opinions to the parents, and apart from helping with diagnosis and assessment he can act as a questioner on behalf of the child and the parents. If for example remedial teaching in a special class has been recommended and has been tried for a reasonable period, it is important to check with the teacher and others concerned whether the child has benefitted or not. The doctor can offer to contact the education authorities on behalf of the parents and child, particularly if antagonisms have arisen. If there are discussions about the child's future education it is important at some stage to include the child in these and not to constantly 'talk over his head'. He needs to know what is happening and why.

Any doctor who sees a number of children with learning difficulties of any type, especially in hospital-based clinics, will soon realise that the majority come from the higher social classes. There are a number of obvious reasons for this, such as the importance attached to learning among some families, the particular ability of some parents to communicate, and the reluctance of others to make a fuss, or the awe in which many parents hold the teacher. Bax (1976) has pointed out that when the handicapped child starts at school he begins to spend as much time with the teachers as with his parents during term time, and if the doctor who is trying to help cannot visit the child's school this is likely significantly to limit the role he can play. He may be unable correctly to assess the child's situation and to integrate the medical aims with those of the teachers. This is a strong argument for as much of this work as possible to take place within the community, with the hospital-based unit mainly supplying a specialist role, as well as being a centre for teaching and research.

CONCLUSIONS

Learning difficulties affect many children and if the disabilities are not recognised early in school life, emotional complications are almost inevitable and these in their turn will delay progress. Much of this is preventable, and although children often overcome their difficulties, it may be at a great cost emotionally and intellectually. The failure to realise potential is difficult to measure but is likely to be large. Doctors must play an increasing part in helping these children; if possible, as members of assessment teams whether these are based in hospitals or in the community.

REFERENCES

Abercrombie M L J 1960 Perception and eye movements. Some speculation on disorders in cerebral palsy. Cerebral Palsy Bulletin 2: 142

Bax M 1976 Back to school. Developmental Medicine and Child Neurology 18: 419

Bax M, Whitemore K 1973 Neurodevelopmental screening in the school entrant medical examination. Lancet 2: 368

Beard R M 1969 An outline of Piaget's developmental psychology for students and teachers. Routledge and Kegan Paul, London

Boder E 1973 Developmental dyslexia: a diagnostic approach based on the atypical reading-spelling patterns. Developmental Medicine and Child Neurology 15: 663

Boucher J 1976 Is autism primarily a language disorder? British Journal of Disorders of Communication 11: 135

Brenner M W, GillIan S, Zangwill O L, Farrell M 1967 Visuo-motor disability in schoolchildren. British Medical Journal 4: 259

Brown J K 1976 Infants damaged during birth. Perinatal Asphyxia. In: Hull D (ed) Recent advances in paediatrics. Churchill Livingstone, Edinburgh

Cashdan A 1969 The role of movement in language learning. In: Planning for better learning. Clinics in Developmental Medicine no 33 William Heinemann Medical Books, London

Childs B 1972 Genetic analyses of human behaviour. Annual Review of Medicine 23: 373

Conners C K 1976 Learning disabilities and stimulant drugs in children: theoretical implications. In: Knights R M, Barker D J (eds) The neuropsychology of learning disorders. University Park Press, London

Critchley E M R 1968 Reading retardation, dyslexia and delinquency. British Journal of Psychiatry 115: 1537

Dare M T, Gordon N 1970 Clumsy children: a disorder of perception and motor organisation. Developmental Medicine and Child Neurology 12: 178

De Hirsch K L 1970 A review of early language development. Developmental Medicine and Child Neurology 12: 87

Dobbing J 1970 Undernutrition and the developing brian. American Journal of Diseases of Children 126: 411

Drillen C M 1972 Aetiology and outcome in low-birthweight infants. Developmental Medicine and Child Neurology 14: 563

Finucci J M, Guthrie J T, Childs A L, Abbey H, Childs B 1976 The genetics of specific reading disability. Annals of Human Genetics 40: 1

Gaze R N 1970 The formation of nerve connections: a consideration of neural specificity ,modulation and comparable phenomena. Academic Press, London

Geschwind N 1965 Disconnection syndromes in animals and man. Brain 88: 237 and 585

Gordon N 1969 A history of Laura Bridgman from American Notes by Charles Dickens. British Journal of Disorders of Communication 4: 107

Gordon N 1979 Neurological processes concerned with communication and their analysis. Child Care, Health and Development 5: 29

Gordon N, Grimley A 1974 Clumsiness and perceptuo-motor disorders in children. Physiotherapy 60: 311

Gordon N, McKinlay I 1980 Helping the clumsy child. Churchill Livingstone, Edinburgh

Griffiths P 1979 An approach to language therapy for children with specific language disability. New Zealand Speech Therapist Journal 34: 14

Gubbay S S 1978 The management of developmental apraxia. Developmental Medicine and Child Neurology 20: 543

Hermann K 1959 Reading disability. Munksgaard, Copenhagen

Kiernon C 1977 Alternatives to speech: a review of research on manual and other forms of communication with the mentally handicapped and other non-communicating populations. British Journal of Mental Subnormality 23: 6

Kinsbourne M 1973 School problems. Pediatrics 52: 697

Laufer M W, Denhoff E 1957 Hyperkinetic behavior syndrome in children. Journal of Pediatrics 50: 463

Lea J 1965 A language scheme for children suffering from receptive aphasia. Speech Pathology and Therapy 8: 58

Markides A 1978 Speech discrimination functions for normal-hearing subjects with AB isophonemic word lists. Scandinavian Audiology 7: 239

McNeil D 1966 Developmental psycholinguistics In: Smith F, Miller G A (eds) The genesis of language. MIT Press, Cambridge, Massachusetts

McNeil D 1974 How to resolve two paradoxes and escape a dilemma. In: Conolly K, Brunner J (eds) The growths of competence. Academic Press, London

Naidoo S 1972 Specific dyslexia. Pitman, London

Ounsted C, Taylor D C 1972 Gender differences: their ontogeny and significance. Churchill Livingstone, Edinburgh

Pasamanick B, Knobloch H 1960 Brain damage and reproductive casualty. American Journal of Orthopsychiatry 30: 298

Pavlidis G Th 1979 How can dyslexia be objectively diagnosed? Reading 13: 3

Peckham C S 1973 Speech defects in a national sample of children aged seven years. British Journal of Disorders of Communication 8: 2

Peters J E, Romine J S, Dykman R A 1975 A special neurological examination of children with learning disabilities. Developmental Medicine and Child Neurology 17: 63

Rutter M L 1970 Psych-social disorders in childhood and their outcome in adult life. Journal of the Royal College of Physicians of London 4: 211

Sladen B K 1970 Inheritance of dyslexia. Bulletin of the Orton Society 20: 30

Stratton P M 1977 Criteria for assessing the influence of obstetric circumstances on later development. In: Chard T, Richards M (eds) Benefits and hazards of the new obstetrics. Clinics in Developmental Medicine, no 64. William Heinemann Medical Books, London

Taylor D C 1969 Differential rates of cerebral maturation between sexes and between hemispheres. Lancet 2: 140

Touwen B C L 1979 Examination of the child with minor neurological dysfunction, 2nd edn. Clinics in Developmental Medicine no 71. William Heinemann Medical Books, London

Townes P L 1982 Fragile X syndrome. American Journal of Diseases of Children 136: 389

Wedell K 1968 Perceptual motor difficulties. Special Education 57: 25

Wepman I M 1973 Auditory discrimination test, revised from IA University of Chicago Press, Chicago

Williams C E 1969 Early diagnosis of deafness and its relation to speech in deaf maladjusted children. Developmental Medicine and Child Neurology 2: 777

Woods G E 1976 The incidence of handicapping conditions in childhood resulting from perintal morbidity. Developmental Medicine and Child Neurology 18: 394

Yule W, Rutter M 1976 Epidemiology and social implications of specific reading retardation. In: Knights R M, Bakker D J (eds) The neuropsychology of learning disorders. University Park Press, London

16

Myelomeningocele

H. B. Eckstein

INTRODUCTION

Myelomeningocele is one of the most frequent congenital abnormalities encountered in paediatric and neonatal practice. Together with anencephaly, it represents the externally visible anomalies of the central nervous system, and the overall incidence for both conditions is around 3 per 1000 live births. This incidence varies from 1.5 per 1000 in the south-east of England to 6 per 1000 in south Wales, Liverpool and Ireland. No satisfactory explanation for the geographical variation has been produced, but social factors may be partly involved in an explanation. Anencephaly is incompatible with life and accounts for about half the abnormalities in this group, while the majority of myelomeningocele infants are live-born and will present problems to paediatricians and many others.

The aetiology of the malformation is not known and is considered to be multi-factorial (Carter 1974). Excessive tea-drinking on the one hand, and the eating or touching of blighted potatoes on the other (Renwick 1972), have been incriminated, but neither has been substantiated as a significant factor. There must be an inheritance factor, as the random chance of any couple having a child with a major CNS abnormality is about 3 per 1000 live births. If the couple have had a previous myelomeningocele or anencephalic child, their chances of having a further such affected child rise tenfold to about 1 in 30, and following two similarly affected children, the chances for the third one having a similar lesion become about 1 in 6. The inheritance does not appear to be X-linked.

The diagnosis of myelomeningocele is patently obvious. There will be an obvious midline defect cranio-spinal axis. 10% of lesions affect the skull and are known as encephaloceles (Ch. 17) and these will not be discussed further in this chapter. Myelomeningocele occurs most often in the lumbo-sacral area and in clinical practice is relatively uncommon in the cervical spine. It is likely, however, that infants with large cervical myelomeningoceles will not survive more than a few minutes after birth, as they will have paralysis of the respiratory muscles and will die of anoxia. In about 5% of infants the lesion is covered by normal-looking skin, and presents simply as a midline swelling on the back. This lesion is defined as a meningocele and is not associated with any neurological deficit. Associated hydrocephalus is unusual with meningocele. In the remainder the defect is either covered by a thin translucent membrane or the opened up and flattened spinal cord is visible and fully exposed on the surface. Immediately after birth this lesion tends to be flat but, if untreated, it becomes elevated in a posterior direction, by the accumulation of cerebrospinal fluid. Presumably the intra-amniotic pressure prevented such fluid accumulation before birth. As the spinal cord becomes elevated the nerve roots can be clearly seen through the translucent membrane extending forwards and downwards. The size of the lesion can vary greatly from 1 or 2 cm to one extending from the mid-thoracic to the sacral spine which can be up to 5 cm or even more across (Figs. 16.1–16.4). Occasionally, there are posteriorly projecting bony spikes arising from the vertebral bodies which split the spinal cord into two, so that there is an associated diastematomyelia (Ch. 17).

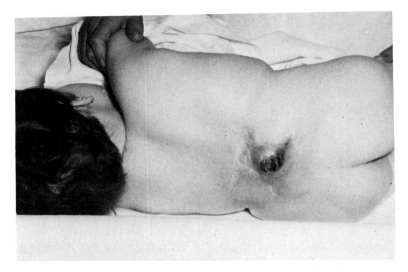

Fig. 16.1 Lumbar myelomeningocele — membrane and open neural plaque clearly seen. Small lesion associated with total paralysis below L2 (age 24 hours). Asymmetry of buttocks suggests vertebral body anomaly

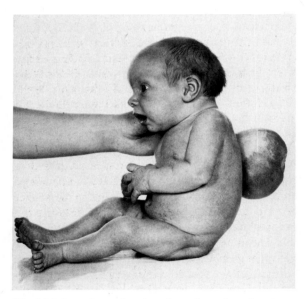

Fig. 16.2 Large lower dorsal myelomeningocele — largely skin-covered. No suggestion of hydrocephalus at age 3 months. Following excision and closure of spinal defect — normal child with normal legs and normal bladder

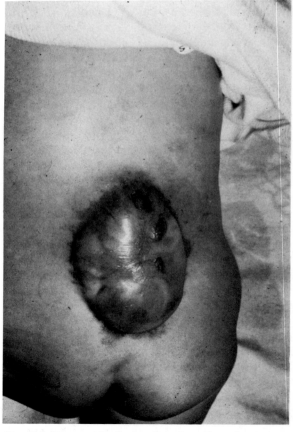

Fig. 16.3 Untreated lumbo-sacral myelomeningocele; note almost complete epithelialisation. Long-term survival likely

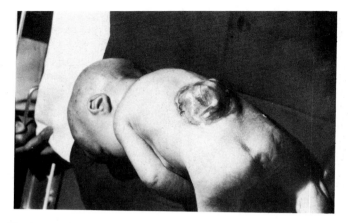

Fig. 16.4 Extensive dorsi-lumbar myelomeningocele with associated gross kyphosis. Simple primary closure impossible. Can be (and was) treated by primary spinal wedge osteotomy and skin closure but today's standards would not be subjected to primary surgical treatment.

NATURAL CONSEQUENCES OF MYELOMENINGOCELE

The neural plaque represents grossly abnormal spinal cord which has often lost its conductive ability well before birth and possibly as a primary malformation. In other cases, with less extensive lesions, there may be surprisingly little loss of nerve conduction at the time of birth. However, as the neural plaque becomes displaced backwards by the accumulation of cerebro-spinal fluid underneath it, the nerve roots become stretched, so that increasing paralysis and anaesthesia must result. The exposed neural plaque is also liable to drying out and to bacterial infection, and both these factors will cause neuronal damage and will increase the paralysis and anaesthesia.

The risk of ascending meningitis resulting from the exposed neural plaque is obvious. If, however, the infant survives (untreated) epithelialisation of the sac will occur; from its periphery it will progress centrally over the next few weeks. Finally the sac will become totally epithelialised, although this process may take between four weeks and six months, depending on the size of the defect. Once complete epithelialisation has occurred, the risk of ascending meningitis is virtually eliminated and the prognosis of the infant changes dramatically in favour of survival.

HYDROCEPHALUS

Hydrocephalus is associated with myelomeningocele in the large majority of patients. Incidence figures quoted in the literature vary from 50% to 90%, and this wide range is undoubtedly the result of the difficulty of diagnosing hydrocephalus (Eckstein & MacNab 1966). If the diagnosis is made entirely on clinical grounds by head circumference measurements, a relatively low figure will be obtained, while in our experience, if the diagnosis of hydrocephalus is based on routine ventriculography in all children with myelomeningocele, then well over 90% will show a significant degree of dilatation of the ventricular system. In clinical practice it is important to differentiate between hydrocephalus per se, which may need no treatment, and *progressive* hydrocephalus, which will require surgical intervention. The downward displacement of the cerebellum and medulla into the upper cervical canal is always present in this situation, and is generally described as the Arnold-Chiari malformation. Although it is likely that the Arnold-Chiari malformation and hydrocephalus develop secondary to the spinal defect, there is as yet no conclusive evidence that this is so and some authors have even suggested that the raised intracranial pressure and hydrocephalus are in themselves a cause of myelomeningocele. The problems of hydrocephalus are dealt with in Ch. 17.

NEUROLOGICAL SEQUELAE OF MYELOMENINGOCELE

1. Paralysis

As already mentioned, myelomeningocele is always associated with a greater or lesser loss of spinal cord conductivity and neuronal activity. Paralysis is an obvious outcome of this situation, and depends on the level of the spinal lesion, its extent, its severity and on possible postnatal damage to the neural plaque. In extensive dorsi-lumbar lesions, there will always be a total paralysis of both lower limbs, which will be completely flaccid but straight. On the other hand, in lesions involving the sacral spinal cord, the nerve supply to the lower limbs is usually normal, but the nerve supply to the pelvic floor, anal and bladder spincters will be impaired, so that the child will have a normal gait but faecal and urinary incontinence. Lower lumbar lesions may result in normally functioning muscles innervated by the first and second lumbar segments but paralysed muscles below that level.

2. Anaesthesia

Just as the motor nerve supply is impaired, so is the sensory nerve pathway. This will result in anaesthesia affecting the skin and will also affect the stretch receptors in muscles, the anal canal and the bladder, so that not only skin sensation, but also postural sense and the ability to appreciate a full rectum or bladder will be lost. In general the neurological levels of motor and sensory denervation are very similar.

3. Deformity

If the lower limbs are totally denervated, they will be perfectly straight but flaccid at birth and will remain so. In this situation, the fitting of calipers later on will present no great problem, and the children can be taught to 'walk.' If innervation of the lower limbs is essentially normal (sacral lesions) the limbs will function normally and there will be no locomotor problem. In the majority of these patients, however, there will be a partial paralysis which will affect certain muscle groups only, so that muscle imbalance will occur, and it is important to realise that this imbalance will have existed in utero for several months before the child is born. Such muscle imbalance results in deformities which include fixed flexion of the hips, hyper-extension of the knees, neuropathic talipes and calcaneus deformity of the feet. The lower limb deformities can, however, be corrected successfully by intensive physiotherapy and stretching of muscles, although at times operative intervention such as tenotomies may be required to straighten the lower limbs. It is, however, essential to realise that the deforming forces persist and the deformity will recur either if the limbs are not permanently splinted or alternatively, if corrective orthopaedic surgery is not undertaken to balance the pull of the various muscle groups. Numerous orthopaedic procedures are practised, of which the psoas transplant is probably the best known (Sharrard 1964). This operation essentially converts the psoas muscle (high innervation) from a hip flexor to a hip extensor, and similar operations can be performed in relation to the knee and ankle joints. With a considerable orthopaedic operative effort and the help of unlimited physiotherapy most of these deformed limbs can be straightened and a useful gait can often be achieved.

4. Incontinence of urine

In the majority of myelomeningocele patients, the nerve supply to the bladder and to the sphincters is lacking, so that urinary incontinence will result. This is most obvious in children with sacral lesions, who are otherwise normal, and on the other hand, there are occasional patients with lumbar or even dorsi-lumbar lesions and almost complete leg paralysis, who have normally functioning bladders. It must be recalled that a myelomeningocele can in no way be compared with a traumatic paraplegia and that often the nerve conduction loss at the neural plaque is a partial and not a complete one, (Stark & Drummond 1971).

5. Incontinence of faeces

The nerve supply to the anal sphincter and rectum is essentially the same as to the bladder and it is not surprising that children who are incontinent of urine will be incontinent of faeces as well. These children have no anal canal sensation and have no functioning external anal sphincter. It must be stressed, however, that the patients have in effect a perineal colostomy and this can usually be trained by suitable diet and drugs to function at a convenient time; faecal incontinence has not been a major problem in our myelomeningocele patients over the years. Provided the motions are normally formed and of normal consistency, these children will achieve a sort of pseudo-continence which is socially acceptable. However, in the event of a gastro-intestinal upset with diarrhoea they will become hopelessly incontinent (Eckstein et al 1970).

6. Obstructive uropathy

Because of partial or total denervation of the bladder, often associated with a partially intact reflex centre in the sacral cord, the synchronisation between the bladder sphincter and the detrusor muscle is lost. As a result, obstruction to urinary outflow develops and detrusor hypertrophy supervenes. Back pressure upon the urinary tract will develop with resultant megaureter and hydronephrosis. Because of the inadequate bladder emptying, urinary stasis results which in turn leads to urinary tract infection. Vesico-ureteric reflux is common in this group of patients and progressive renal damage is to be anticipated in a high proportion as well as urinary incontinence. In clinical practice, these patients should all have an excretory urogram performed on the first admission and this investigation should be repeated at least every second year, so that remedial action (sphincterotomy, urinary diversion, etc.) may be undertaken before there is severe damage to the upper urinary tract. Hypertension in association with pyelonephritis has been described (Lorber & Lyons 1970), but is surprisingly uncommon considering the high incidence of pyelonephritic changes in children with myelomeningocele. Similarly death from renal failure may occur in this group of patients, especially around puberty, but in our experience, this is uncommon (Eckstein et al 1967).

NATURAL FATE OF MYELOMENINGOCELE

In the last few years, the medical profession have assumed and implied that non-treatment of myelomeningocele (no surgery and no antibiotics) will lead to death within weeks or months, or certainly within a year. This concept is undoubtedly wrong.

Evans et al (1974) have reviewed some 500 myelomeningocele patients who had attended The Hospital for Sick Children, Great Ormond Street, before 1958, none of whom had had any surgical treatment in the new-born period and most of whom had had no such treatment at any time. A follow-up some 25 years later showed that although about half the patients had died, there were well over 200 survivors, most of whom had had no treatment at all, or only a urinary diversion. Undoubtedly several of my own patients who have had no treatment whatever have survived for several months or even years. As mentioned earlier, the membranous cover of the myelomeningocele will epithelialise over, and once this has happened, the risk of ascending infection has disappeared. In that situation, the life-expectancy must become much longer, although the problems of urinary tract infection, pyelonephritis and renal failure on the one hand, and the development of pressure sores with spreading infection on the other will take their toll of the survivors in due course. It should be noted that the overall management of so-called untreated patients is much more difficult than that of those who have been treated actively since birth. While many of the untreated patients may die of hydrocephalus, there are many others who survive with large heads and apparently normal brain function.

THE IMPACT ON THE FAMILY

The birth of a baby with myelomeningocele who can usually be guaranteed to have multiple handicaps and numerous problems throughout life, will have a considerable impact upon the family, whether this be a newly-married couple with their first child, or an established family with other children. The arrival of such a handicapped child is inevitably a disappointment, invariably a source of anxiety and only rarely is it regarded as a challenge. Adequate counselling of both parents is essential before the handicapped infant is allowed home, and the services of a skilled social worker are vital for this purpose. In my experience, the social worker and the ward sister of a neonatal surgical unit have always been able to establish a far greater contact with the parents, and even other relatives, than have the doctors.

EXAMINATION OF THE NEONATE WITH MYELOMENINGOCELE

It is important that the infant's temperature is normal at the time of examination. This point is stressed as infants transferred from a maternity unit to a paediatric surgical centre are often hypothermic on arrival for admission, and therefore tend to be inactive and sluggish. It is important to warm the infant gradually in an incubator and to delay full examination until his temperature has reached normal. Hypothermia can, of course, be prevented by covering the infant in gamgee or silver foil and transporting him in a heated incubator in the ambulance. Apart from a standard clinical examination, such as would be performed for any neonate. the head circumference should be checked and recorded and the state of the fontanelle and cranial sutures should be assessed. A palpable and obviously open occipito-mastoid suture at birth is a very real sign of progressive hydrocephalus. The spinal lesion should be examined carefully, and its measurements should be recorded. Once examined it should be covered with a saline-soaked dressing and the use of antiseptics on the neural plaque is to be avoided. Active and passive leg movement and skin sensation of the lower limbs should be checked carefully and the question of muscle charting by a skilled physiotherapist has been dealt with elsewhere in this section. Other congenital abnormalities such as congenital heart disease should be excluded as far as possible. The size, weight and maturity of the baby may all have an important bearing on the choice of management.

THE ATTITUDE OF PARENTS REGARDING TREATMENT

There has been considerable debate amongst paediatricians and paediatric surgeons in recent years, about the involvement of the parents in making a decision whether to operate or not to operate on a child with spina bifida. It has always been my policy to discuss all problems openly with the child's father (the mother is invariably in a maternity unit, often many miles away from a paediatric surgical centre, so that in practice a direct discussion with the mother of the baby is usually not possible. While I have always been anxious to accept the father's views, I have at the same time made it clear that I would not expect a parent to make a final decision regarding surgical treatment or otherwise. Others have suggested that the decision for or against treatment should largely rest with the parents. We have recently reviewed a group of unselected parents and have questioned them about the validity of our concepts. With very few exceptions, the parents agreed that while they would like to be consulted at all times, they felt that it would be totally wrong to ask them to make a final decision relating to operation or otherwise, (Cowie et al 1977). The same review unfortunately revealed that the majority of mothers of myelomeningocele babies had not been seen or consulted by consultant obstetricians or paediatricians immediately after delivery of the handicapped baby, and the source of their information initially has left a great deal to be desired. An improvement in communication is obviously needed here.

INDICATIONS FOR TREATMENT AND 'SELECTION'

A number of historical facts must be appreciated to understand the present-day management of myelomeningocele.

The operation for closure of the spinal defect was first published by Bayer in the *Prague Medical Journal* in 1892 and his operative technique differs in virtually no way from that used by most paediatric surgeons at the present time (Bayer 1892). The very high incidence of progressive hydrocephalus in myelomeningocele has already been mentioned; although many ingenious operations were devised in the last century to deal with hydrocephalus, the results of such surgery were unpredictable, and on the whole unsuccessful. Surgeons therefore felt reluctant to deal with spinal lesions, knowing that the child would develop hydrocephalus, for which there was no treatment. This situation changed in about 1958, when the ventriculo-atrial shunts were introduced, as described by Spitz and Holter and by Pudenz and Heyer almost simultaneously (Scarff 1963, Pudenz 1966). Although the shunts look quite different externally, their essential working parts are almost identical and both shunts were dependent on the recently made discovery of sialastic (Macnab 1966). With the advent of shunt therapy in 1958, hydrocephalus became a treatable condition with an operation which produced a consistently reliable result, even if there were a number of complications. From 1958 to 1962, shunts were used to control hydrocephalus and the myelomeningocele was closed at a later date, usually at around 1 year of age. In 1962 Sharrard et al (1963) presented a paper to the Paediatric section of the Royal Society of Medicine in London. which showed apparently conclusively, that early and emergency closure of the spinal defect produced better results than delayed closure. The authors claimed a lower incidence of ascending meningitis and subsequent brain damage and a decreased amount of nerve loss and paralysis and suggested that there could even be nerve and motor recovery. The majority of paediatric surgeons and neurosurgeons in this country accepted this evidence, and started to treat myelomeningocele as a surgical emergency. A serious attempt was made to close all spinal lesions within 24 hours of birth, and ventriculo-atrial or -peritoneal shunts were inserted if and when progressive hydrocephalus became evident. There were at this stage no ethical or moral implications. With active treatment of all patients, the overall mortality was reduced to about 30% in most of the major paediatric units in the United Kingdom and it is of note that 90% of deaths were within the first year (Eckstein 1973). A treated myelomeningocele child who had survived his first birthday was unlikely to die subsequently. As our experience increased and time passed, it became obvious to most of us involved in myelomeningocele care that the quality of the survivors left a great deal to be desired. We were able to produce a large number of severely handicapped children and the tremendous problems of kyphoscoliosis became obvious. It was, however, not until Lorber (1971), one of the original advocates of early emergency surgery, discussed openly the ethics and morality of routine surgery for all myelomeningocele patients that those involved in their management reviewed the situation critically. Largely as the result of Lorber's work, most paediatric surgical units began to select their myelomeningocele patients for treatment, admittedly on the assump-

tion that the untreated children would die in a short time. While Lorber has specified criteria against emergency surgery (level of lesion, size of lesion, extent of paralysis, extent of deformities, presence of hydrocephalus at birth, etc.) I feel that each individual baby must be assessed individually, and the baby's size and overall fitness must be taken into consideration. If a baby is premature and feeble, this would obviously be a contra-indication, whilst a very healthy overweight baby should be treated, even if there is complete lower limb paralysis and hydrocephalus. In our own experience, about 25% of myelomeningocele patients referred to our unit are not treated actively, but are given routine nursing care. Most of these have died, but there have been notable exceptions. Other centres, such as Dublin, have quoted a non-treatment rate of 75% (Guiney & McCarthy 1981). Selection for treatment poses enormous moral and ethical problems and in the end causes a great deal more work for the surgeon than does routine spinal closure (Robards et al 1975). On the other hand, while the mortality of untreated cases must be around 90%, the survival rate of treated patients has increased to about 85% suggesting and confirming that we are in fact selecting out unsuitable patients, who would in the long run not have survived in any case.

TECHNIQUE OF SURGICAL CLOSURE

Closure of the spinal defect makes the baby more acceptable and attractive to his parents and makes him easier to handle, both by mother and nursing staff. It reduces the risk of ascending meningitis and may preserve motor power and sensation. The actual surgical closure of the spinal defect is not difficult. A general endotracheal anaesthetic is essential and a unit of blood must be available cross-matched, in case of unexpected haemorrhage. An elliptical incision is made around the sac, and the skin is mobilised widely into the flanks by blunt dissection. The membrane is excised completely and a fringe of neural plaque may have to be resected with it. It is essential to leave no part of the covering membrane in situ, as this usually develops into a dermoid cyst later, which could cause pain and increasing neurological deficit by pressure. The open dura mater is easily identified as it is connected to the membranous sac, and the dura can be mobilised and is then closed with interrupted silk sutures. Dural suture is usually feasible, but occasionally in the case of a wide defect, the dura cannot be closed and should simply be left open. Muscle flaps should not be fashioned, as has been recommended in the past, and the skin is finally sutured so as to produce a straight midline scar. If the subcutaneous layer is reasonably tough, a row of subcutaneous sutures can be used, and this reduces the tension on the skin suture line. Drainage of the wound is not necessary. Antibiotic cover of this operation is not normally used. Once the incision has healed, the risk of ascending meningitis has been eliminated.

TEAM MANAGEMENT

Myelomeningocele is much too complex a problem to be dealt with by a single doctor and for its successful management a team of specialists is essential. Many successful spina bifida clinics have evolved in this country and a number of patterns have emerged, which depend on the availability of suitable and in particular of interested members of staff. If a paediatric surgeon is available, he can usually deal with the hydrocephalus, myelomeningocele and urinary tract problems on his own, and from an operative point of view, will require only an orthopaedic surgeon as a colleague. The help and advice of a paediatrician is, however, highly desirable even if it is not available in all centres. The physiotherapist, psychologist and many other paramedical workers are vital members of the treatment team. An appliance fitter will be needed for the older children.

If a paediatric surgeon is not available at the local centre, it is probably best if the entire supervision is looked after by the paediatrician, who will have the help of a neurosurgeon, possibly a plastic surgeon, a urologist and an orthopaedic surgeon. It is however, absolutely essential to have a co-ordinator who can assess the priorities of the different surgical interventions. Adequate secretarial facilities are needed from the outset as such joint clinics or synchronised programmes cannot be effectively organized without close communication and exchange of information between the team members.

FOLLOW-UP ARRANGEMENTS

Unlike the situation with many other congenital abnormalities which can be successfully treated by surgery, the child with myelomeningocele will require regular and life-long follow-up by the various specialists enumerated above. Such arrangements will vary considerably from one hospital to another, but in our own practice spina bifida babies are seen within one month of discharge, three-monthly for the first year, and six-monthly thereafter. The head circumference and valve function are assessed at each visit. A urinalysis should always be done and an excretory urogram should be performed every two years. The follow-up arrangements by the orthopaedic surgeon will depend very much on the degree of deformity and paralysis of the individual child. Suitable arrangements will have to be made when a patient outgrows the paediatric age-group at around 16 years, and this problem is discussed below.

PROBLEMS OF TEENAGE SPINA BIFIDA PATIENTS

While the clinical follow-up arrangements for spina bifida patients present no great difficulties in the paediatric age-group, the problem becomes enormous when these children outgrow their paediatric centre. There are no suitable adult facilities for these multiply handicapped patients and the involvement of various specialists is essential to look after different aspects of the patient. Very few general hospitals have so far provided a satisfactory service for this type of patient, the management of whose many problems is extremely time-consuming. There is an instinctive tendency to have patients with chronic problems seen by the most junior member of the team and this in turn means that the patients are seen by a different doctor every time they attend the clinic. Patients with myelomeningocele should, if possible, be seen by the consultant himself, so that a degree of continuity can be provided in their medical care. A large number of the adolescent spina bifida patients become seriously depressed, so that the help of a psychiatrist may have to be sought.

While schooling facilities for handicapped children have been developed in recent years and are now generally adequate and acceptable, there is a lack of training and education facilities for the school-leaver with paralysis and incontinence and much pioneering work is needed in this field. Provided that adequate training schemes are available for these patients, a significant proportion can ultimately be employed and become independent socially and financially, but with the present state of affairs the large majority of myelomeningocele patients will simply become a burden upon the State and society.

Another problem relating to the over-age spina bifida patient is the question of pressure sores. The development of such pressure sores depends on the circulating pressure of blood and tissue fluids through the capillaries and tissues on the one hand and the weight of the patient on the other. For this reason, pressure sores are most unusual in children, even with extensive paralysis and anaesthesia, but they become an important cause of disability, hospitalisation and surgery in the older patients with myelomeningocele. This is particularly so when these patients, because of their physical inactivity, become overweight. It goes without saying that a serious attempt must always be made to avoid obesity in the spina bifida child and adolescent.

The question of sexual potentiality and the ability to reproduce causes considerable concern to the teenager with spina bifida (Dorner 1977). In general it can be said that females with myelomeningocele can conceive normally and many of them have produced normal children. Males, on the other hand, are likely but not certain to be impotent, and are almost certain to be sterile because of the open bladder neck and retrograde ejaculation. There have been very few documented myelomeningocele fathers, especially if one considers only those with urinary incontinence. Again genetic counselling will be required in this group of patients, at some stage after puberty.

SYNOPSIS OF THE MANAGEMENT OF THE NEUROPATHIC BLADDER

While the large majority of the patients with myelomeningocele will have a neuropathic bladder, it is important to realise that a small but significant number will develop urinary control (Eckstein 1968). It is virtually impossible to predict bladder function in the newborn infant with a meningocele. The importance of regular urinalysis leading to suitable antibiotic treatment in the presence of infection, as well as the importance of regular and repeated excretory urography have already been referred to. For full details of urinary tract management in myelomeningocele patients see Eckstein (1968, 1974) and Stockamp (1977).

1. Bladder expression

The bladder should be manually expressed in all infants with myelomeningocele once the scar on the back has soundly healed. On no account should such expression be performed too soon as it can cause disruption and infection of the incision. Initially expression is aimed at reducing the residual volume of the bladder, and thereby reducing the risk of infection. In older children bladder expression should be attempted as a definitive means of keeping the children socially continent and dry, but to be successful the bladder capacity must be adequate (over 200 ml), there must be no vesico-ureteric reflux, the child must be co-operative and the mother must be willing to devote time to this procedure. Patient teaching by members of the nursing staff is essential for the procedure of expression to be successful. A small but significant number of children can be managed ultimately by such regular bladder expression. The presence of vesico-ureteric reflux (as shown on a cystogram) coupled with urinary infection, is a definite contra-indication to bladder expression as a definitive form of management.

2. Appliances

Urine-collecting appliances can only be used in the male and recent developments have made it possible to use such penile appliances in little boys aged 4 years or more, provided the penis is of a reasonable size (Downs Surgical Co.). These appliances will render the male child socially acceptable, but there may be problems after puberty, and a number of male patients of mine have requested urinary diversion to get rid of their penile appliance! No suitable appliance has been developed for the female.

3. Continuous catheter drainage

This has been recommended by many authors e.g. Minns et al (1980) but has not proved successful in my experience. Indwelling catheters tend to lead to urinary infection, calculus formation, and other problems, and the female urethra especially tends to dilate, so that leakage around the catheter results, and the child remains wet and incontinent in spite of continuous catheter drainage. This method cannot be recommended at present.

4. Drug treatment

Drugs such as Probanthine or Phenyloxybenzamine have been used for the management of the neuropathic bladder with rather unpredictable results but occasionally such drug treatment appears to produce a reasonable degree of continence, and is well worth trying. (For details, see Stockamp 1977).

5. Urinary diversion

Diversion of the urinary stream to a cutaneous stoma has been practised for many years. If the ureters are grossly dilated a cutaneous ureterostomy can be performed; otherwise and more frequently, an intestinal conduit, using either a segment of ileum or colon will have to be utilised. This type of diversion has been used to control urinary incontinence in girls, or for the management of progressive upper tract dilatation and uncontrollable infection as well as incontinence in boys since about 1956. The early results of such cutaneous diversion have been satisfactory but the late (10 years and over) results have been questioned by a number of American authors. Our own results (Stevens & Eckstein 1977), have been eminently satisfactory in a follow-up exceeding 10

years and the procedure has much to commend it, especially in the female.

6. Trans-urethral sphincter resection

The development of the new fibre-light cysto-urethroscopes in paediatric sizes has opened up the possibility of endoscopic resection of the internal or external sphincter. In practice, the internal sphincter (bladder-neck) is usually wide open and requires no surgical interference, and the obstructive element is invariably at the external sphincter level. Endoscopic sphincterotomy may reduce the outlet obstruction and may allow bladder expression in the child in whom expression had not been possible because the outlet resistance had been too high. Alternatively, in the patient with progressive upper urinary tract dilatation due to obstructive forces of the outflow tract, an extensive sphincterotomy will reduce such obstruction and may well lead to a recovery of upper tract dilatation, if this is associated with total incontinence. There is a real and definite place for such endoscopic treatment.

7. Electrical and electronic treatment

The management of bladder dysfunction in neuropathic bladders by implanted electrical pacemakers or other forms of electronic stimulation has proved extremely disappointing, and cannot be recommended at this stage (Caldwell et al 1969, Katona & Eckstein 1974, Nicholas & Eckstein 1975).

8. Intermittent bladder catheterisation

Intermittent catheterisation of a neuropathic bladder as a means of definitive management was advocated by Lapides et al in 1972 and by Lyon et al in 1975. In the ensuing years this form of therapy has been widely acclaimed and accepted as the ideal and standard method of treating neuropathic incontinence, and a further supporting report was published by Hunt (1978). The bladder is catheterised by a parent, medical attendant or, ideally, by the patient herself at regular (usually three hourly) intervals and the child is expected to remain dry and continent in between. Advocates have recommended this technique as universally successful and numerous trials have been performed in recent years. Our own early experience (Eckstein 1979) showed that while this technique was eminently successful in a large number of patients (70%) there were very real contra-indications. The limitations of intermittent catheterisation were referred to by us (Eckstein 1980) and it is important to realise that intermittent bladder catheterisation is not the universal answer. In deciding upon this line of treatment, one must consider the question of mental retardation of the child, the patient and parent compliance in relation to a complicated and time-occupying form of therapy, the problem of extensive caliperisation for paralysis which may make catheterisation in either sex technically difficult, the problems posed by severe spinal abnormality with kyphoscoliosis, where intermittent catheterisation is simply not feasible on purely technical grounds, and in those children who have low sacral lesions and who have maintained some degree of urethral sensation in whom also catheterisation is technically not possible. It would appear, therefore, that while intermittent bladder catheterisation has a great deal to offer in obtaining a pseudo-continence for the child with neuropathic bladder, this form of therapy is not the universal answer in all the patients concerned.

9. Pyocystis

Infection of the non-functioning bladder occurs in 20% of children. These usually present with a 'vaginal discharge' but such a symptom in a girl with urinary diversion is virtually diagnostic in itself of pyocystis. The treatment of choice today is a vesico-vaginostomy (Eckstein & Stevens 1975).

ANTENATAL DIAGNOSIS

Any subsequent editions of this book may well no longer require a chapter on myelomeningocele! The finding of the chemical substance, alphafetoprotein, in the amniotic fluid and even in the blood of mothers carrying a myelomeningocele or anencephalic child has been one of the greatest medical advances in our lifetime (Brock et al 1973). For several years the test on amniotic fluid has been available, and although amniocentesis cannot possibly be used for the routine testing of all pregnant women, it has been used quite justifiably on those mothers who have had a previous spina bifida child. The risks of amniocentesis are relatively small and the reliability of the test is high. As a result of the amniocentesis alphafetoprotein we have not seen any second spina bifida siblings for the past 6 years in our patients, while this was not a uncommon occurrence before that. The alphafetoprotein test on blood is at present becoming standardised throughout the country and will undoubtedly become a routine antenatal investigation. If the test is positive, then pregnancy will be terminated and even if we accept that the test cannot be 100% reliable, there is no doubt whatever that the number of infants born with myelomeningocele (or anencephaly) will become very much smaller over the next few years and from the point of view of the workload of the paediatric surgeon and of the National Health Service in general it will probably no longer be the major problem which it is now. It is likely that myelomeningocele, from being one of the most important crippling conditions causing multiple handicaps affecting virtually every system of the body, will become a problem of mainly historical interest in our own time.

REFERENCES

Bayer C 1892 Zur Technik der Operation der Spina Bifida und Encephalocele. Prager Medizinische Schrift 17: 317

Brock D J H, Bolton A E, Monaghan J M 1973 Prenatal diagnosis of anencephaly through maternal serum — alphafetoprotein measurement. Lancet 2: 923

Caldwell K P S, Martin M R, Flack F C, James E D 1969 An alternative method of dealing with incontinence in children with neurogenic bladders. Archives of Disease in Childhood 44: 625

Carter C D 1974 Clues to the aetiology of neural tube malformations. Developmental Medicine and Child Neurology (supplement) 32: 3

Cowie V, Colliss V R, Eckstein H B 1976 A study of the effect on parents of selection for treatment of spina bifida patients. Developmental Medicine and Child Neurology (supplement)

Dorner S 1977 Problems of teenagers. Physiotherapy 63: 190–192

Eckstein H B, Macnab G H 1966 Myelomeningocele and hydrocephalus, the impact of modern treatment. Lancet 1: 842

Eckstein H B 1968 Urinary control in children with myelomeningocele. British Journal of Urology 40: 191

Eckstein H B 1968 The neurogenic bladder. In: D I Williams (ed) Paediatric urology. Butterworths, London, p 371

Eckstein H B, Scobie W, Long J 1970 Bowel control in children with myelomeningocele. Developmental Medicine and Child Neurology (supplement) 22: 150

Eckstein H B 1973 Die Myelomeningocele: eine Übersicht über das Problem. Zeitschrift für Kinderchirurgerie 13: 17

Eckstein H B 1974 The neuropathic bladder. In: Williams D I (ed). Encyclopaedia of urology, urology in childhood. Springer, Berlin, p 249

Eckstein H B, Stevens P S 1975 The management of pyocystis following ileal conduit diversion in children. British Journal of Urology 47: 630

Eckstein H B 1979 Intermittent catheterisation of the bladder in patients with neuropathic incontinence. Zeitschrift für Kinderchirurgie 28: 408

Eckstein H B 1980 The urinary tract in Spina bifida or the paediatric urologist's dilemma (Casey Holter Memorial Lecture) Zeitschrift für Kinderchirurgie 31: 296

Evans K, Hickman V, Carter C O 1974 Handicap and social status of adults with spina bifida cystica. British Journal of Preventive and Social Medicine 28: 85

Guiney E J, McCarthy P 1981 Implications of a selective policy in the management of spina bifida. Journal of Pediatric Surgery 16: 136–138

Hunt G M, Whithycombe J F R, Whitaker R H 1978 The management of urinary incontinence by intermittent catheterisation in children with myelomeningocele. Zeitschrift für Kinderchirurgie 25: 395

Katona F, Eckstein H B 1974 The treatment of the neuropathic bladder by trans-urethral electrical stimulation: a preliminary report. Lancet 1: 780

Lapides J, Dickno A C, Silber S J, Lowe B S 1972. Clean, intermittent self-catheterisation in the treatment of urinary tract disease. Journal of Urology 107: 458

Lorber J, Lyons V H 1970 Arterial hypertension in children with spina bifida cystica and urinary incontinence.

Developmental Medicine and Child Neurology (supplement) 22: 101

Lorber J 1971 Results of treatment of myelomeningocele. Developmental Medicine and Child Neurology 13: 279

Lyon R P, Scott M P, Marshall S 1975 Intermittent catheterisation rather than urinary diversion in children with meningomyelocele. Journal of Urology 113: 409

Macnab G H 1966 The development of the knowledge and treatment of hydrocephalus. Developmental Medicine and Child Neurology (supplement) 11: 1

Minns R A, Oag J C, Duffy S W, Brown J K, Stark G, McClemont E 1980 In-dwelling urinary catheters in childhood spinal paralysis. Zeitschrift für Kinderchirurgie 31: 387–397

Nicholas J L, Eckstein H B 1975 Endovesical electrotherapy in the treatment of urinary incontinence in spina bifida patients. Lancet 2: 1276

Pudenz R H 1966 The ventriculo-atrial shunt. Journal of Neurosurgery 25: 602

Renwick J H 1972 Hypothesis: anencephaly and spina bifida are usually preventable by avoidance of a specific but unidentified substance present in certain potato tubers. British Journal of Preventive and Social Medicine 26: 67

Robards M F, Thomas G G, Rosenbloom L 1975 Survival of infants with unoperated myeloceles. British Medical Journal 4: 12

Scarff J E 1963 Treatment of hydrocephalus; an historical and critical review of methods and results. Journal of Neurology, Neurosurgery and Psychiatry 26: 1

Sharrard W J W 1964 Posterior ilio-psoas transplantation in the treatment of paralytic dislocation of the hip in children with myelomeningocele. Journal of Bone and Joint Surgery 46B: 426

Sharrard W J W, Zachary R B, Lorber J, Bruce A M 1963 A controlled trial of immediate and delayed closure of spina bifida cystica. Archives of Disease in Childhood 38: 18

Stark G D, Drummond M 1971 Spinal cord lesions in myelomeningocele. Developmental Medicine and Child Neurology (supplement) 25: 1

Stockamp K 1977 neuropathic bladder. In: Eckstein H B, Hohenfellner R, Williams D I (eds); operative pediatric urology. Thieme, Stuttgart p 313

17

Hydrocephalus and congenital anomalies of the nervous system other than myelomeningocele

E. M. Brett

HYDROCEPHALUS

Although the causes of hydrocephalus include many disorders, congenital and acquired, of varied aetiology, the condition is discussed here because of the important contribution of developmental anomalies.

The term hydrocephalus, as the lay expression 'water on the brain' indicates, implies an excess of CSF within the skull. It is used more specifically to denote the presence of an increased amount of CSF under increased pressure with enlargement of the ventricular system. The CSF is largely produced by the choroid plexuses of the ventricles and circulates through the foramina of Monro, third ventricle, aqueduct of Sylvius and foramina of the fourth ventricle to enter the subarachnoid space in the cisterna magna, which is continuous with the spinal sub-arachnoid space. Most of the fluid passes via the basal and ambiens cisterns to reach the subarachnoid space over the surface of the cerebral hemispheres, whence it is absorbed through the arachnoid villi or granulations into the cerebral venous sinuses.

Aetiology

There are therefore three theoretical ways in which hydrocephalus can arise: obstruction to the flow of CSF at any point, overproduction of CSF or failure of its reabsorption. The term 'communicating hydrocephalus' is sometimes used for the two latter situations, and for obstruction within the subarachnoid space (usually referred to as basal cistern block) in contrast to the non-communicating or obstructive variety.

Obstruction to the flow of CSF may result from congenital malformations, neoplasms and inflammatory conditions.

CONGENITAL MALFORMATIONS

Three main malformations are seen:

Aqueduct stenosis occurs in several different anatomical forms. There may be many channels instead of a single one, most of them ending blindly and only one effectively linking the third and fourth ventricles. There may be gliosis round or a membranous barrier within the lumen of the aqueduct. In most cases aqueduct stenosis is sporadic and non-genetic, but rare X-linked cases have been reported often with adducted thumbs. Postmeningitic ependymitis may lead to an acquired form of aqueduct stenosis which is usually transitory.

The Arnold-Chiari malformation. This common abnormality is often associated with hydrocephalus and myelo-meningocoele (Chapter 16). In its mildest form there is downward displacement through the foramen magnum of the medulla oblongata and cerebellar tonsils, and in a severer form similar downward elongation of the fourth ventricle, while the severest form shows downward herniation of the cerebellum through a bony defect (Fig. 17.1). The malformation obstructs the free flow of CSF either directly or secondarily through associated arachnoiditis with adhesions and so causes hydrocephalus. It may also lead to the later development or syringomyelia (see below).

The Dandy-Walker syndrome. This malformation results from occlusion of the exit foramina (of

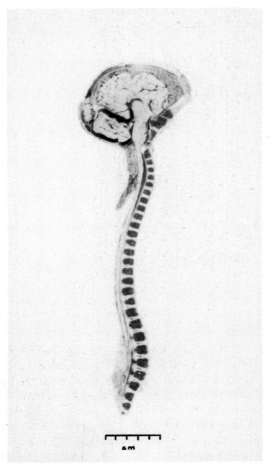

Fig. 17.1 Arnold-Chiari malformation and lumbosacral myelocele in 11-week-old boy. The cerebellar component of the Arnold-Chiari malformation extends down to the level of the 2nd thoracic vertebra. The cranium is small and the falx poorly formed. Other congenital malformations present were a common truncus arteriosus, hypoplastic kidneys and agenesis of left external auditory meatus

Luschka and Magendie) of the fourth ventricle during early cerebral development. There is a small, hypoplastic cerebellum with a greatly distended fourth ventricle and an enlarged posterior fossa (Fig. 17.2). Obstructive hydrocephalus and cerebellar ataxia are the clinical accompaniments.

Bony deformities of the base of the skull, as in achondroplasia and platybasia, may also obstruct the CFS pathways and cause hydrocephalus. Rarely a *vascular malformation*, such as the so-called aneurysm of the great vein of Galen (Ch. 19), may act as a tumour to produce obstructive hydrocephalus.

NEOPLASMS

Tumours, benign and malignant, can readily cause obstruction at various points in the circulation of the CSF. The blockage may be persistent or intermittent. The importance of cerebellar, suprasellar and other neoplasms in causing hydrocephalus is discussed in Ch. 18 and the ball-valve effect of colloid cysts of the third ventricle in causing intermittent raised intracranial pressure is mentioned.

Tumours of non-neoplastic type which can cause hydrocephalus include cystic lesions of the arachnoid, hydatid and other cysts of inflammatory origin, intracerebellar haematomas and the lesions of tuberose sclerosis (Ch. 20).

INFLAMMATORY CONDITIONS

Pyogenic and tuberculous meningitis are often complicated by hydrocephalus as a result of adhesions obstructing the flow of CSF, especially in the basal cisterns and other subarachnoid pathways. Intra-uterine infection with cytomegalovirus or toxoplasma (Fig. 17.3). or subarachnoid haemorrhage, at birth or later, may also cause adhesions and hence hydrocephalus. In many cases of basal cistern block the cause is never determined, but a history of a difficult delivery may suggest that adhesions following subarachnoid bleeding are responsible. Such bleeding is known to be common in the newborn period from the frequent finding at lumbar puncture in sick neonates of blood-stained or xanthochromic CSF. Arachnoid cysts, which may cause hydrocephalus, may also be of inflammatory origin.

Overproduction of CSF by choroid plexus papillomas (Ch. 18) is a very rare cause of hydrocephalus. This is usually of communicating type, but an obstructive element may result from bleeding or from the mass effect of the papilloma.

Theoretically defective reabsorption of CSF could be congenital or acquired. A convincing case for a congenital form was made by Gilles & Davidson (1971) in a report of two boys with communicating hydrocephalus who at autopsy showed a marked diminution of arachnoid granulations with abnormality of the few remaining. Such cases are probably rare. With regard to acquired forms it is

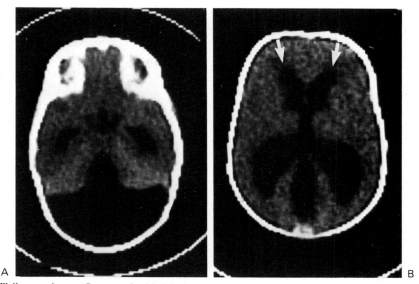

Fig. 17.2 Dandy-Walker syndrome. One-month-old girl with rapidly enlarging head.
CT. Note (A) enlarged posterior fossa, rudimentary cerebellar hemispheres, absence of cerebellar vermis and large 4th ventricle
(B) dilated 3rd and lateral ventricles with frontal periventricular lucencies (arrowed). The dilated 4th ventricle extends up between
the occipital lobes

not easy to assess the contribution of defective reabsorption of CSF after meningitis or subarachnoid bleeding, since these are likely also to cause obstruction to the flow of fluid from basal cistern or other block. Thrombosis of the sagittal and other venous sinuses as a result of dehydrating febrile illnesses or trauma can theoretically lead to communicating hydrocephalus, but is more likely to cause benign intracranial hypertension (Ch. 18).

CLINICAL FEATURES

In some cases of congenital hydrocephalus, usually associated with the Arnold-Chiari malformation, the condition may be suspected by the obstetrician since the large head may fail to descend normally into the maternal pelvis. Radiological or ultrasound examination may enable the diagnosis to be made in utero. Delivery by Caesarean section or other methods may be needed.

The ability of the skull of the infant and young child to expand by sepatation of the sutures when obstruction to the CSF pathways has caused intracranial hypertension has already been mentioned in the context of cerebellar and other tumours. There is no difficulty in recognizing gross enlarge-

ment of the head, but lesser degrees (which one should aim to detect) are easily overlooked unless the head circumference is measured and checked against tables of figures for normal children and, when available, previous figures for the patient. Serial measurement and plotting of the centile group are often needed to confirm that unduly rapid growth of the skull is occurring. An increase of head circumference from a lower to a higher centile should always be treated seriously. The measurements should preferably be taken with a flexible steel tape and must encompass the maximum circumference of the head.

The hydrocephalic head is often abnormal in shape as well as in size, being unduly rounded with the face overshadowed and dwarfed by the large head with its bulging forehead (Fig. 17.4). The skin over the scalp may be shiny with distended veins in the frontal and temporal regions. The temporal fossae may be filled in. The anterior fontanelle is often large, remaining open after the usual age of closure. It may feel tense on palpation and lack the normal transmitted pulsations even when the child is erect. A caveat must be mentioned that dehydration, which may result from vomiting, may cause the fontanelle to be less tense than it would otherwise be. The separation of the cranial sutures

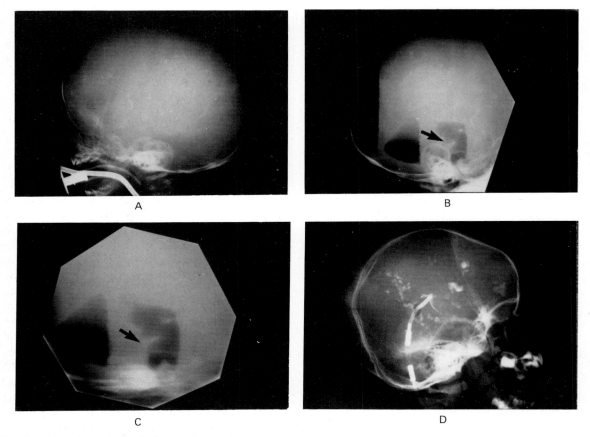

Fig. 17.3 Toxoplasmosis with hydrocephalus.
A. Lateral film of skull. The skull vault is obviously hydrocephalic. Nodular and linear calcification is present in the cerebral hemispheres.
B. Ventriculogram — brow-down lateral film.
One lateral ventricle only contains air and is grossly dilated. The 3rd ventricle is partly filled and also dilated. There is stenosis of the aqueduct (arrow) but the air has passed into the 4th ventricle which is very large (triangular shadow). Its exit foramina are obstructed.
C. Tomogram of (B) showing 3rd and 4th ventricles and stenosed aqueduct.
D. Skull film following relief of hydrocephalus by a Holter shunt system.
The calcification is more dense and extensive.

can sometimes be palpated. The head should be percussed lightly with a flexed finger to assess the percussion note. This is often abnormal when intracranial pressure is raised: in older children it often has a boxy character and in infants resembles the effect of tapping a ripe water melon. Till (1978) stresses the value of holding the child's head with the other hand opposite the point of percussion to detect a reverberation or fluid thrill as a sign of raised pressure.

In suspected hydrocephalus the head should always be transilluminated. For this purpose a completely dark room is needed and a powerful torch which can be applied to the scalp with a tight fitting rubber seal. In severe cases the head may appear translucent, but seldom to the degree seen in hydranencephaly.

It is rare to find papilloedema in young children with hydrocephalus since skull enlargement acts as a safety valve, but retinal haemorrhages and optic atrophy may be seen with varying degrees of visual impairment. Choroidoretinopathy may point to the diagnosis of toxoplasmosis or cytomegalo-virus infection. An important ocular sign in many cases

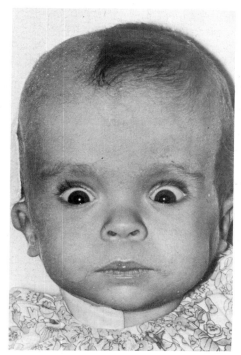

Fig. 17.4 Setting sun sign in 8-month-old girl with hydrocephalus

which should act as a warning is the 'setting sun sign' with downward deviation of the eyes and a rim of sclera visible between the upper edge of the iris and upper lid on either side (Fig. 17.4). This may be intermittent at first. It is seen in other conditions with raised intracranial pressure, and also in kernicterus and in some otherwise normal premature babies.

Other clinical features of hydrocephalus in the infant and young child (apart from those of the causal condition and the other sequelae of the latter) include somnolence, vomiting, failure to thrive, irritability, a shrill cry, and delayed motor and social development or mental deterioration. Retardation in motor milestones is often particularly marked with delay in independent sitting. In some cases the large size of the head is a contributory factor but is often possible to detect an element of cerebellar ataxia as shown by titubation of the head on the trunk and truncal instability.

Mental impairment may be mild or severe. It may be masked in some older children with hydrocephalus by a relatively advanced verbal facility which gives a false impression of intelligence (the 'cocktail party' or 'parrot' syndrome). Variable neurological signs may be found in the limbs with pyramidal features, especially in the legs, and cerebellar ataxia. In early and in mild later cases there may be no symptoms and diagnosis depends on the signs, especially cranial enlargement.

A rare but important sign seen in some cases of obstructive hydrocephalus is the occurrence of bizzare bobbing movements of the head. The term the 'bobble head doll syndrome' is used to describe this situation (Benton et al 1966, Tomasovic et al 1975). The movements, usually of a forward and backward nodding type but sometimes from side to side, are reminiscent of those dolls with weighted heads or of the toy dogs or other animals which some motorists like to place near the rear windows of their cars. Many cases are associated with hydrocephalus due to third ventricular cysts but the movements have also been seen with hydrocephalus secondary to aqueduct stenosis. In two hydrocephalic children the head bobbing preceded by six months any other features of raised intracranial pressure so that it can be a valuable warning sign. The onset of bobbing has been under the age of 10 years in all cases. It can be abolished voluntarily, at least for brief periods. Successful surgical treatment of the hydrocephalus has almost always led to decrease in the abnormal head movements (Russman et al 1975). The published cases were reviewed by Tomasovic et al (1975) who also considered the unresolved question of the pathogenesis of the bobbing. The differentiation of these head movements from those seen in other disorders, including those sometimes seen in cases of congenital nystagmus was discussed by Görke et al (1975) who reported the association of head-nodding with a large cyst of the septum pellucidum in a boy with spinal muscular atrophy.

Hydrocephalus due to aqueduct stenosis may occasionally declare itself in older children with abnormalities of gait and manipulation due to pyramidal and cerebellar dysfunction without gross evidence of raised intracranial pressure or cranial enlargement.

THE DIAGNOSIS OF HYDROCEPHALUS

This involves two separate processes, the recognition and differential diagnosis of hydrocephalus from other conditions, and the discovery of its cause.

a. The distinction between hydrocephalus and other causes of macrocephaly

A large head, or *macrocephaly*, may be due to hydrocephalus, but it may also be caused by subdural effusion or haematoma which is often bilateral and often, but not invariably, associated with a broad somewhat square head rather than a uniformly round head. Localized cranial enlargement may be seen, often in the temporal region, in some cases of cerebral glioma, ependymoma, and other tumours. Bony disorders such as achondroplasia, rickets and osteogenesis imperfecta may be associated with a large skull.

It must be stressed that the actual head circumference at one moment is less important than the *rate* at which it has increased and is increasing. Data on previous head size are unfortunately often lacking. In the first four months of life the normal rate of increase for term infants is 0.4 cm per week. The situation is different in prematurely-born infants of low birth weight in whom the head circumference shows a rapid increase in the first months of up to 1.0 cm per week, a rate similar to that occurring in the last trimester of pregnancy in fetuses delivered at term. Failure to recognize this fact and to make suitable allowance for prematurity by plotting the circumference on charts corrected to the expected date of delivery may cause unnecessary alarm (Sher & Brown 1975a).

The situation is more complex when the preterm infant is medically unwell, needing, for example, prolonged respiratory control or intravenous therapy. The average rate of head-growth in these sick pre-term infants is often much slower, and is approximately half that of term infants. Sher & Brown (1975b) found that only infants with significant medical problems in the neonatal period conformed to, or fell below, the expected pattern of growth. These authors also studied the important phenomenon of 'catch-up' head-growth and its distinction from early hydrocephalus. In a group of 18 pre-terms infants with birth weights between 1000 and 1800 g they found 9 who, after recovery from illness, showed a spurt in head-growth

between the third and seventh postnatal weeks parallel to that of healthy pre-term infants. These children were showing 'catch-up' growth and were all neurologically normal. By contrast 6 sick infants who had initial rates of growth equal to or above those of healthy pre-term children were hydrocephalic, even though their growth curves did not cross percentile lines and they showed no clinical signs of raised intracranial pressure. Three healthy infants with initial rates above the maximum rates for healthy pre-term infants all showed early signs of raised pressure and neurological dysfunction and radiological evidence of hydrocephalus.

The head may also be enlarged because the brain substance itself is larger than normal. In general terms this situation is described as *megalencephaly*. This may result from many different causes. In certain degenerative brain diseases such as Tay-Sachs disease in the later stages, Alexander's and some spongiform leucodystrophies (Ch. 5) the brain is enlarged. In some of the mucopolysaccharidoses (MPS) and in some cases of neurofibromatosis, tuberous sclerosis and achondroplasia the same is true. The associated clinical features usually make the distinction from hydrocephalus fairly simple, although hydrocephalus can complicate some cases of MPS disorder. Megalencephaly is also used in a neuropathological sense for a rare condition without neuronal storage or biochemical disorder and with a normal ventricular system, but with occasional additional structural cerebral anomalies. In these cases non-progressive mental retardation is common.

Lastly a large head may be a benign familial feature (Day & Schutt 1979) and, as in problems of stature, it is wise to measure the head size of both parents (the father is the more usual parent to show a large head in these families).

The *rate* of growth of the head is a most important factor in the recognition of progressive hydrocephalus, but unfortunately previous measurements of the head circumference are often lacking.

b. Investigation of the cause of hydrocephalus

Sometimes examination will show clinical features to suggest the cause (choroidoretinopathy with intrauterine infections, a bruit with an aneurysm of the vein of Galen, myelomeningocele with the

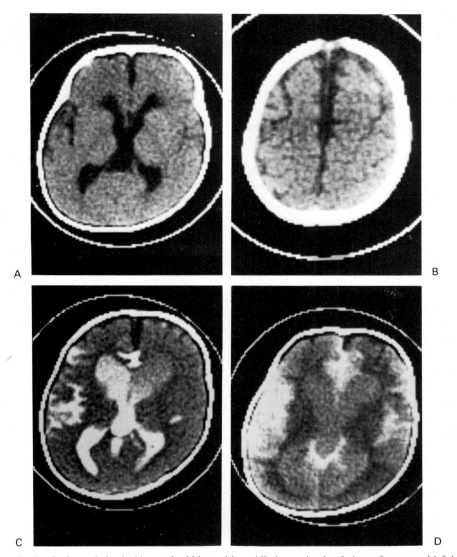

Fig. 17.5 Communicating hydrocephalus in 11-month-old boy with rapidly increasing head circumference and left hemiplegia. CT. Note (A and B) moderate communicating hydrocephalus with widening of left Sylvian and interhemispheric fissure. (C) 1 hour after lumbar injection of Metrizamide, much of the contrast has entered the ventricles while the remainder is in the left sylvian fissure and pericallosal cistern. (D) 6 hours later Metrizamide was still present in the lateral ventricles and diffusing into the cerebral substance. Contrast is held up in the interhemispheric fissures indicating distal obstruction to its flow

Arnold-Chiari malformation), but radiological investigations are needed to define the cause precisely.

Plain skull X-rays of good quality may give helpful information. They may show a thin vault with suture diastasis and other signs of raised intracranial pressure. In aqueduct stenosis they may show a posterior fossa which is shallower than normal. Intracranial calcification may suggest toxoplasmo-sis (Fig. 17.3), a craniopharyngioma, pinealoma or other tumour. More often skull X-rays do not give clues and special X-rays are needed.

Previously contrast radiology with air-encephal-ography, ventriculography and occasionally arteri-ography was needed in most cases to determine the cause of hydrocephalus. When the CT scan is not available these methods may still be needed, but the advent of the scan has made much simpler and safer the differentiation between hydrocephalus and other causes of macrocephaly, the differential diagnosis of hydrocephalus and, stemming from this, its management. In most cases the scan alone gives sufficient information but in some situations, when failure of reabsorption of CSF is suspected, studies of the rate of clearance of injected contrast material (Metrizamide) may provide the answer (Fig. 17.5).

MANAGEMENT OF HYDROCEPHALUS

This will depend on the cause. With tumour, whether neoplastic or otherwise, treatment will consist of its removal when possible or a shunt procedure to bypass the obstruction when it cannot be removed. Certain cystic lesions causing obstructive hydrocephalus, whether developmental or acquired, may be drained surgically with relief of the obstruction.

The assessment of non-neoplastic hydrocephalus and of its treatment is rendered difficult by the common occurrence of spontaneous 'arrest' with cessation in the unduly rapid rate of skull growth. Though poorly understood, this may depend on a restored balance between the production of CSF and its absorption, or possibly recanalization of obstructed CSF pathways. Active hydrocephalus can sometimes recur in a patient in whom arrest had previously occurred either spontaneously or after a shunt procedure. The assessment and management of such cases may be very difficult but is facilitated by the CT scan which can be used serially to detect change in ventricular size. Close co-operation with a surgeon experienced in the paediatric aspects of neurosurgery is highly desirable, but may not always be available. The risks of mental deterioration and, in older children with more rigid skulls, of visual impairment from persistent hydrocephalus must be borne in mind. Even in hydrocephalic children with a poor prognosis for mental and motor development, such as some survivors from bacterial meningitis, surgical treatment may be beneficial by preventing the gross and distressing degrees of head enlargement which may make nursing and daily management most difficult.

The surgical procedures for the relief of hydrocephalus are discussed by Matson (1969), Till (1975) and Eckstein (1977). Most depend on draining CSF from a lateral ventricle to elsewhere in the body. (Coagulation or removal of the choroid plexuses has been used in the past but is rarely practised today). The three main shunt procedures are the ventriculo-atrial shunt (draining the CSF through tubing from the ventricle to the right atrium of the heart), ventriculo-peritoneal shunt (draining it into the peritoneal cavity), and ventriculo-cisternostomy or Torkildsen's operation (draining it to the cisterna magna to bypass an obstruction in the aqueduct or third ventricle). The last method is not suitable when the subarachnoid space is obliterated as in post-meningitic or post-haemorrhagic basal cistern block since the CSF cannot then be adequately absorbed. Various forms of tubing and valves, opening at different pressures, are available.

The main problems with ventricular shunts are infection of the system and blockage. Shunt infection is common, occurring in about 12% of treated children, and is usually due to the *Staphylococcus albus*. A low-grade chronic bacteriaemia results and may cause fever, anaemia, failure to thrive, splenomegaly and, in rare cases, shunt nephritis. Infection requires replacement of the shunt and antibiotic treatment. Blockage of the shunt may occur proximally, from the choroid plexus growing into the ventricular catheter, or distally, when growth of the child results in the catheter withdrawing from the right atrium into the superior vena cava. Blockage from any cause leads to the clinical features of raised intracranial pressure and usually requires replacement of the valve and revision of the shunt. Use of the ventriculo-peritoneal shunt may avoid some of these difficulties including those due to growth, since redundant tubing in the peritoneal cavity can compensate for this.

Neonatal hydrocephalus of mild to moderate degree has been successfully treated in some infants with meningo-myelocoele by compressive head wrapping (Epstein et al 1974, Porter 1975). The method is somewhat controversial. It is thought, when successful, to work by causing accelerated CSF absorption during cranial compression.

Medical treatment with isosorbide (Lorber 1972,

1975) has been successfully used as a purely temporary measure in some children with hydrocephalus due to inflammatory lesions such as meningitis or after surgery for repair of spina bifida. In some cases the need for a shunt may be averted. The serum electrolytes must be measured daily and the drug should be avoided in those with impaired renal function.

In some cases of hydrocephalus it is difficult to know whether the condition is arrested or not, and whether treatment should be arranged. In these cases and in patients treated by shunts who develop the features of raised intracranial pressure monitoring of intracranial pressure may be helpful.

ANENCEPHALY

This grossest of cerebral maldevelopments is the commonest severe malformation found in still-births and is incompatible with more than a short survival. The skull vault is usually absent and the forebrain and midbrain are represented by a spongy mass of vascular tissue containing neural elements and choroid plexus, the *area cerebrovasculosa*. The anterior pituitary gland may be absent or hypoplastic which is thought to explain the invariably small size of the adrenal glands. The eyes are often normal, but with no sign of the optic nerves, and this suggests that there has been disintegration of preformed parts of the brain. Defective closure of the anterior end of the neural tube is probably the primary defect. The cause of this and the reason why the condition is much commoner in girls than in boys are unknown. Excess of vitamin A has produced a similar condition in rat embryos. In man genetic factors are probably involved, since a familial incidence is seen, especially in those of Celtic origin (Ch. 21). Environmental factors may also be involved since a seasonal variation is seen in its incidence.

Prenatal diagnosis is possible when hydramnios, with which it is often associated, has been detected, or when a previous child has been affected. X-rays to show the fetus will often demonstrate anencephaly, and an early diagnosis can be made by measuring the plasma alphafetoprotein in the mother's blood (Brock et al 1974) as in spina bifida. Genetic

counselling should be given since the risk of another child with anencephaly or spina bifida is high (Ch. 21).

Many of the primary or automatic responses may be normal in the anencephalic newborn infant (Gamper 1926), although the placing reaction in the feet and automatic walking may be absent (André-Thomas et al 1944).

HYDRANENCEPHALY

In this rare, sporadically occurring condition the greater part of the cerebral hemispheres are replaced by large membranous sacs filled with CSF. There is some evidence that it may arise as a result of the obstruction to the blood flow in the territory supplied by the internal carotid arteries in fetal life, though the mechanism of this is speculative. The structures supplied by the vertebral arteries are usually spared, so that the basal parts of the temporal and occipital lobes, the hippocampi and amygdaloid nuclei, the cerebellum and brain-stem are present. Transillumination of the skull (Fig. 17.6) may suggest the condition, showing complete passage of light through the skull except at its lower levels. Sometimes a light applied to the back of the head may be seen anteriorly through the child's eyes. The EEG may indicate the presence of some functioning brain tissue and seizures may occur. They were present in four of the seven patients reviewed by Hamby et al (1950). In the child reported by Neville (1972) with infantile spasms starting at 4 months and continuing until her death at $2\frac{1}{4}$ years there was no electrical activity on the EEG and a brain-stem origin for the attacks seemed very likely.

It is important to distinguish hydranencephaly from the more common condition of congenital hydrocephalus, which carries a much better prognosis with treatment. The head may be large at birth and may sometimes show unduly rapid enlargement after birth due to an obstruction at the aqueduct, but shunt procedures as for hydrocephalus are of no benefit in hydranencephaly and should be avoided.

Radiological investigation with ventriculography, air encephalography or the CT scan (Fig. 17.7) usually allow the two conditions to be distinguished.

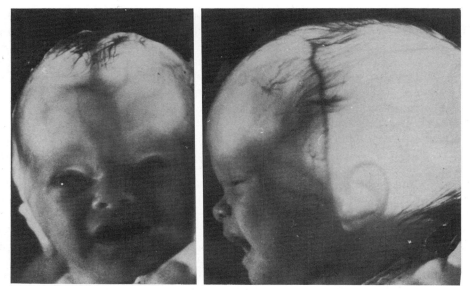

Fig. 17.6 Hydranencephaly — transillumination of head in 12-day-old girl

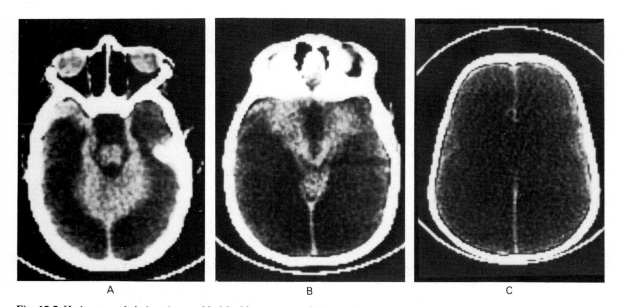

A   B   C

Fig. 17.7 Hydranencephaly in a 6-year-old girl with severe retardation and a large head.
CT. The lateral and 3rd ventricles are grossly enlarged and occupy most of the supratentorial space. The 4th ventricle is not enlarged. The cerebellar hemispheres, midbrain, thalami and basal ganglia appear to be the only significant masses of brain substance. There is possibly a thin mantle of cerebral substance in both temporal regions.

PORENCEPHALIC CYSTS

Large cystic lesions within the substance of the brain have been found in patients with congenital hemiplegia, retardation and other chronic neuro-logical handicaps from the nineteenth century onwards. Heschl (1868), who had earlier proposed the term 'porencephaly' for such lesions, suggested that they might result from reduction of the blood supply to a localized area of brain. Their location and the frequent demonstration at arteriography of occluded anterior or middle cerebral arteries (Naef 1958, Freeman & Gold 1964, Isler 1971) strongly support an ischaemic aetiology. In many cases the cysts probably develop prenatally. Their frequent association with polymicrogyria (Dekaban 1965) suggests that in these cases both originate before the sixth month of gestation. In other cases origin at the time of delivery seems likely from circumstantial evidence and rarely the history suggests a postnatal onset. The sudden development of an acute hemiplegia in a previously normal child may be followed by the demonstration of a porencephalic cyst in the appropriate situation. The CT scan has facilitated the detection of porencephalic cysts which may have previously been missed on air encephalography since many of the lesions do not communicate with the ventricular system (Fig. 17.8).

The cysts may be single or multiple and are normally found in the distribution of the anterior and/or middle cerebral arteries. They may cause localised thinning or bulging of the overlying skull bones and occasionally cause a shift of the lateral ventricles to the opposite side. Despite their enormous size in some cases, they seldom seem to enlarge or to cause further disturbance of neuro-

logical function. Very rarely when pressure within a cyst builds up surgical drainage may be needed.

MULTICYSTIC ENCEPHALOMALACIA OR POLYPORENCEPHALY

In this rare condition both cerebral hemispheres are replaced by multiple cystic spaces. The affected infants are usually abnormal at birth with seizures, hypertonia, irritability and an abnormal cry. Sometimes the fetal movements have been reduced and there is often a history of neonatal asphyxia, which may be the result rather than the cause of the cerebral abnormality. The prognosis is very poor, most children dying within a few weeks or months.

The cause of the condition is obscure and may vary from one case to another. A prenatal cause seems likely in most cases but neonatal asphyxia may have been responsible in the case of Crome (1958). Rarely the disorder has been familial affecting several siblings (Claireaux 1972) but most cases are sporadic. A vascular cause, with destruction of brain tissue due to ischaemia, is possible but the cystic lesions seen at post-mortem are very widespread and do not correspond to any particular

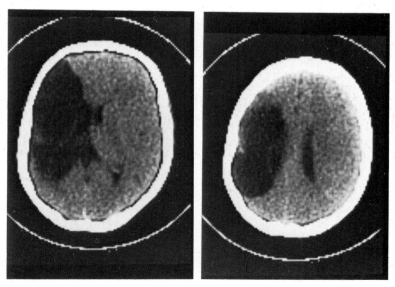

Fig. 17.8 Large left sided porencephalic cyst with left hemiatrophy of skull in a 10 year old boy with a right hemiplegia and right-sided convulsions.
CT. The area of low attenuation in the left hemisphere involves most of the territory of the middle cerebral artery in the frontal and parietal lobe.

areas of vascular supply or drainage, unlike the single porencephalic cysts. Many cases have involved the survivor of twins, the co-twin having died in utero and often being macerated. Aicardi and his colleagues (1972) believe that the twin with encephalomacia may have bled into the other twin, causing the death of the latter and severe damage to its own brain from under-perfusion. They also believe there may be a link between multicystic encephalomalacia and hydranencephaly, since air encephalography in one patient was typical of the former at 4 weeks or age but suggested hydranencephaly at 4 months. Lyen et al (1981) have made a good case for fetal viral encephalitis as the cause in two infants with multicystic encephalomalacia.

Clinically the affected children are neurologically and developmentally abnormal and may be microcephalic. Abnormal transillumination of the head can usually be shown in a dark room as in hydranencephaly. Radiological confirmation is given by air encephalography or CT scan (Fig. 17.9). The EEG usually shows absence of phasic activity and the CSF protein level may be high. In some cases evidence of intrauterine infection with various viruses or with toxoplasma suggest an infective cause.

CRANIUM BIFIDUM

This term covers a group of midline developmental cranial defects which are analogous to the various forms of spina bifida. The overt forms include cranial meningocele and encephalomeningocele (often difficult to distinguish clinically) and occult cranium bifidum is also seen. The word 'encephalocele' is often used to include all these lesions and will be so used here.

The encephalocele is much rarer than its spinal analogue. In one clinic 265 cases of encephalocele were seen compared with 1390 spinal lesions (Matson 1969). The lesion may occur at any site over the vertex or base of the skull, usually in the midline. Most are occipital and these are often associated with various malformations of the midbrain. 195 of Matson's 265 cases were occipital.

There may be a genetic component in some cases of occipital encephalocoele which may alternate in some families or kinships with anencephaly, spina bifida or hydrocephalus. In the very rare Meckel-Gruber syndrome (Smith 1976) a posterior encephalocoele is seen associated with microcephaly, microphthalmia, polydactyly and polycystic kidneys with autosomal recessive inheritance and a very poor prognosis.

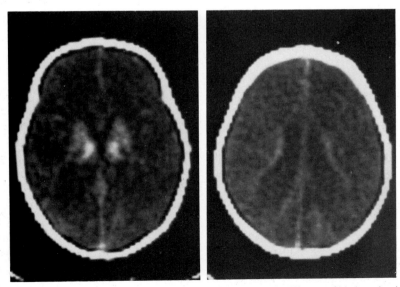

Fig. 17.9 2-month-old girl with polyporencephaly or multicystic encephalomalacia. History of birth asphyxia and generalized fits. Abnormal transillumination of head.

Both cerebral hemispheres are of almost uniform low attenuation of density slightly higher than CSF. Contrast injection caused enhancement of ependymal walls of the lateral ventricles and also of strands of tissue within the cerebral hemispheres.

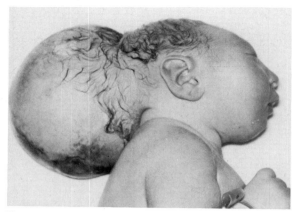

Fig. 17.10 Occipital encephalocoele in newborn baby (note microcephaly)

The occipital lesions may be pedunculated or sessile and may be covered by normal skin or by epithelium only (Fig. 17.10). The scalp over the sac and near it may show vascular abnormalities and the overlying hair may be long and silky. If the sac or the anterior fontanelle are compressed gently pressure can usually be transmitted from one to the other. The size of the sac and that of the head are very variable. A large sac does not necessarily carry a worse prognosis than a small one since its contents may be entirely fluid, whereas a small sac may contain mainly brain tissue. A small skull, however, implies a worse outlook for development. Inspection and transillumination of the sac may help to show whether it contains solid tissue or not, but the anatomy can only be fully defined by X-ray studies, particularly ventriculography or CT scan which will also disclose any structural abnormalities of the cranial contents. This information is needed before the surgical approach can be planned.

In some cases the function of the central nervous system is so abnormal that survival is obviously limited to a matter of hours or days, and in such cases surgical intervention does not seem justified. In all other cases early repair should be the aim in order to facilitate nursing and feeding and to avoid the severe psychological trauma which the gross deformity often causes to the child's mother and father, preventing the bonding process from occurring. With ulcerated and leaking sacs there is a grave risk of infection and meningitis, and urgent repair is needed. The pedunculated sacs with nar-

row stalks are relatively easily dealt with surgically. The prognosis is difficult to assess in the newborn period, just as it is in other malformations of the brain and various encephalopathies in early life. Mental retardation, cerebellar ataxia, other forms of cerebral palsy, visual problems, epilepsy and hydrocephalus may occur as sequelae. Microcephaly and gross neurological abnormality in the newborn period are obvious grounds for pessimism, but in the absence of these guarded optimism is reasonable.

Frontal, nasal and nasopharyngeal encephalocoeles differ from the occipital lesions in seldom showing a genetic component. They are often associated with cerebral malformations such as agenesis of the corpus callosum and single ventricle, and should be regarded as examples of frontonasal dysplasia and as part of the spectrum of the median cleft face syndrome (Opitz 1979). They are rare in Europe and the United States but common in South East Asia and in West Africa. 25 cases were seen in Bangkok in 3 years (Suwanela & Hongsaprabhas 1966). Ocular hypertelorism is invariably present and may be gross. Six of the Siamese patients had microcephaly and two had hydrocephalus. The lesions are usually obvious at birth (Fig. 17.11) but may encroach on the orbit or present as a swelling in the nose causing unexplained nasal obstruction or, rarely, meningitis.

MEGALENCEPHALY

This term, by its derivation, means an abnormally large *brain*, and must be distinguished from macrocephaly, meaning a large *head* (which is not necessarily due to a large brain).

Megalencephaly is sometimes applied to heavy brains with additional structural anomalies (Urich 1976). The latter include heterotopia of subcortical white matter, absence of the corpus callosum, abnormal gyral patterns, polygyria and a diffuse overgrowth of the protoplasmic macroglia. It may be associated with tuberous sclerosis and neurofibromatosis (Ch. 20) and occurs also in some patients with Tay-Sachs disease at a later stage and in some cases of spongiform and Alexander's leucodystrophy (Ch. 5).

Megalencephaly also occurs as a benign familial

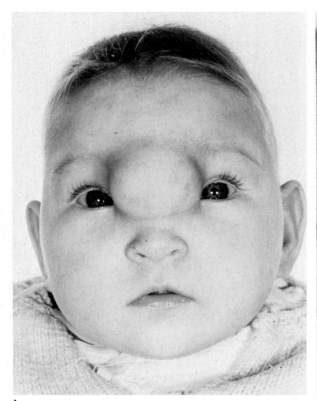
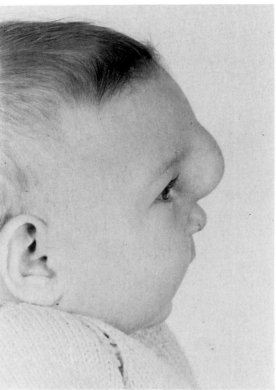

A   B

Fig. 17.11 Frontal encephalocoele. 5 month old girl (A) frontal (B) lateral

feature (Asch & Myers 1976, Day & Schutt 1979). This affects males more often than females, and may be dominantly inherited. Three generations of males were affected in the family reported by Asch & Myers (1976).

Day & Schutt (1979) reported 15 normal children with large heads (circumference more than 0.5 cm above the 98th centile). In most cases in which parental head size was measured one parent (the father in all but one case) was found to have a large head, as were 6 of 17 siblings. The head circumference was large at birth and its rate of growth excessive in most of the cases in which data were available. The size of the ventricles was normal in 14 of the 15 children investigated by CT scan. It is important to recognise the condition in order to avoid unnecessary investigation and anxiety in the case of normal children with large heads. It is probably much commoner than is recognized and its true incidence will not be known until more doctors make a regular practice of measuring the head size of both parents; the fact that it is usually the mother who takes the child to the doctor militates against recognition of the familial nature of the large head.

MICROCEPHALY

Most cases of microcephaly (defined as a head circumference more than two standard deviations below the mean for age and sex) are non-genetic. Many are due to acquired factors operating in pregnancy or early post-natal life. Others are associated with a variety of congenital anomalies and may be genetic or non-genetic. The condition is very rarely familial with autosomal recessive inheritance and without anomalies of other structures. In these cases the very small skull with brow sloping backwards and furrowed scalp is dwarfed by the normal sized face (Fig. 17.12). The brain is grossly reduced in size, usually weighing between 500 and

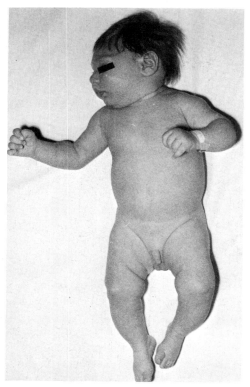

Fig. 17.12 Microcephaly. 10-week-old boy

the brains of mentally retarded children are examined at autopsy. These cannot be diagnosed clinically and are seldom demonstrable radiologically. Their pathology is well reviewed by Urich (1976).

Pachygria (lissencephaly: agyria)

The basic features of this malformation are a reduced number of secondary gyri and an increased depth of grey matter between the smooth areas of the cortex. Extreme cases may show a short and oblique Sylvian fissure as the sole indentation over the outer surface of the cerebrum. (Agyria implies an absence of gyri. The term 'lissencephaly' (literally 'smooth brain') is sometimes used as a synonym for pachygyria or agyria). More often the primary gyri and a few sulci are present. The lamination of the cerebral cortex and the underlying white matter may be grossly abnormal in the affected smooth areas, but normal in the regions where fissures and sulci are present. Heterotopic nerve cells may be found in the centrum semi-ovale and may protrude into the ventricles.

Pachygyria may be unilateral, when it is often associated with a congenital hemiplegia.

600 g and the cerebellum contributes more than its normal share to the total weight. The simplified convolutional pattern is reminiscent of that seen in the higher anthropoid apes with abnormally wide gyri and the architecture shows many minor anomalies affecting the various layers and the size and distribution of cells. Clinically the affected children are severely mentally retarded, but they are less likely to suffer from epilepsy or cerebral palsy than are patients with other forms of microcephaly.

Other recessively inherited syndromes with microcephaly are seen each with diagnostic groupings of associated anomalies marking them off from others. Some, such as the bird-headed dwarf syndrome of Seckel, are more easily recognized than others such as the Smith-Lemli-Opitz syndrome in the female.

ABNORMALITIES OF CORTICAL GYRI

Many anomalies of gyrus formation are seen when

Micropolygyria

In this prenatal anomaly the surface of the cortex appears wrinkled or bossed like morocco leather but sectioning reveals many small convolutions lying near the surface but separated from it because their molecular layers remain fused together so preventing intervening sulci from being formed. The condition may be extensive or limited. When there is bilateral involvement of the central convolutions spastic deplegia is often present and when only one hemisphere is affected a hemiplegia is commonly seen. There is evidence that various prenatal anomalies, including micropolygyria and heterotopias, may be strictly confined to the territories of the main cerebral arteries. Micropolygyria may be present in the cortex overlying a porencephalic cyst and the demonstration at arteriography of occlusion of the middle or anterior cerebral artery in some cases of this kind suggests a vascular aetiology for both lesions.

Agenesis of the corpus callosum

Partial or complete absence of the corpus callosum is among the commonest developmental anomalies of the brain. The corpus callosum, composed of commissural fibres crossing from one cerebral hemisphere to the other, develops between the 12th and 22nd weeks of gestation and factors operating at this stage presumably account for the malformation. There is evidence that some cases may have been caused by maternal ingestion of drugs taken early in gestation as a test of pregnancy. It has also been reported occasionally in association with chromosomal abnormalities including trisomy 18, 13 and 8 (Smith 1976).

The clinical features are very variable. Mental retardation, usually mild to moderate, epilepsy and cerebral palsy often of hemiplegic type are common accompaniments. The head is often enlarged from an early age, sometimes causing suspicion of hydrocephalus. In one patient at least, the large head was associated with cephalopelvic disproportion and with fetal distress requiring emergency Caesarian section. (Ettlinger et al 1972). Often there are facial features suggesting the diagnosis, with ocular hypertelorism (an increased distance between the inner canthi) commonly present (Fig. 17.13) and sometimes a median cleft of the lip, palate or nose.

The diagnosis can be confirmed radiologically. Air encephalograms show elevation of the third ventricle which separates the anterior horns of the lateral ventricles which are themselves elevated and have sharp upward-pointing angles, the so-called rabbit's ear or ox-horn appearance. The CT scan shows the same features in the horizontal plane (Fig. 17.14). Occasionally other abnormalities may be found such as a lipoma or cyst between the cerebral hemispheres, or a porencephalic cyst; a frontal meningocoele was present in one child with partial callosal agenesis (Ettlinger et al 1972).

In the course of investigating children with mental retardation, epilepsy and cerebral palsy callosal agenesis is sometimes diagnosed. The diagnosis is helpful, not only in providing an explanation of sorts for the child's problems, but also in excluding a genetic cause, since most cases are sporadic.

A rare variation on the theme of callosal agenesis is the *Aicardi syndrome* (Aicardi et al 1969, Dennis & Bower 1972.) This syndrome seems not to be genetically determined and all reported infants have been girls with one exception. (Curatolo et al 1980). It comprises a combination of infantile spasms, severe retardation, an unusual form of choroidoretinopathy with a lacunar appearance resembling that of Swiss (Gruyère) cheese (Fig. 17.15)

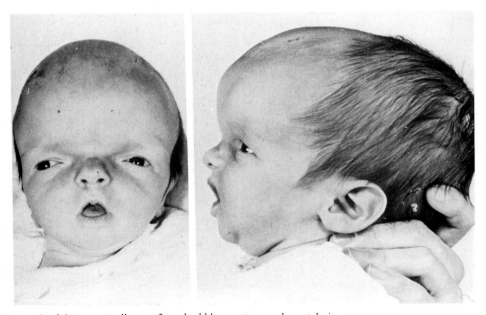

Fig. 17.13 Agenesis of the corpus callosum. 2-week-old boy: note gross hypertelorism

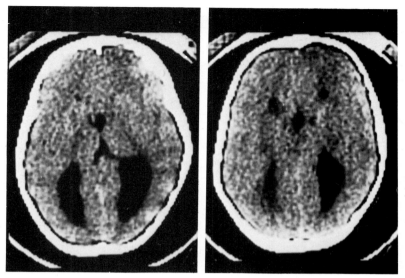

Fig. 17.14 7-year-old girl with agenesis of the corpus callosum. She was moderately retarded and had a large head. CT. Note upward extension of cavity of 3rd ventricle associated with separation of the bodies of the lateral ventricles and flattening of their medial walls. The 4th ventricle is normal

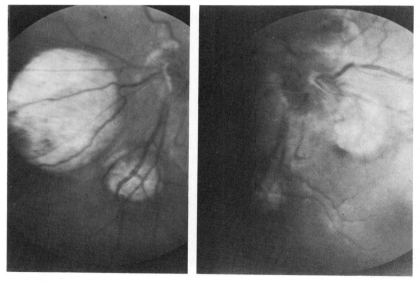

Fig. 17.15 Aicardi's syndrome — note the 'punched out' white areas which represent a retinal pigment epithelial defect without hyperplasia. The left optic disc also has a congenital glial anomaly

and agenesis of the corpus callosum. Though rare, it seems likely that cases are missed since, as Willis & Rosman (1980) have pointed out, the erroneous diagnosis of a congenital infection is sometimes made.

Two rare genetic syndromes are recognised with callosal agenesis. Hereditary partial agenesis of the corpus callosum has been reported with X-linked recessive inheritance affecting five brothers (Menkes et al 1964). All were severely handicapped with seizures within a few hours of birth and three died under the age of two years.

Lastly, an autosomal recessive syndrome with familial callosal agenesis and sensorimotor neuropathy has been reported from Canada (Andermann et al 1976). Originating from an ancestral couple who married in Quebec in 1657, these patients present with psychomotor retardation and a slowly progressive flaccid tetraplegia, have complete absence of the corpus callosum with dysmorphic features, evidence of anterior horn cell disease and absence of sensory action potentials.

SEPTO-OPTIC DYSPLASIA (AGENESIS OF THE SEPTUM PELLUCIDUM WITH HYPOPLASIA OF ONE OR BOTH OPTIC DISCS)

This condition in which abnormalities of the optic nerves, optic chiasm and optic tracts are associated with anomalies of midline structures in the brain was first described in 36 cases by de Morsier (1956). The clinical features are blindness with searching nystagmus and hypoplasia of one or both optic discs. Radiologically there is absence of the septum pellucidum and dilatation of the chiasmatic cistern on air encephalography (Fig. 17.16), and it may be possible to show that the optic nerves are abnormally slender. These features can also be shown by the CT scan (Fig. 17.17). Neurophysiological studies show a normal electroretinogram but abnormal visually-evoked cortical responses.

The optic discs show a characteristic appearance with a double edge, an inner hypoplastic margin and an outer halo. There may also be paucity of the retinal vessels.

Pituitary dysfunction was recognized in this condition by Hoyt et al (1970). Many patients have short stature with inability to secrete growth hormone. This was the case in three of the four children reported by Brook et al (1972), one of whom also had hypoglycaemia.

The septum pellucidum normally begins to develop at six weeks of gestation when differentiation of ganglion cells in the eyes also occurs, so that the factor or factors (at present unknown) responsible for the maldevelopment must operate at this time. The associated endocrine features presumable reflect involvement of the hypothalamus in the midline abnormality.

CYSTS OF THE SEPTUM PELLUCIDUM

The posterior part of the septum pellucidum normally disappears in the course of development. It contains a cavity, the cavum septi pellucidi, which is always present in premature infants but is usually obliterated or remains as a narrow slit in the more mature brain. Sometimes the cavum may persist as a large cavity, demonstrable radiologically. This is usually symptomless but may rarely cause pressure symptoms, if very large, by obstructing the foramina of Monro and causing hydrocephalus which may be intermittent.

Large lesions are sometimes called cysts of the septum pellucidum. One such case was associated with the bizarre movements of the bobble-head doll syndrome in a seven year old boy with spinal mus-

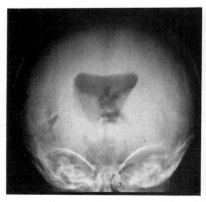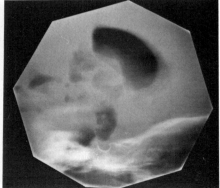

Fig. 17.16 Septo-optic dysplasia in 19-month-old girl. She was blind with small, pale optic discs. Lumbar air-encephalogram. There is a common lateral ventricle with absence of the septum pellucidum. The cerebral substance and optic nerves appeared normal. Note flat roofs of the anterior horns of the lateral ventricles

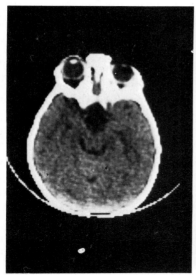 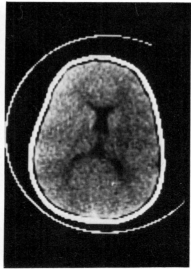

Fig. 17.17 Septo-optic dysplasia. CT

cular atrophy (Görke et al 1975).

An acquired form of cavum septi pellucidi is also seen which is probably of traumatic origin. Though common in punch-drunk veteran boxers, it is happily rare in childhood.

CRANIOSYNOSTOSIS

The growth of the skull is determined by the growth of the brain which more than doubles in weight in the first year of life, so that more than half the postnatal increase in skull circumference occurs in the first twelve months. Skull growth is made possible by the sutures which normally separate the cranial bones from one another at birth, become joined together by fibrous tissue by the fifth or sixth month, but are not normally united by solid bone until late in life. When one or more sutures are obliterated skull deformity results.

Virchow (1851) proposed the term 'craniostenosis' (literally 'a narrow skull') for premature fusion of the cranial sutures but the term 'craniosynostosis' is usually preferred today. 'Virchow's law' defines the effect of premature fusion with prevention of skull growth in a direction perpendicular to the fused suture, resulting in compensatory growth in a direction parallel to this. The cause of craniosynostosis is unknown in most cases, but a small number of familial genetically determined cases are recognized.

The sutures affected by premature fusion are the sagittal, coronal, metopic and lambdoid. Stenosed sutures may be seen singly or in different combinations. The sagittal and coronal are those most often involved. In the two large series of Matson (1969) (519 cases) and Till (1975) (136 cases), from Boston and London respectively, the sagittal suture was the commonest affected with a striking preponderance of males, while coronal stenosis showed a less obvious predilection for females. One or both coronal sutures may be fused. Rarely all the sutures in the vault are involved.

The main clinical features of craniosynostosis are the skull deformity, present in all cases, and the mental retardation, ocular problems and associated congenital defects which may co-exist.

The skull deformity depends on the suture or sutures involved. In the past various graphic terms of Greek origin (oxycephaly, scaphocephaly, brachycephaly, trigonocephaly, turricephaly) have been applied to these deformities, but this terminology is unhelpful, as a similar appearance may occur in the absence of sutural stenosis.

The commonest condition, sagittal craniosynostosis, (Figs. 17.18 and 17.19) is associated with a long, narrow skull, recognizable at birth or soon after, and perhaps the least aesthetically and emo-

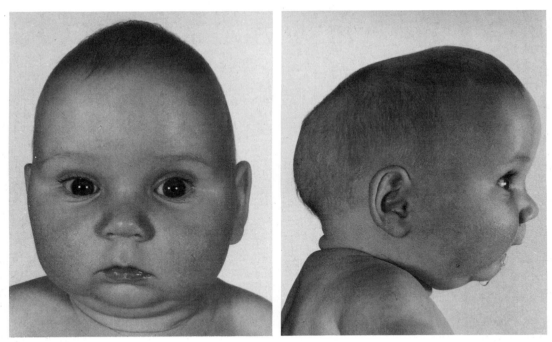

Fig. 17.18 Sagittal craniosynostosis. 4-month-old boy

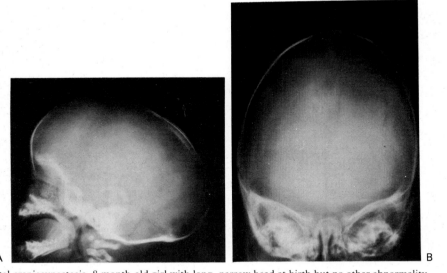

Fig. 17.19 Sagittal craniosynostosis. 8-month-old girl with long, narrow head at birth but no other abnormality.
A. Lateral film. The skull vault is very long. The abnormal length is caused by overgrowth of the parietal bones at the coronal and lambdoid sutures. The great squamo-parietal sutures are relatively high.
B. The skull is narrow. The anterior part of the sagittal suture is visible and the posterior part has closed. There is thickening of the outer table at the site of closure.

tionally distressing of the various deformities. Three to four times as common in boys as in girls, this form of premature stenosis usually occurs in pure culture (though occasionally seen with coronal stenosis) and does not appear to restrict the growth of the brain. Though associated in rare cases with mental retardation (Cohen 1977) it cannot be held directly responsible for this. It occurs very rarely as a dominantly inherited trait. Its main importance is cosmetic, since raised intracranial pressure and ocular problems are not associated.

Bilateral coronal craniosynostosis gives rise to a head which is broad in its lateral dimensions and narrow anteroposteriorly with shallow orbits and usually some proptosis. More important than the cosmetic features are the mental retardation from restricted brain growth, conjunctival and corneal injury associated with proptosis, and optic atrophy resulting from compression of optic nerves or papilloedema in untreated cases. Associated congenital anomalies affecting the face, nose, palate and limbs are particularly common when the coronal suture alone is affected. Several syndromes of combined malformations are seen. Of these Crouzon's syndrome or craniofacial dysostosis, with hypoplasia of the maxilla, and Apert's syndrome or acrocephalosyndactyly are the best known. Both show autosomal dominant inheritance but fresh mutations are common. Cohen (1977) in his review of 37 syndromes with craniosynostosis lists 21 which are genetically determined, autosomal recessive outnumbering autosomal dominant, 3 of chromosomal origin, one teratogenic (due to aminopterin or methotrexate during pregnancy) and 12 of unknown origin. He emphasises that, *for genetic purposes*, syndromes with craniosynostosis should never be classified on the basis of the sutures affected since these may vary among patients with the same syndrome. The intellectual level also varies within the same syndrome.

Synostosis of one coronal suture gives a skull which is asymmetrical anteriorly with flattening of the supra-orbital and anterior temporal regions on the affected side. The ipsilateral eye appears prominent, often giving the child a quizzical expression (Till 1975) (Fig. 17.20).

The rare combined coronal and sagittal stenosis restricts the normal expansion of the brain and may produce a turret-like deformity of the skull, the so-called turricephaly or clover-leaf skull (Fig. 17.21).

More serious still is the equally rare condition with retarded growth and later fusion of all the skull sutures, producing a vault which is normal in shape but small in relation to the base of the skull

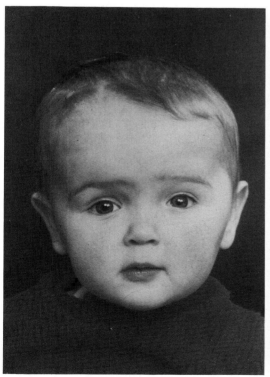 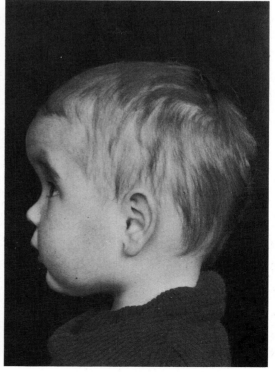

Fig. 17.20 Unilateral coronal craniosynostosis. 20-month-old girl with left coronal suture stenosis. Note her 'quizzical' expression

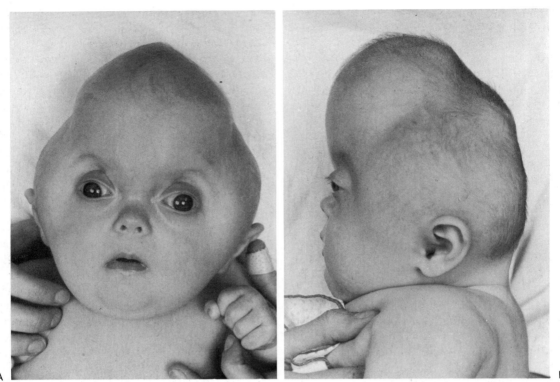

Fig. 17.21 (A and B) Clover-leaf skull or turricephaly in 3-month-old girl with combined coronal and sagittal suture stenosis. Note proptosis.

and the face. There is a sustained but insidious compressing effect on the brain throughout childhood usually without clinical features of raised intracranial pressure, though evidence of this is seen on skull X-rays in the extensive digital markings. Although, purely descriptively, such a skull can be described as microcephalic, it is essential to distinguish it from the common form of microcephaly in which a small brain (the result of malformation, fetal infection or of prenatal, natal or postnatal damage) is associated with slow growth of the skull, the sutures being normal. Early diagnosis is vital as a prelude to early surgical treatment to give the brain space to grow normally.

Metopic suture synostosis is of mainly cosmetic importance.

Surgical treatment

To give the best results surgery must be performed early, whenever possible before three months of age. This is particularly important with bilateral coronal, combined coronal and sagittal and total craniosynostosis. Unfortunately the condition is often diagnosed late. Shillito and Matson (1968) found in their review of 519 cases that only 36% were operated on under 6 weeks of age. Good quality skull X-rays are essential in deciding which sutures are affected. The principle of treatment is to create an artificial suture by a linear craniectomy in the region of the prematurely fused suture, removing a strip of bone and also the pericranium for 2 or 3 cm beyond the edge of the gap in the bone. The edges are covered with a film of polythene or nylon to prevent bony re-union. The cosmetic results are often excellent, especially in sagittal synostosis. The effects on preventing retardation, intracranial hypertension and visual failure are closely related to the age at operation. Sometimes they may appear disappointing when, despite early operation, the child is later mentally retarded. This is often due to associated defects, the synostosis being only one feature (the earliest and most easily recognized) in a syndrome with mental retardation. It is not normally possible to detect in advance those children who will be retarded despite early surgery, and an aggressive approach with early operation in all cases in which it is indicated seems the best policy.

CONGENITAL DERMAL SINUSES AFFECTING THE SKULL

A depression or tract extending inwards from the surface of the skin and lined by stratified squamous epithelium constitutes a congenital dermal sinus. During development the neural ectoderm is separated from the cutaneous ectoderm along the midline of the dorsum of the embryo between the third and fifth week of fetal life. Fusion of the epithelial ectoderm starts in the middle of the embryo and proceeds caudally and cranially so that defects due to incomplete fusion are commonest in the lumbosacral and suboccipital regions. Sinuses may extend to any depth; when there is associated failure of fusion of mesodermal structures they may connect with the cerebellum, fourth ventricle, spinal cord or central canal. They may be very shallow and involve only the deeper layers of the skin. Any point in a congenital dermal sinus, but especially its termination, may be the site of its expansion to form a cyst. These may be multiple or single. They are of two types, *epidermoid cysts* containing only epithelial debris and lined by stratified squamous epithelium and *dermoid cysts* which also contain keratin, sebaceous material and hair and include in their lining hair follicles, sebaceous glands and other dermal elements.

Dermal sinuses of deep or shallow extent are common over the spinal axis, especially in the lumbosacral area and are discussed later.

Those extending into the cranial cavity are much less common but perhaps more important because of the more serious effects which may arise from infection within them. Congenital dermal sinuses are often multiple and may occur at two, three or even four levels, so that the finding of one defect should prompt a search for others.

Ideally all such lesions would be discovered during the routine examination of the newborn baby. The larger lesions are found at that time, but many smaller defects are missed. The clue may lie in a minute dimple or sinus tract in or very close to the midline, usually in the occipital region, often with a few hairs protruding from it. Sometimes a small subcutaneous mass can be palpated beneath, and there may be redness, tenderness or other signs of infection.

The intracranial complications of dermal sinuses include their mass effect, features caused by infection within them, and a combination of the two. Owing to the relationship between dermatomes and spinal cord segments the sinus tracts run caudally and not directly inwards. Most terminate in the posterior fossa, in the cerebellum, fourth ventricle or cisterna magna. Here a dermoid cyst may act as a space-occupying lesion, causing hydrocephalus, ataxia and nystagmus. Infection may result in a cerebellar abscess, again with raised intracranial pressure and ataxia, in meningitis or both. Meningitis related to intracranial dermal sinuses is usually due to *Staphylococcus aureus*, in contrast to that associated with lumbosacral lensions where *E. coli* is usually responsible. In all cases of meningitis the midline of the spine and skull should be carefully examined for a sinus which could be the portal of entry. In the occipital region a lesion may escape detection unless the skin is shaved.

Skull X-rays may show a midline bony defect up to 2 cm in diameter, but the hole may be so small and the tract so oblique that it is not shown on plain films. With a thin skull vault due to raised intracranial pressure the defect is even more difficult to detect. Ventriculography or the CT scan will show enlargement of the lateral and third ventricles in the presence of an occipital dermal sinus and often indicate the mass.

When a sinus has been shown, preventive surgical treatment should aim to excise the tract and associated cyst or cysts. The posterior fossa may need to be explored. Previous infection may have caused adhesions to form. Active infection calls for vigorous antibiotic treatment and a cerebellar abscess needs to be aspirated or drained. When the diagnosis is delayed until after severe infection has occurred the results of surgery are often poor.

SPINA BIFIDA OCCULTA

Embryological considerations

The three primary germ cell layers, ectoderm, mesoderm and endoderm, are early differentiated from a mass of multipotential cells. At a slightly later stage the central neural axis is formed when a groove appears in the ectoderm along the mid-dorsal aspect of the embryo. This groove sinks deeper and its edges, the neural crests, converge and fuse dorsally to form the primitive neural tube. Fusion starts at the midpoint of the embryo and progresses both cranially and caudally, usually being complete about the end of the fourth week after conception. Later the proliferating cells of the neural tube differentiate to produce ultimately the neuronal and supporting elements of the central nervous system and perhaps part of the meninges. Simultaneously mesodermal tissues are organized to form the structures which support and surround the neural axis, such as bone, cartilage, fat, connective tissue, blood vessels and meninges. These complex processes of germ layer differentiation may be disturbed at different levels and to varying extents, producing a wide range of malformations, varying from a symptomless, occult laminar defect of the lumbar spine detectable only radiologically to complete spinal or cranial rachischisis or splitting (spina bifida cystica, discussed in Ch. 16), and cranium bifidum.

Differential growth of the spinal cord and vertebral canal occurs from the third month of gestation onwards leading to changes in their relative positions. The vertebral column and its associated mesodermal structures grow at a more rapid rate than the spinal cord, so that the latter migrates cranially, the greatest change in relation to corresponding vertebral segments occurring at the tail end. At birth the medullary conus lies opposite the third and fourth lumbar vertebra, but by the time growth has ceased it is opposite the first or slightly cranial to this. This differential growth means that the age of the patient influences both the anatomy and the clinical effects of certain malformations of the spinal cord.

The term 'spina bifida occulta' is applied to those cases in which fusion defects of the vertebral column occur without protrusion of intraspinal contents on to the surface of the body, in contrast to spinal rachischisis or spina bifida cystica. The condition is common: X-rays show a minor defect of a lamina or vertebral spine in about one child in four, most often in the lumbosacral region and usually without symptoms. Many cutaneous and subcutaneous abnormalities are found in association with these bony defects, and provide useful pointers to the diagnosis of the disorder which is only 'occult' relative to the dramatic features of the cystic variety. Another important point of distinction from spina bifida cystica is that the Arnold-Chiari malformation and hydrocephalus are not seen in occult spina bifida. Sex differences are also seen, occult spina bifida affecting girls twice as often as boys, whereas spina bifida cystica affects the sexes more or less equally.

The developmental errors seen in spinal dysraphism are many and often multiple, occurring at two or more levels of the neuraxis. Failure of normal separation of ectoderm into its cutaneous and neural components may lead to formation of a dermoid cyst within the spinal cord or adjacent to it. A dermal sinus may link the cyst to the overlying skin providing a route by which bacteria may enter with the risk of meningitis. The spinal cord may be split into two separate parts over a short and occasionally a longer distance, with the cleft between occupied by a bony or fibrous spur. This condition of split cord or *diastematomyelia* may occur alone or be associated with elongation and tethering of the cord. Rarely a split in the cord and duplication of vertebral bodies allows structures of endodermal origin to lie within the spinal cord or adjacent to it in the dorsal region. These lesions, known as *neurenteric cysts* (Bentley & Smith, 1960) may expand or compress the cord and are lined by intestinal epithelium which can secrete trypsin. A common anomaly is a low medullary conus often associated with a tight filum terminale which may interfere with the normal mobility of the cord by anchoring it, making it vulnerable to direct or ischaemic injury in the course of the repeated flexion and extension movements of the spine. Mesodermal anomalies may be seen in the form of fibrous bands connecting the cord to the dura and lipomata attached to the cord and also situated subcutaneously as large soft swellings over the lower back. The external and internal lipomata may be continuous with one another.

The operative findings in 160 children with spinal dysraphism reported by Till (1975) included 292 anomalies. In decreasing order of frequency these were low conus medullaris (100), diastematomyelia (73), (with bony spur present in 24), intradural lipoma (67), extradural tethering bands (35: with intradural extension in 23), dermoid cyst (14) (intradural 9: extradural 5) and neurenteric cyst (3).

Clinical features

The clinical features of occult spina bifida are of four types, cutaneous, orthopaedic, neurological and meningitis. They will be discussed in that order since, though one or the other category may predominate, it is usually the skin features and/ or foot deformities which are detected first and the neurological features may be delayed or, at any rate, undetected, until a later stage.

The cutaneous defects are most often seen in the lumbar region. They may be so large and unsightly as to constitute the presenting symptom at birth, or so small that only a careful search will detect them. They lie in or close to the midline of the spinal axis. They may be hidden in the gluteal cleft where skin dimples and sinus tracts are easily overlooked. There may be signs of inflammation of the skin adjacent to a sinus and sometimes one or more hairs are seen protruding from it. Hairy patches ranging from a small tuft to a luxuriant 'pony tail' (Fig 17.22) are among the commonest skin stigmata. Naevi, vascular or pigmented, and subcutaneous lipomata varying in size from small nodules to large, diffuse swellings are other skin lesions. It is not possible from the cutaneous features to infer which of the possible forms of intraspinal anomaly is present, with the exception that a subcutaneous lipoma is likely to be associated, and often directly connected, with a lipoma within the spinal canal.

Talipes of one or both feet and asymmetry in the size of the feet and legs are often present at birth frequently associated with diminished muscle bulk in the lower leg which may also feel cold and appear discoloured. These features should strongly sug-

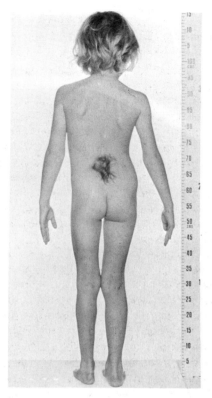

Fig. 17.22 Spina bifida occulta — 7-year-old girl with 'pony tail'. Note wasting of left leg

gest the possibility of spinal dysraphism and prompt a careful search for cutaneous anomalies.

The associated neurological disorders are of two main kinds: those affecting movement or sensation in the legs and those related to control of bladder or rectal sphincters. In Till's (1975) series of 160 children 72% had abnormal development of one or both legs and 24% had disorders of micturition. There may be obvious weakness of one or both legs at birth or in early infancy, but this may be overlooked until some months have passed. The weakness is usually greater distally than proximally. The age of independent sitting is usually not delayed and it may only be at the start of the second year of life when the child first attempts to walk that weakness is detected. An abnormal gait is then noted, often with a unilateral limp, and examination shows deformity of one or both feet, with reduced muscle bulk in the lower leg and sometimes shortening of the limb. Changes in tendon reflexes, which may be increased or decreased, an extensor plantar response and reduced sensation in the leg may be found. Sometimes medical advice may not be sought until some years have passed, even when a limp has been present from an early age, because the disability is mild. In such cases it is often the increased demands for agility made at primary school age, or even the greater demands of competitive sports at secondary school age which show up the difficulty and prompt referral. In some cases, as with all milder neurological deficits, medical help has been sought and reassurance been wrongly given through failure to think of the diagnosis or fully to examine the child.

These situations must be distinguished from that in which a neurological deficit appears for the first time in a hitherto normal child, and from that in which a recognized deficit becomes worse. A careful history may be needed to distinguish between these various possibilities, and in some cases it may be difficult to do so. Deterioration may appear at any age but is common at the ages when growth spurts occur.

Sphincter disturbances due to spinal dysraphism may, if mild, be overlooked in the same way as leg weakness, until the age when toilet-training is normally achieved. Sphincter function may deteriorate with regression in bladder and bowel control in a child who was previously 'clean and dry'. Though spinal dysraphism is not a common cause of such regression it is important to detect it since, although sphincter function rarely improves after surgical treatment of the spinal anomaly, further deterioration may perhaps be avoided and impairment in renal function prevented or lessened. Borzykowski & Neville (1981) have stressed the severity of the bladder problems which can result from spinal dysraphism in children. Four of their patients were referred with orthopaedic problems, but were found to have bladder abnormality as their major disability. All had unstable, variably thickened, small bladders. Their bladder impairment was thought to be due to a partial lesion of lumbosacral innervation, rather than to an upper motor neuron lesion.

Another rare, but very important, presentation of spinal dysraphism is with bacterial meningitis in children with a dermal sinus extending to the dura. These may occur at any level and may be multiple.

The finding of *any* midline defect over the spine should lead to a careful search for another defect, including the occipital region and the skin in the depths of the gluteal cleft. This is particularly important in children who have had more than one attack of meningitis.

Radiological features:

In all cases in which the clinical features suggest spinal dysraphism good quality X-rays of the entire spine should be taken. Various bony abnormalities are seen. These are rarely diagnostic of the precise anomaly affecting the spinal cord but a midline bony spur is pathognomonic of diastematomyelia (Fig. 17.23); this is often associated with narrow disc spaces and malformed vertebral bodies at the same level. Hemivertebrae, fused and malformed laminae, a widened spinal canal and abnormal spinal curvatures over affected segments are other radiological defects, with spina bifida affecting vertebrae to varying degrees.

The finding of such bony anomalies with cutaneous stigmata makes spinal dysraphism extremely likely, even if there is no detectable neurological deficit. The only practical way to establish the diagnosis is by myelography which is logically the next step. The purpose of this test is to define the anatomy as clearly as possible with a view to considering whether surgical intervention is feasible and advisable. The natural history of spina bifida occulta shows that in most children who develop urinary incontinence or lower limb problems *after infancy* the harmful effects of the spinal condition are long delayed. Early treatment should therefore prevent at least some of these. Previously deterioration in leg or bladder function was taken as the indication for myelography, but improvement in these functions after surgery is unusual, so that it is logical to adopt a more aggressive attitude in the hope of preventing deterioration.

Myelography for this purpose is carried out with air or metrizamide by injection into the cisterna magna. The lumbar route should be avoided since the lumbar subarachnoid space is often obliterated or partly occupied by the spinal cord. The results will show the structural abnormalities present and usually indicate whether spinal exploration is advisable.

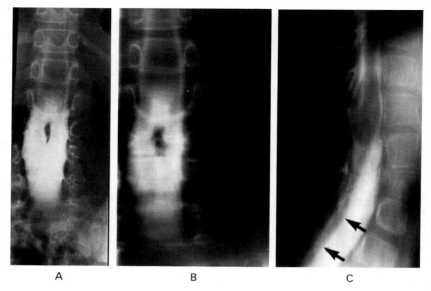

Fig. 17.23 Diastematomyelia. 7-year-old girl with progressive thoracolumbar scoliosis first noticed at the age of 1 year. She had a hairy naevus in the lumbar region and congenital anomalies of some ribs on the left side.

A. Antero-posterior film of metrizamide myelogram. There is a bony spur at the level of the third lumbar vertebra and the conus divides into two halves at the level of the second lumbar vertebra, the halves passing on either side of the spur.

B. The conus is well shown and is swollen due to the presence of a cyst. The two halves of the conus are shown on either side of and below the bony spur. Nerve roots emerge from them and they do not appear to unite.

C. Lateral tomogram of myelogram. The bony spur is at the level of the hypoplastic vertebral body. Disc spaces above and below it are narrow. The bony spur and its dural sheath is shown as a filling defect of the contrast column. The two halves of the conus are elongated and extend down into the sacral canal (arrows). The conus above the split is confirmed to be enlarged.

It is essential that parents should understand that the purpose of surgery is to prevent deterioration in function and not to cure or improve function which is already impaired. Occasionally improvement is seen post-operatively, but this is a bonus not to be counted on.

Till's (1975) experience of surgery in a large series of children has been encouraging. In a follow-up period of up to eight years no patient who was neurologically normal when operated on had developed lower limb or sphincter disorder. However, two patients with extensive lumbosacral lipoma were harmed by surgery, from damage to nerve roots embedded in the fatty tissue. When an intraspinal lipoma is demonstrated radiologically or at laminectomy, surgical discretion is probably the better part of valour.

THE KLIPPEL-FEIL SYNDROME

In this usually sporadic disorder the main anomaly is fusion of the cervical vertebrae, sometimes with hemivertebrae and other defects (Fig. 17.24). About two-thirds of the patients are female. A solid mass of bone may replace the cervical spine with only three or four vertebral elements recognizable. The posterior wall of the spinal canal is usually defective or absent in its upper part giving rise to spina bifida occulta.

Clinically the neck is very short and may appear to be absent. All neck movements are grossly restricted. This immobility predisposes to fractures of the neck, so that minor trauma may be hazardous to the patient who is also liable to develop a spastic paraplegia which may progress to a tetraplegia. Mirror movements of the hands may be associated with the anomaly, so that the two hands are incapable of executing movements independently. These movements may constitute a serious handicap in some patients, and are sometimes mistaken for ataxia or other forms of involuntary movement (Ch. 10).

Other defects which have been associated with

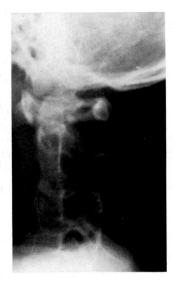

Fig. 17.24 Klippel-Feil syndrome in 11-year-old girl. There is complete fusion of the axis and the third cervical vertebra which shows partial fusion with the fourth

the Klippel-Feil anomaly are deafness, congenital heart disease, cleft palate, scoliosis, defects of ribs, Sprengel's shoulder and mental retardation.

Progressive weakness of the limbs should suggest the possibility of spinal cord compression and the need for myelography and decompressive laminectomy.

AGENESIS OF THE SACRUM AND COCCYX WITH MYELODYSPLASIA

Rarely the sacrum and coccyx fail to develop as may the sacral or lumbosacral segments of the spinal cord (Fig. 17.25). Clinically there is weakness of both legs with sensory defects and incontinence of urine and sometimes of faeces as well. The condition may readily be suspected by simple palpation which fails to detect the normal bony prominences, yet the diagnosis in some cases has been remarkably delayed.

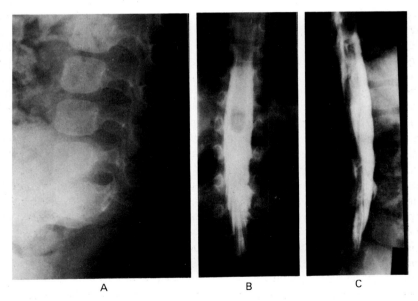

A   B   C

Fig. 17.25 Sacral dysgenesis with low conus. 22-month-old girl with congenital talipes on right, weakness of legs and double incontinence.

A. Lateral film. Lower spine. Four normal lower lumbar vertebrae are shown while the lowermost vertebra is the only part of the sacrum present.

B. Myelogram. Antero-posterior view. The conus is at the level of D12 and is abnormal in shape. The subarachnoid space just reaches the fifth lumbar vertebra. There are relatively few roots within the cauda equina and their pouches are asymmetrical. The lowest roots visible are the fifth lumbar roots and there is no sign of any sacral root pouches.

C. Myelogram. Lateral film. This confirms that the conus is bulbous and that there is a small number of roots within the subarachnoid space. Termination of the theca at L5 is well shown.

SYRINGOMYELIA

Syringomyelia, like hydrocephalus, is an anatomical diagnosis and occurs in different forms with varying aetiology. Although often regarded as a disorder of adult life, it can present at any age between childhood and senescence and may well confront the paediatrician or paediatric neurologist.

The anatomical basis of the condition is a cavitating lesion within the cervical and/or upper dorsal segments of the spinal cord. The fluid within the syrinx, as the lesion is called, is usually in continuity with the CSF in the fourth ventricle and the term communicating syringomyelia is applied to this situation. Less often syringomyelia is non-communicating, with no continuity between these two spaces.

There have been many theories and heated debate on the origin of communicating syringomyelia, but in recent years the 'hydrodynamic theory', developed by Chiari in relation to the anomalies associated with his name, has gained most adherents. The subject is well reviewed by Foster (1975). Gardner and his colleagues in Cleveland, Ohio, have stressed the association between the less severe degrees of the Arnold-Chiari malformation and syringomyelia. They have developed the thesis over many years (e.g. Gardner 1973) that partial obstruction to the outflow of CSF from the ventricular system, produced by a developmental anomaly at the level of the foramen magnum, with communication between the fourth ventricle and the central canal of the spinal cord causes the latter to become progressively dilated. This hydromyelic dilatation dissects through the wall of the cavity to become the syrinx or syringomyelia. Gardner's theory has been supported in Britain by the Newcastle school (Barnett et al 1973) and by Williams (1971).

The mechanism of the expanding force is still debated. Gardner considers it is due to long-continued arterial pulsation in the spinal fluid, while Williams believes that the changes in CSF pressure causing the syringomyelic dilatation are due to sudden increases in central venous pressure such as occur with straining, coughing and sneezing. These could cause filling of the spinal epidural veins and partial evacuation of the spinal subarachnoid space into the head. This would be followed, in the erect position, by a recovery phase with CSF dropping back into the spinal sac and some of it being directed by the valvular effect of the cerebellar herniation into the central canal.

In addition to developmental anomalies at the foramen magnum and in the posterior fossa, acquired abnormalities such as basal arachnoiditis, posterior fossa tumours and cysts, may also give rise to communicating syringomyelia. Williams (1977) obtained a history of difficult labour in over half of a series of syringomyelia patients and suggested that this might have caused cerebellar ectopia and arachnoiditis which had later led to syrinx formation.

Clinical features of communicating syringomyelia

Sensory loss of 'dissociated' type, with loss of pain and temperature sensation and retention of light touch, may be found in one or both upper limbs, often associated with severe pain, absence of deep tendon reflexes in the arms, and weakness and wasting of the small hand muscles. The loss of pain appreciation may lead to a mutilating arthropathy, a kind of Charcot joint. The legs may be involved in a spastic paraplegia from affection of the pyramidal tracts. Upward extension of the syrinx into the brain stem (syringobulbia) may produce cranial nerve and cerebellar signs. A minority of patients with syringomyelia have abnormally short necks (which should suggest the possibility of an anomaly of the foramen magnum or craniocervical junction). Scoliosis is found in about 20% of patients.

Hydrocephalus is recognized in some patients with communicating syringomyelia. It may be arrested, active or treated. Fisher et al (1977) have reported three cases in which syringomyelia was demonstrated years after communicating hydrocephalus had been treated by a lumbo-ureteral shunt at a few months of age. The mechanism of the syrinx formation was not clear, but in two cases arachnoiditis was perhaps responsible.

Investigations

These are mainly radiological. Plain X-rays of the cervical spine may show widening of the antero-posterior diameter of the spinal canal or abnormalities of the craniovertebral junction, but a

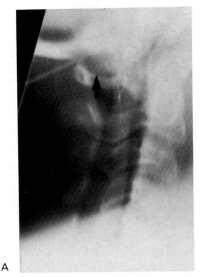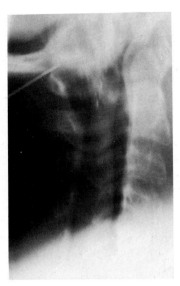

A   B

Fig. 17.26 Hydromyelia and ectopia of cerebellar tonsils in 11-year-old boy. Cisternal air myelogram.
A. Air has been injected through a needle inserted into a narrow cisterna magna compressed by the ectopic cerebellar tonsils (arrow). The cervical cord is very large.
B. Also shows the 4th ventricle extending down to the foramen magnum.

radiologically normal spine does not exclude communicating syringomyelia.

Skull X-rays may show signs of arrested hydrocephalus or 'basilar impression', but are normal in most cases.

Myelograpic examination of the craniovertebral junction is the definitive investigation. It is essential to screen the metrizamide (or air if this is used) in the supine as well as the prone position, since only in supine can cerebellar tonsillar ectopia be demonstrated (Fig. 17.26). When air is used for myelography a collapsing cystic dilatation of the cord can be shown, so distinguishing communicating cysts from non-communicating syringomyelia and spinal cord tumours.

The whole body scanner may help in some cases to demonstrate a cyst within the cord, and is indeed the only non-invasive radiological method disclosing a non-communicating syrinx.

Non-communicating syringomyelia

In a minority of cases the cavity within the spinal cord does not communicate with the fourth ventricle. Such non-communicating syringomyelia may follow trauma. It may also occur with spinal cord tumours, both intramedullary and extra-

medullary and occasionally with arachnoiditis confined to the spinal cord. The whole body scanner, as mentioned above, can demonstrate a non-communicating intraspinal cavity.

In the skilled hands of an experienced neuroradiologist percutaneous aspiration of a syrinx, with or without injection of metrizamide, can sometimes give helpful information. The chemical and cellular content of the aspirated fluid should be studied since an intraspinal cavity may occasionally occur as part of a neurenteric cyst, in some cases of which trypsin can be shown in the fluid.

Surgical treatment

Many surgical procedures have been tried, mostly designed to relieve the pressure within the distended syrinx. They include decompressive laminectomy, posterior fossa craniotomy, removal of the posterior rim of the foramen magnum, aspiration of the contents of the cyst, myelotomy with attempts to 'marsupialize' the syrinx, and insertion of ventriculo-atrial shunts. The results of these procedures have been disappointing. More encouraging results have been obtained by Gardner and by others by decompressing the exit foramina of the fourth ventricle by separation of the prolapsed cerebellar tonsils. This will disclose the obex or opening of the central canal in the floor of the fourth ventricle which can then be occluded with a small piece of muscle. The procedure may be technically difficult since if the muscle plug is too loosely inserted it is ineffective and if it is pushed in firmly enough to create a water-proof seal there is a risk of inducing apnoea. Another surgical approach has been to cut the filum terminale, so allowing the CSF to drain out of the end of the central canal. If a syrinx is present in the cord at this level a tube can be inserted upwards into it to promote drainage of CSF.

Significant improvement has been reported after surgery in many patients with cure of symptoms in some cases, but the results have often been disappointing.

MOEBIUS' SYNDROME

Congenital bilateral facial weakness of lower motor neuron type with internal strabismus is sometimes seen as a sporadic occurrence in the syndrome described by Moebius. The clinical picture is of a mask-like expressionless face with bilateral external rectus palsies (Fig 17.27). Intelligence is usually normal despite the dull facial appearance, but mental retardation is present in a minority of affected children. Occasionally there is involvement of the other oculomotor nerves and of lower cranial nerves including the twelfth with complete external ophthalmoplegia and a small, immobile tongue. The condition is asymmetrical in a few cases. Skeletal abnormalities occur in a third or more of patients with Moebius' syndrome, and include talipes, syndactyly, smallness of limbs and occasionally absence of pectoralis major muscle.

Feeding problems at birth and in infancy may be severe, often aggravated by the micrognathia which may be associated.

The few detailed necropsy studies made suggest that the underlying defect is hypoplasia or agenesis of the cranial nerve nuclei concerned. In some children facial mobility increases with age so that by school age the condition is happily less of a social embarrassment.

Moebius' syndrome must be distinguished from various congenital myopathies, particularly dystro-

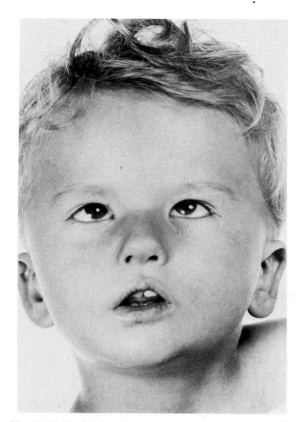

Fig. 17.27 Moebius' syndrome. 2½ year-old boy

phia myotonica, facioscapulohumeral muscular dystrophy and myasthenia gravis, from acquired facial palsy due to birth trauma, and from the syndrome of congenital suprabulbar paresis (see below).

CONGENITAL SUPRABULBAR PARESIS

In this rare syndrome described by Worster-Drought (1974) there is thought to be relative 'agenesis' or 'hypogenesis' of the cortico-bulbar tract running from the motor cortex to the tenth and twelfth cranial nerve nuclei. The clinical picture differs from that in Moebius' syndrome in that the orbicularis oris is usually the only facial muscle affected, the upper part of the face and the external ocular muscles being normal, while there is variable involvement of the tongue, pharynx and soft palate, so that dysarthria and feeding difficulty are prominent. There is great difficulty in rounding the lips and in protruding the tongue, which does not show wasting or fasciculation. Excessive dribbling is often the main complaint. The jaw jerk is usually exaggerated and there is often a 'snout' reflex in which tapping the upper or lower lip elicits a contraction of orbicularis oris. The severity of the condition varies and in milder cases speech is comprehensible and salivation can be controlled. There is a definite tendency towards spontaneous improvement.

Worster-Drought found in a series of 200 patients that the distribution curve of intelligence was markedly skewed towards the lower end of the scale, 78 having IQs under 80, and only 6 being in the superior range. The ability of the duller children to cope with their problems and co-operate in the necessary speech therapy is much less than that of the brighter patients. Surgical procedures tried in an attempt to reduce drooling and improve speech have included bilateral ligation of Stensen's duct, removal of the submandibular glands and palato-pharyngoplasty.

REFERENCES

Aicardi J, Chevrie J J, Rouselle F 1969 Le syndrome spasmes en flexion, agénésie calleuse, anomalies chorio-retiniennes. Archives françaises de Pédiatrie 26: 1103

Aicardi J, Goutières F, Hodebourg de Verbois A 1972 Multicystic encephalomalacia of infants and its relation to abnormal gestation and hydranencephaly. Journal of Neurological Sciences 15: 357–373

Andermann E, Andermann F, Carpenter S, Karpati G, Eisen A, Melancon D et al 1976 Familial agenesis of the corpus callosum with sensorimotor neuropathy: a new autosomal recessive syndrome originating in Charlevoix County. Journal Canadien des Sciences Neurologiques. Scientific Programme of the 11th Canadian Congress

André-Thomas, Lepage F, Sorrel-Déjèrine Mme 1944 Examen anatomoclinique de deux anencéphales protubérantiels. Revue neurologique 76: 173–193

Barnett H J M, Foster J B, Hudgson P 1973 Syringomyelia. Saunders, London

Bentley J F R, Smith J R 1960 Developmental posterior enteric remnants and spinal malformations. Archives of Disease in Childhood 35: 76–86

Benton J W, Nellhaus G, Huttenlocher P R, Ojemann R G, Dodge P R 1966 The bobble head doll syndrome. Neurology 16: 725

Borzykowski M, Neville B G R 1981 Neuropathic bladder and spinal dysraphism. Archives of Disease in Childhood 56: 176–180

Brock D J H, Bolton A E, Scrimgeour J B 1974 Prenatal diagnosis of spina bifida and anencephaly through maternal plasma-alpha fetoprotein measurement. Lancet 2: 767

Brook C G D, Sanders M D, Hoare R D 1972 Septo-optic dysplasia. British Medical Journal 3: 811

Claireaux A E 1972 Multicystic encephalomalacia. Developmental Medicine and Child Neurology 14: 662

Cohen M M 1977 Genetic perspectives in craniosynostosis and syndromes with craniosynostosis. Journal of Neurosurgery 47: 886–898

Crome L 1958 Multilocular cystic encephalopathy of infants. Journal of Neurology, Neurosurgery and Psychiatry 21: 146

Curatolo P, Libutti G, Dallapiccola B 1980 Aicardi syndrome in a male infant. Journal of Pediatrics 96: 286–287

Day R E, Schutt W H 1979 Normal children with large heads — benign familial megalencephaly. Archives of Disease in Childhood 54: 512–517

Dekaban A 1965 Large defects in cerebral hemispheres associated with cortical dysgenesis. Journal of Neuropathology and Experimental Neurology 24: 512

De Morsier G 1956 Etudes sur les dysraphies cranio-encéphaliques III. Agénésie du septum lucidum avec malformation du tractus optique. La dysplasie septo-optique. Schweizer Archiv für Neurologie und Psychiatrie 77: 267

Dennis J, Rosenberg H, Alvord E 1961 Megalencephaly, internal hydrocephalus and other neurological aspects of achondroplasia. Brain 84: 427–443

Dennis J, Bower B D 1972 The Aicardi syndrome. Developmental Medicine and Child Neurology 14: 382

Eckstein H B 1977 Hydrocephalus in operative surgery. In: Nixon H H (ed) Paediatric surgery, 3rd edn. Butterworths, London

Epstein F, Wald A, Hochwald G M 1974 Intracranial pressure during compressive head wrapping in treatment of neonatal hydrocephalus. Pediatrics 54: 786–790

Ettlinger G, Blakemore C B, Milner A D, Wilson J 1972 Agenesis of the corpus callosum: a behavioural investigation. Brain 95: 327–346

Fischer E G, Welch K, Shillito J 1977 Syringomyelia following lumbo-ureteral shunting for communicating hydrocephalus. Report of three cases. Journal of Neurosurgery 47: 96–100

Foster J B 1975 Syringomyelia In: Matthews W B (ed) Recent advances in clinical neurology. Churchill Livingstone, Edinburgh

Freeman J M, Gold A P 1964 Porencephaly simulating subdural hematoma in childhood. A clinical syndrome secondary to arterial occlusion. American Journal of Diseases of Childhood 107: 327

Gamper E 1926 Bau und leistungen eines menschichen mittelhirnwesens (arhinencephalie mit encephalocele) zuglich ein beitrag zur teratologie und fasersystematik. Zeitschrift für Neurologie 102: 154 and 104: 49

Gardner W J 1973 The dysraphic states from syringomyelia to anencephaly. Excerpta Medica, Amsterdam

Gilles F H, Davidson R I 1971 Communicating hydrocephalus associated with deficient dysplastic parasagittal arachnoidal granulations. Journal of Neurosurgery 35: 421

Görke W, Pendl G, Pandel C 1975 Spinal muscular atrophy in a boy with head-nodding resulting from a large septum pellucidum cyst. Neuropädiatrie 6: 190

Hamby W B, Kraus R F, Beswick W F 1950
Hydranencephaly: clinical diagnosis; presentation of 7
cases. Pediatrics 6: 371–383

Heschl R 1868 Neue fälle von porencephalie.
Vierteljahrschrift für Praktikale Heilkunde 100: 40

Hoyt W F, Kaplan S L, Grumbach M M, Glaser T S 1970
Septo-optic dysplasia and pituitary dwarfism. Lancet 1: 893
(letter)

Isler W 1964 Acute hemiplegias and hemisyndromes in
childhood. Clinics in Developmental Medicine Nos 41/42,
S I M P, Heinemann, London

Lorber J 1972 The use of isosorbide in the treatment of
hydrocephalus. Developmental Medicine and Child
Neurology 14 (suppl 27): 88

Lorber J 1975 Isosorbide in treatment of infantile
hydrocephalus. Archives of Disease in Childhood
50: 431–436

Lyen K R, Lingam S, Butterfill A M, Marshall W C,
Dobbing C J, Lee D S C 1981 Multicystic
encephalomalacia due to fetal viral encephalitis. European
Journal of Pediatrics 137: 11–16

Matson D 1969 Neurosurgery of infancy and childhood, 2nd
edn. Charles C Thomas, Springfield, Illinois

Menkes J H, Philippart M, Clark D B 1964 Hereditary partial
agenesis of the corpus callosum. Biochemical and
pathological studies. Archives of Neurology 11: 198

Naef R W 1958 Clinical features of porencephaly. Archives of
Neurology and Psychiatry 80: 133

Neville B G R 1972 The origin of infantile spasms: evidence
from a case of hydranencephaly. Developmental Medicine
and Child Neurology 14: 644

Opitz J M 1979 Median cleft face syndrome In: Bergsma D
(ed) Birth defects compendium, 2nd edn. Published for
National Foundation March of Dimes by Alan R Liss, New
York

Porter F N 1975 Hydrocephalus treated by compressive head
wrapping. Archives of Disease in Childhood 50: 816–818

Russman B S, Tucker S H, Schut L, 1975 Slow tremor and
macrocephaly: expanded version of the bobble-head doll
syndrome. Journal of Pediatrics 87: 63–66

Schreier H, Rapin I, Davis J 1974 Familial megalencephaly or
hydrocephalus? Neurology 24: 232–236

Sher P K, Brown S B 1975a A longitudinal study of head
growth in pre-term infants. I. Normal rates of head growth.
Developmental Medicine and Child Neurology 17: 705–710

Sher P K, Brown S B 1975b A longitudinal study of head
growth in pre-term infants. II. Differentiation between
'catch-up' head growth and early infantile hydrocephalus.
Developmental Medicine and Child Neurology 17: 711–718

Shillito J, Matson D D 1968 Craniosynostosis: a review of 519
surgical patients. Pediatrics 41: 829–853

Smith D 1976 Recognizable patterns of human malformation.
In: Major problems in Clinical Pediatrics W B Saunders
Company, Philadelphia, vol VII

Suwanwela C, Hongsaprabhas C 1966 Fronto-ethmoidal
encephalomeningocele. Journal of Neurosurgery 25: 172

Till K 1975 Paediatric neurosurgery for paediatricians and
neurosurgeons. Blackwell Scientific Publications, Oxford

Till K 1978 Cerebellar tumours in children. Journal of
Maternal and Child Health Oct 1978: 326–332

Tomasovic J A, Nellhaus G, Moe P G 1975 The bobble-head
doll syndrome: an early sign of hydrocephalus. Two new
cases and a review of the literature. Developmental
Medicine and Child Neurology 17: 777–792

Urich H 1976 Malformations of the nervous system. Perinatal
damage and related conditions in early life. In: Blackwood
W, Corsellis J A N (eds) Greenfield's neuropathology.
Edward Arnold, London

Virchow R 1851 Ueber den cretinismus, namentlich in
Franken, und ueber pathologische Schaedel formen.
Verhaltensphysiologische Medizinische Gesellschaft

Williams B 1971 Further thoughts on the valvular action of
the Arnold-Chiari malformation. Developmental Medicine
and Child Neurology (supplement) 25: 105–112

Williams B 1977 Difficult labour. A cause of communicating
syringomyelia. Lancet 2: 51–53

Willis J, Rosman N P 1980 The Aicardi syndrome versus
congenital infection: Diagnostic considerations. Journal of
Pediatrics 96: 235–239

Worster-Drought C 1974 Congenital suprabulbar paresis.
Developmental Medicine and Child Neurology. Spastics
International Medical Publications and William Heinemann
Medical Books, London, Supplement 3, vol 16, no 1

18

Intracranial and spinal cord tumours

E. M. Brett

INTRACRANIAL TUMOURS
INTRODUCTION

Intracranial tumours in children are among the commonest paediatric tumours, being second only to leukaemia. Yates (1968) in a study of one million children under 15 years of age in the Manchester region found an average annual incidence of 17 gliomas, compared with 29 cases of leukaemia. Till (1975) has calculated that in the United Kingdom there are probably from 180 to 200 children newly diagnosed each year as having intracranial tumours, and in the USA 680 new cases.

These tumours occur with almost equal frequency in childhood from early infancy onwards. They differ from those in adults in type and location. In childhood the commonest type seen is the glioma, which makes up about 75% of childhood series compared with about 45% in adult surveys. In children under 12 years of age some 55% of intracranial neoplasms arise below the tentorium cerebelli, whereas in older patients supratentorial tumours predominate. The series of 575 patients from the Hospital for Sick Children, Toronto, however, showed a slight preponderance of supratentorial sites (Harwood-Nash & Fitz 1976), perhaps reflecting a change in patterns of referral due to more aggressive investigation of children with suspect symptoms.

However, these generalizations are seen to be misleading when the figures are analysed according to age of admission of the children. Harwood-Nash and Fitz in Toronto found distinct differences between various age groups. In the first year of life there were equal numbers of supratentorial and infratentorial neoplasms, the preponderance of astrocytomas in the supratentorial compartment being counterbalanced by that of ependymomas and medulloblastomas infratentorially. By 4 years of age infratentorial tumours predominated due to a sudden increase of cerebellar astrocytomas, medulloblastomas and ependymomas. The situation changed again at the age of 8 with a slight majority of supratentorial neoplasms due to an increase in cerebral astrocytomas.

The midline location of cerebellar gliomas which are common in early life often causes early obstruction to the circulation of the CSF and raised intracranial pressure without localizing neurological signs. However, the ability of the skull in infancy to expand as the sutures separate may delay the onset of the clinical features of raised intracranial pressure, so that an enlarging head may for a time be the sole clue, making early detection difficult. Measurement of the head circumference is especially important for this reason, and diagnostic X-ray procedures assume great importance in suspected cases.

Till (1975) in a series of 303 consecutive cases of intracranial neoplasm in children under 13 found the commonest symptoms to be headache, vomiting, unsteadiness and impaired consciousness.

Headache due to intracranial hypertension is usually felt over the vertex or frontally and is often associated with and relieved by vomiting. Both symptoms are often mild and intermittent at first and are commonly most severe in the morning, improving after breakfast, with the result that they may not be taken seriously for some time. When he has a headache the child tends to be silent and still; he will sob rather than cry noisily in order to avoid increasing the pain. Pressure headaches are rarely present for more than a year without diagnosis because the causal conditions usually produce dramatic signs and symptoms before that time. In infants who cannot complain of headache it may be manifested only by their irritability. Absence of headache does not exclude intracranial tumour. Vomiting occurs readily in children with raised pressure, usually associated with headache. Vomiting alone without other features of intracranial hypertension is rarely due to a neurosurgical condition with the important exception of a pontine tumour in which an irritative lesion of brainstem centres may be responsible. Papilloedema is often absent in children with intracranial neoplasms because of the 'safety-valve' effect of expansion of the young skull from suture separation. Its absence should never be taken as excluding the diagnosis. In Till's series 45% of children with intracranial tumours showed no papilloedema, while in the 103 supratentorial tumours it was absent in 56%. Retinal haemorrhages may be seen in infants and young children with raised pressure. In young children with suspected intracranial hypertension it may be difficult to see the optic discs and retinae, and mydriatic eye drops are often used to dilate the pupils to facilitate the examination. This is dangerous and is contra-indicated, since it deprives the examiner of the valuable information to be gained from pupil reactions if the child's condition worsens and radiological and neurosurgical intervention are needed.

Raised intracranial pressure from tumours, cerebral oedema (which is often associated with it) and other causes may result in herniation or displacement of the swollen cerebellum or cerebral hemisphere. With increased pressure in the posterior fossa herniation of the cerebellar tonsils through the foramen magnum may occur, compressing the cervicomedullary junction and causing impairment of the control of respiration and heart rate. Raised pressure above the tentorium cerebelli may cause uncal herniation with downward displacement of the medial part of the temporal lobe through the tentorial opening and compression of the mid-brain with disturbances of the pupillary reactions and other third nerve features.

Ataxia, often truncal and associated with titubation, was common in Till's series, occurring in 61% of those with posterior fossa tumours. Its assessment in young children may be difficult. A head tilt is seen in a few children with posterior fossa neoplasms and this sign should always be treated with respect. The head is held with the occiput inclined towards the shoulder on the side of the tumour. The sign is seldom seen with midline cerebellar tumours. Sometimes there is stiffness and pain in the neck. A similar but painless head tilt may occur as a result of strabismus due to sixth nerve palsy, perhaps as an attempt to correct the separation of the images.

Signs of raised intracranial pressure on plain skull X-rays are seen in most cases. The main radiological features of intracranial hypertension are as follows:

a. In infancy, widening of the skull sutures, a width of 3 mm or more being regarded as significant. (In the first 2 weeks of life the sutures are usually wide.) Beyond infancy suture diastasis is less commonly seen as they become more tightly knit end, when it occurs, it usually indicates that raised pressure has been present for some time.

b. Abnormal digital markings, the impression of the cerebral gyri on the inner table of the skull. Digital markings are a normal feature of children's skull X-rays, but they become more obvious if the vault is thin, as it often is in the presence of raised pressure. The markings are normally not found above the level of the parietal eminence but with high pressure they extend up to the sagittal suture or to the midline in the frontal bones. Increased digital markings are seldom the only radiological sign of raised pressure.

c. In older children, rarefaction of the lamina dura in the pituitary fossa. If there is obstructive hydrocephalus the dilated third ventricle causes enlargement of the pituitary fossa and erosion of the dorsum sellae and posterior clinoid processes.

The classical triad of headache, vomiting and papilloedema was absent in 25% of Till's patients with raised intracranial pressure from all causes, but it is reassuring that in only 2% were headache, vomiting, papilloedema, *and* skull X-ray changes *all* absent. The value of clinical assessment and plain skull X-rays is therefore clear, and their neglect explains the unfortunate fact that the diagnosis of raised pressure is often long delayed.

A brief account follows of the commoner types of intracranial neoplasm seen in childhood.

MEDULLOBLASTOMA

This tumour is commonest in the first decade of life and rare in adolescence: it has been reported in the newborn period. It is commoner in boys than girls in a ratio of about 2 : 1. The tumour accounted for 21% of all intracranial tumours in Till's series and for 33% of all posterior fossa neoplasms. A small proportion of the total medulloblastomas arose above the tentorium.

The medulloblastoma is a soft, very invasive and rapidly growing glioma, arising from undifferentiated neural cells, perhaps from 'rests' of embryonic cells called medulloblasts, which may occur anywhere in the brain but are commonest in the roof of the fourth ventricle. It is here that the tumour usually arises, extending towards the dorsum of the cerebellar vermis and growing into the lumen of the fourth ventricle to fill it completely and block its exit foramina. Metastatic 'seeding' is common throughout the subarachnoid pathways, downwards to involve the spinal meninges and nerve roots and upwards to affect the basal cisterns and ventricular system. The tumour is soft, friable and fairly vascular without a clear line of demarcation from normal tissue. Microscopically it is very cellular and composed of small, round or oval cells in no definite pattern with frequent mitotic figures.

Ataxia and raised intracranial pressure are the main clinical features. These are not specific to this tumour and the pathology cannot be predicted on clinical grounds. Since it is a midline lesion the ataxia is rarely unilateral, and usually affects either the limbs on both sides or the trunk alone with a tendency to fall backwards or forwards. The features of raised pressure with headache and vomiting, with or without papilloedema and usually with radiological signs are non-specific but usually dramatic. The children are often iller when first seen than those with other intracranial tumours, and often look wasted despite a history of usually less than three months duration. The head may be enlarged with an abnormal percussion note. The limbs, especially the legs, often show hypotonia and hyporeflexia and the knee jerks are often pen-

dular. Meningeal deposits from seeding usually occur late in the history but may be an early feature: cranial nerve palsies, multiple and often symmetrical, affect the eighth and fifth nerves particularly, and there may be spinal cord compression with paraplegia or spinal nerve root infiltration with root pains, spinal tenderness and areflexia.

The CSF should not be examined routinely since lumbar puncture may be dangerous in the presence of raised pressure. It may be justified as part of a radiological procedure. [When available the CT scan (Fig. 18.1) will usually allow the diagnosis to be made making ventriculography unnecessary]. High cell counts are seen with lymphocytes and tumour cells in mitosis. The protein level is often raised and the sugar may be reduced or absent.

When the diagnosis is strongly suspected on clinical and radiological grounds, a posterior fossa exploration is indicated, often preceded by a period of ventricular drainage. The tumour must be examined at operation to exclude a more benign lesion such as an astrocytoma. Complete surgical removal is not possible but as much as feasible should be removed to re-establish the free flow of CSF and to take a biopsy. Removal is partly by suction and partly by dissection. The tumour is very sensitive to radiotherapy, which should be given not only to the tumour site, but also to the whole brain and spinal cord as prophylaxis against spread by growth and seeding. This usually prolongs life and makes it more comfortable for the child and less distressing for his family. The ultimate prognosis, formerly regarded as very bad, has improved in recent years. A survival of more than 10 years from surgery was achieved in 29% of patients in the series of Bloom et al (1969). It seems likely that survival for a period equal to the age of the child at diagnosis plus nine months implies that recurrence will not occur and that the tumour has been eradicated. McIntosh (1979) in a review of 87 consecutive cases of medulloblastoma diagnosed at The Hospital for Sick Children, London, in the 10-year period 1965–74, following the patients up until death or 1 January 1978, found that only one patient survived in the first 5-year period and is a 'cure'. In the second 5-year period 17 (41%) patients presenting are alive and, of these, 11 are 5-year survivors. The improved outcome in the second quinquennium is due partly to surgical advances

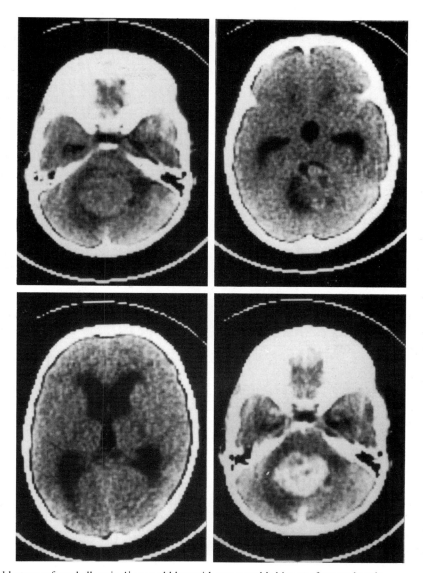

Fig. 18.1 Medulloblastoma of cerebellum in 4½-year-old boy with one month's history of unsteady gait.
Note large midline posterior fossa mass, surrounded by low attenuation and enhancing with contrast. It encroaches upon and displaces the fourth ventricle

and partly to more effective use of radiotherapy. The contribution of immunotherapy and chemotherapy has still to be assessed.

ASTROCYTOMA

The astrocytoma in childhood is among the most favourable intracranial tumours in any age group. It affects the two sexes equally. It is a slowly grow-

ing tumour, far more benign than in adult life and usually occurring in the posterior fossa. The malignant cerebral hemisphere astrocytoma seen in adult life is rare in childhood.

Like the medulloblastoma the astrocytoma of childhood arises in or near the midline of the cerebellum but often extends into the cerebellar hemisphere on either side. It has a remarkable tendency to the formation of cysts which may become much larger than the solid portion of the tumour which is usually attached to one part of the cyst wall. The cyst contains a clear yellow fluid rich in protein. About one-third of astrocytomas show no cyst macroscopically, and these solid tumours include most of the more malignant lesions. Microscopically the tumour shows astrocytes diffusely arranged in a loose stroma.

The clinical features are similar to those of the medulloblostoma and a pre-operative diagnosis cannot be made with certainty, though radiological features may be very suggestive when a cyst is shown. With the astrocytoma the history is often longer and the child appears less ill at first referral than with the medulloblastoma, but exceptions abound and undue reliance should not be placed on this feature. Periods of relative remission are commoner with this tumour than with other gliomas. Unilateral or asymmetrical ataxia and head tilt are often seen when one cerebellar hemisphere is affected and nystagmus is more likely in such cases. Features of raised intracranial pressure develop in time with papilloedema, often chronic,

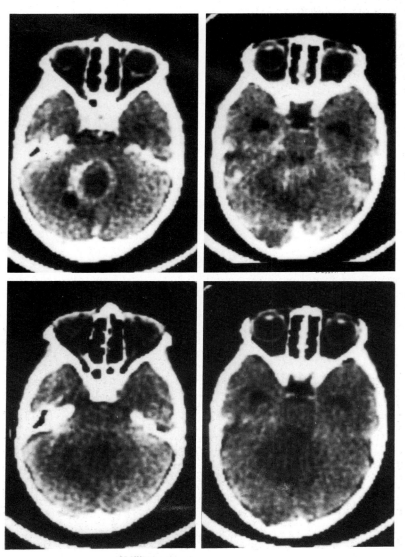

Fig. 18.2 Cystic cerebellar astrocytoma in 4-year-old boy with short history of headache and vomiting, papilloedema and minimal truncal ataxia. Note low attenuation mass with irregular ring enhancement

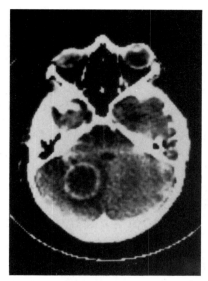

Fig. 18.3 Cystic astrocytoma in left cerebellar hemisphere with hydrocephalus. 14-year-old girl with 5-month history of headache and vomiting.
CT. Note large area of low attenuation in left cerebellar hemisphere with rim enhancement. Surrounding low attenuation represents oedema. The fourth ventricle was displaced to the right, and the lateral and third ventricles were dilated

signs of raised pressure and also thinning and expansion of the occipital bone on the side of the tumour (Fig. 18.4). This feature suggests a slowly growing unilateral mass and a high probability of an astrocytoma. This can be confirmed by special X-rays. Ventriculography is helpful but the CT scan may be more informative, showing the presence of a cyst (Fig. 18.2 and 18.3).

Total surgical removal is often possible since in cystic lesions only the mural nodule need be removed as the cyst wall does not usually contain tumour cells. In more solid lesions and those involving the brain-stem or mid-brain excision may be dangerous or impossible. In 254 patients with cerebellar astrocytoma in Till's (1975) series only partial removal was possible in 103 cases, but the prognosis was often good with 50 patients alive at follow-up and 32 of these in good health after 10 years. Radiotherapy of astrocytomas is considered unhelpful by many authorities.

EPENDYMOMA

This tumour is rarer than the astrocytoma and medulloblastoma in childhood and is unusual in arising as often above the tentorium as below it. The posterior fossa ependymoma tends to cause raised intracranial pressure as it arises in the floor of the fourth ventricle. Stiffness of the neck and shoulders are sometimes complained of with downward extension of the tumour into the cervical

in most cases. The degree of hydrocephalus produced is often greater than with the medulloblastoma since it is often more chronic. Though non-invasive and not causing seeding, the tumour may extend into the brain-stem or mid-brain producing cranial nerve palsies and long tract signs.

Plain skull X-rays may be very helpful, showing

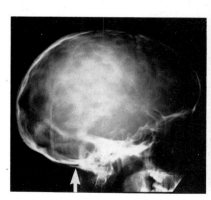
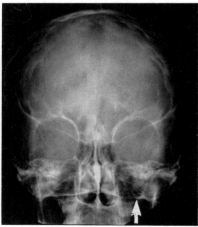

Fig. 18.4 Plain skull X-rays in same patient showing large vault with increased digital markings and minor separation of sutures as signs of raised intracranial pressure. The left side of the posterior fossa is slightly thinned (arrowed)

spinal canal. Lower cranial nerve involvement is also seen, with weakness of the face, pharynx and tongue.

As with other posterior fossa tumours a pre-operative diagnosis is seldom possible, though small flecks of calcification on plain skull X-rays may be suggestive, and surgical exploration is needed. Though total removal is rarely feasible because of the tumour's continuity with the floor of the fourth ventricle, partial removal will often re-establish the circulation of the CSF and relieve hydrocephalus. Radiotherapy is needed post-operatively, but need not be given to the rest of the neuraxis except in the more malignant cases when seeding may occur as with the medulloblastoma.

Cerebral hemisphere ependymomas tend to cause focal neurological symptoms such as convulsions or hemiplegia. They are often cystic and may

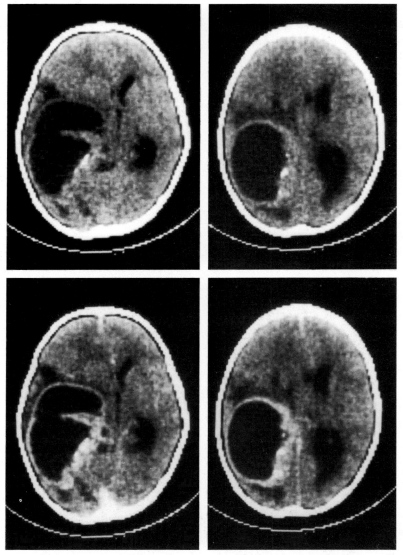

Fig. 18.5 Ependymoma of left cerebral hemisphere in 22-month-old girl with symptoms of raised intracranial pressure
CT shows large mass in region of left trigone and temporal horn extending up into the left parietal region. There is irregular rim enhancement round its margins, moderate surrounding oedema and mass effect with midline shift. There was also thinning and expansion of the left side of the skull vault.

cause local expansion of the skull (Fig. 18.5) which may be the presenting symptom.

CEREBELLAR HAEMANGIOBLASTOMA

Single or multiple haemangioblastomas are seen in the rare condition Von Hippel-Lindau disease, which is often dominantly inherited and sometimes included among the so-called phakomatoses (Ch. 20). Haemangioblastomas are also found affecting the brain-stem, spinal cord and retinae. (The cerebellar lesion takes the form of a cyst with a single mural nodule of haemangioblastoma or a more solid mass with many small cysts.) The condition may present in childhood. Progressive ataxia and features of raised intracranial pressure are seen and the finding of retinal lesions, which are present in only about 20% of cases, will confirm the diagnosis. The whole family should be examined to detect other cases. Surgical removal of the cerebellar lesion may be possible.

BRAIN STEM OR PONTINE GLIOMA

Diffuse infiltrative gliomas in the brain stem are common in children, but the diagnosis is often long delayed because increase in intracranial pressure may not occur until a late stage. Their histology is usually undetermined in life, since biopsy is hazardous, but they must be regarded effectively as malignant because of their situation in an area where even a small lesion can cause progressive cranial nerve palsies and long tract signs and where surgical excision is therefore not possible. Diffuse irregular infiltration of the brain stem by abnormal glial tissue is seen on histological examination.

The maximum incidence is between five and eight years of age. The presentation is usually with multiple, progressive palsies of lower cranial nerves, initially unilateral but soon becoming bilateral. The sixth, seventh, ninth, tenth and twelfth nerves are those most often affected in decreasing frequency. Fifth and eighth nerve involvement may occur but may be less easily detected than the dramatic internal strabismus and facial weakness caused by sixth and seventh nerve palsies. When facial palsy is bilateral it is sometimes overlooked. Pyramidal tract involvement occurs early with hyperreflexia followed later by limb weakness. Often a hemiplegia develops first but later bilateral spastic problems arise. The history is often dated by parents from a fall, so that the effects of the fall and a head injury may be suspected, but it seems likely that the fall has been merely a symptom of

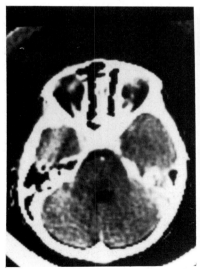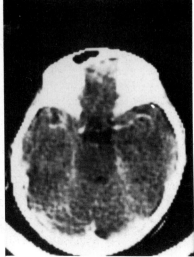

Fig. 18.6 Brainstem tumour in 11-year-old boy with 6-month history of increasing neurological deficit, bilateral 6th and 7th nerve palsies and pyramidal signs.
CT. The pons is swollen and of low attenuation. There was no enhancement after contrast injection

the incipient lower limb weakness or of the ataxia which also often develops.

The features of raised intracranial pressure develop only at a late stage, so that absence of headache, drowsiness and papilloedema is in favour of the diagnosis. By contrast, vomiting may be an early symptom, due perhaps to a local irritative effect on brain-stem centres. Irritability, too, may be a striking early feature.

Plain skull X-rays are usually unhelpful as they do not show signs of raised pressure until very late. Previously lumbar air encephalography (LAEG) was needed to make the diagnosis, or ventriculography in cases with raised pressure. The CT scan is nowadays often adequate to demonstrate the tumour, provided low enough cuts are made (Fig. 18.6), but sometims LAEG is needed for confirmation and occasionally vertebral angiography to exclude a vascular lesion such as an angioma. Deterioration in the child's condition may follow air studies and previous treatment with dexamethasone may be advisable to help to reduce oedema of the brain-stem.

Surgical intervention is not advisable since removal of this infiltrating tumour is clearly impossible and biopsy is dangerous. When hydrocephalus is present at a late stage a shunt procedure may be justified but radiotherapy may sometimes alleviate the features of raised pressure. Radiotherapy is the treatment of choice and is often combined with dexamethasone treatment. It will often improve the patient's condition dramatically, so that a child with a totally expressionless flaccid face, internal squint, dysphagia and gait disorder may improve sufficiently to return to school and enjoy life again. The remission is unfortunately usually limited to some months, but the period of survival has been trebled (Panitch & Berg 1970,) and many of the months of life gained are happier for the child and his family. The ultimate prognosis is still poor, with the average survival under four years. Cases of brain-stem tumour showing recovery or longer survival may well be examples of brain-stem encephalitis or of some other non-neoplastic pathology, perhaps vascular.

CRANIOPHARYNGIOMA (RATHKE'S POUCH TUMOUR OR SUPRASELLAR CYST)

Embryologically the pituitary gland has two components, one from the buccal epithelium (Rathke's pouch) and another from the primitive diencephalon. Squamous cell rests from Rathke's pouch may come to rest in the pars tuberalis of the pituitary and the proliferation of these ectopic cells is thought to give rise to the craniopharyngioma. The tumour is non-neoplastic and composed of solid masses of epithelial tissue and cysts filled with ker-

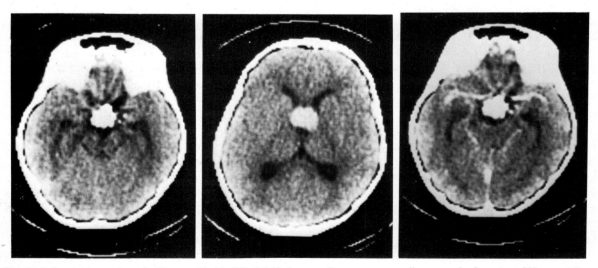

Fig. 18.7 Craniopharyngioma in 10-year-old girl. CT. Calcified suprasellar tumour extending up to the foramina of Monro and causing hydrocephalus

atin, cellular debris and crystals of cholesterol. It expands as a result of multiplication of cells with desquamation and liquefaction of the products, situated as a rounded lesion above the diaphragma sellae. This expansion compresses neighbouring structures and impairs their function.

The tumour grows slowly and rarely produces symptoms before the age of four years though it is probably present from birth or earlier in some cases and has occasionally caused symptoms in the newborn period (Azar-Kia et al 1975). Though it is extracerebral its situation above the sella turcica can produce several different effects from involvement of various structures. Obstruction of the third ventricle or of one or both foramina of Monro may cause raised intracranial pressure and hydrocephalus. Compression of the optic chiasma, nerves or tracts leads to various visual field defects, most commonly bitemporal hemianopia from chiasmal involvement. Optic atrophy may occur with pallor of the optic discs and visual impairment. Pituitary function may be disturbed with delayed skeletal growth and sexual maturation. Easy fatiguability, a low basal metabolic rate and blood pressure and, in advanced cases, panhypopituitarism may result. Hypothalamic disturbance may cause drowsiness, obesity and diabetes insipidus. Raised intracranial pressure may be long delayed so that its dramatic features may often lead to investigation and diagnosis when other effects such as visual failure are far advanced. Delayed development of secondary sexual characteristics may be a striking symptom in children of pubertal age and over, but genital underdevelopment in younger patients is often overlooked. Endocrine dysfunction may also produce insidious symptoms which are not detected until more dramatic features prompt careful assessment.

Skull X-rays are a valuable and frequently diagnostic investigation, sadly often delayed until a late stage. In Till's (1975) patients with craniopharyngioma these had never failed to show some abnormality. Calcification was seen in or above the sella, in 98% of cases, a much higher proportion than in adults. The calcification is often diagnostic, indicating the circular outline of the tumour. The sella is often enlarged or distorted and its floor may have a J or, better, an omega Ω shape. The posterior clinoid processes may be eroded and there may be radiological signs of raised intracranial pressure including diastasis of skull sutures. The exact size and location of the tumour may be shown by lumbar air encephalography or by the CT scan (Fig. 18.7). Laboratory investigations may show a low fasting blood sugar level, flattened glucose tolerance curve and abnormal thyroid, pituitary and adrenal cortical function.

Pre-operatively detailed assessment of endocrine function should be made whenever possible. A morning blood sample should be taken for measurement of cortisol, thyroxine, prolactin, electrolytes and osmolality. The osmolality of an early morning specimen of urine should be measured. An accurate fluid balance chart should be started before operation.

Surgical treatment is needed. Total removal is possible in half or more cases but the close proximity of the tumour to the pituitary, hypothalamus and optic pathways and the mortality sometimes associated with attempted total removal often prevent this. Aspiration of the contents of cysts is helpful and may allow the flow of CSF to be re-established with relief of hydrocephalus and improvement sometimes in vision. Treatment with adrenal cortical steroids is needed in the pre-operative period (covering air-encephalography which may cause deterioration with hypotension and endocrine imbalance), and during and after operation. Post-operatively diabetes insipidus and a salt-losing syndrome may develop and these and other endocrine problems require vigorous and vigilant management. Radiotherapy is often given after surgery or when surgery is not feasible; it seems more effective with cystic than with solid tumours and may work by reducing the rate of fluid formation. Recurrence of craniopharyngioma is seen unfortunately in many cases of subtotal removal and in some in which it was thought the tumour had been removed in toto. Further operation can again relieve acute problems such as hydrocephalus, but the prognosis is poor after recurrence (Katz 1975).

Careful endocrine replacement treatment may be needed after the post-operative period. Diabetes insipidus may persist and can be treated with synthetic preparations administered by nasal spray in older children or injections of pitressin tannate in oil in younger patients. Thyroxine may be needed for hypothyroidism and human growth hormone in some cases with persistent retardation of growth. Some children require prolonged treatment with corticosteroids.

GLIOMA OF THE OPTIC PATHWAYS

The optic nerve arises as an outgrowth from the brain and contains glial cells. Gliomas may arise within the nerves themselves, the optic chiasm and the optic tracts. These tumours account for about 4% of intracranial tumours and are of great concern to the paediatrician, paediatric neurologist and neurosurgeon since 75% of them occur in children under the age of 12 (Matson 1969). Many of them may be congenital, though not detected until some time after birth. There is an important association between neurofibromatosis and these tumours, as there is with acoustic neuromas in older patients. *Café au lait* skin patches in a child with nystagmus or visual failure should therefore focus attention on this possibility. The tumour grows very slowly and is confined within the nerve sheath, so that it may show little change over many years. Its slow growth often results in long delayed recognition and it may be very extensive by the time symptoms and signs lead to diagnosis.

Anatomically the tumour may arise in different parts of the optic pathways: its origin may be very anterior, within the orbit, from the retro-orbital part of the optic nerve, from the chiasma and even from behind the chiasma where it merges into the hypothalamic astrocytoma.

The intraorbital glioma often presents with progressive non-pulsatile proptosis of one eye without abnormalities of eye movements. Vision is usually reduced but this may not be recognized until severe loss has occurred since the child may be unaware of it and adjust to the gradual onset of blindness. If the tumour is confined to the orbit papilloedema may be seen. When it extends backwards optic atrophy may result from pressure on neurons.

With intracranial gliomas loss of visual acuity is the common presentation. It is often asymmetrical or unilateral and accompanied by primary optic atrophy and often by spontaneous nystagmus of ocular type. Such nystagmus, especially when unilateral or asymmetrical, should raise suspicion of an optic nerve glioma. Visual field defects of various kinds may be present, though difficult to demonstrate in the young child.

When the neoplasm extends to other structures various other deficits may arise. Compression of the third ventricle may impede the CSF circulation and

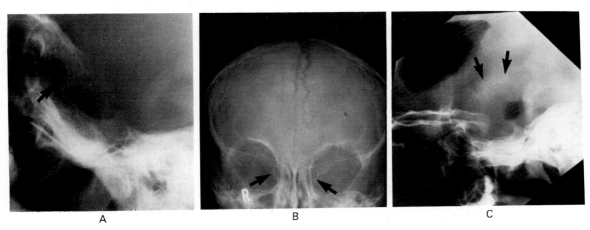

A   B   C

Fig. 18.8 Optic chiasm tumour in 4 year 9 month-old girl with visual impairment and 8-week history of nausea, vomiting and headache. Found to have bilateral papilloedema and sixth nerve palsies.
  A. Lateral view of pituitary fossa. The fossa is enlarged. The dorsum sellae is short, its upper part and the posterior clinoid processes being eroded. There is erosion of the pre-sellar sphenoid (arrowed) tuberculum sellae, sulcus chiasmaticus and planum sphenoidale and the optic struts are visible. The lamina dura of the whole of the fossa is osteoporotic.
  B. Postero-anterior film. The sutures are wide. The optic foramina are so large that their lateral margins are visible (arrowed) within the orbit.
  C. Ventriculogram. The lateral ventricles are dilated. The upper surface of the tumour is encroaching on the 3rd ventricle (arrowed).

cause hydrocephalus. Hypothalamic involvement may lead to the diencephalic syndrome (see below) in which there is gross emaciation, sometimes despite an increased appetite, and a head circumference which may be normal or enlarged. Other hypothalamic effects include diabetes insipidus and precocious sexual development.

Plain skull X-rays (Fig. 18.8) may show the changes of raised intracranial pressure and a J or Ω shaped sella with excavation beneath the anterior clinoid processes. Special views should be taken to show the optic foramina. Tumours of the optic nerve cause enlargement of these on one or both sides and thinning of their bony edges. The neoplasm itself may be defined by lumbar air encephalography but ventriculography may be needed when there is hydrocephalus and when distortion of the third ventricle impedes the upward passage

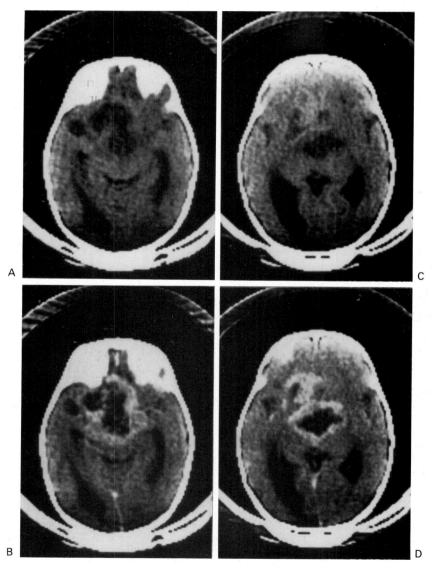

Fig. 18.9 Optic nerve glioma with hydrocephalus. 2 years 8 month-old boy with 3-month history of visual failure, failure to thrive and ataxia. CT. Note large mass of multilobular outline and mixed attenuation in upper part of pituitary fossa, suprasellar and sub-frontal region. It obliterates the third ventricle and extends between the lateral ventricles. There was erosion of the tuberculum sellae, left anterior clinoid and left orbital apex

of air. The CT scan will usually allow the lesion to be clearly shown with less risk (Fig. 18.9).

Management must depend on the anatomy of the tumour. Exploration is needed when the radiological evidence does not clearly show extension back from the optic nerve or chiasm. The chiasm is inspected and, if it is normal, the nerve may be cut across behind the tumour which may be radically excised with the eye when the globe is involved. Operative removal is impossible with tumours involving the hypothalamus and radiotherapy is then needed. Hydrocephalus can be dealt with by a shunt procedure. In Till's (1975) series survival has varied from one to over 17 years.

OTHER SUPRASELLAR TUMOURS

The craniopharyngioma and some optic pathway gliomas are two examples of expanding lesions situated above the sella turcica, but other rarer conditions in the same site may produce a similar clinical picture by involvement of neighbouring structures. These include gliomas arising in the floor of the third ventricle and extracerebral lesions within the skull such as arachnoid cysts, hamartomas and leukaemic deposits, as well as lesions arising in the base of the skull and spreading intracranially (sarcoma, neuroblastoma, eosinophilic granuloma and some carcinomas).

The clinical features of these varied lesions are similar to those of the craniopharyngioma. Thus disordered function of the optic nerves, hypothalamus or pituitary may be seen, and the CSF circulation may be obstructed.

More specific features may result from tumours of the median eminence of the hypothalamus which may cause precocious puberty. The hamartoma, a tumour composed of mature normal neurons, is the commonest such lesion, but astrocytoma, teratoma or ectopic pinealoma may also be found in cases of precocious puberty.

Tumours of the pituitary gland are much rarer in childhood than in adult life. Cushing's syndrome in childhood, itself a rare condition, is occasionally due to a basophil adenoma. Pituitary tumours may cause raised intracranial pressure and visual field defects.

THE DIENCEPHALIC SYNDROME

In some children with tumours in the hypothalamic region and the floor of the third ventricle a dramatic syndrome is seen with profound emaciation (Fig. 18.10) despite a good appetite and calorie intake (Russell 1951). The patients look well and may be overactive with a mood of elation. These findings may be present for some time before the tumour betrays itself by the appearance of abnormal neurological signs. Bain et al (1966), among others, have described the diencephalic syndrome of early infancy due to silent brain tumours. Their three patients, all boys in the first year of life, were emaciated, pale, overactive and excessively alert, and two were euphoric. No abnormal neurological signs were found apart from nystagmus in one patient but the air encephalogram in all three showed space-occupying lesions involving the floor of the third ventricle and astrocytomas were found

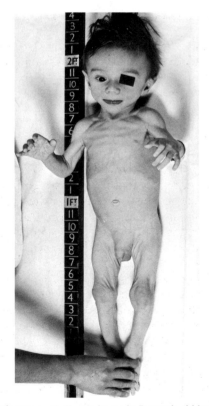

Fig. 18.10 Diencephalic syndrome in 7-month-old boy with astrocytoma. Note severe emaciation and alert expression.

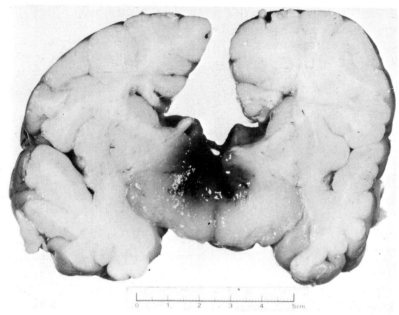

Fig. 18.11 Grade III astrocytoma in 5-month-old girl with diencephalic syndrome. Coronal section of brain at level of hypothalamus which is completely replaced by an enormous grey tumour showing some haemorrhage

in the two who had craniotomies. The syndrome may be seen with tumours arising elsewhere and involving the hypotholamus (Fig. 18.11) including some cases of optic pathway glioma.

CEREBRAL HEMISPHERE GLIOMAS

These tumours are rarer in childhood than infratentorial neoplasms, and they may produce little disturbance and few signs in early life. They only cause raised intracranial pressure at a late stage, in contrast to the midline cerebellar tumours. Personality changes and headache, often without vomiting, may be early symptoms. For these reasons their recognition may be long delayed. Progressive neurological deficit may result, such as a hemiplegia, dysphasia or visual field defect. Seizures may be due to a cerebral glioma, and may sometimes be the only symptom for some years: nineteen of the 23 children with cerebral gliomas reported by Page et al (1969) had experienced convulsions for half their lives or longer before their tumours were recognized. Temporal lobe epilepsy in children is far less often due to neoplasms than in adults, but

cases are seen from time to time of slowly growing gliomas being detected after many years of such seizures. Sometimes the EEG indicates this possibility by showing a focus of slow wave activity. Plain skull X-rays sometimes show changes with local expansion of the skull vault, signs of shift of midline structures away from the lesion and, at a later stage, signs of raised intracranial pressure. Rarely calcification is seen. The CT scan will usually detect gliomas readily (Fig. 18.12). In children with epilepsy, however, including focal seizures, it is unlikely to show a tumour unless there are clinical features suggesting this (Brett & Hoare 1969).

The cerebral hemisphere ependymoma, which is often cystic causing local skull expansion, has been mentioned earlier.

HAMARTOMAS OF THE CEREBRUM

These developmental tumours consisting of apparently normal mature cells are found occasionally when children with focal neurological symptoms, especially seizures, are investigated. They are probably an important cause of temporal lobe epilepsy

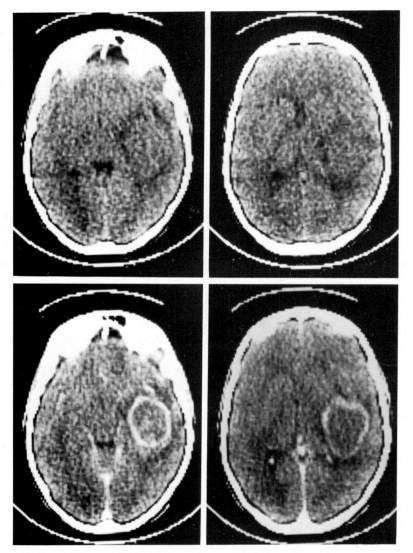

Fig. 18.12 Left temporal glioma. 10-year-old girl with short history of headache and vomiting.
CT. Scan shows large mixed density mass in posterior two thirds of right temporal lobe with irregular rim enhancement and a little surrounding oedema.

in childhood, having been found in about 20% of the temporal lobes removed surgically by Falconer (1971) (Ch. 12). They may appear as calcified lesions on plain skull X-rays but since the introduction of the CT scan they are sometimes shown by this investigation when plain X-rays and even lumbar air encephalography have been normal (Fig. 18.13). These lesions may well be much commoner than is recognized.

TERATOMAS AND TERATOID TUMOURS

Certain intracranial tumours of non-malignant type arise as a result of delayed or continued growth of originally multipotential or undifferentiated cells misplaced early in embryonic life. The craniopharyngioma, already discussed, comes into this category.

One group of these congenital lesions, the tera-

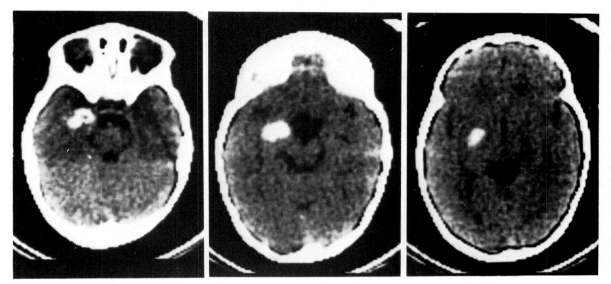

Fig. 18.13 Hamartoma of left temporal lobe in 2-year-old girl with history of right-sided fits from 6 months of age. (She later underwent a subtotal left temporal lobectomy with complete cure of her epilepsy)
CT. Note calcified tumour in left temporal lobe without mass effect. It showed no enhancement with contrast injection

tomas and teratoid tumours, contains epithelial ectodermal elements sometimes with tissues of mesodermal and endodermal origin in addition. All these lesions are cystic, at least in part, and all contain spaces lined by epithelium with liquid or degenerated tissue products within them. Matson (1969) has classified them into three subgroups. The simplest contains only stratified squamous epithelium undergoing keratinization (the epidermoid cyst or cholesteatoma). More complex are cysts lined with squamous epithelium but also containing collagenous elements such as hair, sebaceous glands and other components of normal skin (the dermoid cyst). The rarest of these tumours, the teratomas, contain elements of all three germ layers and are complex structures with mature tissues of mesodermal and endodermal as well as ectodermal origin.

The clinical features of these non-invasive lesions are caused by local pressure on neural structures or CSF pathways, and their onset may be insidious since they usually grow only slowly. They occur mainly in the midline, particularly the pineal area, third ventricle and suprasellar region. In the region of the pineal hydrocephalus from obstruction of the sylvian aqueduct and loss of upward gaze from pressure on the quadrigeminal plate are common

effects. Third ventricular lesions may show themselves only by raised intracranial pressure. Suprasellar lesions may produce visual loss, visual field defects, precocious puberty, diabetes insipidus and also hydrocephalus. Pre-operative distinction between the three tumour types is difficult unless dense calcification is seen on X-rays suggesting the presence of bone or teeth in a teratoma. The treatment is surgical excision, which should be as complete as the situation allows. Radiotherapy is not indicated unless malignant changes are seen in removed tissue.

THE PINEALOMA

This tumour is rare in children under 12 years of age. When it is suspected because of hydrocephalus, paralysis of upward gaze, ptosis and pupillary changes in a young child, the lesion usually proves to be of some other kind such as a teratoma or an astrocytoma. The true pinealoma contains a mixture of two cell types, a large, pale cell and a small, dark, lymphoid-like cell. Surgical removal is difficult and hazardous, and treatment must often consist of a shunt procedure for hydrocephalus followed by radiotherapy.

PAPILLOMA OF THE CHOROID PLEXUS

This benign tumour is commoner in childhood than at other ages and in children is usually within a lateral ventricle. It is thought to result in excessive secretion of CSF causing a communicating type of hydrocephalus and may also cause obstructive hydrocephalus by occluding the third or fourth ventricle or blocking off the occipital or temporal horn of one lateral ventricle. It may also cause intraventricular haemorrhage. Choroid plexus papillomas formed 3% of the 750 cases of intracranial tumours in children in Matson's (1969) series. These 23 patients had an average age of under two years and the oldest was 12. The commonest presenting symptom was vomiting and the commonest

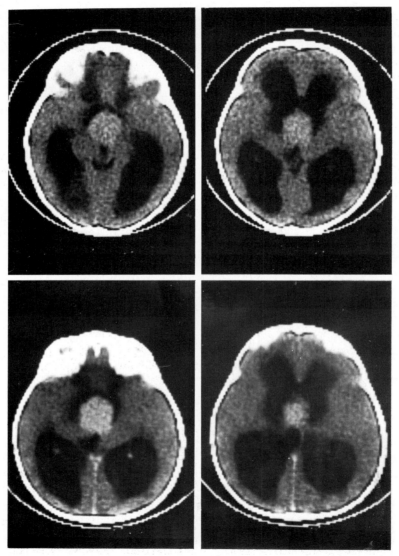

Fig. 18.14 16-month-old girl with papilloma of the choroid plexus and hydrocephalus. She had had ataxia for 3 weeks and vomiting for one week.
CT. Note well-defined lobulated mass of high attenuation lying within the 3rd ventricle. (C and D) Post-contrast films show enhancement of the mass

sign an enlarged head, but the clinical features are non-specific and Matson has emphasized that lack of diagnostic symptoms and signs is the most consistent clinical feature. Evidence of raised intracranial pressure was present by the time of hospital admission in all cases, but in one-third the only abnormal findings were enlargement of the head and separation of the skull sutures. Most children were referred for investigation of hydrocephalus. The pressure of the CSF was usually raised to between 300 and 600 mm, and the protein level was increased in over two thirds of cases. The spinal fluid was often xanthochromic. Plain skull X-rays usually show only signs of raised pressure, but air-encephalography and the CT scan (Fig. 18.14) confirm the diagnosis. The hydrocephalus is usually of communicating type, the whole ventricular system being diffusely enlarged. The lateral ventricle which contains the papilloma may be larger than its fellow and there may be a slight shift of midline structures to the normal side.

The tumours are soft and very vascular. Malignant change in childhood is rare.

Treatment is by surgical removal when possible and radiotherapy is not indicated in most cases.

The outlook in patients who survive the removal of benign papillomas is usually good.

MENINGIOMA

This tumour, very common in young adults, is excessively rare in children. Matson (1969) encountered three cases under the age of 14 years. In recent years at the Hospital for Sick Children, Great Ormond Street, a girl of 14 was seen with visual failure due to chiasmal compression which proved to be due to a meningioma of the planum sphenoidale. Figure 18.15 shows the CT scan of an 11-year-old girl with a tentorial meningioma.

ACOUSTIC NEUROMA

This is another tumour found almost exclusively in adults, but it has occasionally been seen in childhood and should be suspected when features suggesting a cerebello-pontine angle tumour (disturbed seventh and eighth nerve function) occur in a child with stigmata of neurofibromatosis (Ch. 20).

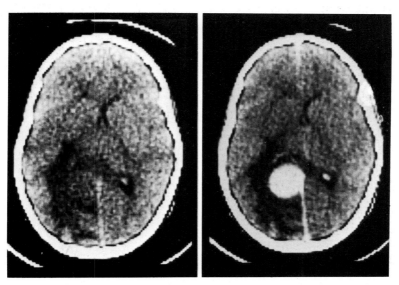

Fig. 18.15 Tentorial meningioma in 11-year-old girl with complaint of left-sided headache. Note small area of density almost identical to that of brain on left side of tentorium and contiguous with the falx (A). There is marked associated oedema and mass effect and the lesion shows homogeneous enhancement after contrast injection (B). (The tumour was removed and the child is well)

CONGENITAL BRAIN NEOPLASMS

The age of diagnosis of intracranial neoplasms in no way reflects the age at which their microscopic onset occurred. The average time from first complaint or clinical clue until hospital admission in 164 cases of brain tumour in childhood (Odom et al 1956) was 11½ months. Many cases diagnosed in the first year of life or even later are probably congenital and occasional cases are seen in which congenital hydrocephalus is treated surgically in the newborn period without detailed radiological studies and the cerebellar neoplasm responsible is only recognized much later.

Arnstein and co-workers (1951) defined as congenital brain neoplasms those presenting before 60 days of age. Many such cases are reported. Wei & Norman (1972) studied 75 children with brain neoplasms seen under 2 years of age at Toronto Sick Children's Hospital over 52 years. 26 cases occurred in the first year of life (13 supratentorial and 13 infratentorial) and 49 presented in the second year (17 supratentorial and 32 infratentorial). Astrocytomas were the commonest supratentorial neoplasm. Infratentorially ependymomas were the commonest followed by medulloblastomas and astrocytomas. Other tumours in this series were brain-stem glioma (3) and undifferentiated malignant neuro-ectodermal neoplasm (5). A congenital origin is likely for many cases of early onset craniopharyngioma, choroid plexus papilloma and some other tumours.

NON-NEOPLASTIC TUMOURS AFFECTING THE BRAIN

Many non-neoplastic space-occupying lesions within the skull can affect the brain. These may cause raised intracranial pressure and other features suggestive of neoplasms. They may be associated with focal neurological deficits or may even be clinically 'silent'. These lesions include subdural haematoma and effusion, chronic juvenile subdural effusion, cerebral abscess, hydatid cysts, intracerebral and intracerebellar haematoma and tuberose sclerosis. Many of these are discussed in other chapters but it seems appropriate to consider the first two conditions here.

SUBDURAL HAEMATOMA AND EFFUSION IN INFANCY AND CHILDHOOD

Hark ye, good parents, to my words true and plain,
When you are shaking your baby, you could be bruising his brain,
So, save the limbs, the brain, even the life of your tot,
By shaking him never, never and not.
Caffey (1972) *On the theory and practice of shaking infants.*

This non-neoplastic space-occupying lesion is common in childhood, and frequently less serious than the subdural haematoma of adult life which often carries a grave prognosis because of the associated injury to the brain. The management of acute subdural haematoma is discussed in Ch. 19.

The term implies an accumulation of fluid between the dura and arachnoid membranes overlying the cerebral hemispheres. Rarely the fluid is pure blood, as in an acute haematoma due to head injury, but much more often — due to the common delay in diagnosis — it is a watery fluid, varying in colour from pale yellow to dark brown and containing little or no blood (usually less than 500 000 red cells per cubic mm). The term subdural *effusion* is more appropriate for such a collection. It is often bilateral and may extend widely over both hemispheres, but is sometimes loculated and unilateral. The fluid collection is contained within a vascular outer membrane up to 0.5 mm thick beneath the dura and a thin, filmy membrane over the arachnoid. The protein content is always high, usually between 0.5 and 6.0 g per 100 ml, an important point of distinction from cerebrospinal fluid and fluid in other cystic structures. The fluid and membranes around it are similar whatever the aetiology of the effusion, and it seems likely, from studies with radioactively-labelled albumin, that a change in membrane permeability allows albumin to escape from the plasma into the subdural space so that more fluid is drawn into it by osmosis. The striking preponderance of males in all published series is unexplained.

Aetiology

The aetiology is often uncertain but trauma, accidental or non-accidental, is the commonest recognized cause. In Till's (1968) series of 116 cases of subdural haematoma and effusion in infancy, trauma was involved in 40%. In 5% meningitis was an aetiological factor. The remaining 55% had no known antecedent disease. The relative importance of trauma and meningitis is likely to vary in different series, according to the type of problem referred to the neurosurgical centre concerned. The clinical features of the post-meningitic subdural effusion, usually following meningitis due to *Haemophilus influenzae* or the pneumococcus, have been discussed in Chapter 22. Rarely blood disorders such as haemophilia and leukaemia can cause subdural haematoma and effusion. They may also rarely result as an iatrogenic event from the rapid reduction of raised intracranial pressure which may follow a shunt procedure for hydrocephalus or removal of a posterior fossa tumour. Air-encephalography has occasionally caused a subdural effusion to develop. Menkes' syndrome and Moya-Moya disease are other rare associations.

Clinical features

These are not specific and the presentation may be insidious so that the diagnosis is often long-delayed. In this disorder, as with meningitis and spinal cord tumours, a high index of suspicion in the clinician is essential. There is little difficulty when there is a clear history of recent head injury or meningitis, but the absence of a history of trauma does not exclude it.

In the series of 106 babies with subdural effusions from the Hospital for Sick Children, Great Ormond Street, reported by Till (1975), vomiting was the commonest symptom and a tense anterior fontanelle the commonest sign, both occurring in 67 infants. The other common symptoms, in decreasing order of frequency, were seizures (57), a complaint of a tense fontanelle (45), impaired consciousness (23) and irritability (12). The commoner *signs* in the series, after a tense fontanelle, were signs of raised pressure on skull X-rays (50), retinal or subhyaloid haemorrhages (48), enlarged head (33), fractured bones other than skull (17) and fractured skull (13). Some of these features are more helpful in indicating the likely diagnosis than others. Fractured long bones or ribs or a skull fracture give proof of injury, as do bruises, wheals, scars and burns, all of which must be looked for

in the careful scrutiny of the skin which should be routine in all sick children. Retinal or subhyaloid haemorrhages are particularly useful since they usually imply a recent rapid rise in intracranial pressure. Their presence should be taken as evidence that the child has subdural effusions until this has been disproved. Another common, though non-specific, finding is anaemia, due probably to a combination of blood loss and dietary deficiency; 40% of the children in Till's series had a haemoglobin level of less than 10 g/100 ml.

Subdural effusions are one of the commonest and most important (because treatable) lesions in cases of non-accidental injury ('the battered baby syndrome') and whenever trauma is suspected they must be carefully searched for, together with other evidence of trauma. They may result from repeated shaking of an infant (Caffey 1972). The possibility of their developing later in a child known to have sustained trauma to the head must also be kept carefully in mind as his progress is followed. Here, as with hydrocephalus, serial measurement of the head circumference is essential; this may sometimes be the only clue in a child whose clinical progress seems reasonably good. When subdural effusions develop in a child who has had previous injury to the head it is sometimes difficult to know whether these indicate further trauma or have evolved spontaneously and insidiously from the original injury. The CT scan is a valuable aid in following up such cases.

Diagnosis and treatment

Transillumination of the skull may suggest the presence of a subdural collection, and the finding of a localized area of electrical silence on the EEG may do the same. Previously radiological demonstration of the effusion required arteriography (or air-encephalography), but the advent of the CT scan has made its detection and management much easier. A common finding on CT is an interhemispheric subdural haematoma. Zimmerman et al (1978) found these lesions in the parieto-occipital region in 17 of 28 abused children who presented with neurological symptoms. This could be correlated with injury due to severe shaking, with the presence of retinal haemorrhages and with the absence of obvious stigmata of 'battering'. Later CT in these children showed cerebral infarction in the affected area in half the cases and cerebral atrophy in all. The CT scan may also demonstrate retinal haemorrhage.

Lumbar puncture may be helpful, showing frankly blood-stained or pink CSF or, in cases of longer duration, a yellow fluid. Red blood cells and a raised protein level are often found.

When the CT scan is not available the diagnosis may depend on tapping the subdural spaces to obtain fluid for examination. Though reasonably safe in experienced hands, the procedure is not free from morbidity and should not be undertaken lightly. Firm restraint of the baby swaddled in a sheet with all his limbs anchored is achieved by a nurse whose forearms on either side of his trunk and head act as a further splint. The anterior fontanelle should be needled at least 1 cm from the midline to avoid the sagittal sinus. The tapping should be done on both sides since effusions are commonly bilateral. When fluid is obtained it should not be rapidly aspirated but released slowly. The fluid should be examined for colour, protein, cell count and culture. A subdural effusion rarely contains less than 0.5 g of protein per 100 ml, whereas the CSF usually contains far less than this. It is helpful to confirm the diagnosis after the initial tap by injecting 5 or 10 ml of air into each subdural space. Later lateral X-rays of the skull with the baby's brow first up and then down will define the limits of the spaces. This is helpful in deciding whether repeated aspiration may suffice to obliterate the space or not. Till (1975) has found that a depth of over 1.5 cm implies that simple aspiration will not eradicate the effusion.

In the past the commonest surgical approach was by craniotomy and removal of the subdural membranes. This was often difficult so that they could not be totally removed. The modern approach is to shunt the fluid from the subdural space to the pleural space by a tube placed subcutaneously. The fluid will usually drain for some weeks allowing the compressed brain to expand and the subdural space to become obliterated. After six to 12 weeks the catheter can be easily removed (Till 1968).

The long-term management of the child with subdural effusion depends partly on the cause, where known. Cases due to non-accidental injury require careful follow-up. The social and psychological appraisal of the parents, and the weighing up of the risk of further injury, are of great importance. A team approach is needed with the help of experienced social workers and provision of support to the parents. It is often necessary for the Police to be involved, but in general a punitive attitude should be avoided. These problems, some of the most difficult encountered by the paediatrician who must consider his responsibility to the child, the parents and the community, are the subject of wide debate. They are discussed, among other publications in Helfer & Kempe (1968) and Franklin (1975 and 1977).

Prognosis

Unfortunately the outlook for infants with subdural effusion from all causes is not bright, since only about half of them develop normally. From 5 to 15% die later, often from repeated trauma. In the survivors the nature of the illness causing the effusions seems to determine the outcome rather than the size and duration of the effusion itself. Severe meningitis or gross, often repeated, contusions and damage to the brain itself may severely affect cerebral function. Hydrocephalus is a common association of subdural effusion due to trauma or meningitis. It may be transient or persistent, and is usually due to basal cistern occlusion.

Fits in later life are probably due to the causal condition rather than the effusion.

Mental retardation, often associated with microcephaly, is the most serious sequela and is common. Some 10% are 'ineducable' with IQs below 50, and 20% are educationally subnormal (Till 1968). Cerebral palsy of spastic type and tetraplegic or hemiplegic distribution is another serious sequela.

CHRONIC JUVENILE SUBDURAL EFFUSION

A condition previously regarded as a 'relapsing juvenile subdural haematoma' or a chronic juvenile subdural 'hygroma' or 'hydroma' was reassessed by Robinson (1964) as being probably due to a developmental anomaly affecting the temporal lobe. In this condition apparent agenesis of the fronto-temporal region of the brain on one side is associated with expansion of the anterior and lateral boundaries of the middle cranial fossa. Robinson suggested that the underdevelopment of this region of the brain leaves a locally capacious subarachnoid space and that this has the secondary effect of causing expansion of the overlying skull by increased pulsation.

The condition affects males four times as often as females and the patients usually present between the ages of 5 and 21 years, though occasionally it is silent, being found incidentally at autopsy. Headache is the commonest complaint and is often accentuated by trivial head injury. Some patients have convulsions. Asymmetry of the head is present from an early age, even in the newborn period. Examination shows a hard, non-tender bulging of the temporal region on one side (Fig. 18.16) sometimes with elevation of the eyebrow and a mild degree of exophthalmos. Intelligence is usually normal and no abnormal neurological signs are present until complications occur.

It is the complication of bleeding with subdural haematoma resulting often from quite trivial trauma which usually brings the condition to light. This may need surgical evacuation.

The striking bulging of the skull must be distinguished from that due to a neoplasm affecting the skull, an expanding brain tumour and neurofibromatosis. Appropriate X-ray studies will help to make the distinction.

CEREBRAL ARACHNOID CYSTS

These benign cysts, probably of developmental origin, are occasionally found while investigating children with hydrocephalus. A series of fourteen children in whom hydrocephalus proved to be due to a cyst of the posterior fossa or subarachnoid cisterns was reported by Harrison (1971). Five of the patients showed ataxia of the limbs or gait and visual abnormalities were present in seven. Ataxia and visual problems were particularly common with cysts in the suprasellar region, and these two fea-

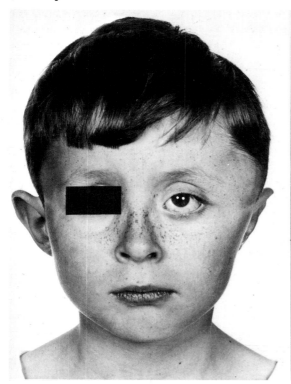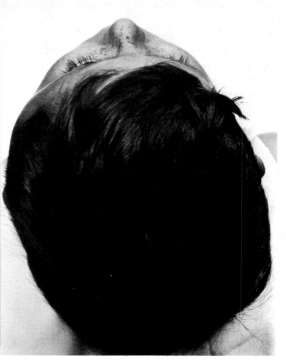

Fig. 18.16 8-year-old boy with L-sided chronic juvenile subdural effusion. Note expansion of skull

tures may be commoner with hydrocephalus due to arachnoid cysts than in cases due to other causes. No other clinical features distinguished these cases.

Pneumography showed hydrocephalus in all fourteen patients and in all but one case the features of basal cistern block. Suprasellar cysts were associated with a filling defect in the floor of the third ventricle. In some cases this was shown to vary in size, indicating the cystic nature of the lesion, and was sometimes large enough to block the foramen of Monro. Cysts in the region of the quadrigeminal plate cistern caused displacement of the aqueduct downwards and forwards and a forward shift of the posterior end of the third ventricle. Cysts in the posterior fossa could not be distinguished radiologically from other space-occupying lesions.

Histologically most of the cysts examined showed glial tissue with an ependymal-like lining. There was no evidence of neonatal haemorrhage, infection or trauma from the history and many cases showed other signs of maldevelopment such as agenesis of the corpus callosum and porencephalic cysts. In all but one case basal cistern block was also present and it seems likely that this and the arachnoid cysts represent maldevelopment of the subarachnoid space.

Local drainage and opening of the cysts often seemed to control the hydrocephalus even though basal cistern block was present in most cases. In other patients an additional shunting procedure was needed.

CEREBRAL OEDEMA

Cerebral oedema is defined as an increase in brain volume due to an increase in its water content (Fishman 1975). It is commonly associated with raised intracranial pressure although either may occur alone. It may be mild or severe, localized or widespread, acute or chronic. When severe, cerebral oedema may result in focal or generalized dysfunction of the brain, uncal or tonsillar herniation and failure of respiration and circulatory control.

Until recently cerebral oedema could usually only be suspected from the clinical picture or from the finding of a shift of brain structures or of small ventricles on air encephalography or arteriography.

Use of the CT scan now allows oedema to be detected by the appearance of decreased radiodensity (low attenuation) due to the high water content. Oedema is often shown by the scan in the neighbourhood of neoplasms (Fig. 18.15), infarcts and inflammatory lesions such as cerebral abscess or herpes encephalitis, and this oedema may be partly responsible for their effects on adjacent structures, while diffuse oedema may be shown with similar lesions and may explain their occasional association with more widespread neurological dysfunction.

The occurrence of brain oedema is such an important factor in the complex equation of many neurological and neurosurgical disorders of childhood that a short discussion of its pathogenesis and management is needed.

TYPES OF CEREBRAL OEDEMA

It is now recognized that cerebral oedema can be classified into several separate categories (Fishman 1971, Miller 1978). *Vasogenic* oedema, the commonest form, is due to increased permeability of endothelial cells in cerebral capillaries, the 'tight' junctions between the cells opening up and allowing the escape of protein-rich plasma filtrate into the extracellular fluid which is increased in volume. This type of oedema particularly affects the cerebral white matter. The causes include brain tumour, abscess, infarction, haemorrhage, trauma, lead encephalopathy, and purulent meningitis. Displacement of the cerebral hemisphere and herniation may result. The clinical features include those of raised intracranial pressure, altered consciousness and focal neurological deficits, and there is often focal slowing of the EEG. Treatment with corticosteroids is often helpful and osmotic therapy with hypertonic solutions (mannitol, isosorbide and glycerol) may be useful in the acute stage.

In *cytotoxic* cerebral oedema all the cellular elements of the brain (neurons, glia and endothelial cells) may undergo rapid swelling with reduction in the volume of extracellular fluid. Hypoxia, as with asphyxia or cardiac arrest, purulent meningitis and certain rare toxins are among the causes of this type of oedema, which affects grey and white matter alike and is associated with generalized slowing of the EEG. Changes in consciousness, with stupor or coma, are the main clinical features. Focal deficits, such as hemiplegia, may result from cerebral infarction. In patients with cerebral arterial occlusion vasogenic and cytotoxic oedema often co-exist. Steroid therapy is probably ineffective for the cytotoxic form of oedema but may be helpful for the associated vasogenic element. Mannitol is often effective in cytotoxic oedema.

A third type of cerebral oedema, *interstitial* oedema, is seen in obstructive hydrocephalus, with an increase in the water and sodium content of the periventricular white matter due to the movement of CSF through the ependyma. The CT scan may show localized areas of low attenuation round the walls of the lateral ventricles, known as periventricular lucency. Myelin lipids in this periventricular zone may disappear rapidly as the hydrostatic pressure builds up. Successful shunt procedures can reverse this situation.

A fourth type of cerebral oedema, the *hydrostatic* variety, results when increased intravascular pressure is transmitted to the capillary bed due to lack of a compensatory increase in cerebrovascular resistance with an outpouring of water into the extracellular space. This may result from direct trauma to the brain, excessive arterial hypertension, hypercapnia or hypoxaemia. It may also complicate craniotomy when a rise in intravascular pressure is not balanced by an equivalent increase in extravascular pressure. Hydrostatic oedema affects the white matter and is generally diffuse, unlike the vasogenic type which is often focal.

A fifth variety, *hypo-osmotic* oedema, occurs with the intracellular accumulation of water diffusely in grey or white matter as a result of low plasma osmolality. It is often associated with hyponatraemia, such as occurs with inappropriate secretion of antidiuretic hormone (ADH) or with excessive infusion of intravenous solutions low in sodium, a hazard to beware of in the correction of hypernatraemic dehydration.

THE MANAGEMENT OF CEREBRAL OEDEMA

This depends on recognizing the cause or causes, whenever possible, and on anticipating and avoiding those factors which favour the production of oedema and impede its resolution (Miller 1978). The use of intracranial pressure (ICP) monitoring is a valuable weapon but is not available in all centres. James et al (1975) have reviewed intracranial subarachnoid pressure monitoring in children.

GENERAL PRINCIPLES

These have been well reviewed by Miller (1978). Severe hypoxaemia and hypercapnia, both potent cerebral vasodilators, should be corrected promptly, and volatile anaesthetic agents such as halothane should be avoided because of their vasodilating effect. Arterial blood pressure should be monitored and maintained in the normal range. Hypertension, however, may be a compensatory response to increased ICP in some patients, so that its reduction may reduce perfusion pressure and lead to ischaemia. It is in situations such as this that ICP monitoring can be most helpful.

Fluid intake should be restricted to 60% of the normal daily requirement.

SPECIFIC TREATMENT

Hyperventilation. Reduction of the arterial partial pressure of carbon dioxide (P_{CO_2}) causes an increase in cerebrovascular resistance and a consequent decrease in cerebral blood volume and fall in ICP. This slows down the rate of oedema formation and speeds up reabsorption of the excess fluid in the white matter. The P_{CO_2} should be maintained between 25 and 30 mm Hg since levels below 20 may be associated with a change to anaerobic glycolysis in the brain. Hyperventilation may also help in cases of raised ICP due to cerebrovascular engorgement rather than to true cerebral oedema. The blood vessesls in oedematous areas may not be able to respond fully to changes in P_{CO_2} but their response is not predictable and hyperventilation should be given a trial when the situation warrants it.

Hyperbaric oxygen is another method of inducing cerebral vasoconstriction in the hope of reducing cerebral oedema but its benefits are less well established.

CSF drainage. An indwelling ventricular catheter allows drainage of CSF against a positive pressure of 15 mmHg. The resultant reduction in ICP improves cerebral perfusion and encourages the absorption of oedema fluid. Drainage of CSF by lumbar puncture is contra-indicated (with few exceptions) in patients with cerebral oedema since it may cause tonsillar or tentorial herniation and may leave the supratentorial ICP unchanged.

Hypertonic solutions are helpful in cytotoxic oedema, in some cases of mixed cytotoxic and vasogenic type, and hydrostatic cases. Mannitol in a 20% solution is the most widely used agent. It is given intravenously in a dose of 1.5–2 g/kg body weight over about 10 minutes to produce the maximum osmotic gradient. A 'rebound effect' is sometimes seen, with the ICP rising above its original level as the effect of the drug wears off. Monitoring of the ICP is desirable for the best results and the serum osmolality should be watched carefully when mannitol is given frequently. It is not advisable to give it more often than once every 3 or 4 hours.

Isosorbide and glycerol are less widely used agents.

Steroid treatment is most effective in vasogenic cerebral oedema, particularly the focal and chronic type such as that surrounding a tumour or an abscess. It may be very helpful in the management of brain stem tumours. With more diffuse and acute lesions it is less helpful. Dexamethasone is a widely used drug. It may be given intravenously or intramuscularly in a dose of 0.25 mg/kg initially and continued either parenterally or orally in a dose of 0.25–0.5 mg/kg per day in 4 divided doses.

Other drugs

Acetazolamide may be of limited value in lowering ICP by reducing the rate of CSF formation.

Frusemide is another diuretic drug which can reduce ICP and decrease cerebral oedema.

BENIGN INTRA-CRANIAL HYPERTENSION

A syndrome with raised intracranial pressure without any space-occupying lesion or obstruction to the CSF pathways has been recognized since 1893. Its frequent association with otitis media, which was thought to cause thrombosis of the major lateral venous sinus, led Symonds (1931) to suggest the name otitic hydrocephalus (inappropriate because the lateral ventricles are not usually enlarged). The term 'pseudotumor cerebri' has also been used. Foley (1955) introduced the term 'benign intracranial hypertension' for cases of unknown cause, but this has since come to be applied both to otogenic and other cases. The cause of the raised intracranial pressure is uncertain. It has been ascribed by some to vascular engorgement and by others to interstitial cerebral oedema; biopsy material from ten patients showed intracellular and extracellular oedema (Sahs & Joynt 1956).

The many aetiological factors involved in adult patients with the condition include obesity, pregnancy, mild head injury and infections. The condition is not common in children, in whom many other causes have been recognized. Grant (1971) analysed a series of 79 cases in infancy and childhood seen at the Hospital for Sick Children, Great Ormond Street, between 1953 and 1970. He found an equal sex incidence, in contrast to adult series in which females predominate. The commonest predisposing factor was chronic middle-ear disease, present in 39%. Often an exacerbation of otitis media preceded or coincided with the onset of intracranial hypertension. Systemic steroid therapy for asthma, arthritis and epilepsy and corticosteroid treatment for eczema was implicated in four cases. Tetracycline may have been a factor in another case. Mild head injuries seemed related to the condition in three children and hypocalcaemia in another. Headache was the commonest presenting symptom (57%) and single complaint (71%). Diplopia with sixth nerve palsies, blurred vision, vomiting and other symptoms were also presenting features. In 95% of cases the optic discs showed abnormalities ranging from blurred margins to gross papilloedema and haemorrhages. Lateral rectus palsy, bilateral or unilateral, occurred in 23 cases, slight ataxia in 7, and extensor plantar responses in 6. Plain skull X-rays were abnormal in 34 cases with suture separation in 17. Ventriculography or lumbar air encephalography were performed in most cases and showed normal or small ventricles in the majority. The children were all treated conservatively. None required surgical decompression for visual deterioration. The diagnostic lumbar puncture which 31 patients underwent seemed to have a therapeutic effect. Repeated lumbar punctures were needed in a few children. The range of CSF pressure was from 140 to 550 mm CSF. The outcome was good in all cases. One child had a recurrence of intracranial hypertension three years after the first, but the second attack resolved quickly.

There is an impression that in recent years the number of children seen with the syndrome has decreased and that fewer cases are related to chronic ear infections. Severe otitis media has become rarer than it was ten to twenty years ago. An important cause of the syndrome recently recognized is withdrawal of steroid treatment. Seven cases were reported by Neville & Wilson (1970) in which withdrawal of cortical steroids or ACTH, given for various disorders, was followed by the development of headache, vomiting and papilloedema, often with retinal haemorrhages. This is particularly likely to occur when steroid treatment has been prolonged. In such cases the withdrawal should be gradual and spread out over at least one month. When features of intracranial hypertension develop it is advisable to resume treatment with a half to a third of the original dose and to reduce the dose gradually over two to three months. Cases have even occurred when topical steroid applications for eczema have been stopped. Tetracycline and Nalidixic acid are other iatrogenic causes of the syndrome.

The management of benign intracranial hypertension has been made much easier by the CT scan. The diagnosis is one of exclusion, and it is particularly important to exclude intracranial tumours. Fortunately the condition is usually self-limited and without sequelae, but in cases with prolonged raised pressure vision is at risk. Corticosteroid treatment with dexamethasone is often effective. Repeated lumbar punctures have also been used in treatment. Surgical decompression was sometimes necessary in the past, but is rarely needed nowadays, perhaps due to the decrease in cases due to severe ear infections.

LEAD ENCEPHALOPATHY

Sources of lead

Plumbism in children is usually due to the continued ingestion of inorganic lead compounds. Since these are poorly absorbed from the gut, poisoning requires a prolonged period of repeated exposure. The main hazards for children are putty and paint pigments, but other sources are toys made of lead (now rare), lead nipple shields, soft water conveyed in lead pipes, lead-glazed ceramic vessels and the burning of storage battery cases as fuel. Atmospheric pollution in the neighbourhood of smelting works and factories making lead batteries is another potential source, the importance of which is reviewed by Rutter (1980). 'Surma', a cosmetic containing lead sulphide, is a special hazard for the children (of both sexes) of immigrants to Britain from India and Pakistan (Ali et al 1978, Lobo 1978). This is applied to the rim of the eyelid daily from the first weeks of life, and is washed by tears through the naso-lacrimal duct into the throat, swallowed and absorbed. Lobo explains the absence of harmful effects in India and Pakistan by the fact that the material used there, called Kajal, is made of non-toxic soot from oil-lamps and vegetable dyes, whereas in Britain unscrupulous businessmen have concocted Surma from lead-sulphide as a simple and profitable alternative. Though now banned from sale in Britain, it is still imported by travellers and tragedies may still occur from its use.

With lead-containing paints and some other sources pica, or perverted appetite, is a major factor, children with exaggerated oral activities being at special risk. These include retarded children in whom the stage of oral exploration is prolonged, normal toddlers and some other disturbed children of normal intelligence. Lobo (1978) in his Luton survey of Pakistani immigrant families found that lack of toys and the use of Surma were important factors. Chisholm (1970) has stressed the three factors of the high-risk child, the high-risk dwelling (old and poorly maintained with lead paint on window-sills and other surfaces) and the high-risk mother, depressed, immature, overwhelmed or unaware. Barltrop & Killala (1969), in a survey of paint samples from 56 homes, found the lead content was related to the age of the building and the social class of the family. 53% of samples contained over 1% of lead. Paints from pre-1855 homes contained 5% of lead. Paint applied several decades previously, even if covered by layers of later, safer paint, was still a potential hazard.

Clinical features and management

The early symptoms of lead poisoning in childhood may be mild and non-specific, with anorexia, constipation, vomiting, apathy, irritability, poor coordination and loss of recently gained skills. Symptoms may wax and wane, and so may be explained away as due to recurrent infections. Iron-deficient anaemia is almost always present.

The clinical picture may suggest a posterior fossa tumour or tuberculous meningitis. Parents are not likely to volunteer a history of pica, since they do not appreciate its importance, so this feature should always be enquired for. Iron deficiency anaemia is almost always present.

Acute encephalopathy is the most serious symptom and is commonest between 15 and 30 months of age. It usually presents with convulsions and altered consciousness. Papilloedema is not common because suture separation allows the skull to expand. Viral encephalitis is the most popular wrong diagnosis if lead encephalopathy is overlooked and a history of pica or other lead exposure is not obtained. Most affected children are anaemic. The blood may show basophilic stippling but this is not invariable. The urine may or may not contain coproporphyrins. Evidence for lead may be found on X-rays of the abdomen, showing opaque material, or X-rays of the knees and wrists, with dense lead lines at the growing ends. If lumbar puncture is performed (and it is hazardous) the pressure is usually high with a pleocytosis of up to 30 cells per cubic mm and a more impressive elevation of protein to between 70 and 300 mg/100 ml. More specific confirmation is given by the finding of a raised blood lead level. The upper limit of normal in urban populations is about 36μg/100ml. Levels of over 80 are usually found in acute lead encephalopathy.

The prognosis of acute encephalopathy due to lead is bad with a high mortality and morbidity. This is true in the developed and undeveloped countries alike. Three deaths occurred in London children within one month in 1970 (Alexander & Delves 1972). In all cases paint scrapings had been regularly ingested, but in one child Surma applied to the face containing more than 10% of lead by weight was thought to be responsible. Six cases of acute lead encephalopathy in black children in South Africa with two deaths were reported by Harris (1976), three of which at least were due to burning battery cases. In all these cases the diagnosis was made late. The hazards of unrecognized lead exposure from a similar source were shown in a recent report on two families from rural North Carolina (Dolcourt et al 1981). Recycling exhausted automobile storage batteries to recover the lead and burning the discarded battery cases for fuel were the factors involved. One child developed encephalopathy leading to permanent brain damage. The importance of an 'occupational family history' is shown by the fact that the great grandfather of the index patient worked in a small scale operation to recover lead from exhausted batteries and that the family had burned two truck-loads of discarded batteries in their stove.

Lead encephalopathy carries a poor prognosis for those who survive the acute illness. Smith et al (1963) found that, 5 years after acute lead intoxication, recurrent convulsions and focal EEG abnormalities occurred only in those children who had suffered from frank encephalopathy.

Early diagnosis, based on clinical suspicion and rapid confirmation, are essential for effective treatment. X-rays of long bones and abdomen may give immediate evidence while blood tests will take longer. Urine lead determinations may be less reliable than blood levels because of impaired renal function caused by the lead. Normal urine levels in children range from zero to 400 mg per litre. In doubtful cases a stimulation test with intramuscular versenate (calcium disodium edetate) can be helpful when excretion of lead in an amount greater than 500 mg per litre results.

Adequate chelation therapy should be started as an emergency when the diagnosis seems likely, since delay while awaiting the results of blood tests is hazardous. Chisholm (1970) gives guide-lines for the choice of chelating agents. Treatment with Baledta (2–3 dimercapto-1-propanol edathamil calcium disodium) should be started at once in hospital for 5 to 7 days. Since the chelating drugs promote the absorption of lead present in the gut, this should be removed by small saline enemas. Seizures must be controlled by intravenous diazepam or paraldehyde by the rectal or intramuscular route.

Renal and cardiac involvement and inappropriate antidiuretic hormone secretion can complicate the problems of lead encephalopathy, so that fluids should be limited to the daily urine output plus insensible fluid loss, unless there is dehydration. An indwelling bladder catheter is needed. Endotracheal intubation is advisable to ensure an adequate airway. Mannitol, dezamethasone or a combination of the two are used in an attempt to reduce cerebral oedema.

SPINAL TUMOURS

In relation to intracranial tumours, neoplasms involving the spinal cord and spinal canal are rare in childhood. In Matson's (1969) experience they were outnumbered by intracranial tumours by more than 5 to 1, and in that of Till (1975) by more than 10 to 1. Despite this their importance is in some ways greater for the paediatrician than that of brain tumours because of their greater potential for causing early neurological dysfunction due to spinal cord compression, ischaemic effects or lesions within the cord itself, and because prompt surgical treatment can often improve the outlook substantially. There is a much greater tendency to overlook the possibility of a spinal cord tumour than of a brain tumour. The initial diagnosis was erroneous in about 70% of Matson's (1969) series of 115 cases, with poliomyelitis leading the field. Many paediatricians have seen cases in which a diagnosis of 'hysteria' or 'functional disorder' has been made in a child with spinal cord tumour. With this diagnosis above all a high index of suspicion is essential. Spinal cord compression is a more serious emergency than raised intracranial pressure, yet it still risks being treated in a dilatory fashion.

Since the exact site and pathology of the suspected tumour can seldom be known before investigation and surgical exploration, it is appropriate to consider together the many and varied processes which may affect the spinal cord directly or indirectly, by disruption of its substance, by compression and distortion and by impairment of its blood supply. In addition to neoplasms these include leukaemic infiltration, lymphoma, epidural haemopoietic tissue in thalassaemia, arteriovenous malformations, teratomas, and congenital developmental lesions such as dermoid sinuses and cysts and benign intraspinal arachnoid cysts. (Duncan & Hoare 1978).

The presenting clinical features of these lesions will depend on their anatomical site in terms of cord level and whether they are extradural, intradural but extramedullary or intramedullary. As a rough guide most intraspinal tumours in childhood occur in the thoracic region with about 25% in the cervical region and fewest of all in the lower lumbar and sacral canal. About half of childhood intraspinal tumours are extradural, spreading from nearby bone or through intervertebral foramina. About one quarter are intradural but extramedullary. Tumours in these two sites tend to cause diffuse, rather than focal, dysfunction resulting from cord compression, although involvement of nerves in the intervertebral foramina may produce focal sensory symptoms (pain or paraesthesia with a girdle distribution) or lower motor neuron weakness. Intramedullary tumours, mostly gliomas, contribute the remaining quarter. These may produce localized motor or sensory deficits early on, or remain remarkably silent until a late stage, depending partly on their pathology and their level. Cervical tumours may cause lower motor neuron weakness early in the upper limbs and upper motor neuron features in the legs. Localized neck pain or torticollis are common with tumours in this region. Tumours in the thoracic region may produce few symptoms for some time apart from pain in the back and scoliosis, so that persistent pain and deformity of the spine, however mild, must be taken seriously. Younger children have difficulty in describing pain and may show irritability as the sole evidence of it. Those who can describe it may report that the pain is aggravated by physical effort, coughing, sneezing, straining and flexion of the neck or back.

Regression in bladder or bowel control occurs in about one third of children with spinal cord tumours and is a most important symptom to be taken seriously. Enuresis is commoner than faecal incontinence. Sphincter problems are usually missed in the younger child who has yet to gain control. Unfortunately their significance may also be overlooked in older children who have been clean and dry but relapse, since urinary frequency and incontinence are common symptoms in childhood and may be attributed to psychological factors or urinary infections. Urinary retention with overflow should be assumed to be due to spinal cord compression until proved otherwise; it should never be attributed to psychological causes without thorough investigation. When due to spinal cord compression it is an indication for urgent decompression since with every hour that passes the chances of recovery of bladder function decrease.

The examination findings include abnormalities of tendon reflexes, paralysis of flaccid, spastic or mixed type, muscle wasting, sensory changes, scoliosis, kyphosis, torticollis and localized spinal tenderness. Abnormalities of the tendon reflexes are particularly helpful in younger and unco-operative children, as are extensor plantar responses. Sensory testing in young children is often difficult but a sensory level to pinprick can often be detected, and sometimes hyperaesthesia is found at the level of a thoracic cord lesion. Careful attention to the abdominal reflexes may suggest a level in the lower thoracic region if some of these are absent or 'fatigue' easily. Localized tenderness over one or more spinous processes may be helpful in finding the level of a lesion. The spine should be examined carefully for any visible or palpable paravertebral mass or signs of spina bifida. Cutaneous stigmata of neurofibromatosis (café au lait patches) should be looked for. Hepatic enlargement may suggest a neuroblastoma. Signs of infection in the skin may suggest the possibility of an extradural or intradural abscess. Evidence of trauma may suggest direct or indirect injury to the spinal cord, including the possibility of a haematoma causing cord compression or of haematomyelia.

Table 18.1 (from Till 1975 and personal communication 1982) shows the types and incidence of spinal cord tumours in his own and in three previous series.

The importance of neuroblastoma, which contributes over 10% of the combined series, is shown by the paradoxical statistic that although only about 2% of all children with neuroblastoma present with signs of spinal compression (Bragg & Linden 1969), this disease is the commonest cause of paraplggia in childhood, accounting for 30% in some series (Lepintre et al 1969).

THE INVESTIGATION AND MANAGEMENT OF SPINAL CORD TUMOURS

This should be planned urgently but with care, bearing in mind the implications of the possible findings on investigation. It is desirable for the investigations, which may need to be followed quickly by exploratory laminectomy, to be carried out in a centre with full neurosurgical facilities and in close consultation with a neurosurgeon and a neuroradiologist. Plain spine X-rays, which should include the *whole* spine with anteroposterior and lateral views, should be examined most carefully since retrospective scrutiny post-operatively has often shown minor changes which were previously missed. Widening of the interpedicular distance and sagittal diameter of the spinal canal may indicate an expanding intraspinal mass (Fig. 18.17). The pedicles may be deformed and decalcified. The size of the interventricular foramina should be assessed. Enlargement of a foramen may indicate an expanding lesion within it and outside the spinal canal: this is seen particularly with neurofibroma.

The value of lumbar puncture and CSF examination in investigating a case of suspected spinal tumour is limited. True, the index of suspicion may be increased by the finding of a raised CSF protein or a xanthochromic fluid, and occasionally tumour cells may be found. There is a grave risk, however, of damage to the cord at the site of compression with increased neurological deficit due probably to slight downward displacement of the cord and tumour after CSF is withdrawn. Thus the volume of fluid removed must be small and it must be withdrawn very slowly. A major drawback is that the chances of successful lumbar myelography during the week following the lumbar puncture are poor and precious time may be lost by the enforced delay.

Table 18.1 Types and incidence of spinal cord tumours in childhood from three previous series and from Till (1975 and personal communication 1982)

Report and number of cases	Till	Matson 1969	Rand & Rand 1960	Hamby 1944	Total
Intramedullary gliomas					
Astrocytoma	4	24	9		
Ependymoma	8	6	8	44	135
Unclassified			3		
Ependymoblastoma	2				
Unverified	28				
Extramedullary					
Meningioma	5	3	2	10	
Neurofibroma	6	6	5	23	60
Extradural					
Sarcomas (all types)	4	2	10	51	142
Neuroblastoma	32	24	5	6	
Ganglioneuroma	1	3	1		
Ganglioglioma	3				
Other types					
Dermoid cyst	3	14	2	37	56
Abscess (intramedullary)	1	5			6
Medulloblastoma (presenting as spinal tumour)	4	4	4		12
Pinealoma (presenting as spinal tumour)	2				2
Aneurysmal bone cyst	3		1		4
Bronchogenic cyst	1				1
Hamartoma	1	1			2
Angioma	1			7	8
Arachnoid cyst	3				3
Syrinx	1				1
Exostosis	2				2
Benign osteoblastoma			3		3
Neurenteric cyst	4	2			6
Teratoma	1	13	1		15
Ewing's tumour	1		2		3
Lymphoma	1				1
Rhabdomyosarcoma	1				1
Retinoblastoma			2		2
Chloroma			1		1
Haemangioma of vertebra		3	2		5
Lipoma		7	4	10	21
Metastatic tumour		18			18
Miscellaneous				26	26
Total	123	135	65	214	537

The need for close consultation with the neurosurgeon is thus clear: it is, after all, he who has the responsibility for operating and it is desirable that the surgical approach should be made at a time and in the circumstances of his own choosing, rather than as an urgent procedure following a lumbar puncture undertaken without adequate thought.

The definitive investigation is myelography (Fig. 18.17). It may demonstrate the lesion in de-tail by the lumbar approach, but in cases of complete CSF block only the lower end may be shown, and in some such cases its upper limit must then be defined by cisternal myelography. It may be necessary in some cases to undertake an exploratory laminectomy at once when there is a risk of deterioration, but in many cases this can be safely deferred for a few days. Inspection of the lesion will allow the surgeon to decide whether to

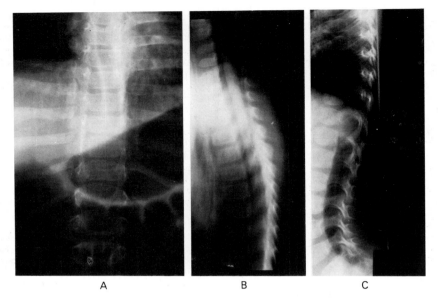

A   B   C

Fig. 18.17 Intramedullary spinal cord tumour (poorly differentiated glioma) in 22-month-old boy.
A. Antero-posterior film of the dorsal spine. The spinal canal is widened from D7 to L1 inclusive. The pedicles are thin and their medial borders flat.
B. Air myelogram. The spinal cord is normal in the cervical and upper dorsal region. The subarachnoid space is not visible in the lower dorsal region due to swelling of the spinal cord.
C. Air myelogram. The lumbar subarachnoid space is filled with air and the lower end of the swollen cord is outlined at D12

attempt to remove it in whole or in part, and to insert a needle in the midline of the cord to detect a cystic cavity in the case of intramedullary lesions which clearly cannot be removed but in which drainage may improve function.

The prognosis after operation will clearly depend on the pathology, size and degree of removal of the lesion. The relief of cord compression achieved by laminectomy may produce marked improvement in function whatever the pathology. The outlook for children with intramedullary glioma treated by decompression and radiotherapy may be remarkably good with prolonged survival.

REFERENCES

Alexander F W, Delves H T 1972 Deaths from acute lead poisoning. Archives of Disease in Childhood 47: 446–448
Ali A R, Smales O R C, Aslam M 1978 Surma and lead poisoning. British Medical Journal 2: 915–916
Arnstein L H, Baldrey E, Naffziger H C 1951 Case report and survey of brain tumors during neonatal period. Journal of Neurosurgery 8: 315
Azar-Kia B, Krishnan R R, Schechter M M 1975 Neonatal craniopharyngioma. Case report. Journal of Neurosurgery 42: 91
Bain H W, Darte J M M, Keith W S, Krayff E 1966 The diencephalic syndrome of early infancy due to silent brain tumors: with special reference to treatment. Pediatrics 38: 473
Barltrop D 1973 Chronic neurological sequelae of lead poisoning. Developmental Medicine and Child Neurology 15: 365–366

Barltrop D 1975 Chemical and physical environmental hazards for children. In: Barltrop D (ed) Paediatrics and the environment. Fellowship of Postgraduate Medicine
Barltrop D, Killala N J P 1979 Factors influencing the exposure of children to lead. Archives of Disease in Childhood 44: 476–479
Bell W E, McCormick W F 1978 Increased intracranial pressure in children. Diagnosis and treatment, 2nd edn. Vol III in series, Major problems in clinical pediatrics. W B Saunders, Philadelphia
Bicknell J, Clayton B E, Delves H T 1968 Lead in mentally retarded children. Journal of Mental Deficiency Research 12: 282–293
Bloom H J G, Wallace E N K, Henk J M 1969 The treatment and prognosis of medulloblastoma in children. American Journal of Roentgenology 105: 43
Bragg K U, Linden G 1969 Neuroblastoma in childhood. American Journal of Diseases of Childhood 118: 441–450

Brett E M, Hoare R D 1969 An assessment of the value and limitations of air encephalography in children with mental retardation and with epilepsy. Brain 92: 731–742

Caffey J 1972 On the theory and practice of shaking infants. American Journal of Diseases of Children 124: 161–169

Chisholm J J 1970 Poisoning due to heavy metals. In: Coleman A B, Alpert J J (eds) Pediatric clinics of North America: poisoning in children, vol 17 no 3. W.B. Saunders, Philadelphia, London, Toronto

Dolcourt J L, Finch C, Coleman G D, Klimas A J, Milar C 1981 Hazard of lead exposure in the home from recycled automobile storage batteries. Pediatrics 68: 225–231

Duncan A W, Hoare R D 1978 Spinal arachnoid cysts in children. Radiology 126: 423–429

Falconer M A 1971 Genetic and related aetiological factors in temporal lobe epilepsy. Epilepsia 12: 13–31

Fishman R A 1975 Brain edema. New England Journal of Medicine 293: 706

Foley J 1955 Benign forms of intracranial hypertension. Toxic and otitic hydrocephalus. Brain 78: 1–41

Franklin A W (ed) 1975 Concerning child abuse. Papers presented by the Tunbridge Wells Study Group on Non-Accidental Injury to Children. Churchill-Livingstone, Edinburgh

Franklin A W (ed) 1977 The challenge of child abuse. Proceedings of a Conference sponsored by the Royal Society of Medicine, 2–4 June 1976. Academic Press, London, Grune and Stratton, New York

Grant D N 1971 Benign intracranial hypertension: a review of 79 cases in infancy and childhood. Archives of Disease in Childhood 46: 651–655

Harris I 1976 Lead encephalopathy. Case reports. South African Medical Journal 50: 1371–1373

Harrison M J G 1971 Cerebral arachnoid cysts in children. Journal of Neurology, Neurosurgery and Psychiatry 34: 316–323

Harwood-Nash D C, Fitz C R 1976 Brain Neoplasms. In: Neuroradiology in infants and children. C.V. Mosby, Saint Louis, ch 11

Helfer R E, Kempe C H (eds) 1968 The battered child. University of Chicago Press, Chicago

Katz E L 1975 Late results of radical excision of craniopharyngioma in children. Journal of Neurosurgery 42: 86

Lobo E de H 1978 Children of immigrants in Britain. Their health and social problems. Hodder and Stoughton, London

McIntosh N 1979 Medulloblastoma — a changing prognosis? Archives of Disease in Childhood 54: 200–203

Matson D 1969 Neurosurgery of infancy and childhood, 2nd edn. Charles C Thomas, Springfield, Illinois

Neville B G R, Wilson J 1970 Benign intracranial hypertension following corticosteroid withdrawal in childhood. British Medical Journal 3: 544–556

Odom G L, Davis C H, Woodhall B 1956 Brain tumors in children: clinical analysis of 164 cases. Pediatrics 18: 856

Page L K, Lombroso C T, Matson D D 1969 Childhood epilepsy with a late detection of cerebral glioma. Journal of Neurosurgery 31: 253–261

Panitch H S, Berg B O 1970 Brain stem tumors of childhood and adolescence. American Journal of Diseases in Childhood 119: 465–472

Robinson R G 1964 The temporal lobe agenesis syndrome. Brain 87: 87

Russell A 1951 A diencephalic syndrome of emaciation in infancy and childhood. Archives of Disease in Childhood 26: 274

Rutter M 1980 Raised lead levels and impaired cognitive/behavioural functioning: a review of the evidence. Suppl. no 42 to Developmental medicine and child neurology, vol 22 no 1. Spastics International Medical Publications in association with William Heinemann Medical Books Ltd, J B Lippincott Company, Philadelphia, London

Sahs A L, Joynt R J 1956 Brain swelling of unknown cause. Neurology 6: 791–803

Smith H D, Baehner R L, Carney T, Majors W J 1963 The sequelae of pica with and without lead poisoning. A comparison of the sequelae five or more years later. I: Clinical and laboratory investigations. American Journal of Diseases of Children 105: 609–616

Symonds C P 1931 Otitic hydrocephalus. Brain 54: 55–71

Till K 1968 Subdural haematoma and effusion in infancy. British Medical Journal 3: 400

Till K 1975 Paediatric neurosurgery for paediatricians and neurosurgeons. Blackwell Scientific Publications, Oxford

Wei P, Norman M G 1973 Brain tumours in children under two years. Paper presented at the Eleventh Annual Meeting of the Canadian Association of Neuropathologists, Kingston, Ontario, October 1972

Yates P O 1968 Tumours in children. In: Recent Results in Cancer Research, 13. Springer-Verlag, Berlin

Zimmerman R A, Bilaniuk L T, Bruce D, Schut L, Uzzell B, Goldberg H I 1978 Interhemispheric acute subdural hematoma: a computed tomographic manifestation. Neuroradiology 16: 39–40

19

Vascular disorders including migraine

E. M. Brett

Various vascular lesions and disorders of the cerebral circulation affecting the nervous system in childhood will be considered in this chapter. Many of these have been mentioned elsewhere in the context of particular symptoms (epilepsy, cerebral palsy, mental retardation) but they deserve discussion in greater depth from a pathological, diagnostic and therapeutic viewpoint.

The clinicopathological features resulting from these conditions fall into 4 main groups:

1. Acute hemiplegia and certain other acute neurological deficits;
2. Spontaneous intracranial haemorrhage;
3. Rarer manifestations of congenital vascular malformations (space-occupying effects, 'steal' syndromes, etc.);
4. Migraine.

The many pathological conditions of varied aetiology giving rise to these features will be described first and the clinical syndromes related to them will then be discussed.

AETIOPATHOLOGICAL CONDITIONS

Arteriovenous malformations of the cerebral cortex (sometimes known as arteriovenous angiomas or aneurysms)

There are congenital lesions due to persistence of the normal embryonic arteriovenous shunts with failure of development of the capillary network normally separating arteries and veins. Lack of the capillary bed allows blood to be shunted very rapidly through the lesion. The feeding artery or arteries are dilated and tortuous breaking up into many smaller arteries which pass directly to thin-walled venous channels. These in turn drain into the sagittal or transverse sinuses, the Galenic system or both. The lesions are usually shaped like a wedge with its base on the surface of the brain and its apex extending towards the lateral ventricle. They are commonest in the territory of the middle cerebral artery.

The condition may present in infancy with congestive heart failure due to the enormous size of the arteriovenous shunt (Silverman et al 1955, Holden et al 1972). A loud cranial bruit may be audible and contrast radiography of the heart may allow the intracranial lesion to be detected. Davidson & Falconer (1973) have reported the case of a 6-year-old boy with epilepsy and cardiomegaly due to a cerebral arteriovenous malformation removal of which reduced his cardiac output from 7 to 3 litres per minute.

In older children in several series (Matson 1969, So 1978) the commonest presentation (seen in over two-thirds of cases) has been with spontaneous intracranial haemorrhage, usually with severe headache and vomiting followed by deep coma. The bleeding is most often into the cerebral substance itself and the clinical features may vary with the site of the malformation, hemiplegia being common. Less often the bleeding is subarachnoid, when the symptoms may be milder with headache and neck stiffness. Subdural bleeding may occur from rupture of a surface lesion.

The second commonest childhood presentation is with focal fits due to ischaemic scarring or gliosis. Focal headaches may also occur. In some children ischaemia of the cerebral cortex causes progressive intellectual deterioration. No neurological abnormality may be present but in more than half the cases an intracranial bruit is audible over the skull vault and eyeballs. This can usually be distinguish-ed from the soft bruit heard in many normal young children. Occasionally the bruit can be heard with the unaided ear applied to the skull, and in rare cases parents have been woken by the noise from their child's head. Another rare presentation is with transient focal deficits such as hemiplegia or aphasia due to a 'steal' effect with a so-called aneurysm of the great vein of Galen, blood being temporarily shunted away from one hemisphere.

The same lesion may act as a tumour blocking the CSF pathways and causing hydrocephalus.

The diagnosis is made radiologically. Plain skull X-rays may show enlarged venous channels on the inner table of the skull. Air encephalography may be unhelpful, but the CT scan will usually show the lesion provided enhancement is carried out (Fig. 19.1, 19.3). Cerebral arteriography is needed to define the situation clearly in order to plan a surgical approach (Fig. 19.2).

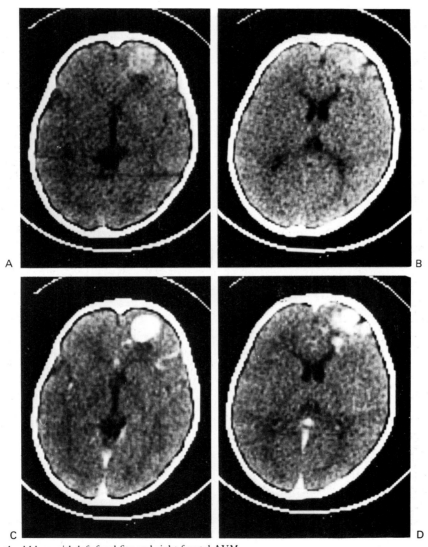

Fig. 19.1 20-month-old boy with left focal fits and right frontal AVM.
CT. Note areas of abnormal density in right frontal pole. Most show the density of circulating blood, but there is an area of low attenuation close to the dilated anterior horn of the lateral ventricle. Contrast injection caused enhancement of the dense lesion and showed two large vessels, a feeding artery (C) and draining vein (D)

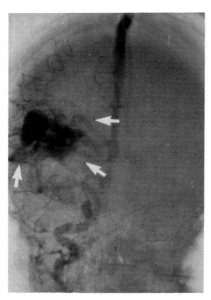

Fig. 19.2 Right carotid angiogram in same patient shows AVM with superficial feeding branches from right middle cerebral artery (arrowed) and draining veins medially (arrowed)

The risk of re-bleeding in those who present with haemorrhage is 25% within 5 years. In a series of 36 children with cerebral arteriovenous malformations at the Hospital for Sick Children, Great Ormond Street (So 1978) there were 10 deaths in a follow-up period averaging 6.2 years, at least 8 of these being from further haemorrhage. A combination of seizures and bleeding seemed a bad prognostic sign. 5 children with subarachnoid haemorrhage later developed communicating hydrocephalus which required shunting.

The total mortality rate after the first bleed in 33 patients aged between 7 and 20 years with arteriovenous malformations causing subarachnoid haemorrhage was 21.2%. (Sedzimir & Robinson 1973). The rate was 12.1% for the first haemorrhage. Recurrent bleeding occurred in 41.3% of cases with a mortality rate of 25% for the subsequent haemorrhage.

Surgical treatment must be considered whenever possible. It gives good results when all the involved vessels can be dissected and excised. In Matson's (1969) series of 34 children with arteriovenous malformations, 14 were well after excision, up to 15 years later, 8 were well without surgery, and 11 had died. In So's (1978) series 23 children were operated on. Complete excision of the lesion was possible in 8 cases, 5 were inoperable except for evacuation of haematoma and in 10 attempts were made to clip the feeding arteries. This procedure

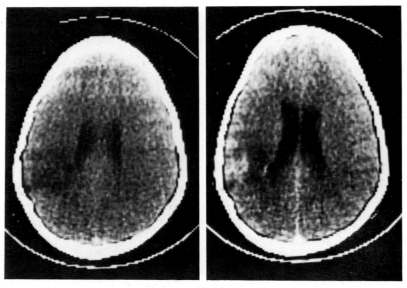

Fig. 19.3 Partially thrombosed arteriovenous malformation in 10-year-old boy with recent acute right hemiplegia and almost complete recovery.
CT. Scan shows low attenuation in left superior temporal and inferior parietal regions showing superficial enhancement with contrast and no mass effect.

seemed to improve the prognosis. The results of radiotherapy are difficult to assess.

Intracranial arterial aneurysms

These saccular lesions, thought to be due to a congenital defect in the media of the arterial wall, are rarer in children than in adults. In five separate series from Britain and North America (Matson 1969, Patel & Richardson 1971, Sedzimir & Robinson 1973, Amacher & Drake 1975, Harwood-Nash & Fitz 1976) there were 156 cases of ruptured intracranial arterial aneurysms between the ages of 6 months and 20 years. Most of the patients were older children or adolescents. There were 89 males and 67 females, the male preponderance being greatest in Matson's series.

Some idea of the relative rarity of these lesions in childhood and adolescence as compared with adult life is given by the two larger series (Patel & Richardson 1971, Sedzimir & Robinson 1973) of 58 and 50 cases in total series (all ages) of 3000 and 1066 respectively.

Despite their rarity there are several important respects in which these lesions presenting in the young differ from those in older patients.

Situation

Most of the lesions in the younger patients are supratentorial as in adults, but a high proportion of the former have been on the carotid termination or the anterior cerebral artery complex in contrast to the situation in older patients. Thus in 20 of Patel and Richardson's cases (38%) the ruptured aneurysms were on the terminal part of the carotid artery compared with an over-all incidence of 3 to 5% in adults with subarachnoid haemorrhage (Richardson 1969).

Multiple aneurysms

These were present in only 6 of the 156 cases in the combined series, a much lower figure than in adults.

Presentation

Most of the patients in the five series of younger patients with ruptured intracranial aneurysms were well until they presented with spontaneous intracranial bleeding. This may be massive with coma and grossly blood-stained CSF or milder producing severe pain in the neck and head and signs of meningeal irritation with less blood in the CSF and later xanthochromia. It may give rise to intracerebral haematoma and be associated with acute hemiplegia or other focal neurological deficit. Focal or generalized convulsions may occur.

Focal features caused by the direct mass effect of aneurysms which have not bled are uncommon, but brain stem compression resulted from aneurysms of the basilar trunk and vertebral artery in two cases (Amacher & Drake 1975).

Associated findings

Intracranial aneurysms are known to be associated with coarctation of the aorta, but there were only 7 cases of coarctation in the combined series. These were all among the 58 patients of Patel and Richardson, making up 12% of their series. A rarer association is with congenital bilateral polycystic kidneys, and there were two cases with these among the patients of Patel and Richardson.

Hypertension is not uncommon after subarachnoid haemorrhage as a *result* of the bleeding, but it must also be considered as a contributory *cause*. In all cases coarctation and renal lesions should be excluded.

Very rarely intracranial bleeding proves to be due to rupture of a mycotic aneurysm. These may be multiple. In most such cases there is evidence of infection elsewhere.

Prognosis

This seems to be much better in younger than in older patients. Matson noted a marked tendency towards spontaneous improvement in his patients. He believed that early recurrent bleeding was rare and that delay in operation was advisable until clinical improvement had occurred. Proved recurrent haemorrhage occurred in 8 of Patel and Richardson's 58 patients, in most cases between 3 days and 6 weeks after the first bleed, but in two cases after a lapse of 5 years. Six of these 8 patients died. The total mortality was 30% compared with a mortality in adults of over 50%. Mortality was related to the condition of the patients at the time of surgical intervention, being 7% in alert patients and 38% in those who were stuporose or comatose. A similar mortality rate (28%) was noted by Sedzimir and Robinson.

Incidence of cerebral infarction and atherosclerosis

Necropsies were performed on 15 of the 18 patients who died in the series of Patel and Richardson. Cerebral infarction was seen in only one case, in which clipping of the terminal internal carotid artery had caused haemorrhagic infarction in the distribution of both anterior cerebral arteries. Four of these 15 patients had shown evidence of vasospasm on angiography but none of these had evidence of cerebral infarct. These findings contrast with the high necropsy incidence (60%) of cerebral infarct in adults with ruptured intracranial aneurysms.

Atherosclerosis was found in 4 of the 15 necropsies but only involved cerebral arteries in one case.

The low incidence of infarction and atherosclerosis may partly account for the relatively better prognosis of ruptured intracranial aneurysm in young patients as compared to that in adults.

Management

The condition must first be thought of if it is to be diagnosed. Its rarity in childhood often results in delayed diagnosis. If there is a history of a recent head injury this may prejudice the initial clinical assessment so that the possibility of bleeding from an aneurysm is overlooked. Amacher & Drake (1975) reported two fatal cases with antecedent head injury in one of which the fall causing the trauma may well have been due to rupture of the aneurysm.

The CT scan is a valuable tool and will often show blood within the ventricles or subarachnoid space as well as an intracerebral haematoma (Fig. 19.5). In many cases it will demonstrate the responsible aneurysm, but angiography is needed to define the lesion precisely as a prelude to surgery (Fig. 19.4). The possibility of multiple and of mycotic aneurysms must be considered, though both are rare, and associated disorders such as

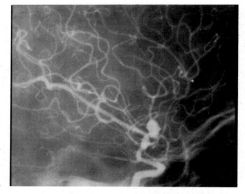

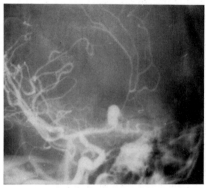

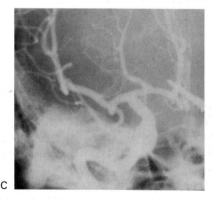

Fig. 19.4 Subarachnoid haemorrhage. Anterior communicating artery aneurysm in 13-year-old boy.

A. Lateral film of right carotid angiogram showing a large bilocular aneurysm and spasm of the carotid syphon.

B. Oblique film which confirms the anatomical site of the aneurysm and shows narrowing of the anterior cerebral artery due to spasm.

C. Oblique film (post-operative). A clip has been placed across the neck of the aneurysm. There is no longer any spasm.

coarctation and polycystic kidneys should not be overlooked.

When the CT scan is available a diagnostic lumbar puncture is not necessary. In most cases the

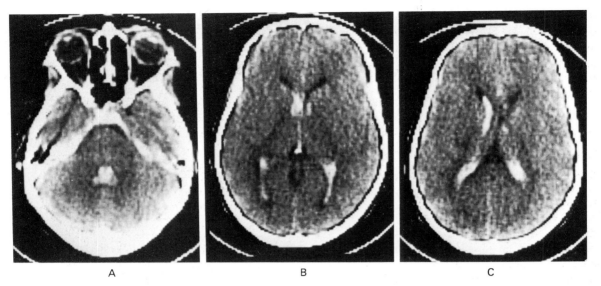

Fig. 19.5 Same patient. CT showing intraventricular and subarachnoid haemorrhage.
A. Clotted blood in 4th ventricle.
B. Clotted blood in lateral ventricles, left more than right, in the 3rd ventricle and in the inter-hemispheric fissure.
C. Clotted blood in lateral ventricles and inter-hemispheric fissure.

appearances of blood in the scan are characteristic. When there is doubt whether the diagnosis is meningitis or subarachnoid haemorrhage, examination of the CSF is of course essential.

Cerebral arterial occlusion

Thrombotic arterial occlusion may occur in infants and children as a result of trauma, infection and cardiac disease. Rarer causes are haematological disorder (sickle-cell disease, polycythaemia, idiopathic and thrombotic thrombocytopenic purpura), collagen-vascular diseases (lupus erythematosus, periarteritis nodosa) and metabolic conditions (diabetes mellitus, homocystinuria). Atheroma of cerebral arteries is rare in childhood, in contrast to adult life.

Moyamoya disease

A particular syndrome of progressive cerebral arterial occlusive disease in children and young adults has been increasingly recognized as a cause of acute hemiplegia and other acute focal neurological deficits since cerebral angiography has been more widely used. First described in the Japanese and for a time thought to be confined to them, it is now known to affect all races. The condition is sporadic and non-genetic in most cases and there are no pathological clues to its cause, predisposing factors such as infection, hypertension, atheroma etc. being absent.

It is a syndrome of the young, 50% of cases occurring in patients under 10 and 70% under 20 years of age. The youngest patient in the series of Harwood-Nash & Fitz (1976) was 6 months old and most were under 4 years.

A common presentation is with an acute hemiplegia, transient dysphasia or other acute deficit with or without seizures. Often only one episode occurs and recovery from this may be complete or partial. In some cases the prognosis is excellent but in others rapid deterioration with repeated acute episodes leads to death. There is a clear but poorly understood association with neurofibromatosis (Hillal et al 1971, Levisohn et al 1978). The CT scan often shows an infarct or an area of localised brain swelling, but the diagnosis can only be made angiographically (Fig. 19.6). There is progressive, often bilateral occlusive disease starting in the supraclinoid internal carotid arteries and spreading to involve the trunk of the anterior and middle cerebral arteries, sometimes the posterior communicating and proximal posterior cerebral arteries and

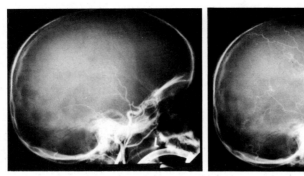

Fig. 19.6 Moya Moya disease in 5-year-old girl with short history of episodic weakness of right hand who later developed a right hemiplegia.
Left carotid angiogram. Sequential lateral films show very narrow internal carotid artery with occlusion below the bifurcation. The posterior communicating artery fills. Telangiectasia in the basal ganglia is typical of 'Moya Moya' type of anastomosis. There are transdural anastomoses from meningeal arteries including the falcine artery to cortical branches of the anterior and middle cerebral arteries.
Antero-posterior film shows that much of the frontal transdural anastomosis is to anterior cerebral artery branches on the right side, indicating proximal disease of the right internal carotid artery.

finally the basilar. The distal parts of the main cerebral arteries are usually unaffected. The condition may become bilateral. A collateral circulation develops through unusual pathways, since the circle of Willis, being involved early, cannot provide relief channels. Perforating branches in the region of the basal ganglia, leptomeningeal arterial anastomoses and other links across the subdural space between the external and internal carotid arteries (*rete mirabile*) are seen. The Japanese term *moyamoya* which means something hazy, like a puff of smoke, refers to the appearance of the fine net-like collaterals. The transdural anastomoses may rupture causing a subdural haematoma to form; this has been found in some cases at autopsy. It seems probable that the arterial lesions develop within a fairly short period of weeks or months, and it is difficult to know why symptoms do not occur earlier. It seems possible that the condition may remain symptom-free since the typical appearances have sometimes been shown on angiography in patients with no relevant symptoms.

Medical treatment with anticoagulants and other agents is usually unhelpful. Vascular surgery offers better hope of success, and Japanese workers have been particularly active in this field. Cervical sympathectomy and superior cervical ganglionectomy have been tried in some patients. Suzuki et al (1975) found that angiographic improvement was seen in most cases examined within the first two

months after surgery but was not maintained when the angiograms were repeated more than six months post-operatively. However, clinical improvement seemed to continue over a long period of time. Anastomosis of the superficial temporal to the middle cerebral artery and encephalo-myo-synangiosis, in which the temporal muscle is placed on the surface of the brain, have also been tried. Neurological deterioration has often occurred after the former procedure, while the latter may be complicated by focal seizures. A new surgical approach, encephalo-duro-arterio-synangiosis, has been tried by Matsushima et al (1981) with good results. The aim is to promote the natural tendency present in the disease to develop a collateral circulation by transplanting a scalp artery with a strip of galea, leaving the distal as well as the proximal arteries intact, to a narrow linear dural opening made under an osteoplastic craniotomy. The method is relatively simple and may well become the treatment of choice.

Cardiac disease in relation to cerebral thrombosis, embolism and abscess

Cerebral thrombosis is common in children with cyanotic congenital heart disease, usually occurring in those under two years of age, and caused by increased viscosity of the blood with polycythaemia or hypoxia. Tyler & Clark (1957) showed that it only occurred with a low arterial oxygen content or a red blood cell count above 8 million per cu mm. Iron deficiency anaemia also contributes to the risk of cerebral thrombosis in children with cyanotic heart disease. The same risk factors also predispose to intracranial venous thrombosis. Their avoidance greatly reduces the chances of thrombosis occurring. In children over two years a cerebral abscess tends to occur rather than arterial thrombosis.

Children with heart disease are also at risk of cerebral emboli which may cause an acute hemiplegia or other neurological deficit. Emboli may result when mural thrombi form in the presence of atrial fibrillation and other arrhythmias in cyanotic congenital heart disease and rheumatic fever. Rarely paroxysmal auricular tachycardia may cause cerebral embolism. Embolization from cardiac vegetations in children with bacterial endocarditis and the rare cardiac myxomas are other causes of acute hemiplegia.

Intracranial venous thrombosis

Venous thrombosis within the skull may be sterile or infected (thrombophlebitis). The sterile variety occurs in cyanotic heart disease, severe dehydration, trauma, sickle cell anaemia and diabetic coma. Infected thrombophlebitis is usually caused by focal infection in the head, particularly otitis media and mastoiditis in which a purulent thrombosis of the transverse sinus may occur. The cavernous sinus may become thrombosed when there is infection of the tonsils, pharynx and nasal and paranasal cavities. Encephalopathic features such as fever, headache, vomiting and altered consciousness are common, and may suggest an actual infectious encephalitis. Focal neurological features such as an acute or subacute hemiplegia or tetraplegia may be added when cerebral veins are involved. In some cases the clinical picture resulting from venous sinus thrombosis is one of 'benign intracranial hypertension' (Ch. 18).

Septic thrombophlebitis has become less common and less severe since antibiotics have been used. In Isler's (1971) series of children with acute hemiplegia it accounted for only three cases. These were proved angiographically. The incidence of venous thrombosis is difficult to determine since radiological proof is rarely sought.

ACUTE HEMIPLEGIA

The clinical features of acute hemiplegia in childhood have been discussed in Chapter 11. There is nothing specific about the aetiology of the condition which is caused by a wide variety of disorders and is often idiopathic. The earlier terms 'Marie-Strümpell encephalitis' and 'polioencephalitis' implied an infective element in its causation but, though some cases are related directly or indirectly to infection, many are mediated by vascular mechanisms. The proportion of cases of known origin is increasing at the expense of the idiopathic as newer techniques of investigation (cerebral arteriography and CT scanning) are increasingly exploited.

The difficulty sometimes found in deciding whether a case of childhood hemiplegia is congenital or of acute onset postnatally has been mentioned (Ch. 11). In most cases the catastrophic onset of weakness leaves little room for doubt. The circumstances of onset vary with the aetiology. Acute hemiplegia may develop in a setting of trauma, dehydration, infection, status epilepticus, congenital heart disease, migraine, leukaemia and other factors. The clinical picture in these varied conditions will differ greatly with hemiplegia as the only common factor.

The best study of acute hemiplegia in childhood is that of Isler (1971) from Zürich, who surveyed the clinical and radiological data on 116 cases, assigning them to many aetiopathogenetic groups. Isler's analysis of the causes in his series is shown below (Table 19.1).

Vascular causes were prominent. They may also have operated in some of the cases of encephalitis and other cerebral diseases. Only one case of subdural haematoma was formed, a lower figure than in some other series.

All but one of Isler's 10 patients with acute hemiplegia due to arteriovenous malformations suffered intracranial haemorrhage (intracerebral or subarachnoid). Saccular arterial aneurysms contributed only two cases.

Among the 31 cases with arterial occlusion the largest subgroup was of 12 children who showed spontaneous occlusion in the region of the internal carotid territory or its large branches, no cause being found. By contrast, in all 4 cases of occlusion

Table 19.1 The causes of acute hemiplegia in 111 cases (from Isler 1971)

1. *Vascular malformations*	21
Arteriovenous malformations	10
Saccular arterial aneurysm	2
Cerebral venous aneurysm	3
Dissecting aneurysm	2
Cerebral microangioma	4
2. *Arterial occlusions*	31
Focal arteritis	2
Fibromuscular hyperplasia	1
Moya-Moya disease	2
Arteriosclerosis	1
Hypertension	2
Traumatic vascular occlusion	2
Embolism	2
Spontaneous cerebral arterial occlusion	12
Fetal cerebral arterial occlusions	3
Vasospasm	4
3. *Venous occlusions*	
Venous thrombosis	3
4. *Cerebral diseases*	46
Post-ictal hemiplegia	22
Pre-ictal hemiplegia	2
Encephalitis	18
Cerebral abscess	1
Intracranial tumours	2
Multiple sclerosis	1
5. *Subdural haematoma*	1
6. *Migraine accompagnée*	9

of the internal carotid artery in the neck a definite aetiology was present (probable homocystinuria, throat infections in 2 cases and perforating injury to the left internal carotid artery in the throat).

Other surveys have varied in the aetiological factors found. Among 86 children with acute hemiplegia seen over a 21-year period (Gold & Carter 1976) trauma accounted for 11 cases, CNS infections for 11 and cardiac disease for 10. Five children had sickle cell disease (Ch. 23) and 4 had a vascular malformation. In 25 cases neither an aetiological nor radiological diagnosis could be made. Systemic lupus erythematosus accounts for a few cases (Ch. 23).

Trauma

Trauma, a common occurrence in childhood, can cause acute hemiplegia by various mechanisms. Head injury can readily result in bleeding into the epidural or subdural spaces or into the cerebral substance itself with acute hemiplegia as a result.

The history of trauma may be lacking or suppressed but the associated change in consciousness caused by direct damage to the brain should suggest what has happened. A skull fracture and superficial signs of injury will strengthen the suspicion.

Another mechanism is that of thrombosis of the internal carotid artery caused by non-penetrating injury to the paratonsillar area (Bickerstaff 1964a) when a child who is carrying a foreign body in his mouth falls forward so that the object is driven backwards. The offending object is often a pencil or a stick but many others have been involved. There is usually a latent period of up to 24 hours between the time of the injury and the onset of the hemiplegia, since time is needed for thrombosis to develop in the injured artery. As a result the trauma may have been forgotten or its significance overlooked. Bickerstaff (1964a) has stressed the need to perform arteriography early in order to detect minor changes of narrowing and irregularity in the middle cerebral and internal carotid arteries which may not be seen some weeks later.

Traumatic thrombosis of the extracranial part of the internal carotid artery from injury to the head or neck may cause a hemiplegia (Frantzen et al 1961). Overextension of the neck with rotation of the head may result in sudden stretching of the artery against the upper cervical vertebrae. Apart from thrombosis, emboli may enter the cerebral circulation from the injured artery. A latent period of up to 24 hours is usual between the time of trauma and the hemiplegia, as with injury to the artery via the mouth.

Rarer mechanisms by which trauma can cause acute hemiplegia include air embolism, as a complication of surgery or cardiac catheterization, and fat embolism complicating fractures of long bones.

Infections

Infections are common antecedents of acute hemiplegia in childhood operating, like trauma, by various mechanisms.

Encephalitis of direct viral origin does not often cause hemiplegia, as it usually affects both hemispheres. Herpes simplex encephalitis (Ch. 22) is an important exception, since the lesions are often focal in older children; clinical, EEG and CT scan findings often suggest focal pathology which makes this form of encephalitis very likely. Fever, seizures and altered consciousness are common associated symptoms of encephalitis due to herpes simplex and to other viruses less often responsible. CSF changes include a raised protein level and cell count initially with polymorphs and later with lymphocytes. The diagnosis of herpes simplex encephalitis is particularly important since it can be treated. The serological findings are often unhelpful as the antibody titre may be slow to rise in the CSF. Brain biopsy may be the quickest way to a diagnosis (by culture of the virus) but when there is a high index of suspicion it is reasonable to start specific treatment with acyclovir (if available) while awaiting the results of investigations.

Post-infectious encephalitis due to measles, mumps, rubella, varicella and influenza may cause a hemiplegia, as may vaccination against small pox and rabies.

Bacterial meningitis may cause acute hemiplegia by thrombosis in cortical veins or arteries. The diagnosis is usually straightforward except in some cases of partially treated meningitis. Severe infections with dehydration may produce hemiplegia by the same mechanism. Severe tonsillitis may be complicated by thrombosis of the adjacent internal carotid artery leading to a hemiplegia in the same way as trauma in this region (Bickerstaff 1964a).

The importance of convulsions and status epilepticus as a precursor of acute hemiplegia are stressed by many authors (Gastaut et al 1960, Aicardi et al 1969, Isler 1971). Gastaut and his colleagues applied the term 'hemiconvulsions — hemiplegia-epilepsy (HHE) syndrome' (Ch. 12) to this relationship. Aicardi and his colleagues in a review of 122 infants and children with acute hemiplegia found that 89 had status epilepticus at the time of its onset and 33 had no seizures. They noted a worse prognosis with post-convulsive hemiplegia with frequent residual mental retardation and epilepsy. The median age of these children was 16 months (similar to that of children with febrile convulsions) and 90% were under three years. Arteriography, performed in 31 cases, showed no vascular occlusion and the only abnormality was cerebral swelling or atrophy. By contrast the patients without seizures at the onset had a better prognosis, a later age of onset and showed vascular occlusion in one-third of the cases investigated angiographically.

SUBARACHNOID HAEMORRHAGE

Bleeding into the subarachnoid space may be massive or slight, and transient, continuous or repeated depending on its aetiology. The clinical features vary with its severity, from coma or even death resulting from a massive bleed to a milder illness with headache, pain and stiffness of the neck and sometimes also of the back, convulsions or hemiplegia. The bleeding may be accompanied by intracerebral haemorrhage in which case the illness tends to be more severe. Most patients have been well until the sudden onset of symptoms with the bleeding, which may come on at rest or during exercise.

An analysis of spontaneous subarachnoid haemorrhage in four series including their own, totalling 8413 patients was made by Sedzimir & Robinson (1973). 321 (3.8%) of the patients were aged 0 to 20 years. Analysis of the aetiology showed striking differences between these younger patients and those of all ages. The proportion of aneurysms was lower in the juvenile cases (36.13%) compared with the total group (56.69%) while that of arteriovenous malformations was much higher in the younger (27.41%) than in those of all ages (6.53%). No lesion was found to account for the bleeding after detailed angiographic studies in about the same proportion of cases (a little over one third) among the younger and the total age group patients. In Sedzimir and Robinson's series the proportion of unexplained juvenile cases was lower than in other series, probably because their angiographic studies were more vigorous, including vertebral angiography if bilateral carotid angiography showed no lesion, and the studies were often repeated. A 'cryptic' malformation may not be demonstrated on initial or even serial angiography. This was the case in a 17-year-old boy in whom angiography showed a lesion after a second bleed 11 years later.

The total mortality rate after the first bleed in 33 patients aged between 7 and 20 years with arteriovenous malformations causing subarachnoid haemorrhage was 21.2%. (Sedzimir & Robinson 1973).

The rate was 12.1% for the first haemorrhage. Recurrent bleeding occurred in 41.3% of cases with a mortality rate of 25% for the subsequent haemorrhage.

MIGRAINE

Migraine, a common disorder in adults, may have its onset in childhood. In children its frequency is lower than in the general population in which it is thought to affect about 10%. Accurate assessment of its incidence in childhood is difficult, especially in the earlier years when symptoms may differ from classical hemicrania. In children of school age in Uppsala, Sweden, Bille (1962) found that migraine occurred in 4%, increasing in frequency with age. In the age group 7–9 years the frequency was 2.5%, with almost equal numbers of boys and girls. In children aged 10–12 years it was 4.6% and at 13–15 years 5.3%, with an increasing proportion of girls in the older age groups.

Bille in his survey adopted the following criteria for the definition of migraine: paroxysmal headaches separated by free intervals, and at least two of the following four: unilateral pain, nausea, visual aura and a family history of migraine in parents or siblings. By convention cases of headache due to demonstrable intracranial disease are excluded, and the diagnosis of migraine is thus one of exclusion and should only be made after reasonable steps have been taken to rule out structural disorders. The aetiopathogenesis of migraine is not well understood but vascular changes in arteries inside and outside the skull underlie the various symptoms, these vessels being abnormally labile and liable to constriction and dilatation under the influence of various factors. The aura or initial symptoms of an attack which precede the headache seem to be due to ischaemia from spasm of intracranial arteries. Thus visual symptoms result from ischaemia of the occipital cortex with a 'fortification spectrum' of flashing lights or zig-zag patterns or from retinal or visual pathway ischaemia with hemianopic field defects or scotomata. Weakness and/or sensory disturbances with paraesthesiae affecting the limbs on one side, the face or tongue, and transient dysphasia result from spasm of middle cerebral artery branches. Headache usually follows the fading away of these premonitory symptoms. Often unilateral and throbbing, it is due to dilatation of branches of the external carotid artery or swelling of their walls. These vascular changes may be related to serotonin, noradrenalin and other compounds, alterations in which may be mediated by many different factors, including diet (chocolate, cheese and various foodstuffs), hormonal and psychological stress. In the individual case a clear relationship can often be seen to a particular item of food, to menstruation or to recurrent stresses at home or at school. The triggers involved in provoking migraine attacks are almost as many and varied as the factors precipitating seizures in children with epilepsy, yet in both these common paroxysmal disorders attacks may occur without recognized provocation.

There is little difficulty in diagnosing migraine in a classical case in an older child. The attacks are often more frequent, but shorter, than in adults and the headaches may be bilateral for some years before becoming unilateral. As with epilepsy a clear history of a visual or other aura may be difficult to obtain in young children, so that one must depend on the parents' account of events. As with epilepsy, however, it is always worth asking a child to describe his symptoms. Bille noted that children in the Uppsala study often seemed unaware that they had had prodromal symptoms until these were drawn to their attention and they became more observant of later attacks. The commonest prodromal symptom in this series was aura, occurring in half the children, but paraesthesiae, increased irritability, yawning and indefinable feelings also preceded the migraine attacks. Older children will attempt to draw their visual aura when encouraged (Dalton & Dalton 1979), just as children with temporal lobe epilepsy may be able to draw the more complex visual hallucinations experienced in their attacks. Nausea and vomiting are very common and the headache often ceases with the onset of vomiting. The migraine attack has been described as 'something between a headache and seasickness', and many migraine children are liable also to severe travel sickness. Photophobia and dislike of noise (phonophobia) are also common symptoms and most children, like adults, want only to lie down in a dark, quiet room during an attack. Hallucinations of distorted body image ('the syndrome of Alice in Wonderland', Todd 1955), taste, smell or hearing, are much rarer in children than in adults with migraine.

Examination of the nervous system is normal between attacks, but may show transient deficits in the course of an attack. Ophthalmoscopic examination is needed to exclude signs of raised intracranial pressure and auscultation over the skull and eyes is advisable in order to detect a bruit which may suggest an intracranial arteriovenous malformation or aneurysm.

Investigations in a typical case of migraine need not be rigorous. Skull X-rays are advisable and demonstration of their normality is often of therapeutic benefit in allaying the anxieties of parents which may have been communicated to the child. CT scanning allows exclusion of a structural brain abnormality and the authoritative reassurance which can then be given is often tactically helpful in management. The EEG is often abnormal but not diagnostic (see Ch. 24).

Complicated migraine (migraine accompagnée)

This term is applied to the rare cases of migraine in which a neurological deficit of a kind which usually occurs in an attack as a transient feature is more prolonged and may occasionally persist indefinitely. The three main varieties are hemiplegic, including alternating hemiplegia, ophthalmoplegic and basilar migraine.

Hemiplegic migraine

In this variant there is hemiplegic weakness of sudden onset, often with sensory changes, which may last for several days and may affect the left or the right side at different times. There is often a family history of similar attacks in one or other parent. The prognosis is usually good with complete recovery after a few hours or days but some patients have been left with a persistent weakness. Sometimes included in this group are patients who experience episodes of unilateral sensory disturbance without weakness.

Rosenbaum (1960) in a review of 5 cases of hemiplegic migraine noted two distinct clinical patterns. The first was very similar to ordinary migraine except that the visual aura was replaced by more serious signs of neurological deficit — hemiplegia, unilateral sensory loss and aphasia. In the second type headache could precede the aura and the signs were usually prolonged for hours or days. Serial EEGs suggested that there was an initial vasoconstriction followed by focal oedema of the brain.

Glista et al (1975) have reported a family with hemiplegic migraine in ten patients in three generations. In three of these the attacks followed minor injuries to the head. Trauma to the head was important in the 5 cases of 'Footballer's Migraine' provoked by blows to the head reported by Matthews (1972), one of whom was a 12-year-old boy who developed blurred vision followed by numbness of the right hand and speech difficulty and later by severe headache with rapid recovery. In a review of 40 Swiss cases of complicated migraine, Rossi et al (1980) found that 38 had paraesthesiae usually on one side of the body or part thereof, while 9 had weakness either restricted to the arm or a hemiplegia. The attacks of complicated migraine tended to cease in adult life and none of the 25 patients followed up showed any neurological deficit.

Alternating hemiplegia

A severe syndrome of alternating hemiplegia starting in infancy is recognized as a form of complicated migraine (Verret & Steele 1971, Hosking et al 1978). The fourteen children in these two series all developed symptoms under three years of age, mostly under eighteen months. Their attacks lasted between 12 hours and three weeks. Most had a family history of migraine. Seizures occurred in some cases and the EEG was abnormal in many with excess of slow waves. Detailed radiological investigations with angiography in 9 patients gave normal results and biochemical studies were negative.

Headache occurred in association with the hemiplegia in 4 of the children in the Toronto series (Verret & Steele 1971), being contralateral in two and diffuse in the others, but it was only complained of by the oldest patient in the series of Hosking et al (1978), as she grew older. Many of the younger children appeared miserable in their attacks, suggesting that they may also have had headache.

The prognosis of this rare condition is poor; low intellectual status and evidence of progressive neurological deterioration were present in many of the 14 patients.

Ophthalmoplegic migraine

This condition, first named by Charcot in 1890, was brought to prominence more recently by Bickerstaff (1964b) in a report of 11 cases.

The clinical picture is of infrequent but recurrent attacks of severe pain starting in or above one eye, spreading to the vertex on this side, accompanied by vomiting and lasting 24 to 48 hours. As the pain subsides towards the end of this time, the ipsilateral eyelid starts to drop and within another 24 to 48 hours a complete third nerve palsy has developed with dilatation of the pupil. In severe attacks the fourth and sixth nerves are also affected, giving a complete unilateral ophthalmoplegia. The pain ceases completely but the ocular palsy persists for between three days and several weeks, then clearing up rapidly and completely. Recurrent attacks usually affect the same side but occasionally the opposite one, a helpful point of distinction from cases of ophthalmoplegia due to aneurysm or other structural lesions.

Nine of Bickerstaff's 11 patients were boys, in contrast with the sex ratio in common migraine. All had their first attack under the age of 17 years, and 8 between 5 and 11.

Carotid and vertebral angiography and air encephalography were carried out in most patients. Although no gross abnormality was found, the carotid artery showed a localized constriction in and below the region of the cavernous sinus in one case with return to normal after clinical recovery. Similar appearances were seen in four other cases. These may result from oedema in the vessel wall constricting its lumen and affecting the nearby oculomotor nerves either by local pressure or interference with their vasa nervorum. The prognosis appears good, the attacks tending to diminish with increasing age.

Basilar artery migraine

Bickerstaff (1961) has described cases of migraine in which features of brain-stem dysfunction predominate. The symptoms consist of bilateral loss of vision or flashing lights, ataxia, vertigo, dysarthria, tinnitus and dysaesthesia followed by occipital headache. The attacks lasted between 2 and 45 minutes. The syndrome was commonest in adolescent girls in whom it was related to menstruation, and there was a family history of migraine in close relatives in 28 of the 34 patients. Bickerstaff stressed the occurrence of other more classically migrainous attacks in the patients, their rapid return to complete normality and the positive family history as important diagnostic points. Similar features have been reported by Golden & French (1975) in 8 children, mostly girls presenting under the age of four years.

Investigation in the complicated forms of migraine is concerned with excluding underlying structural abnormalities, especially vascular. Plain skull X-rays should be taken. When symptoms of brain-stem dysfunction or ataxia predominate brain-stem and cerebellar lesions should be excluded and the CT scanner will usually achieve this. Neurometabolic disorders such as syndromes with hyperammonaemia may occasionally suggest basilar migraine. Angiographic investigations in most patients with complicated migraine are unhelpful. Pearce & Foster (1965) found two angiomas in 33 patients investigated by angiography. Both patients were adults with symptoms starting at 17 and 29 years of age and neither had hemiplegic or ophthalmoplegic migraine.

Ophthalmoplegic migraine may be confused with ophthalmoplegia due to myasthenia gravis, in which the pupil is normal. The Tolosa-Hunt syndrome of recurrent painful ophthalmoplegia (Tolosa 1954) due to peri-arteritic lesions of the carotid artery in its intracavernous course, is rare in children. Terrence & Samaha (1973), who reported two childhood cases, found no previously reported case under ten years of age. In both their cases there was marked improvement on steroid therapy. One patient showed a mononuclear pleocytosis in the CSF and carotid and vertebral angiography gave normal results.

Acute confusional states in childhood migraine

Rarely children with migraine and, less often, children with no previous history of migraine, may suffer from episodes of agitated confusion lasting from several minutes to 20 hours, (Gascon & Barlow 1970, Emery 1977, Ehyai & Fenichel 1978). The children reported have been aged between 5 and 16 years. In most cases the attacks have been preceded by classical migraine symptoms, but a few patients (Emery 1977) have given no clear history of preceding headache but have suffered a mild head injury some hours before the onset of the confusional state. In 4 of the 13 cases in the three series above 'acute confusional migraine' (as Ehyai and Fenichel have termed it) was the first manifestation of migraine. Diagnostic difficulty is inevitable in such cases and a family history of migraine may be a helpful clue.

During the attacks the children are confused and disorientated and show agitation with a mixture of apprehension and combativeness. The episodes usually end in a deep sleep with return to normal on waking. In some cases the attacks have tended to recur, but have often been replaced by typical migraine after some years. The mechanism of these episodes may be cerebral ischaemia affecting one or both hemispheres. An episode of 'transient global amnesia' in a 13-year-old boy with a 3-year history of recurrent headache was thought to have a similar basis with brief vasoconstriction of arteries supplying hippocampal structures (Jensen 1980).

Migraine variants and related symptoms in childhood

The diagnosis of any syndrome in young children may be made difficult by the problems of discovering exactly what symptoms they experience, since they usually cannot describe these accurately. The fact that a child does not complain of headache in his attacks does not mean that it is absent (experience with temporal lobe epilepsy in children shows that as they grow older and more articulate they often describe complex subjective sensations which they have experienced periodically for years). Vahlquist & Hackzell (1949) in their study of 31 cases of migraine of early onset found that headache was not mentioned under the age of two years, but that attacks of pallor and intense vomiting sometimes began as early as one year of age. The attacks were usually shorter, the prodromal signs less marked and nausea more intense than in adults.

In most migraine attacks in older children headache and other classical features occur, but occasionally headache is not prominent and the picture is one of recurrent abdominal pain and vomiting. In children with the 'periodic syndrome' described by Kempton (1956) there is a tendency for the abdominal symptoms to decrease as the child matures and for headache to become more prominent in his attacks. Hammond (1974) studied the late sequelae of recurrent vomiting of childhood in 12 patients aged 17 to 27 years who had suffered from severe cyclical vomiting as children. She found that the symptoms tended to persist into adult life, and that 8 of the patients had migraine, 5 of them having developed headaches in their early teens. The natural history of recurrent abdominal symptoms in many children justifies their being regarded as a 'larval' form of migraine. (The term 'abdominal migraine' is sometimes used but is inexact and better avoided). It would be wrong, however, to consider all children with recurrent abdominal pain and vomiting as 'apprentice migraineurs', though the possibility must be considered.

The interesting problem of the relationship between migraine and epilepsy has been debated for a century or more (Jackson 1876, Gowers 1907, Lennox & Lennox 1960, Whitty 1972). Jackson believed cases of migraine to be sensory epilepsies, but Gowers considered the relationship indirect, with epilepsy following migraine in some cases or rarely preceding it. In individual children it may be difficult initially to decide whether paroxysmal symptoms are epileptic or migrainous. Epileptic attacks may involve abdominal pain and rarely headache. Migraine attacks may occasionally be associated with loss of consciousness and a convulsion, probably due to syncope. Concurrence of migraine and epilepsy in the same patient is quite common. Lennox & Lennox (1960) found that 11% of 1600 epileptics also had migraine, while 6.5% of 415 patients presenting primarily with migraine also had epilepsy. In the epileptic group there was a history of migraine in 9.6% of parents and 1.6% of siblings, while in the migraineurs 0.7% of parents and 1.6% of siblings had epilepsy. The two conditions have often been noted together in monozygous twin pairs.

EEG evidence as to the relationship is somewhat conflicting. Dysrhythmias occur in many patients with migraine. Hockaday & Whitty (1969) in a study of 560 patients found that 61% showed an abnormal EEG, the rate being higher in those with a lateralized non-visual aura and lowest in those with basilar migraine. Dysrhythmia was common in patients whose migraine began when they were young.

An EEG study of patients with recurrent abdominal pain starting in childhood by Papatheophilou et al (1972) showed electrical abnormalities of a type usually associated with epilepsy in 22%, but follow-up of 14 patients 12 to 14 years later showed that all had become symptom-free and only one patient (with spike and wave in his original EEG) had developed epilepsy. The authors believe that EEG abnormalities other than spike and wave should not be taken as evidence of epilepsy in children with recurrent abdominal pain. The equation 'abdominal pain plus an abnormal EEG equals epilepsy' receives no support from this study and it is unfortunate when the label of epilepsy is wrongly applied to any child on EEG rather than sound clinical grounds.

The prognosis of childhood migraine

The outlook for cessation of attacks in children with migraine is quite good. Bille (1962) found at follow-up of his migraine children 6 years after the first interview that 35 to 50% had become symptom-free. No clear prognostic factors were found. In cases with early onset Vahlquist & Hackzell (1949) found the frequency of attacks was usually decreasing at follow-up. It is not known what proportion of children who become symptom-free may have a later recurrence, but the experience of some adult patients suggests that it may be considerable. At the time of puberty attacks often improve but may become worse. Migraine may start at this time, especially in girls.

The management of migraine

A detailed history and examination is needed in every case in order to exclude any more serious cause for the symptoms and to discover provoking factors, particularly dietary or stresses at school or at home with a view to altering these. Often intense anxiety is felt by parents who may believe, perhaps because of experience of illness in a relative or neighbour, that the child has a brain tumour, leukaemia or disseminated sclerosis. If these fears are seen to be considered seriously and allayed by examination and simple investigations, the emotional tension may be greatly reduced and the child's attacks improve with reassurance alone. Migraine is a common enough ailment for most parents to be familiar with it as a paroxysmal disorder without serious underlying disease and the diagnosis even carries a certain cachet (probably because of the unfounded view that it affects the more intelligent rather than duller members of society).

Changes may be needed at home or at school if particular stressful situations are acting as triggers for attacks. Liaison with a school medical officer may help when a clash of personalities between a teacher and a child causes repeated stress to the latter expressing itself as migraine. Sometimes the rather perfectionistic attitude of the child himself and the need to do well in school (a need often consciously or unconsciously stressed by ambitious parents) are important factors calling for tact in attempting to modify them. A good rapport between the physician and the child and his parents will allow the former to fulfill his role as teacher in a tactful yet effective way.

Adequate sleep and regular meal times should be ensured since lack of sleep and hypoglycaemia can provoke attacks. 'Moderation in all things' should be the life-style of those liable to migraine, as it is also in epilepsy.

The drug treatment of migraine in children involves that of the attacks and, in selected cases, regular prophylactic treatment. Mild attacks will often respond to simple analgesics such as aspirin or paracetamol. If vomiting is severe oral medication is often useless. When an aura occurs regularly the attacks can often be aborted or shortened by ergotamine tartrate given orally, rectally or parenterally as promptly as possible, in a dose of one to two mg. The drug causes vasoconstriction and so may prevent the vasodilatation which underlies the headache phase of the migraine attack. If there is persistent vomiting despite ergotamine a phenothiazine drug, such as chlorpromazine given rectally (12.5 to 25 mg) may bring relief. Rest in a quiet, dark room is essential and the child should *not* be allowed to resume strenuous activities as soon as the attack abates.

Preventive treatment may be non-specific with drugs, such as diazepam or phenobarbitone, which may help by their tranquillizing effect, or more specific, with anti-migraine agents. These include ergotamine tartrate given regularly and Clonidine (Dixarit®) 0.025 mg twice daily. Propanolol has been reported (Ludvigsson 1974) to have an excellent prophylactic effect on migraine in school children in a dose of 1 mg/kg three times daily. Methysergide (Deseril®) is often very effective in the prophylaxis of migraine in adults, but its many side-effects, including retroperitoneal fibrosis, make it a drug to be used in children with caution and as a last resort. In girls whose migraine is related to their periods a diuretic such as acetazolamide may be helpful if given two days before the expected onset.

THE NEUROLOGICAL COMPLICATIONS OF SEVERE HYPERTENSION IN CHILDHOOD

The incidence of arterial hypertension in children and adolescents is not clearly defined. Between 1 and 11% of all children have been assessed by various authors as having a greater than optimal blood pressure (Dillon 1979). Hypertension is probably greatly underdiagnosed in childhood since routine measurement of the blood pressure (BP) is unfortunately sadly neglected, by contrast with the more ideal (one hopes) situation with adults. Hypertension in children has often been present for some years before it is detected as a result of complications. The investigation of hypertension in childhood is more rewarding than in adults since the

chances are greater that a treatable cause will be found. Lloyd Still & Cottom (1967) in a series of 55 children with hypertension seen at the Hospital for Sick Children, Great Ormond Street, found that the commonest cause was pyelonephritis, present in 35 cases and invariably associated with evidence of vesico-ureteric reflux. Glomerulonephritis accounted for 6 cases and other causes for 14.

Of 54 children with severe hypertension reported by Lloyd Still & Cottom, 18 had neurological complications. Some of the complications of childhood hypertension will be discussed.

Acute hemiplegia

Two of the 111 cases of acute hemiplegia in childhood reported by Isler (1971) were associated with severe hypertension, due to renal causes in one case and to aortic stenosis in the other which was associated with two attacks of subarachnoid haemorrhage. Both children made a complete recovery. In some cases of this kind the CT scan has shown a 'fibre-splitting' haemorrhage in the internal capsule which has later resolved.

Hypertensive encephalopathy

Episodes of headache, convulsions and altered consciousness without hemiplegia may occur in some children with severe hypertension. This is sometimes seen as an iatrogenic effect in children on corticosteroid treatment. The raised BP and the retinal arterial changes help to distinguish this situation from benign intracranial hypertension due to corticosteroid withdrawal (Ch. 18). Of the 54 children reported by Lloyd Still & Cottom (1967), 12 had convulsions while headaches occurred in 20. 11 of the 100 children with severe and persistent hypertension reported by Gill et al (1976) had hypertensive fits. In 9 cases these occurred with untreated hypertension and only two children had fits while under treatment.

Some atypical aspects of hypertensive encephalopathy in childhood have been discussed by Del Giudice & Aicardi (1979) who described four patients whose misleading focal symptoms created difficult problems of differential diagnosis. The patients were aged between 5 and 17 years. One child had peculiar periodic EEG features consistent with herpes simplex encephalitis. Another had a complex syndrome suggesting a psychiatric condition with ocular features pointing to upper brainstem involvement. In the third patient ventriculography suggested a cerebellar space-occupying lesion but no such lesion was found at operation. The fourth patient, a boy with the Guillain-Barré syndrome, developed coma, seizures and decerebrate movements which could have been wrongly attributed to a associated encephalopathy of the same aetiology as the polyneuropathy, if its hypertensive origin had not been recognized. Hypertension in the Guillain-Barré syndrome is not uncommon and the blood pressure should be carefully monitored so that hypertensive encephalopathy can be swiftly treated if it occurs.

Facial palsy in hypertension

The association between hypertension and lower motor neuron facial palsy was first noted by Moxon in 1869, and is now well recognized in children and adolescents. Paine (1957) in a survey of 47 children with facial palsy of postnatal onset found 2 with hypertension. Lloyd et at (1966) found 7 patients with facial palsy among 35 children with severe hypertension seen over a 10-year period at The Hospital for Sick Children, Great Ormond Street. Facial palsy was the presenting feature in 3 cases. Its onset usually coincided with a rise in the BP and it tended to improve when this was controlled. It was always unilateral, being right-sided in 4 cases and left in 3. Its duration varied from weeks to months and two patients had a second attack coinciding with an exacerbation of their hypertension. In all cases the diastolic BP exceeded 120 mmHg and there was left ventricular hypertrophy. The hypertension was of renal origin in 6 of the 7 cases. The paralysis is probably due to haemorrhage into the facial canal. The memorable statistic that facial palsy occurs in 11% of children with severe hypertension and that 11% of all cases of lower motor neuron facial palsy in children are caused by hypertension underlines the importance of measuring the BP in all children with facial palsy. It seems probable that many cases of unexplained facial palsy are due to undetected hypertension.

Hypotensive treatment

Neurological problems may arise in the course of reduction of severe hypertension in childhood. 3 examples were reported by Hulse and his colleagues (1979). All 3 children had severe renal hypertension and, while being treated with hypotensive agents, developed severe and permanent visual loss due to optic nerve infarction. One child also developed an ischaemic transverse myelopathy. All 3 children had probably been hypertensive for a considerable time. Reduction of BP in such cases should be gradual and cautious, since the auto-regulatory mechanism to maintain blood-flow may be set well above that in non-hypertensive subjects. Generalized vasculitis occurs in severe hypertension and probably contributed to these ischaemic problems.

Hypertension as a symptom of acute neurological disease in childhood

Severe hypertension may occasionally occur transiently in the course of acute neurological disease in children, a situation very different from those previously discussed.

5 cases in children aged between 4 months and 6 years were reported by Eden et al (1977). The neurological diagnoses were cerebellar astrocytoma, pontine glioma, scalds encephalopathy, occipital meningocoele with hydrocephalus and asphyxial brain damage with cardiac arrest. Paroxysmal rises in BP occurred in 4 cases, the pressure showing normal resting levels and transient increases up to 250/180. Pallor was common. The intracranial pressure was not raised. The duration of the condition varied between 4 days and 6 weeks. Fits, coma and extensor hypertonus occurred in all 5 cases.

All patients showed hyponatraemia or reduced serum osmolality at the time of the hypertension and studies of plasma and urine osmolality in two of them suggested inappropriate antidiuretic hormone activity.

The hypertensive episodes were controlled with diazoxide in a dose of 5 mg/kg body weight by rapid intravenous injection. Diazepam was also useful, especially if the child were convulsing, and is a good first drug for control of the acute situation.

The authors postulate that the mechanism of the hypertension is a loss of integration between control of blood volume and capacity of the vascular bed. They stress the need to monitor the BP in all acute neurological diseases in children since detection and correction of hypertension can prevent aggravation of the neurological condition. Hypertension in the context of acute neurological disease appears to be a bad prognostic sign.

A rare but important neurological disease associated with hypertension is acute porphyria (Ch. 4).

Vascular effects of head injury — extradural and subdural haematoma

Subdural haematomas resulting from trauma have been discussed in Chapter 18. Brief mention will be made of extradural haematoma, a serious condition which may quickly be lethal if not recognized and evacuated, so that all who deal with children should be alert to it and able to arrange effective treatment. A concise account is given by Grant (1979) in a wider discussion of acute neurosurgical emergencies in childhood.

Children, especially babies and infants, may rapidly deteriorate after a head injury, though initially seeming to have suffered no harm. A minor degree of trauma may be enough to cause serious damage to the brain, and trauma should always be enquired for in all neurological illnesses of childhood. When in doubt as to whether to admit a child to hospital after a head injury, it is wise to err on the side of caution and safety. Any child with loss of consciousness, however brief, after a head injury, or with a skull fracture, and any child remaining or becoming drowsy after the injury deserves admission.

With extradural bleeding, which may follow mild trauma such as a fall or a kick on the head at football, there may be no immediate sequelae or there may be loss of consciousness for a short time followed by apparent recovery for a few hours. This lucid interval may be marked by increasing headache and drowsiness. These symptoms worsen and the child becomes comatose if the situation is not relieved. Limb weakness of hemiplegic distribution may appear and the pupil on the injured side may dilate and respond only sluggisly to light, later becoming fixed. Bradycardia, rising blood pressure and respiratory problems may develop, suggesting raised intracranial pressure. Plain skull X-rays may show a fracture crossing the markings of the middle meningeal vessels or one of the major venous sinuses.

The situation as described above is very dangerous, and urgent treatment is needed if irreversible damage to the brain-stem is to be avoided. Transfer

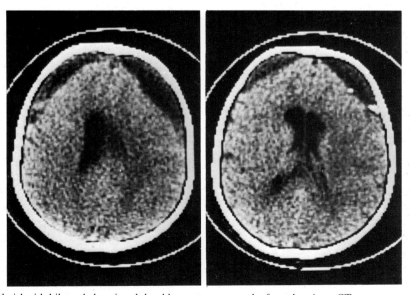

Fig. 19.7 8-year-old girl with bilateral chronic subdural haematomas over the frontal regions. CT

to a neurosurgical centre may be hazardous because of the time involved, so that surgery must be undertaken at once by *whatever surgeon is available*, while more specialized help is summoned. A 4 cm incision is made over the fracture site or point of external trauma, or, if these markers are missing, midway between the external auditory meatus and posterior limit of the orbital margin. The pericranium is incised and a burr-hole made through which the extradural clot will begin to extrude if the diagnosis is correct.

With acute subdural, as opposed to extradural, bleeding deterioration is usually less rapid but urgent surgical relief may be needed. The cerebral hemisphere is more likely to be damaged in subdural bleeding than extradural, and the clinical picture is more variable and the site of the haematoma less predictable. If time does not permit transfer to a neurosurgical centre, surgery must be undertaken by a general surgeon in order to find and drain the haematoma. A minimum of three burr-holes, frontal, temporal and posterior parietal are needed. If no haematoma is found on the side explored, the search must be extended to the other side. It should be remembered that many subdural haematomas are bilateral (Fig. 19.7).

REFERENCES

Aicardi J, Amsili J, Chevrie J J 1969 Acute hemiplegia in infancy and childhood. Developmental Medicine and Child Neurology 11: 162

Amacher A L, Drake C G 1975 Cerebral artery aneurysms in infancy, childhood and adolescence. Child's Brain 1: 72–80

Bickerstaff E R 1961 Basilar artery migraine. British Medical Journal 1: 15–17

Bickerstaff E R 1964a Aetiology of acute hemiplegia in childhood. British Medical Journal 2: 82–87

Bickerstaff E R 1964b Ophthalmoplegic migraine. Revue neurologique 110: 582–588

Bille B 1962 Migraine in school children. Acta paediatrica scandinavica 51: (suppl) 136

Charcot J M 1890 Sur un cas de migraine ophtalmoplégique (paralysie oculomotrice périodique). Progrès Médicale 18, 2me sér, T 15, 83–86, 99–102

Court D 1941 Malignant hypertension in childhood. Archives of Disease in Childhood 16: 132–139

Dalton K, Dalton M 1979 Clinical aspects of migraine in young children. Journal of Maternal and Child Health 6: 6

Davidson S, Falconer M A 1973 Cerebral arteriovenous malformation causing cardiac enlargement and epilepsy: correction after operation. British Medical Journal 1: 754

Del Giudice E, Aicardi J 1979 Atypical aspects of hypertensive encephalopathy in childhood. Neuropädiatrie 10: 150–157

Dillon M J Recent advances in evaluation and management of childhood hypertension. European Journal of Pediatrics 132: 133–139

Eden O B, Sills J A, Brown J K 1977 Hypertension in acute neurological diseases of childhood. Developmental Medicine and Child Neurology 19: 437–445

Ehyai A, Fenichel G M 1978 The natural history of acute confusional migraine. Archives of Neurology 35: 368–369

Emery E S 1977 Acute confusional state in children with migraine. Pediatrics 60: 110–114

Frantzen E, Jacobsen H H, Therkelsen J 1961 Cerebral artery occlusions in children due to trauma to the head and neck. A report of 6 cases verified by cerebral angiography. Neurology 11: 695–700

Gascon G, Barlow C 1970 Juvenile migraine, presenting as an acute confusional state. Pediatrics 45: 628–635

Gastaut H, Poirier F, Paynan H, Salamon G, Toga M, Vigouroux M 1960 HHE syndrome: hemiconvulsions, hemiplegia, epilepsy. Epilepsia 1: 418

Gill D G, Mendes Da Costa B, Cameron J S, Joseph M C, Ogg C S, Chantler C 1976 Analysis of 100 children with severe and persistent hypertension. Archives of Disease in Childhood 51: 951–956

Glista G G, Mellinger J F, Rooke E D 1975 Familial hemiplegic migraine. Mayo Clinic Proceedings 50: 307

Gold A P, Carter S 1976 Acute hemiplegia of infancy and childhood. Pediatric Clinics of North America 23 (3): 413–433

Golden G S, French J H 1975 Basilar artery migraine in young children. Pediatrics 56: 722–726

Gowers W R 1907 The borderland of epilepsy. Churchill, London

Grant D N 1979 Acute neurosurgical emergencies. In: Black J A (ed) Paediatric emergencies. Butterworths, London, ch 27

Hammond Josephine 1974 The late sequelae of recurrent vomiting of childhood. Developmental Medicine and Child Neurology 16: 15

Harwood-Nash D C, Fitz C R 1976 Abnormalities of the cerebral arteries. In: Neuroradiology in infants and children, C V Mosby, Saint Louis, ch 14

Hepner W R 1951 Some observations on facial paresis in the newborn infant: etiology and incidence. Pediatrics 8: 494

Hillal S K, Solomon G E, Golp A P, Carter S 1971 Primary cerebral occlusive disease in children. II. Neurocutaneous syndromes. Radiology 99: 87

Hockaday J M, Whitty C W M 1969 Factors determining the electroencephalogram in migraine: a study of 560 patients according to clinical type of migraine. Brain 92: 769

Hockaday J M 1979 Basilar migraine in childhood. Developmental Medicine and Child Neurology 21: 455–463

Holden A M, Fyler D C, Shillito J, Nadas A S 1972 Congestive heart failure from intracranial arteriovenous fistula in infancy. Clinical and physiological considerations in eight patients. Pediatrics 49: 30

Hosking G P, Cavanagh N P C, Wilson J 1978 Alternating hemiplegia: complicated migraine of infancy. Archives of Disease in Childhood 53: 626

Isler W 1971 Acute hemiplegias and hemisyndromes in childhood. Clinics in Developmental Medicine nos 41/42, SIMP, Heinemann, London

Jackson J H 1876 In: Taylor J (ed) 1931 Selected writings of John Hughlings Jackson. Hodder and Stoughton, London, p 153

Jensen T S 1980 Transient global amnesia in childhood. Developmental Medicine and Child Neurology 22: 654–667

Kempton J J 1956 Periodic syndrome. British Medical Journal 1: 83–86

Lennox W G, Lennox M A 1960 Epilepsy and related disorders. Churchill, London

Levisohn P M, Mikhael M A, Rothman S M 1978 Cerebrovascular changes in neurofibromatosis. Developmental Medicine and Child Neurology 20: 789–793

Lloyd A V C, Jewitt D E, Lloyd Still J D 1966 Facial paralysis in children with hypertension. Archives of Disease in Childhood 41: 292–294

Lloyd Still J, Cottom D 1967 Severe hypertension in childhood. Archives of Disease in Childhood 42: 34–39

Ludvigsson J 1974 Propanolol used in prophylaxis of migraine in children. Acta neurologica scandinavica 50/1: 109–115

Matson D 1969 Neurosurgery of infancy and childhood, 2nd edn. Charles C Thomas, Springfield, Illinois

Matsushima Y, Fukai N, Tanaka K, Tsuruoka S, Inaba Y, Aoyagi M et al 1981 A new surgical treatment of moya moya disease in children: a preliminary report. Surgical Neurology 15: 313–320

Matthews W B 1972 Footballer's migraine. British Medical Journal 2: 326

Moxon W 1869 Apoplexy into canal of Fallopius in a case of Bright's disease, causing facial paralysis. Transactions of the Pathological Society of London 20: 40

Paine R S 1957 Facial paralysis in children. Review of the differential diagnosis and report of ten cases treated with cortisone. Pediatrics 19: 303–316

Papatheophilou R, Jeavons P M, Disney M E 1972 Recurrent abdominal pain: a clinical and electroencephalographic study. Developmental Medicine and Child Neurology 14: 131

Patel A N, Richardson A E 1971 Ruptured intracranial aneurysms in the first two decades of life. A study of 58 patients. Journal of Neurosurgery 35: 571–576

Pearce J M S, Foster J B 1965 An investigation of complicated migraine. Neurology 15: 333–340

Richardson A 1969 Subarachnoid haemorrhage. British Medical Journal 4: 89–92

Rosenbaum H E 1960 Familial hemiplegic migraine. Neurology 10: 164

Rossi L N, Mumenthaler M, Vassella F 1980 Complicated migraine (migraine accompagnée) in children. Clinical characteristics and course in 40 personal cases. Neuropädiatrie 11: 27–35

Sedzimir C B, Robinson J 1973 Intracranial hemorrhage in children and adolescents. Journal of Neurosurgery 38: 269–281

Silverman B K, Brecker T, Craig J, Nadas A A 1955 Congestive failure in the newborn caused by cerebral arteriovenous fistula. American Journal of Diseases of Childhood 89: 539

So C S 1978 Cerebral arteriovenous malformations in children. Child's Brain 4: 242

Suzuki J, Takaku A, Kodama N, Sato S 1975 An attempt to treat cerebrovascular 'moyamoya' disease in children. Child's Brain 1: 193–206

Terrence C F, Samaha F J 1973 The Tolosa-Hunt syndrome (painful ophthalmoplegia) in children. Developmental Medicine and Child Neurology 15: 506

Todd J 1955 The syndrome of Alice in Wonderland. Canadian Medical Association Journal 73: 701

Tolosa E 1954 Periarteritic lesions of the carotid siphon with the clinical features of a carotid infraclinoid aneurysm. Journal of Neurology, Neurosurgery and Psychiatry 17: 300

Tyler H R, Clark D B 1957 Incidence of neurological complications in congenital heart disease. AMA Archives of Neurology and Psychiatry 7: 17–22

Vahlquist B, Hackzell G 1949 Migraine of early onset: a study of 31 cases in which the disease first appeared between one and four years of age. Acta paediatrica scandinavica 38: 622

Verret S, Steele J C 1971 Alternating hemiplegia in childhood: a report of eight patients with complicated migraine beginning in infancy. Pediatrics 47: 675

Whitty C W M 1972 Migraine and epilepsy. Hemicrania 4 (1): 3

20

Neurocutaneous syndromes

E. M. Brett

Syndromes involving genetic and developmental anomalies in structures of ectodermal origin are of great importance to the paediatrician since they present with clinical features affecting the central and peripheral nervous system, the eye and the skin. The cutaneous stigmata are often present at an early age, even at birth and may allow the diagnosis to be made before neurological symptoms have developed.

The disordered development of cerebral tissue, which varies from one syndrome to another, probably arises between the eighth and twenty-fourth week of gestation at a stage of very active cell proliferation and migration. The term 'phakomatoses' is sometimes used for the whole group of disorders. It was introduced by Van der Hoeve (1921) in reference to the retinal tumours often seen in tuberous sclerosis. Similar lesions are occasionally seen in neurofibromatosis, but rarely in other members of the group, so that its use as a generic term seems inappropriate.

The genetically determined members of this group are classically inherited in autosomal dominant fashion, but there is a high mutation rate and in some disorders the expressivity is very variable. Thus siblings of an affected child may show only cutaneous features of the disease, which they can nonetheless transmit to half of their offspring. A parent of an index case may also show minimal skin signs, which are easily overlooked unless a careful search is made. The cutaneous stigmata of these disorders usually become more prominent with increasing age, making diagnosis easier, but in one disease, incontinentia pigmenti, the naevi disappear after childhood.

There is debate about the inclusion of certain disorders in this group. Ataxia-telangiectasia (Ch. 8) and the Von Hippel-Lindau syndrome (Ch. 18) are discussed elsewhere, although sometimes classified among the phakomatoses.

Only some of the commoner and more important neurocutaneous syndromes are considered here. Other works, such as Vinken & Bruyn (1972) and Smith (1976) may be consulted for a more comprehensive list.

TUBEROUS SCLEROSIS (BOURNEVILLE'S DISEASE: EPILOIA)

This disorder, with protean manifestations, makes an important contribution to chronic neurological handicap in children and adults, with mental retardation, epilepsy and cerebral palsy as common symptoms. This was recognized first by Bourneville (1880) in his *Contribution à l'étude de l'idiotie*, a report of a three-year-old girl with epilepsy, retardation and hemiplegia. Viscera and other structures may also be affected with occasional serious symptoms of a non-neurological kind. Its frequent inheritance as an autosomal dominant character gives the disease important genetic implications. A comprehensive review of the disorder is given by Gomez (1979).

Neurological features

The neurological presentation is usually with mental retardation, epilepsy or a combination of the two. Occasionally the child shows delayed development from birth and may later develop seizures. A common presentation is with infantile spasms at between four and seven months of age, the child having either appeared developmentally normal previously or shown some evidence of delay. The onset of the spasms, as in cases of other or unknown causation, is usually associated with a loss of social responsiveness and marked slowing in subsequent development (see Ch. 12). The EEG typically shows the gross disturbance known as hypsarrhythmia, and treatment with conventional anticonvulsants is often disappointing in its results, though nitrazepam or clonazepam may prove helpful. The response to ACTH or steroids is often gratifying with cessation of attacks and improvement in the EEG and development, but the ultimate outcome tends to be bad in terms of intelligence level and later problems with epilepsy.

Tuberous sclerosis must always be considered in the aetiology of childhood seizures. These may begin in later childhood or even adolescence in a child who has been previously regarded as entirely normal.

Examination of the eye grounds may show a retinal phakoma, a raised, mushroom-like lesion present either near the optic disc, sometimes overlying it, or more peripherally (Fig. 20.1). These lesions can develop as early as a few months of life. They were detected in 20 cases in a series of 100 children with tuberous sclerosis seen at the Hospital for Sick Children, Great Ormond Street (Pampiglione & Moynahan 1976), but may be present in a higher proportion of older patients. They are usually symptomless.

Blockage of one foramen of Monro or of the aqueduct of Sylvius by a strategically placed nodule may cause obstruction to the flow of CSF and thus a rare but important presentation of the disease is with symptoms of raised intracranial pressure. If the diagnosis of tuberous sclerosis has been made previously, this possibility should come promptly to mind, but in other cases careful examination of the skin for stigmata of the disease and of the eye grounds for a phakoma will enable it to be made. A rarer neurosurgical complication is the neoplastic transformation of a long-standing benign nodule or tumour into an astrocytoma or glioblastoma. Four cases of brain tumours in tuberous sclerosis were reviewed recently by Tsuchida et al (1981).

Cutaneous features

The best known, but not the earliest, skin manifestation of the disease is adenoma sebaceum, a papular, acneiform rash over the 'butterfly area' of the face. This is rarely detectable under the age of two years and may not be sufficiently developed to

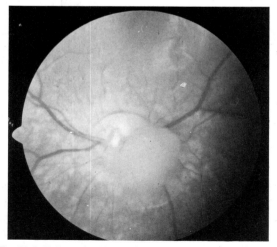

Fig. 20.1 Tuberous sclerosis. Retinal phakoma — 5-month-old boy

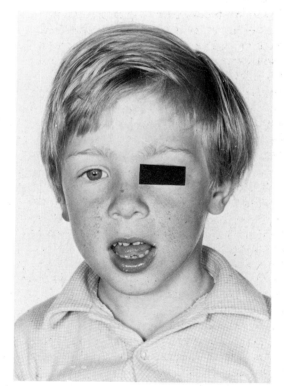

Fig. 20.2 Tuberous sclerosis. Adenoma sebaceum — 5-year-old boy

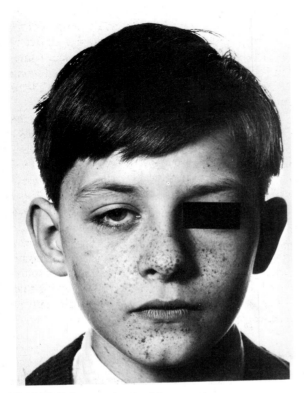

Fig. 20.3 Tuberous sclerosis. Adenoma sebaceum — more marked lesions in 11-year-old boy

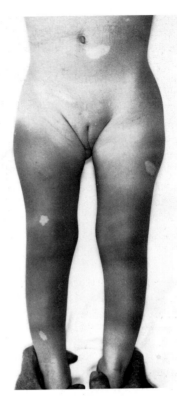

Fig. 20.4 Tuberous sclerosis. Amelanotic naevi in 2-year-old girl

be diagnostic until later (Figs. 20.2 and 20.3). It was present in 53% of cases by the age of 5 years and in 100% by 35 in one series (Bundey & Evans 1969). The lesions increase year by year and may become large, unsightly, wart-like protrusions. Microscopically they consist of an overgrowth of sebaceous glands, connective tissue and small blood vessels.

These lesions are diagnostic though occasional difficulty is found in distinguishing them from acne vulgaris in adolescents. In younger children adenoma sebaceum is either absent or insufficiently developed for reliance to be placed on it. The earliest skin lesions of tuberous sclerosis, which are diagnostic and present from infancy and perhaps from birth, are achromic or amelanotic naevi, pale leaf-shaped lesions in which pigmentation is absent so that they contrast with the normal surrounding darker skin (Gold & Freeman 1965, Crichton (Figs. 20.4, 20.5 and 20.6). [Histologically the naevi contain melanocytes but despite this little or

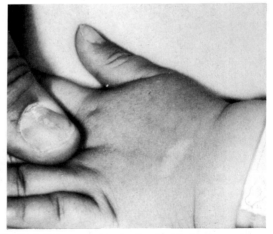

Fig. 20.5 Tuberous sclerosis. Amelanotic naevus on dorsum of L. hand. 16-month-old girl

no melanin is produced (Fitzpatrick et al 1968), suggesting a metabolic block]. They vary in size from 3 to 60 mm or more, and occur on the trunk and limbs and occasionally on the face. Mothers

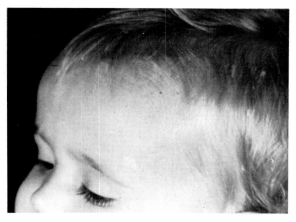

Fig. 20.6 Tuberous sclerosis. Amelanotic naevus on forehead. 16-month-old girl

examination fails to show them, a search should be made with ultraviolet light (Wood's lamp) before they can be considered absent. There is a tendency for the lesions to become darker with age, sometimes with a punctate appearance of brown dots on a white ground. The naevi must be distinguished from the scars of chicken pox or trauma.

Other rarer cutaneous signs of the disease are the 'shagreen patch' or 'peau de chagrin', a raised, irregular, rough area of skin usually over the lumbar region (Fig. 20.7) where it will be missed if the patient is not completely undressed) and the subungual fibroma, a fleshy outgrowth on a finger or toe made up of a mixture of fibrous and angiomatous tissue (Fig. 20.8) The latter is uncommon in children, but is a helpful sign of the disease in a parent of an affected child indicating classical dominant inheritance. *Café au lait* patches and vascular naevi are both commoner in tuberous sclerosis than in the general population, occurring in about 5% of cases, but are not diagnostic.

have often noticed these pale patches on their child's skin and have sometimes asked about them in the newborn period, only to be reassured that they were unimportant. More often they are first discovered later when the child is examined because of seizures or retardation. The lesions are more easily detected in white-skinned races during the summer months when they contrast more starkly with the adjacent sun-tanned skin. They must be looked for carefully and if a naked eye

Visceral abnormalities

The kidneys are affected in tuberous sclerosis more often than other viscera with an estimated frequency of 80%. Polycystic disease of the kidneys

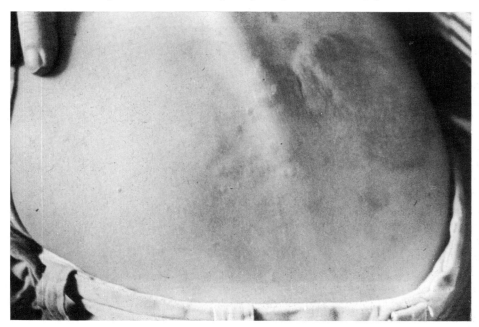

Fig. 20.7 Tuberous sclerosis. Shagreen patch in lumbar region — 12-year-old boy

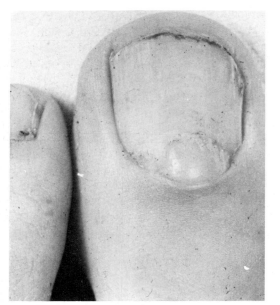

Fig. 20.8 Tuberous sclerosis. Subungual fibroma in mother of patient

is common, but adenoma, fibroma, myoma, lipoma, angioma and teratoma are also found. Cardiac lesions may be found with rhabdomyomata which may be solitary, multiple or diffuse.

Pulmonary involvement with numerous small cysts is seen more often in females than in males,

and may cause pneumothorax. Rarely the thyroid, liver, adrenal and other organs may contain hamartomas.

The neuropathology of tuberous sclerosis

The weight of the brain may be normal or moderately reduced. It is occasionally increased and tuberous sclerosis is a rare cause of megalencephaly. The pattern of convolutions over the cerebral hemispheres is usually normal, but may be altered by the presence of the 'tubers' or sclerotic patches which give the disease its name. Their pallor and hardness contrast with the surrounding convolutions. These lesions vary in size, seldom exceeding 20 mm in diameter but they show greatly increased numbers of astrocytic nuclei with scanty neurons whose lamination is disordered. Large, bizarre 'giant cells' may be found in the lesions and sometimes also in the cortex or white matter. Dense fibrillary gliosis is seen in the outer part of the molecular layer, particularly near the central parts of the tubers, and may also occur in the white matter. Calcification, varying in size from microscopic to massive 'brain stones' is often present in the tubers. Small subependymal tumour-like nodules are often seen projecting from the walls of the lateral ventricles into their cavities in a manner

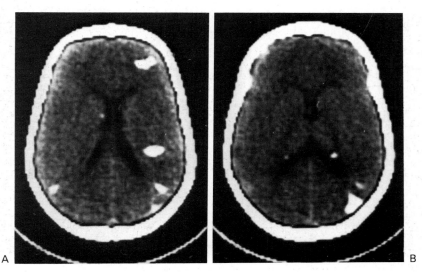

A   B

Fig. 20.9 Tuberous sclerosis in 8-year-old girl with mild retardation and seizures and a past history of infantile spasms. Her identical twin sister is similarly but more severely affected by the disease.
CT. Note (A) typical calcified nodule in wall of left anterior horn and several large parenchymal nodules, a less common feature of this condition, (B) the calcified nodules in the trigone are tubers and should not be confused with choroid plexus.

suggestive of 'candle guttering'. They are occasionally found in the cerebellum or brain-stem. Their diameter varies from that of a pinhead to a centimetre or more. They consist of collections of large round or oval cells mingled with fibrillary glial tissue and sometimes show calcification. Lesions near the foramen of Monro or mouth of the aqueduct of Sylvius may block these openings causing obstructive hydrocephalus. The retinal phakoma has a similar structure involving mainly the nerve cell layer of the retina. It may increase in size and sometimes disorganize the eye by doing so, but probably does not develop malignant change.

Radiological investigations

These are the most helpful form of investigation since demonstration of calcified lesions in the subependymal region or deeper in the brain sub-

stance will confirm the diagnosis in many cases in which the neurological and cutaneous features suggest it. Calcification is rarely visible on plain skull X-rays in very young children, but may be detected earlier by the CT scan (Fig. 20.9). Air-encephalography was formerly used to show the characteristic 'candle-guttering' protrusions into the lateral ventricles, (Fig. 20.10) but this is seldom necessary since CT scanning has become available. The finding of intracranial calcification in a parent of an affected child is helpful confirmation that the disease has been inherited in dominant fashion and not arisen as a new mutation. Intravenous pyelography is advisable in an affected child in a search for associated renal anomalies.

Genetic considerations

Tuberose sclerosis is classically inherited as an

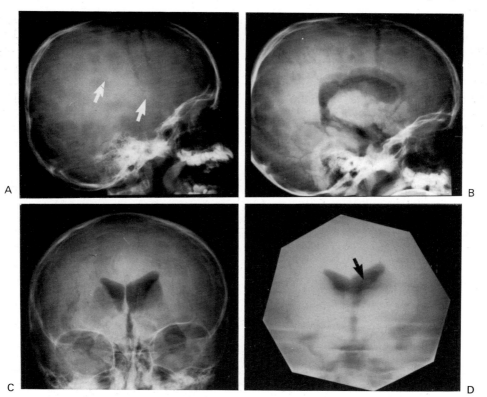

Fig. 20.10 Tuberose sclerosis in 6-year-old girl.
A. Lateral film of skull showing faintly calcified nodules (arrow).
B. Lateral film of encephalogram showing nodules projecting into the lateral ventricles.
C. Antero-posterior film of encephalogram showing two nodules in the left lateral ventricle.
D. Antero-posterior tomogram confirms the presence of the nodules in the left lateral ventricle.

autosomal dominant trait, but most cases are considered to be examples of new mutations since neither parent shows any evidence of the disease. An important study of 71 patients attending three London hospitals (Bundey & Evans 1969) showed affected relatives in an earlier generation in 10 families, while in the remaining 61 cases (86%) the parents showed no signs of the disorder, the condition being attributed to a new mutation. No family with two affected siblings was seen in this series without one parent having adenoma sebaceum, but a previous case was reported with a shagreen patch as the sole cutaneous manifestation in a man who had three children with probable tuberous sclerosis (Bundey et al 1970). For genetic counselling detailed examination of the skin of both parents is essential to detect heterozygotes. Inadequate examination has often led to reassurance being wrongly given to a parent who has later had another affected child. Parents should also be examined ophthalmoscopically for phakomata, and when possible by skull X-rays or CT scan for intracranial calcification, though these tests are unlikely to be positive when the skin is normal.

A remarkable exception to the general rule that an affected parent always shows stigmata of tuberous sclerosis is the recently reported case (Wilson & Carter 1978) of a family with two affected siblings both of whose parents were normal clinically and had normal CT scans.

NEUROFIBROMATOSIS (VON RECKLINGHAUSEN'S DISEASE) (Von Recklinghausen 1882)

The main features of this disorder are cutaneous pigmented lesions and multiple tumours arising from elements of the peripheral and central nervous system due to dysgenesis of the primitive ectoderm.

It is inherited as an autosomal dominant, and its incidence is difficult to determine accurately since estimates tend to be based on series biassed in favour of severe cases with gross cutaneous, neurological or orthopaedic complications. The many cases in which skin stigmata are the sole manifestation are largely overlooked except when identified during examination of relatives of an index case presenting with more serious problems. The criteria for the minimum cutaneous signs of the disease will also affect its apparent incidence. The characteristic café-au-lait patches are common in normal people, but when few in number are unlikely to be significant. Crowe et al (1956), from a careful statistical study, concluded that any person with more than six café-au-lait spots exceeding 1.5 cm in broadest diameter should be presumed to have neurofibromatosis. Whitehouse (1966) considered five or more spots necessary for the diagnosis. Crowe et al (1956) estimated the frequency to be between 1 in 2500 and 1 in 3000 births. A preponderance of males over females in a ratio of 2 : 1 has been noted in many series.

Cutaneous features

The café-au-lait patch, a light brown, macular pigmented lesion, is the hallmark of the disease (Fig. 20.11). These lesions may occur anywhere but

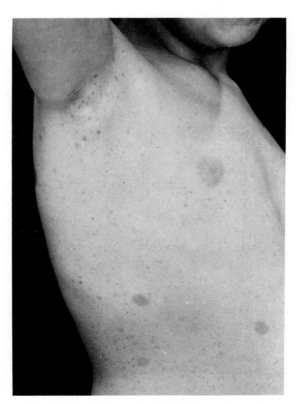

Fig. 20.11 Neurofibromatosis. Café au lait patches and axillary freckling in 11-year-old girl

are most numerous over the trunk. They are present from an early age but tend to increase in number with increasing years. Brown axillary 'freckling' (Fig. 20.11) is thought to be a useful early sign of neurofibromatosis (Crowe 1964). Cutaneous and subcutaneous tumours usually develop in later childhood, occurring in the distribution of cutaneous nerves, particularly on the trunk. Plexiform neurofibromas associated with localized hypertrophy of subcutaneous tissues seem commoner over the limbs. The tumours may increase in size and number with increasing age and in adults, but rarely in children, give rise to bizarre and unsightly 'elephantiasis' with enlargement of the trunk or extremities.

Neurological features

The varied neurological manifestations of the disease are mainly related to the effects of the various tumours, which may be intracranial or intraspinal in site or involve peripheral nerves. Rarely several sites may be involved. Other neurological features, the cause of which is less clear, are mental retardation, seizures and precocious puberty. Skeletal deformities such as scoliosis may cause secondary neurological dysfunction. The rare association noted between neurofibromatosis and cerebral vascular disease (Hilal et al 1971, Levisohn et al 1978) (Ch. 19) has been mentioned.

One of the most important associations in children is with optic pathway gliomas (Ch. 18). The finding of café-au-lait patches on the skin of a child with failing vision or unilateral nystagmus makes the diagnosis of an optic nerve or chiasma glioma very likely. Acoustic neuromas, tumours of the eighth nerve, though extremely common in adults with neurofibromatosis, are rare in children. The same is true of meningiomas, which are often multiple and associated with bilateral acoustic neuromas. The association between cerebral hemisphere gliomas and neurofibromatosis is also much commoner in adults than in children. However, a few families in which many members have neurofibromatosis and acoustic neuromas, unilateral or bilateral, have been recognized. Fabrikant and his colleagues (1979) reported three such kindreds with two or three generations affected. In most cases the acoustic neuroma presented after the age of 30 years, but in some the onset was at 16 or 17 years. One patient also suffered from a meningioma. Increased levels of a nerve-growth factor with low to normal function were found in these patients.

Plexiform neurofibromas of the fifth nerve are occasionally seen in children. They may distort the skull and sinuses and cause protrusion of the orbit (Fig. 20.12). A commoner abnormality seen in neurofibromatosis is a unilateral defect of the sphenoid bone, anterior clinoid process and occasionally sella turcica associated with enlargement of the middle cranial fossa and pulsating exophthalmos.

The association between cerebral hemisphere gliomas and neurofibromatosis, which is common in adults, is rarely seen in childhood.

Intraspinal tumours in children show a frequent association with neurofibromatosis and the presence of the skin lesions should suggest the diagnosis in any child with features of progressive spinal cord dysfunction. Delay in diagnosis is all too common with disastrous results for cord function. The skin stigmata may allow an early diagnosis to be made before cord compression has caused serious damage. Intraspinal neurofibromas occur at all levels of the cord, especially the thoracic region (Ch. 18). They may affect the cauda equina and may be multiple. The tumour often grows outwards from within the spinal canal through the intervertebral foramen as a 'dumb-bell' tumour. The clinical features are those of spinal cord compression with localizing signs of weakness and reflex changes at the level of the lesion and pyramidal and other long tract signs below it. Multiple tumours of the cauda equina give rise to pain, paralysis and loss of reflexes depending on the roots affected. Intramedullary neoplasms are also associated with neurofibromatosis: ependymomas and, less often, astrocytomas have been reported in this situation. Rarely syringomyelia has been seen in such cases. The radiological features of these varied lesions are similar to those seen in cases without neurofibromatosis.

Peripheral nerve involvement in von Recklinghausen's disease is uncommon in childhood; the ulnar and radial nerves are those most often affected.

Mental retardation occurs in neurofibromatosis

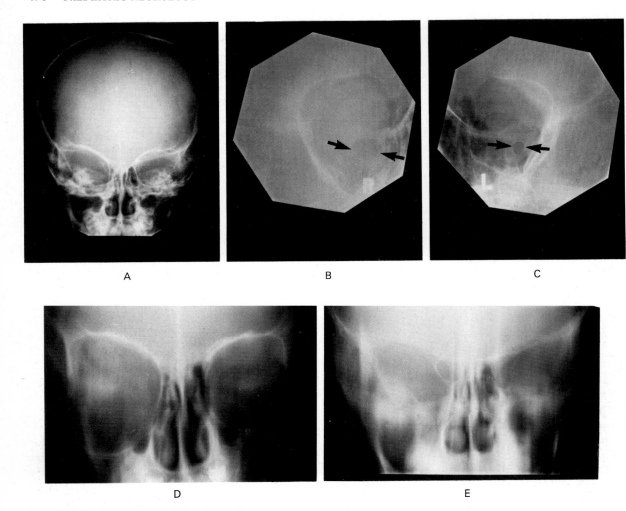

Fig. 20.12 Neurofibromatosis of right 5th nerve.
A. Postero-anterior film of the skull shows enlargement of the right orbit
B. Enlarged right optic foramen
C. Normal left optic foramen for comparison
D. Tomogram showing large right orbit
E. Tomogram showing lateral wall of the enlarged optic foramen.

with a much greater frequency than in the general population. It is usually mild to moderate in degree and non-progressive. Its exact cause is unclear and investigations seldom provide an explanation. Hamartomatous lesions and heterotopia of glia and neurons may be responsible. Mental deterioration in a child with neurofibromatosis should raise the suspicion of a cerebral glioma. Seizures, with or without retardation, are another association, for which an explanation is often not found on investigation. The possibility of a neoplasm or of pro-

gressive occlusive cerebral arterial disease (Moya Moya disease) (Ch. 19) should be considered.

Various bony lesions in neurofibromatosis may cause neurological dysfunction. A severe angular scoliosis due to dysplasia of vertebral bodies may cause spinal cord compression. Thoracic meningocoeles, usually without neurological deficit, are another association. A unilateral defect in the postero-superior wall of the orbit is also seen, presenting with a pulsating exophthalmos.

STURGE-WEBER SYNDROME (ENCEPHALOFACIAL OR ENCEPHALOTRIGEMINAL ANGIOMATOSIS)

In a report in 1879 of a patient with hemiplegia, epilepsy and a facial naevus flammeus, Sturge suggested that the neurological features would prove to be due to a similar naevoid condition affecting the brain. This was confirmed later when leptomeningeal angiomatosis and cortical calcification were shown radiologically and at operation. Weber, whose name is included in the eponymous title, suggested the descriptive term 'encephalofacial angiomatosis'.

The Sturge-Weber syndrome is a rare disorder, usually occurring sporadically, though dominant and recessively inherited cases are recorded. Both sexes and all races are affected, though cases are more easily overlooked in coloured patients and probably under-reported.

The naevus is congenital and allows the diagnosis to be made at birth. It affects the face, invariably involving its upper part over the forehead and usually also the cheek, side of the nose and upper lip in a distribution corresponding partially, but not completely, to that of the first and second divisions of the trigeminal nerve (Fig. 20.13). It is usually unilateral but bilateral distribution is commoner than is realised; it was present in one-third of 22 cases seen at the Hospital for Sick Children, Great Ormond Street (Boltshauser et al 1976) The medial border of the naevus may fall short of or cross the midline of the face. The philtrum of the upper lip is often spared. The eye and lip may be involved on the affected side. The naevus is flat and red,

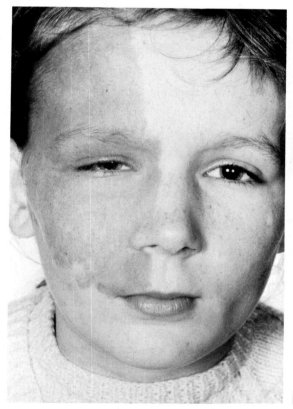
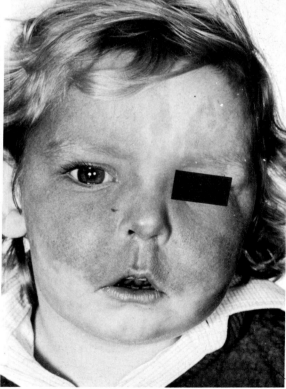

A

B

Fig. 20.13 Sturge-Weber syndrome
A. Unilateral facial naevus
B. Bilateral facial naevus

being sometimes described as port-wine in colour. It is usually easily distinguished by its distribution from other commoner types of red naevus. One theory explains it as due to a persistence of the primordial vascular plexus of the embryo, an arrangement of primitive blood vessels which is the earliest stage in the development of the arteries and veins of the head. At the stage of development when the primordial plexus appears the ectoderm which will later form the skin of the upper face overlies that part of the neural tube destined to form the occipital and adjacent parts of the cerebral cortex, the areas most often involved in the angiomatosis. Separation of the cutaneous and deep elements of the vascular malformation occurs as a result of later growth of the cerebral hemispheres. Occasionally flame-like naevi are present over the trunk and limbs as well as the face. Very rarely cases are seen with the typical radiological and neurological features of the syndrome, but without a facial naevus.

Neurological features

The main neurological features of the syndrome are those common to all cerebral abnormalities of early onset — seizures, developmental retardation and cerebral palsy, in the form of a spastic hemiplegia. Convulsions are usually the earliest neurological symptom, and are rarely absent. They commonly begin in the first year of life, often in the newborn period, and seldom later than two years of age. They are often abrupt and catastrophic in onset and the child may suffer a severe setback in his development after the first episode. A hemiplegia may be detected for the first time after the onset of seizures and may progressively worsen after each subsequent bout. The fits are commonly unilateral and contralateral to the naevus but may become generalized. A visual aura is surprisingly rare, despite the frequent involvement of the occipital lobe and the common finding of a hemianopia. The seizures may prove intractable with frequent status epilepticus, and progressive deterioration is common in such cases. Mental retardation becomes more obvious as time passes and as fits recur, and the hemiplegia may also become more severe. The reasons for this worsening are not absolutely clear but may be due in part to the effects of the seizures

themselves. The cyanosed appearance of the angiomatous vessels noted at operation in one child (Alexander & Norman 1960) suggests that the greatly increased oxygen and energy requirements of discharging neurons during seizures cannot be met. Localized hypoxia may well explain the necrosis of laminar distribution found in the cortex. Areas of electrical silence may be shown by the EEG over the affected lobe or lobes, and electrocorticography shows circumscribed areas of low potential.

Ophthalmological features

Raised intra-ocular tension is found in about one-third of cases of the Sturge-Weber syndrome with buphthalmos, probably due to an antenatal rise of tension within the globe, and glaucoma. This aspect of the disease is easily overlooked and needs attention to prevent visual impairment.

A homonymous hemianopic field defect is very common, though often missed.

Radiological findings

The pathognomonic X-ray feature is intracranial calcification with a double contour, like a railway-line, showing a gyriform distribution. This is commonest in the occipital and parietal regions. It is not visible on plain skull X-rays in early life but becomes detectable and denser at later ages (Fig. 20.14). It can be shown earlier by the use of the CT scan (Fig. 20.15 and 20.16). The calcification lies in the outer part of the cortex. It is usually unilateral on the side of the naevus, but 21 cases have now been reported with bilateral calcification. In 4 recently reported cases (Boltshauser et al 1976), the naevus was bilateral in two. Microcephaly developed in three of these children suggesting that this may be a useful sign of bilateral cerebral involvement.

Atrophy of an affected hemisphere may be suggested by the finding of a smaller hemicranium on one side, with an enlarged frontal sinus and mastoid, and confirmed by air encephalography or CT scan. Carotid arteriography may show slowing of circulation in the angiomatous vessels.

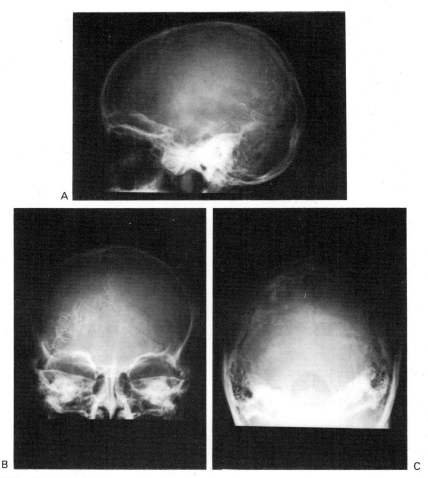

Fig. 20.14 Sturge Weber Syndrome in 8 year old girl.
Skull films A. Lateral view
      B. P.A. view
      C. Half-axial view
Calcification characteristic of this condition is present in the right parieto-occipital region. It consists of parallel lines in the configuration of gyri. Note hemiatrophy of the skull

Pathological findings

The affected hemisphere is often atrophic and shows areas of leptomeningeal angiomatosis most often over the occipital lobe but sometimes over the temporal and parietal regions. The vessels in these areas are closely packed and thin-walled, and densest in the sulci. Intracerebral calcification is seen with several different patterns: concretions are seen in the outer cortical layers, the larger lumps of calcium being more superficial, and this produces the gyriform calcification seen on X-rays. 'Droplet' incrustation of the smaller blood vessels is also seen. The calcium is mainly in the form of phosphate and carbonate. The iron content of affected cortex was not increased in five lobectomy specimens studied by Alexander & Norman (1960).

Treatment

This is largely symptomatic with drug treatment for epilepsy, appropriate education and physio-

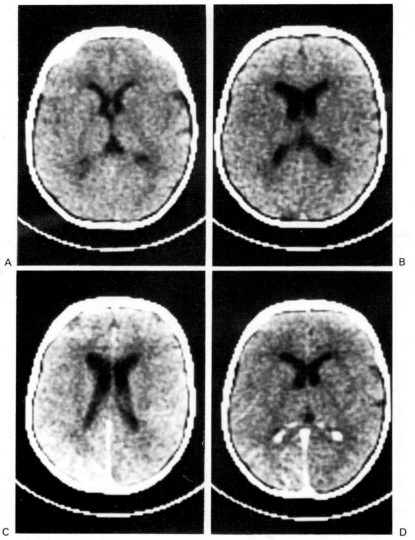

Fig. 20.15 Sturge-Weber syndrome in 8-month-old boy. CT pre-contrast scans (A and B) show no calcification or hemiatrophy and no focal tissue abnormality. Post-contrast scans (C and D) show linear enhancement in the cortex and white matter of left temporo-parieto-occipital region due to telangiectasia. Such appearances usually disappear when calcification appears

therapy and orthopaedic management for the hemi-plegia.

The progressive deterioration, often in associa-tion with seizures, makes their prevention a matter of great importance. Unfortunately, they are often very difficult to control. For this reason a surgical approach with lobectomy was favoured in the past in the hope of preventing deterioration and this may still be justified in selected cases, though improvements in anticonvulsant drugs and moni-toring of drug levels have made it less often

necessary than before. Surgery should not be considered in cases with bilateral hemisphere involvement.

INCONTINENTIA PIGMENTI (BLOCH-SULZBERGER SYNDROME)

This rare disease is confined almost exclusively to females and combines distinctive skin lesions with neurological and ocular features. Though rare, it

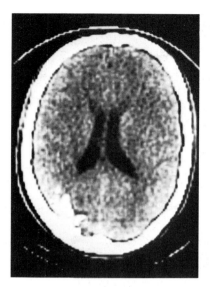

Fig. 20.16 Sturge-Weber syndrome in 15-year-old boy. CT shows calcification in left parietal cortex extending down into the sulci. There was no enhancement with contrast

is probably commoner than reports would suggest since the fading of the skin lesions with increasing age removes an important diagnostic clue.

Skin features

Erythematous and bullous lesions are present at birth or appear in the first weeks of life, being most marked on the trunk and limbs. The fluid in the bullae contains many eosinophils and the peripheral blood also shows an eosinophilia in early infancy. Rupture and crusting of the bullae occur and are followed later by the characteristic pigmentation. Brown lesions are seen distributed as if splashed onto the skin with a paint-brush. These lesions gradually fade, clearing completely by the end of the second decade. The older child may show only a few remnants of the naevi (Fig. 20.17) and her mother usually shows none at all, though she often remembers having many lesions as a

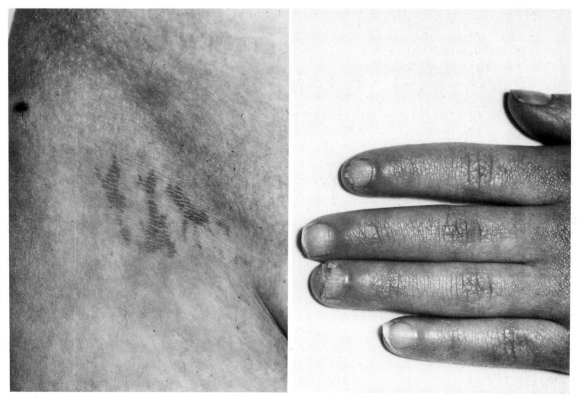

A

B

Fig. 20.17 Incontinentia pigmenti (A) residual naevus in groin; (B) dystrophic fingernails

child. Histologically the skin shows breaches in the basement membrane with melanin granules in the dermis, whence the fanciful name 'incontinentia pigmenti'. The finger and toe nails, teeth and hair may show dystrophic changes. It seems likely that all these ectodermal abnormalities develop in the second trimester of gestation.

Neurological aspects

Neurological features occur in 30 to 40% of cases and include spasticity, with hemiplegia or tetraplegia, developmental retardation and seizures. Spastic cerebral palsy was found in 15 of the 145 cases reviewed by Pfeiffer (1959). Fits may occur in the newborn period when the prognosis for development is worse. The degree of mental retardation may be severe and associated with microcephaly, moderate or mild. Some patients are of normal intelligence. The condition is not progressive, although children with intractable seizures may show some deterioration in function.

Ocular features

Ocular abnormalities are found in about 30% of affected girls. They include a mass in the posterior chamber, which may suggest a glioma or retrolental fibroplasia, but which is not malignant. In the first reported patient of Bloch the right eye was enucleated at one month of age, presumably on suspicion of a malignant neoplasm. It is clearly important to recognize these lesions for what they are, as with the phakomata of tuberose sclerosis.

Neuropathological findings

In the case of O'Doherty & Norman (1968), a severely affected girl who died of pneumonia aged seven weeks, the left cerebral hemisphere showed micropolygyria and areas of focal necrosis, and the brainstem an abnormally small left medullary pyramid.

Treatment is symptomatic. The severe early skin lesions may be controlled by cortical steroids. Anticonvulsants, physiotherapy and orthopaedic management are needed for the seizures and cerebral palsy.

Genetics

The overwhelming predominance of affected females in pedigrees and evidence of previous skin lesions in their mothers may be explained by X-linked dominant inheritance with lethality in the affected male who suffers spontaneous abortion or dies very early in pregnancy. The genetic implications make early diagnosis very important.

The disease is very unusual in the behaviour of the skin lesions which disappear with age, rather than persisting or increasing as in the other neurocutaneous syndromes. If the patient's mother does not remember her own earlier skin lesions and if there is no affected *younger* sister to show more impressive naevi, it is easy to overlook the significance of scanty residual skin lesions in a girl.

A similarly named but different neurocutaneous syndrome has been reported by Ito (1952) as 'incontinentia pigmenti achromians' with areas of cutaneous hypopigmentation which may increase with age. Neurological symptoms may occur but the disorder is quite distinct from incontinentia pigmenti as described above, in that it affects males and females alike and does not show melanin in the dermis. For these reasons, it seems appropriate to use another name and the term 'hypomelanosis of Ito' has been suggested (Jelinek et al 1973).

THE SJÖGREN-LARSSON SYNDROME

This recessively inherited syndrome combines ichthyosis with mental retardation and spastic paralysis. Sjögren and Larsson estimated its incidence as one in 10 000 births in the area of northern Sweden in which their 28 cases were found. These 28 patients represented 14 siblings and the consanguinity rate in their families was high.

The cutaneous hallmark is ichthyosis, which is usually congenital and is known as congenital ichthyosiform erythrodermia. Hyperkeratosis and scaling of the skin are widespread over the trunk and limbs and may involve the hands and feet. Facial lesions are usually mild. The skin is thick and patterned like leather, often with a 'fish-scale' appearance.

The neurological features are mental retardation which seems invariable and is often severe, and spastic diplegia with symmetrical involvement of both sides more marked in the legs than the arms. In about 75% of reported cases walking has been impossible without support and many patients are chair- or bed-bound. Seizures of various kinds are common. Pigmentary degeneration in the macular region occurs in about 25% of patients.

The main neuropathological features noted in the few autopsied cases are degeneration and loss of neurons in the cortex and basal ganglia, demyelination in cerebral white matter, corticospinal and vestibulospinal tracts and Purkinje cell loss with focal atrophy in the cerebellum.

KLIPPEL-TRENAUNAY SYNDROME (HAEMANGIECTATIC HYPERTROPHY OF A LIMB)

In this disorder a complex angiomatous malformation is present over a limb or part of it, associated with hypertrophy of the affected part. Vascular effects include ischaemic ulcers and, rarely, cardiac failure if the malformation is very large. Mental retardation is relatively common in this syndrome which has affinities with the Sturge-Weber syndrome, thought distinct from it. A few patients have been reported who were thought to have features of both conditions. One such patient also had hydrocephalus (Meyer 1979).

LINEAR NEVUS SEBACEUS (FEUERSTEIN'S SYNDROME)

A sebaceous naevus with yellow nodules over the face or scalp was recognized in the late nineteenth century by Jadassohn. Later the triad of a linear midline sebaceous naevus with mental retardation and seizures was recognized by Feuerstein & Mims (1962). Further cases have since been reported of this combination which seems to represent a distinct neurocutaneous syndrome affecting both sexes equally and without a familial incidence. Seizures, which may begin in the newborn period and usually under one year of age, are of various kinds

including grand mal, Jacksonian attacks and infantile spasms (Lovejoy & Boyle 1973). A child with the triad of naevus sebaceus, retardation and salaam seizures with the additional features of a staphyloma of the eye, an enlarged clitoris and a cardiac arrhythmia was reported by Tripp (1971), who suggested that this enlarged syndrome should be called 'the skin, eye, brain and heart syndrome'. Hemimacrocephaly was present at birth in an infant delivered by Caesarian section because of cephalopelvic disproportion who developed seizures on the fourth day of life and had an extensive midline naevus sebaceus (Boltshauser & Navratil 1978).

PROGRESSIVE HEMIFACIAL ATROPHY (PARRY-ROMBERG SYNDROME)

Unilateral progressive atrophy of the superficial

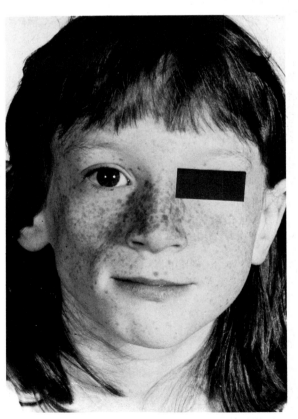

Fig. 20.18 Parry-Romberg syndrome. 10-year-old girl with hemificial atrophy on right

facial tissues (subcutaneous and fatty tissue, muscle and sometimes cartilage and bone) is the hallmark of this rare and disfiguring malady of unknown aetiology (Fig. 20.18). Though of principal importance to cosmetic surgeons, it is associated with neurological symptoms in up to 15% of cases and thus deserves inclusion in a survey of the neurocutaneous syndromes. It is non-genetic and affects both sexes with a female to male ratio of 3 to 2. Good reviews are given by Rogers (1963) and Poskanzer (1975).

Facial features

The hemifacial atrophy usually begins in the first or second decade with a progressive course of between two and ten years after which it seems to reach a plateau. The final state may be of mild or severe atrophy. In a few cases the atrophy is bilateral (39 of the 772 cases in Rogers' series, 1963). Atrophy usually starts at a focal point of the face or head, often with a small area of increased or decreased pigmentation. Discolouration or depigmentation of the hair on the scalp or face may precede other features, and alopecia is also seen. The disorder does not progress indefinitely and does not lead to complete atrophy of the tissues. The grossest degree of atrophy is sometimes called 'coup de sabre' a term originally applied to severe scleroderma of one side of the face, from its resemblance to the scar that might result from a sabre cut. The atrophy is paramedian in its origin and development, not extending to the midline but starting about two finger breadths lateral and parallel to the median (Wartenberg 1945). Intervention by the plastic surgeon cosmetically to improve the facial appearance must be deferred until the atrophy has ceased to progress.

Neurological features

Cerebral symptoms are present in about one in six patients, mainly convulsions and mental retardation. A girl reported by Wartenberg (1945) had the onset of right-sided facial atrophy at the age of seven years and developed left-sided sensory and motor Jacksonian attacks and generalized convulsions at 15 with mild left-sided spastic paralysis. A boy who developed right-sided atrophy at ten years of age later developed Jacksonian fits in the opposite arm. Cerebral calcification was reported in two children with progressive facial hemiatrophy (Merritt et al 1937), one of whom had fits from the age of three with scleroderma 'en coup de sabre' on her forehead and face.

NEUROCUTANEOUS MELANOSIS

Malignant melanoma of the leptomeninges is occasionally associated with giant benign hairy naevi and this syndrome is known as neurocutaneous melanosis. In the case of a 14-month-old boy with a short history of vomiting and evidence of hydrocephalus the initial clinical and radiological diagnosis was aqueduct stenosis (Harper & Thomas 1974). The child died soon after insertion of a shunt and at autopsy the meninges were thickened and opaque. Histologically the subarachnoid space was diffusely infiltrated by tumour with features typical of malignant melanoma. Where invasion of neural tissue had occurred there was a distinctive perivascular arrangement of the melanoma cells. The cutaneous lesions were regarded as benign and no primary tumour or visceral metastases were found.

REFERENCES

Alexander G L, Norman R M 1960 The Sturge-Weber syndrome. John Wright and Son, Bristol
Boltshauser E, Navratil F 1978 Organoid nevus syndrome in a neonate with hemimicrocephaly. Neuropädiatrie 9: 195–196
Boltshauser E, Wilson J, Hoare R D 1976 Sturge-Weber syndrome with bilateral intracranial calcification. Journal of Neurology, Neurosurgery and Psychiatry 39: 429–435

Bourneville D M 1880 Contribution à l'étude de l'idiotie-sclérose tubéreuse des circonvolutions cérébrales: idiotie et épilepsie hémiplegique. Archives de Neurologie 1: 69–91, 670, 671
Bundey S E, Dutton G, Wells R S 1970 Tuberose sclerosis without adenoma sebaceum. Journal of Mental Deficiency Research 14: 243

Bundey S, Evans K 1969 Tuberose sclerosis: a genetic study. Journal of Neurology, Neurosurgery and Psychiatry 32: 591–603

Crichton J U 1966 Infantile spasms and skin anomalies. Developmental Medicine and Child Neurology 8: 273–278

Crowe F W 1964 Axillary freckling as a diagnostic aid in neurofibromatosis. Annals of Internal Medicine 61: 1142–1143

Crowe F W, Schull W J, Neil J W 1956 A clinical, pathological and genetic study of multiple neurofibromatosis. C C Thomas, Springfield, Illinois

Fabricant R N, Todaro G, Eldridge R 1979 Increased levels of a nerve-growth-factor cross-reacting protein in 'central' neurofibromatosis. Lancet 1: 4–7

Feuerstein R C, Mims L C 1962 Linear nevus sebaceus with convulsions and mental retardation. American Journal of Diseases of Childhood 104: 675–679

Fitzpatrick T B, Szabo G, Hori Y, Simone A A, Reed W B, Greenberg M H 1968 White leaf-shaped macules. Archives of Dermatology 98: 1–6

Gold A P, Freeman J M 1965 Depigmented nevi, the earliest sign of tuberous sclerosis. Pediatrics 35: 1003–1005

Gomez M R (ed) 1979 Tuberous sclerosis. Raven Press, New York

Harper C G, Thomas D G T 1974 Neurocutaneous melanosis. Journal of Neurology, Neurosurgery and Psychiatry 37: 760–763

Hilal S K, Solomon G E, Gold A P, Carter S 1971 Primary cerebral arterial occlusive disease in children. II. Neurocutaneous syndromes. Radiology 99: 87

Ito M 1952 Studies on melanin. XI. Incontinentia pigmenti achromians, a singular case of nevus depigmentosus systematicus bilateralis. Tohoku Journal of Experimental Medicine 55: (suppl.) 57

Jelinek J E, Bart R S, Schiff G M 1973 Hypomelanosis of Ito ('incontinentia pigmenti archromians'). Archives of Dermatology 107: 596

Levisohn P M, Mikhael M A, Rothman S M 1978 Cerebrovascular changes in neurofibromatosis. Developmental Medicine and Child Neurology 20: 789–793

Merritt K K, Faber H K, Bruch H 1937 Progressive facial hemiatrophy. A report of two cases with cerebral calcification. Journal of Pediatrics 10: 374–395

Meyer E 1979 Neurocutaneous syndrome with excessive macro-hydrocephalus (Sturge-Weber/Klippel-Trenaunay syndrome). Neuropädiatrie 10: 67–75

O'Doherty N J, Norman R M 1968 Incontinentia pigmenti (Bloch-Sulzberger syndrome) with cerebral malformation. Developmental Medicine and Child Neurology 10: 168–174

Pampiglione G, Moynahan E 1976 Tuberous sclerosis syndrome: clinical and EEG studies in 100 children. Journal of Neurology, Neurosurgery and Psychiatry 39: 666–673

Pfeiffer R A 1959 Das Syndrom Der Incontinentia Pigmenti Bloch-Siemens. Munchener Medizinische Wochenschrift 101: 2312

Poskanzer D C 1975 Progressive hemifacial atrophy (Romberg's Disease) In: Vinken P J, Bruyn G W (eds) Handbook of Clinical Neurology. North Holland Publishing Company, Amsterdam, American Elsevier, New York, vol 22

Recklinghausen F von 1882 Über die Multiplen Fibrome der Haut und Ihre Beziehung zu den Multiplen Neuromen. Hirschwald, Berlin

Rogers B O 1963 Progressive facial hemiatrophy: Romberg's disease. A review of 772 cases. Proc. 3rd Internat. Congr. Plastic Surgery. Amsterdam, Excerpta Medica 105 (66): 681–689

Sjögren T, Larsson T 1957 Oligophrenia in combination with icthyosis. Acta psychiatrica scandinavica 32 (suppl 113): 1–108

Smith D 1976 Recognizable patterns of human malformation, Vol VII in series: Major Problems in Clinical Pediatrics. W B Saunders, Philadelphia

Sturge W A 1879 A case of partial epilepsy, apparently due to a lesion of the vaso-motor centres of the brain, Transactions of the Clinical Society of London 12: 162

Tripp J H 1971 A new 'neurocutaneous' syndrome (skin, eye, brain and heart syndrome). Proceedings of the Royal Society of Medicine 64: 23–24

Tsuchida T, Kamata K, Kawamata M, Okada K, Tanaka R, Oyaka Y 1981 Brain tumors in tuberous sclerosis. Report of 4 cases. Child's Brain 8: 271–283

Van der Hoeve J 1923 Eye diseases in tuberous sclerosis of the brain and in Recklinghausen disease. Transactions of the Ophthalmological Society of the United Kingdom 43: 534–540

Vinken P J, Bruyn G W (ed) 1972 The phakomatoses. Handbook of clinical neurology. North Holland, Amsterdam, American Elsevier, New York, vol 14

Wartenberg R 1945 Progressive facial hemiatrophy. Archives of Neurology and Psychiatry 54: 75–96

Whitehouse D 1966 Diagnostic value of the café-au-lait spot in children. Archives of Disease in Childhood 41: 316–319

Wilson J, Carter J 1978 Genetics of tuberose sclerosis. Lancet 1: 340 (letter)

21

Genetics in relation to neurological disorders

C. O. Carter

There are four types of genetic determination of neurological disease: excess or deficiency of one or more chromosomes; gene mutations; an accumulation of minor genetic variation leading to genetic predisposition to develop malformation or disease; maternal-fetal genetic incompatibility. The fourth type is of largely historic interest since the occurrence of kernicterus due to Rhesus incompatibility may now be prevented.

CHROMOSOMAL ANOMALIES

Chromosomal anomalies are conveniently classified into autosomal, that is involving chromosomes 1 to 22, and sex-chromosomal. The two sources of chromosomal anomaly are: non-disjunction, a failure of a pair of chromosomes to separate at the reduction division in gamete formation leading to the presence of an extra chromosome, called trisomy (for example trisomy 21), or the absence of a chromosome, called monosomy; and breakages leading to a balanced exchange of chromosomal material or partial trisomy or monosomy.

Autosomal anomalies

It is a general characteristic of autosomal anomalies that they affect brain development and cause mental retardation as well as causing multiple physical abnormalities. This is to be expected as even a partial trisomy will result in the presence of many gene loci in triplicate and a dosage effect of many of these, with perhaps a 50% increase in the gene product and hence a disturbance of many metabolic processes. Conversely monosomy will lead to a per-

haps 50% reduction in the level of the gene products with an even greater disturbance in many metabolic processes.

Most autosomal anomalies cause miscarriage and only three complete autosomal trisomies commonly come to term, those of 21, 18 and 13. The frequency of trisomy 21 (Down's syndrome) at birth is about 1 in 700 and of the other two substantially less, about 1 in 10 000. About two thirds of patients with trisomy 21 now survive to school age and constitute about a third of all severely subnormal children in that age-group. The more severe anomalies associated with trisomy 18 (Edward syndrome) and 13 (Patau syndrome) usually lead to death in infancy. Complete autosomal monosomies almost always lead to miscarriage. A few examples of monosomy 21 in live births have been reported but the patients have died in infancy. Among syndromes associated with partial monosomies are those of the short arm of 5 (cri-du-chat syndrome), the short arm of 4, the long arm of 13, the short arm of 18, the long arm of 18 (De Grouchy & Turleau 1977). Some partial trisomies are also well delineated, for example of the short arm of chromosome 9 (De Grouchy & Turleau 1977). The approximate birth frequency of autosomal anomalies in live births is summarised in Table 21.1 (Carter 1957a).

Table 21.1 Autosomal anomalies in live-born per 1000 births

Trisomy 21	1.4
Trisomy 18	0.1
Trisomy 13	0.05
Other	0.05
Unbalanced structural	0.5

Prevention and genetic counselling

The primary prevention of autosomal anomalies, that is by the prevention of non-disjunction and chromosome breakage, is not in sight. Secondary prevention, by the offer of screening for the presence of chromosomal anomaly in the fetus, by culture of amniotic cells followed by the offer of abortion, is already practicable in high risk pregnancies. Such pregnancies include those at relatively late maternal age and those where the mother has already had one trisomic child. The risk of trisomy 21 in births to mothers aged 40 years and over is at least 1%, and about a third of all children with trisomy 21 are born to mothers over 35 of age. Also those where a mother has had one child with trisomy 21. For them the recurrence risk is about 1%, probably irrespective of their age. Where a translocation of autosomes is involved, there will be a relatively high risk of a partial trisomy or monosomy in children and a strong indication for amniocentesis. For example where a mother has a translocation between the long arm of 14 and 21 the loss of the minute short arms of these two chromosomes appears to cause no clinical abnormality; but she has a risk of transmitting the conjoined 14/21 chromosome as well as her normal 21 and so having a child with effective trisomy 21. In practice the risk appears to be about 1 in 10, and perhaps about 1 in 20 where the father has the translocation.

Sex-chromosomal anomalies

Anomalies of the sex-chromosomes have substantially smaller effects on development, including that of the brain, than do anomalies of the autosomes. The two reasons for this are that the small Y chromosome appears to have no genes on it, apart from a masculinising gene or genes, and that any X chromosome in excess of one becomes inactive early in fetal life.

The approximate birth frequency of sex chromosomal trisomies is summarised in Table 21.2 (Carter 1977a).

The low birth frequency of monosomy of the sex chromosomes, XO, depends on the fact that more than 95% of fetuses with this genotype abort. Those that are live born have Turner's syndrome. The intelligence distribution of these girls is near normal, though they probably have a tendency to reduced performance on tests of visuospatial ability. The sex-chromosomal trisomies on the other hand do not tend to miscarry and hence have relatively high birth frequencies. The girls with XXX genotype probably have a shift of distribution of intelligence quotient about 10 points to the left, with a mean of about 90 points; but only a minority are mentally retarded. The boys with the XXY genotype (Klinefelter syndrome) have a similar lowering of mean intelligence quotient and also an increased likelihood of behaviour disorders. This may however be a secondary effect of the testicular hypoplasia and preventable by androgenic therapy. The boys with the XYY genotype have a tendency to behaviour disorder which is not yet fully evaluated. About 2% of men in hospitals for the criminally insane are found to have two Y chromosomes, and this is about 20 times the birth frequency of the condition. There is a smaller increase among the inmates of ordinary prisons. This increase would appear to depend in part on a shift to the left of the distribution of intelligence quotient, associated with an undue degree of impulsiveness and disregard for the likely consequences of their actions. Structural anomalies of the sex-chromosomes may give rise to partial trisomies and monosomies. Mosaicism is common with sex-chromosome anomalies, for example XY/XXY, XO/XX, or even XO/XX/XXX.

Prevention and genetic counselling

The frequency of the XXX and XXY genotype, but not the XYY, is influenced by maternal age and so screening at late maternal age will detect them

Table 21.2 Sex-chromosomal anomalies in live-born per 1000 births

Male	
XYY	1.0
XXY	1.0
Mosaics	0.5
Female	
XXX	0.6
XO	0.05
Mosaics	0.2

as well as the autosomal trisomies. This raises difficult questions of ethics. The best procedure is probably for the physician to inform the parents of the finding and to give them as accurate a picture as he can of the prognosis for the child, so that they may make their own decision on termination. Current follow-up studies of children with sex-chromosomal anomalies detected at birth will improve knowledge of the prognosis. No large scale studies are available to give an empirical recurrence figure after the birth of a child with sex-chromosomal anomalies, but the risk is probably not high. The children of patients with XXX and XXY genotype appear to be usually normal, while men with the XXY and women with the XO genotypes are sterile.

An interesting recent discovery is that in about one third of the families in which there are mentally retarded males in an X-linked pattern of inheritance the patients have a characteristic fragile site at the bottom end of the long arm of their X chromosome (Turner & Opitz 1980). This is seen in 20 to 40% of cells when the lymphocytes are cultured in a folic acid deficient medium. The IQ of these boys is variable from severely retarded to merely dull. A macroorchidism is usually obvious after puberty. Other features often present are a moderately enlarged skull in childhood, but not in adult life, a prominent jaw, a prominent forehead and some midfacial hypoplasia. Females heterozygous for this X-chromosome may be intellectually retarded though to a lesser degree. The frequency of this condition is not yet established, but it may account for up to 10% of severe mental retardation in males.

MONOGENIC DISORDERS

Two main types of genes are recognised: (a) structural genes whose function is to produce specific proteins or parts of specific proteins (for example the α and β peptides of the haemoglobin molecule); (b) regulator genes whose activity controls the activity of one or more structural genes. All genes are present in every cell in the body, but in the course of tissue differentiation individual genes are switched on and off. At birth most tissues have their own specific pattern of actively functioning

structural genes. A mutation of a structural gene may result in the production of an altered protein, with perhaps altered or reduced function, or of a reduced amount of normal protein. Mutation of genes whose function is to regulate the activity of structural genes might in theory influence the activity of several structural genes, but no clear example of this is known in human genetics.

It is a useful generalisation that: where a mutant gene is dominant, in the sense that it produces a significant clinical effect in those heterozygous for the gene, then the product of the gene is likely to be a protein concerned in structure, for example collagen or a cell-membrane protein; where a mutant gene is recessive, in the sense of producing no significant clinical effect in the heterozygote but only in homozygotes, the protein product of the gene is usually an enzyme. A mixture of normal and abnormal structural protein is likely to be functionally inefficient. In contrast, since enzymes are highly active, a loss of 50% of the normal amount of enzyme is likely to disturb function only if the enzyme system is put under stress (for example as in the phenylalanine loading test for heterozygotes for the gene for phenylketonuria). Since less is known of the chemistry of structural proteins than of enzymes the precise biochemical defect is known in few dominant disorders, but in many recessive inborn errors of metabolism. X-linked mutant genes will be expressed in hemizygous males, with their single X-chromosome; but may or may not produce a clinical effect in heterozygous females, where there is one normal gene functioning at the relevant gene locus. The majority of biochemical syntheses involve several steps and it is not unexpected that dominant, recessive and even X-linked forms of a disease may occur and also that there may be more than one recessive form. These different forms may depend on enzyme defects of closely related steps in a synthesis, as in Sanfilippo A and B disease; different mutations at the same gene locus, as in the Hurler and Scheie variants of mucopolsaccharidoses; defects in the enzyme or of a co-factor as in classical phenylketonuria and the variant which does not respond to a diet low in phenylalanine.

In contrast to chromosomal non-disjunction and structural changes of chromosomes, gene mutations are rare events. Typical mutation rates expressed as mutations per individual gene locus per generation tend to be between 1 in 100 000 and 1 in 1 000 000. In the case of serious diseases which substantially reduce reproductive fitness it is to be expected that the birth frequency of the disease will be some small multiple of the mutation rate. The theoretical birth frequencies in a 'population in equilibrium' where M is the mutation rate, and the reproductive fitness of those with the disease is nil, are for dominant 2M, for recessives M, and for X-linked conditions $1\frac{1}{2}$M (or 3M in males). With dominants the relationship is direct, with X-linked conditions fairly direct. But with recessives the mutant gene may be transmitted for many generations in heterozygotes before it affects a homozygote, so that there is scope for much departure from the theoretical equilibrium. Where reproductive fitness is not zero, but a fraction represented by 'f', then the expressions for birth frequency at equilibrium become $\frac{2M}{1-f}$, $\frac{M}{1-f}$, $\frac{1\frac{1}{2}M}{1-f}$, for dominants, recessives and X-linked recessives respectively. In practice 'f' is at or near zero for most recessive and X-linked conditions. It is only those dominants which may on occasion have relatively mild clinical effects, for example neurofibromatosis, and those which often have late onset, for example Huntington's chorea which have a significant degree of reproductive fitness.

Dominant conditons

There are a large variety of dominant conditions affecting the central nervous system. Some of the best known, because most frequent, are listed in Table 21.3 with the estimated frequency per thousand births (Carter 1977b). The higher the reproductive fitness of those affected the more generations on average each mutant gene will persist and the expression B (birth frequency) = $\frac{2M}{1-f}$ may also be written B = 2pM where p is the mean persistence in generations of the mutant gene. Where reproductive fitness is $\frac{1}{2}$, about half the patients will be sporadic cases, about a quarter will involve 2 generations, and about a quarter will involve 3 or more generations. In a consecutive series of cases of tuberose sclerosis (Bundey & Evans 1969) 61 out of 71 (86%) appeared to be affected as a result of fresh mutation.

Table 21.3 Estimates of birth frequencies of some more common dominants affecting the nervous system in European-derived populations per 1000 live-births

Huntington's chorea	0.5
Neurofibromatosis	0.4
Myotonic dystrophy	0.2
Dominant form of congenital deafness	0.1
Dominant form of childhood onset blindness	0.1

A general feature of dominant conditions is that they show considerable variation in age of onset and severity. Dystrophia myotonica may have an onset in childhood and, though rarely, so may Huntington's chorea. Where this variation is mostly between families it is likely to be due to different mutant genes, perhaps at different, perhaps at the same gene locus. Where the variation is mostly within families different mutant genes will rarely be involved, and the most plausible suggestion is that such variation may depend on polymorphism at that gene locus, that is that there are several alternative 'normal' alleles at that gene locus, and the balance between mutant gene and 'normal' gene differs according to which allele is present in the individual heterozygote. It is noteworthy that when a parent passes a dominant mutant gene on to a child he is excluded from transmitting the normal allele on the other chromosome. In the case of dystrophia myotonica analysis of age of onset suggests that there are at least two mutant genes involved; one causing onset between 0 and 20 years, the other onset from 20 years (Bundey 1972); though the particularly early onset of some cases has led to the suggestion of some direct intrauterine influence from the mother (Harper 1975) on some of the fetuses that carry the gene.

Prevention and genetic counselling

No method is yet know of reducing the frequency of gene mutation below the natural level. Cases due to fresh mutation are unpredictable and at present unpreventable. Genetic counselling, that is warning patients of the 1 in 2 risk to their children, can however result in a planned reduction in reproductive fitness and so substantially reduce the number of second and third or more generation cases. Direct prenatal diagnosis is not yet available for any dominant disorders. It may well come first from the discovery of close linkage of the gene loci involved to marker gene loci. The presently known linkage, between the gene locus for dystrophia myotonica and that for saliva secretor status, gives useful information in only a minority of families and gives odds at best of 9 : 1 for or against an affected fetus because of the 10% cross-over between the two loci. In genetic counselling with some dominant conditions, before giving a low risk of recurrence in later sibs of an apparently sporadic case, it may be important to examine both parents carefully for minimal signs of the disease and to allow for the possibility that one or other parent may yet develop signs of the disease. In the case of tuberose sclerosis it appears to be the case that a parent who carries the gene will almost always show at least the facial skin lesions of the disorder. In the case of early onset dystrophia myotonica in a child, if one or other parent has transmitted the gene he or she will almost invariably show some signs of it. The characteristic lenticular opacities are probably the earliest sign.

Recessive disorders

There are a large number of recessive disorders affecting the central nervous system. Specific enzyme deficiencies have already been recognised in many of these. The usual progression of discovery is: first the clinical identification of a disease, then the recognition that its inheritance is recessive, then the identification of an excess accumulation of a metabolite either in blood plasma or in a cell, and finally the identification of the specific enzyme deficiency. Recessive disorders, understandably, tend to have an earlier onset and be more uniform in clinical expression than are dominants.

The more common recessive disorders affecting the central nervous system with their estimated birth frequencies (Carter 1977b) in Europeans are listed in Table 21.4.
Phenylketonuria has an especially high frequency in Europeans, with a peak in Ireland (1 to 5000), Tay-Sachs disease a high frequency (1 in 3000) in Ashkenazi Jews, Juvenile Gaucher's disease in Sweden, Tyrosinosis in French Canadians.

Table 21.4 Estimates of birth frequencies of some more common recessives affecting the nervous system in European-derived populations per 1000 live-births

Phenylketonuria (classical)	0.1
Neurogenic muscle atrophies	0.1
Recessive forms of congenital deafness	0.2
Recessive forms of childhood onset blindness	0.1
Recessive forms of non-specific severe mental retardation	0.5

There are two possible explanations for such local high frequencies, a local selective advantage of the heterozygote and chance. Heterozygote advantage has been conclusively demonstrated only for the haematological disorder sickle-cell anaemia, the advantage being resistance to malignant tertian malaria, and high frequencies of thalassaemia probably also depend on heterozygote resistance to malaria. More localised high frequencies of particular recessive disorders are probably chance events. In a population founded by a few individuals any gene present in one of the founders will start with a high frequency, for example 1% if the founding stock was 50 individuals. Over many generations this frequency would be expected to fall by selection against homozygotes. But one of several such genes might increase in frequency by fortuitous high fertility of heterozygotes. Such a founder effect and drift is, for example, undoubtedly the explanation of the high frequency of tyrosinosis in French Canadians. In the case of Tay-Sachs disease in Ashkenazi Jews a case has been made for heterozygote advantage, but this is perhaps unnecessary. In the case of phenylketonuria the relatively high frequency appears to hold, though at various levels, throughout Europe (with Finland an exception) and there is a stronger case for invoking heterozygote advantage rather than chance alone.

Prevention and genetic counselling

Fresh mutation plays almost no part in the immediate causation of recessive disorders. In almost all cases both parents will be heterozygote carriers of the mutant gene concerned. It follows that, in contrast to the situation with dominants, most instances of recessive disease are in theory predictable and therefore preventable, once carrier detection is feasible. At present, however, parents at risk of having affected children because they are both carriers of mutants at the same gene locus are usually only recognised when they have had an affected child. Once detected and informed of the risk to further children they may plan no more, or plan more only with the safeguard of prenatal screening. But with the current pattern of small families this will prevent less than a fifth of all cases of recessive disorder. The prospects for prevention are much improved once carrier detection by a widely applicable screening procedure becomes possible. With autosomal recessive conditions this may follow the discovery of the specific biochemical abnormality in the disease. Where this is an enzyme defect the level of activity in heterozygous carriers is usually about halfway between that in the affected homozygotes and normal individuals. Screening of the population before marriage, for example as part of the school medical service, will detect carriers and allow them the opportunity of avoiding marriage to another carrier of the same mutant gene, or if they do marry another carrier of asking for prenatal screening even for the first pregnancy. Such screening of a population is appropriate where a particular recessive disorder is common in a particular population. Screening programmes have already been initiated in several American and Canadian cities among the Ashkenazi Jewish community for Tay-Sachs disease.

X-linked conditions

There are about a score of X-linked conditions affecting the central nervous system. For only a few of these is the specific biochemical defect known.

The distinction between dominant and recessive is hardly applicable to X-linked conditions because of the phenomenon of X-chromosome inactivation early in fetal life. The effect of this is that women heterozygous for a mutant gene on the X-chromosome are mosaics, with some cells having the X-chromosome with the mutant gene active and some cells having that with the normal gene active. Tissues made up of uni-nuclear cells will include portions with the deficiency due to the altered function of the mutant gene alternating with portions with normal function. In conditions in which the areas with the defect are visible, for example X-linked

ectodermal dysplasia and ocular albinism, the alternating patches are a few millimetres in diameter. There are few X-linked conditions in which the heterozygous carrier female is significantly affected clinically, but in several because of the mosaicism a relatively crude clinical or laboratory test will be useful in detecting carriers before the precise biochemical defect has been discovered. Further, the degree of abnormality in the carrier female is likely to be variable, since the proportion of abnormal cells will show chance variation from one individual to another and may at times differ significantly from the expected average value of about 50%. This situation is quite distinct from that in carriers of autosomal recessive mutant genes where, as far as is know, there is no inactivation and any effect of the mutant gene on function will affect every cell in the body.

The two most frequent X-linked conditions affecting the central nervous system are listed in Table 21.5 with their estimated frequencies per thousand births.

Prevention and genetic counselling

As with dominant conditions, cases due to fresh mutation are unpredictable and therefore at present unpreventable. Where the reproductive fitness is zero and the mutation rate equal in the two sexes the proportion of cases due to such fresh mutation will be one third (vide supra) with the remaining two thirds born to carrier mothers. About half these carrier mothers are themselves affected as a result of fresh mutation and therefore would be detected only by a screening programme. The other half of carrier women have the mutant gene from their own mothers and so may have an affected brother or sister's son, which may lead to their identification as carriers before they have had an affected son. Where reproductive fitness is not zero a higher proportion of patients will be affected

Table 21.5 Estimates of the birth frequency in males of the more common X-linked conditions affecting the nervous system in European-derived populations per 1000 live-births

Muscle dystrophy — X-linked Duchenne type	0.3
X-linked non-specific severe mental retardation	0.1

by mutant genes originating two or more generations back.

Genetic counselling for X-linked conditions depends essentially on estimating the likelihood that a woman is a carrier. If she is, then the risk of a son being affected is 1 in 2 and the risk of a daughter being carrier is 1 in 2. A woman who is the daughter of an affected male is an obligatory carrier. A woman who has an affected son and another affected relative is almost certainly a carrier. A woman who has had two affected sons is also almost certainly a carrier. A woman who has one affected son and no other sons has, assuming equal mutation rates in the two sexes, a priori a 2 : 1 probability of being a carrier, though this may drop to close to 1 : 1 if she has many unaffected brothers and sisters who have had unaffected sons. If a woman has unaffected sons as well as the affected boy the chances that she is a carrier may drop substantially below one. For example if a woman has had 3 unaffected sons, as well as the patient, her chances of being a carrier could drop from 2 : 1 to 2 x $(\frac{1}{2})^3$: 1, that is 1 : 4 or 1 in 5. These estimates of the likelihood from the pedigree may be combined with estimates from any laboratory tests for the carrier state. For example in the severe X-linked form of Duchenne dystrophy the estimation of creatine kinase in the mother's plasma will often give a useful probability for or against the carrier state (Emery 1969, Dennis & Carter 1978). Prenatal diagnosis is available for only a few X-linked conditions and unfortunately not yet with certainty for Duchenne muscular dystrophy; creatine kinase levels in fetal blood obtained by fetoscopy do not appear to be helpful. Sex determination is however reliable on amniotic cells and a carrier woman who is pregnant may be happy for the pregnancy to continue if the fetus is female, but wish for a termination if it is male. In contrast, in the case of the Lesch-Nyhan syndrome

prenatal diagnosis of an affected male is reliable. Encouraging indications are also present that in Menkes syndrome prenatal diagnosis is reliable.

MULTIFACTORIAL CONDITIONS

The most important conditions with multifactorial aetiology in the field of paediatric neurology are the neural tube malformations. Family studies show that anencephaly, encephalocele and spina bifida cystica are aetiologically related.

Large-scale family studies in Britain (Carter 1974) show that the proportion affected of sibs of index patients with anencephaly or spina cystica is of the order of 4 to 6% (some ten times higher than the proportion affected in all births); but that the relative risk is somewhat higher where the birth frequency is lower. The findings in surveys in South Wales, Glasgow and Metropolitan London are summarised in Table 21.6.

Cytogenetic studies show that the presence of any chromosomal abnormality in such patients is exceptional except in those aborted in the first trimester. A small proportion of cases are monogenically determined, for example cases of the recessive Meckel (or Gruber) syndrome in which encephalocele is associated with polycystic kidney and ulnar polydactyly. Such cases should be treated separately in any aetiological analysis. A purely intrauterine environment hypothesis to account for the observed family concentration is made unlikely by evidence accumulating that there is an increased risk to paternal as well as maternal half-sibs of index patients, by an apparently low proportion affected of co-twins of index patients, and by the accumulating evidence (Carter & Evans 1973) that the children of patients surviving into adult life with spina bifida are perhaps as often affected as are sibs of index patients.

Table 21.6 Spina bifida and anencephaly. Sibs affected in three large family studies

Area	Malformation in population %	Malformation in sibs		Relative proportion sib/population
		Proportion	%	
South Wales (1956–62)	0.767	81/1563	5.18 ± 0.56	× 6.8
Glasgow (1964–68)	0.563	51/904	5.64 ± 0.77	× 10.0
London (1965–68)	0.295	66/1484	4.45 ± 0.54	× 15.1

If further studies of a larger sample show that the proportion of children affected is as high as that of sibs this makes even modified recessive inheritance unlikely, leaving the alternatives of modified dominant and polygenic inheritance with a threshold. These two latter hypotheses cannot easily be distinguished for a condition which has a birth frequency as high as the neural tube malformations in Britain. For some other malformations with a lower birth frequency, for example cleft lip ($\pm$ cleft palate) the polygenic hypothesis fits better the frequencies observed in second and third degree relatives than does dominant inheritance with low penetrance. The two hypotheses however have much in common if it is assumed that the penetrance of a major gene is affected by genetic variation at other loci.

The part played by environmental factors (Carter 1974) is indicated by a higher birth frequency of the neural tube malformations in the children of men in semi- and unskilled occupations, by secular trends in birth frequency, by seasonal variation in birth frequency (in Britain the highest frequency is for conceptions in spring), by geographical variation in birth frequency even within relatively homogeneous population such as that of the United Kingdom. None of these clues however has yet led to the identification of specific environmental factors.

Prevention and genetic counselling

The empiric risk figures may be used in genetic counselling, for example 6% where the birth frequency is 7%, 4% where it is 3%, and perhaps 2% where it is only 1.5%. There are indications that where parents have already had two affected children, or where an affected parent has already had one affected child, the risk rises to 10 to 12% (Carter 1974). Wherever the risk is, say, 1% there is a case for offering the mother screening by ultrasound and the measurement of α-fetoprotein in amniotic fluid. However all but about 5% of patients occur sporadically and here detection in utero must depend on routine screening of all pregnancies. Screening by estimations of α-fetoprotein in maternal serum at 17 weeks of gestation is achieving considerable success, at a very low cost in false positives. This may in time be replaced by expert ultrasound examination of all pregnancies. True prevention of the malformation is only likely to come when the full aetiology is elucidated, both the individual predisposing genes and the environmental triggers, and susceptible fetuses may be protected from the environmental factors which must also be involved. There are encouraging indications that vitamin supplements may reduce the rate of recurrence (Smithells et al 1981).

REFERENCES

Bundey S, Carter C O 1972 Genetic heterogeneity for dystrophia myotonica. Journal of Medical Genetics 9: 311–5

Carter C O 1974 Clues to the aetiology of neural tube malformations. Developmental Medicine and Child Neurology 16 (suppl 32): 3–15

Carter C O 1977a The relative contribution of mutant genes and chromosome abnormalities to genetic ill-health in man. In: Scott D, Bridges B A, Sobels F H (eds) Progress in genetic toxicology, Elsevier/North Holland, Amsterdam, p. 1–14

Carter C O 1977b Monogenic disorders. Journal of Medical Genetics 14: 316–20

Carter C O, Evans K 1973 Children of adult survivors with spina bifida cystica. Lancet 2: 924–6

Carter C O, Evans K, Till K 1976 Spinal dysraphism: genetic relationship to neural tube malformations. Journal of Medical Genetics 13: 343–50

De Grouchy J, Turleau C 1977 Clinical atlas of human chromosomes. John Wiley, New York

Dennis N R, Carter C O 1978 Use of overlapping normal distributions in genetic counselling. Journal of Medical Genetics, 15: 106–8

Emery A E H 1969 Genetic counselling in X-linked muscular dystrophy. Journal of Neurological Sciences 8: 579–87

Harper P S 1975 Congenital myotonic dystrophy in Britain. II. Genetic basis. Archives of Disease in Childhood 50: 514–21

Smithells R W, Sheppard S, Schorah C J, Seller M J, Nevin N C, Harris R et al 1981 Vitamin supplementation for neural tube defects. Lancet 2: 1425

22

Infections of the nervous system

W. C. Marshall

Great advances have taken place in health care in recent decades and the development of immunising agents together with the discovery of a wide range of antimicrobial substances have contributed much to this success. Yet infections of the nervous system remain common life-threatening conditions with great potential for permanent damage in survivors. Gotschlich (1978) has estimated that in the life of a cohort of 1000 newborns bacterial meningitis will develop in at least 6 children, one of whom will die and two will be left with serious permanent neurological defects.

These infections are a formidable challenge to the clinician who must recognise the conditions in their earliest stages for optimal results of treatment. With infrequent exceptions, the many different types of meningitis and encephalitis are clinically indistinguishable. Hence the microbiologist must be provided with appropriate specimens for the identification of the infecting organism. At the time of presentation other causes of a non-infective nature often have to be considered; consequently investigative procedures such as radiology, hae-matology, biochemistry and toxicology are often required. On the establishment of an infective aetiology many of these will be needed to aid in the management of the patient.

In the early phases of an acute infection of the brain and/or the meninges the pathophysiological effects may undergo rapid changes and the clinician must be alert to recognise and indeed should attempt to anticipate these changes. Throughout this period communication with the parents may be extremely difficult. They will often expect answers to questions related to both the short and long-term prognosis but most of these cannot be answered with accuracy in the individual patient.

The nervous system may be invaded by any micro-organism; all carry the potential to evoke an inflammatory response of one type or another so that all known organisms may be the cause of infection of the brain and its surrounding structures. Merely to list the many pathogens would not be helpful, for such lists fail to indicate important factors in individual infections such as the age of the patient, seasonal variations and geographical con-

Table 22.1 Bacterial meningitis in children under 15 years (England and Wales 1976–78[a])

Year	Organism	<1 Year	1–4 Years	5–9 Years	10–14 Years	Total
1976	*N. meningitidis*	117	181	53	39	390
	H. influenzae	103	165	17	1	286
	S. pneumoniae	28	27	24	14	93
1977	*N. meningitidis*	76	92	44	28	240
	H. influenzae	98	220	13	1	332
	S. pneumoniae	38	25	21	18	102
1978	*N. meningitidis*	107	74	33	25	239
	H. influenzae	99	147	11	4	261
	S. pneumoniae	34	40	25	17	116

[a] Based on reports to Communicable Disease Surveillance Centre by P.H.L.S. and other laboratories

siderations. The latter are well illustrated by the arbovirus infections. Other environmental aspects of importance include socio-economic factors, overcrowding and contact with birds and animals.

BACTERIAL INFECTIONS

Bacterial infections are divided for aetiological, clinical and management purposes into infections occurring in the newborn and the first two months of life and those occurring in the remainder of infancy and childhood. In the former there is an extremely wide range of bacteria, but the majority are gram negative bacilli, usually *Escherichia coli*. However in recent years group B β-*haemolytic streptococci* have emerged as major pathogens. In some areas they are the leading cause of neonatal meningitis.

Later in infancy and in childhood the majority of infections are caused by *Haemophilus influenza type b*, *Neisseria meningitidis* and *Streptococcus pneumoniae*. In the United States Mortimer (1973) has estimated that the risk of meningitis occurring in a child by five years of age is between 1 : 400 and 1 : 2500. The meningococcus is the commonest organism isolated from the CSF from patients beyond the neonatal period in the United Kingdom (Table 22.1) whereas *Haemophilus influenzae* is the commonest in the United States and Australia.

Goldacre (1976) has calculated from his study of meningitis in a region in the United Kingdom with a population of 4 million that the risk of acute meningococcal infection was 1 : 1090 and of *H. influenzae* meningitis 1 : 1500 by 10 years of age. Bacterial meningitis was commoner in the first week and first month of life than any subsequent week or month, and in the first year of life than any subsequent year. In the newborn the incidence was 0.26 per 1000 live births. The cases and deaths by organisms and by age groups of the common causes

in this study are shown in Table 22.2.

The most frequent route of infection is via the blood stream. Direct invasion may occur because of congenital defects, most commonly meningomyelocoele. It is important to examine the back and skull for midline defects such as dimples or the entrance to a dermal sinus connecting with the meninges. Traumatic rupture of the anatomical defences or direct spread from infections in contiguous tissues, such as the ears and sinuses may also occur. Surgical treatment of hydrocephalus by shunt or drainage and lumbar or ventricular puncture are further possible routes of infection. In any of these circumstances the types of bacteria are legion but staphylococci, haemolytic and non-haemolytic streptococci, *Pseudomonas aeruginosa*, proteus, and klebsiella-aerobacter species are most common.

Children with recurrent bacterial meningitis require investigation to exclude anatomical defects, for example congenital dermal sinuses or defects in the region of the cribriform plate, ear and the base of the skull. Congenital or acquired defects in the immune system may be the basis for the recurrent infection. The child who has had his spleen removed or who has sickle cell disease is especially vulnerable (Overturf et al 1977). However, recurrence of infection following cure should be distinguished if possible, from relapse, that is, reappearance of clinical and laboratory features within three weeks of completion of therapy, and recrudescence which Schaad et al (1981) have defined as reappearance during treatment of the infection together with symptoms and signs after sterilisation of the CSF has been demonstrated. Relapse and recrudescence are more likely to occur in children under two years of age, and the former is probably due to the presence of a meningeal or parameningeal focus whereas the later is usually caused by inappropriate therapy.

The use of humidifiers and mechanical ventila-

Table 22.2 Acute bacterial meningitis: cases and deaths by age group and organism (Goldacre 1976)

| | No. of cases (deaths) | | | | | |
	<1 mth	1–12 mths	1–4 yrs	5–9 yrs	Total	Case fatality
N. meningitidis	0 (–)	106 (14)	113 (13)	42 (2)	266 (29)	10.9%
H. influenzae	2 (0)	54 (5)	117 (5)	20 (1)	193 (11)	5.7%
S. pneumoniae	2 (1)	27 (4)	26 (3)	12 (3)	67 (11)	16.4%

tion in the newborn poses additional hazards, and infection from these sources as well as sinks, suction apparatus and other infants and staff (Thong et al 1981) is well recognised. If two or more cases occur in a nursery, particularly if the organism is an unusual one, such a source should be suspected. Anaerobic bacteria, especially *Bacteroides fragilis*, may cause meningitis, albeit infrequently (Nelson 1976).

Clinical features

The clinical features of bacterial meningitis vary with age. In an older, previously healthy child an illness consisting of mild to moderate fever, headache, vomiting and nausea, some disturbance of sensorium, possibly generalised but rarely focal seizures makes acute bacterial meningitis very likely. Coma and opisthotonus are late signs but semi-coma may be postictal in origin. There will be stiffness of the neck and sometimes the back as well. Kernig's and Brudzinski's signs may be present. On the other hand the very earliest signs and symptoms may be misleading. Mild irritability and reluctance to flex the neck in a child who is 'not his usual self' may be the sole manifestations. Sudden onset as a 'febrile convulsion' is infrequent but is more likely to occur in younger children, many of whom may show no signs of meningitis (Ratcliffe & Wolf 1977). Although there may be some disagreement the consensus of opinion, supported by several studies (Rutter & Smales 1977, Wolf 1978) is that lumbar puncture is not indicated as a routine procedure in children with febrile convulsions.

It is in the very young that difficulties arise in clinical recognition. In the absence of the 'typical' signs of meningitis as described in the older child, meningitis should be suspected in an infant who is unwell, especially if he is irritable. Low grade fever, vomiting, confusion or convulsions should increase the suspicion of meningitis and a valuable clue may be increased tension of the anterior fontanelle. Papilloedema is extremely rare. Unless an adequate explanation can be found for these symptoms and signs in an infant examination of the cerebrospinal fluid (CSF) is mandatory.

The neonate, and in particular the premature infant, presents the greatest problem in clinical

Table 22.3 Clinical signs of meningitis in 255 new-born infants (after Klein & Marcy 1976)

Raised temperature	61%
Lethargy	50%
Anorexia or vomiting	49%
Respiratory distress	47%
Apnoea	7%
Irritability	32%
Jaundice	28%
Bulging or full fontanelle	28%
Diarrhoea	17%
Neck stiffness	15%

diagnosis. Bacterial meningitis should be included in the differential diagnosis of any newborn who is unwell. The history of the pregnancy and the type of delivery may indicate an 'at risk' baby; birth weight is important for the incidence of neonatal meningitis was 0.37 per 1000 births above and 1.36 per 1000 live births below 2500 g (Overall 1970). Prolonged rupture of the membranes or difficult obstetric manipulations, the presence of congenital malformation and the male sex, should increase suspicion. The frequency of clinical features in 255 newborn with meningitis is shown in Table 22.3. Davies (1977) has drawn attention to the very small infant who may be receiving feeds intravenously or by intragastric tube; the common symptoms of anorexia and vomiting may not be apparent in such infants.

Laboratory diagnosis and investigations

The diagnosis is obtained from examination of cerebrospinal fluid; the tests to be carried out should be carefully planned in case of the need to extend the investigations should a bacterial infection not be confirmed at the initial examination. Microscopy to determine the number and type of cells, Gram's stain, culture and estimation of glucose and protein are the initial minimal requirements. Care should be taken in preparing the CSF and Murray & Hampton (1980) have suggested that the optimal conditions necessary for the recovery of bacteria from the CSF deposit consist of centrifugation at 1500 × G for 15 minutes. An extra volume of fluid will be required for tests to detect the presence of bacterial antigens or for indirect tests for bacterial infection should they be available. Virological investigations (culture and/or antibody estimation) should also be planned.

Table 22.4 A guide to changes in CSF in bacterial and some other forms of meningitis

Type	Leucocytes (mm³)	Glucose (mmol/l)	Protein (gm/l)
Bacterial	100 to ⩾ 50 000. May be lower, even acellular, in very early stages of disease	usually 1.1–1.6 but can be less than 0.5 in severe infections	mild to moderate increase but higher levels may occur in the neonate
Tuberculous	25 to 100 but can be as high as 500. Lymphocytes usually greater than 80% but 50% or more may be polymorphonuclears in the early stages	usually reduced below 2.2–2.7 but may be in low range of normal in early stages	moderate increases to 2 but very high levels if block in flow of CSF is present
Viral	25 to 500 — lymphocytes predominate but polymorphonuclears, which are usually less than 10%, may be 50% or more in early stages	normal but some reduction below 2.2 especially if the leucocyte count is very high e.g. in mumps meningitis	mild increase
Fungal	0 to 500 with predominance of lymphocytes	levels similar to those found in tuberculous meningitis but may be normal	moderate increase rarely greater than 5

A guide to the changes in the CSF in bacterial and some other infections is shown in Table 22.4. The detection of some bacterial capsular polysaccharides in CSF is possible by means of the relatively simple technique of counter immunoelectrophoresis (CIE). Results can be available in less than an hour and testing of serum and urine for the bacterial antigen may increase the chance of diagnosis (Feigin et al 1976). However it is of practical value only in *H. influenzae*, pneumococcal and meningococcal infections and requires pure antisera of high potency. Occasionally cross reactions with some other Gram-negative bacteria may occur. It may be of value in some patients who have already received antibiotics. The same principle is used in the technically more simple test in which antibody coated latex particles are used to detect antigen (Whittle et al 1974). Quantitation of the antigen may be performed as it has been suggested that patients who have very large amounts of bacterial antigen in the CSF are more likely to have neurological sequelae.

Cultures of blood, nose and throat swabs should always be made. The organisms responsible for the common types of bacterial meningitis can frequently be isolated from blood even if antimicrobials have been already administered. It may be useful to examine the buffy-coat from blood by Gram's stain; bacteria may be visible if there is a heavy infection.

A dilemma presents if the CSF contains both polymorphonuclear cells and lymphocytes without identifiable bacteria on Gram's stain. The problem is to distinguish between pyogenic meningitis in which the bacteria can no longer be identified because of treatment, and meningitis caused by viruses or other micro-organisms such as *Myobacterium tuberculosis*. CIE has a small overall false negative rate. The limulus amoebocyte lysate test requires great attention to the method and only detects endotoxin produced by Gram-negative bacteria. For many years it had been known that there is an increase in the concentration of lactate in the CSF in bacterial meningitis. Increased lactate levels are found in pyogenic and tuberculous meningitis as well as in mycoplasma infections (Controni et al 1977, Brook et al 1978). It has been reported by Pavlakis et al (1980) that calculation of the CSF anion gap may be useful if methods to determine lactate levels are not available.

Elevated levels of lactate can also be found in conditions with increased intracranial pressure or reduced oxygen supply to the brain. This test does not replace standard procedures of microscopy and culture and indeed it has been suggested that measurement of lactate levels does not contribute significantly to the management of children with suspected meningitis (Rutlidge et al 1981). However, Gould and colleagues (1980) found it to be useful in monitoring response to treatment in some patients.

Other investigations and management

The child with meningitis should have the following tests carried out; full blood count, electrolytes, urea and creatinine, osmolality of urine and serum. The specimen for blood glucose estimation should be taken immediately prior to the lumbar puncture. The importance of measurement of serum electrolytes, together with osmolality of serum and urine, is the common occurrence of the syndrome of inappropriate antidiuretic hormone activity which occurs in over 80% of patients (Feigin & Dodge 1976). Increased plasma concentration of arginine vasopressin has been demonstrated in such patients with hyponatraemia (Kaplan & Feigin 1978).

Transillumination of the skull should be performed as well as X-rays of the skull and chest. A tuberculin test should also be performed. Electroencephalography may be useful in the event of complications. Computerised tomography of the brain may be of value in showing subdural effusions, brain swelling, infarcts and hydrocephalus and should be performed if there is persistence of fever, seizures or a full fontanelle, the presence of hemiparesis or alteration in the mental state (Stovring & Synder 1980) (Fig. 22.1). This procedure has also provided new insights into the pathogenesis of some of the complications.

In the event of failure to establish the diagnosis of bacterial infection, viral cultures of nose and throat secretions, urine and faeces should be set up. A portion of CSF should have been set aside for viral cultures. A serum specimen for tests for antibody to viruses and immunoglobulin estimation should be taken.

The specific treatment of bacterial meningitis is based on the selection of an antimicrobial agent to which the organisms are susceptible and which reaches the CSF in concentrations sufficient to kill, or at least inhibit the growth of the organisms. This will only be achieved if adequate plasma concentrations of the drugs are attained or if they are instilled directly into the CSF. If this is necessary, it should be noted that injection into the CSF by lumbar puncture is very unlikely to result in adequate concentration in the ventricles as Kaiser & McGee (1975) have demonstrated with aminoglycosides.

Chloramphenicol, sulphonamides and trimethoprim have the greatest capability to enter the CSF; levels of 30–60% of plasma levels are found. Inflammation of the meninges will enhance the penetration of a number of drugs including the penicillins and will also inhibit the active transport system which removes ionised drugs such as penicillin from the CSF. This transport mechanism can be blocked by probenicid (Lietman 1978). The levels of aminoglycosides which are found in CSF (10–20% of plasma levels) are far too low to be effective. This has encouraged their instillation directly into the CSF.

The early cephalosporins have proved to be unsatisfactory for treatment and are not recommended. The newer agents cefotaxime and moxalactam enter the CSF in adequate amounts and are proving to be valuable drugs (Landesman et al 1981). Tetracyclines have been shown to penetrate reasonably well but they are rarely used in infants and children for other reasons. Erythromycin, clindamycin and lincomycin do not achieve satisfactory levels in the CSF.

Although it can be argued that there are theoretical disadvantages of the use of a bacteriostatic and bacteriocidal drug in combination there are studies which do not show antagonism between ampicillin and chloramphenicol; evidence of synergy has been found in some instances (Feldman 1978). The Committee on Infectious Diseases of the American Academy of Pediatrics (1977) recommends the use of both drugs in the treatment of *H. influenzae* meningitis until the sensitivity of the organism is known, when one of these drugs may be stopped.

Until the emergence of sulphonamide-resistant strains of *N. meningitidis*, triple therapy (chloramphenicol/penicillin/sulphonamide) was recommended for the treatment of bacterial meningitis of unknown aetiology in children beyond the neonatal period; the vast majority of cases could be considered to be due to one of the three 'primary' meningitides — *H. influenzae*, *S. pneumoniae* and *N. meningitidis*. The commonest cause for 'bacterial meningitis of unknown aetiology' is probably the result of the administration of antibiotics before meningitis is suspected and the CSF is obtained. This is most likely to occur when the infection is

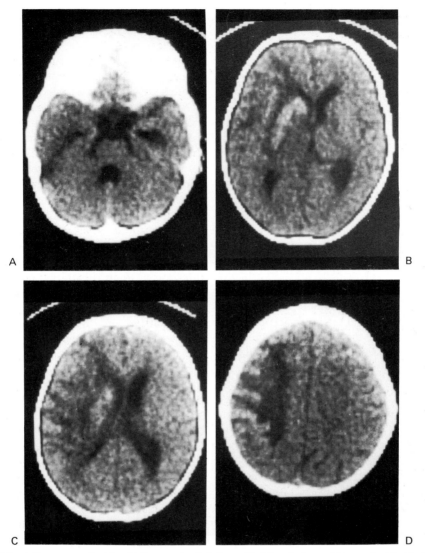

Fig. 22.1 *Haemophilus influenzae* meningitis with haemorrhagic infarct of left hemisphere. A 9-month-old girl who developed left-sided fits and hemiplegia 3 days after commencement of therapy. CT scan was performed 48 hours later.

The 4th, 3rd and lateral ventricles are moderately dilated. The basal cisterns and right hemisphere sulci are wide. There is an extensive area of mixed attenuation in the basal ganglia and left frontal and parietal lobes with mass effect (compression of the left lateral ventricle and displacement of the 3rd ventricle and septum pellucidum to the right). The appearances are of an infarct and the high attenuation indicates haemorrhage within it.

caused by *N. meningitidis* and to a lesser extent *S. pneumoniae*. *H. influenzae*, on the other hand, can often be cultured from CSF of patients who have been pre-treated (Feigin 1981). At the present time, ampicillin and chloramphenicol should be used in these circumstances, but as β-lactamase-producing strains of *H. influenzae* are increasing the use of chloramphenicol alone would be logical provided that chloramphenicol-resistant strains of the bacteria remain very rare.

The antibacterial drugs should be given by the intravenous route for as long as practical but at least for 5–7 days and the total duration of treatment should be 10–14 days. Treatment of neonates with Gram-negative meningitis should continue for 21–28 days after the CSF has been sterile.

The practice of examining the CSF to determine if bacteriological cure has occurred in children with the common forms of meningitis is a matter of personal choice based on experience. In patients who make a rapid response to treatment it is probably not necessary; however recurrence of fever or irritability are indications to re-examine the CSF. Examination at the end of treatment in pneumococcal meningitis may be an advisable practice, though unnecessary in meningococcal or H. influenzae meningitis. Examination of the CSF should be repeated in infections with unusual organisms at all ages and for infections in the neonate and very young infant.

In the early stages of treatment all fluids should be given by the intravenous route and restricted to 50–60% of the daily requirements until the serum sodium levels are normal. This approach presents a serious dilemma when the patient is in shock as excess fluids should be avoided because cerebral oedema may be increased; it is probably one of the major factors in causing death or permanent brain damage (Connor & Minielly 1980). There is no evidence that corticosteroids are helpful in reducing cerebral oedema in acute bacterial meningitis (de Lemos & Haggerty 1969) and they are not recommended (Fishman 1982).

Menkes (1979) has postulated that the infection causes increased cerebral glycolysis. The resulting suboptimal amounts of glucose may be responsible for some cortical neuronal damage. He has suggested that increasing the supply of glucose may remove a potentially correctable cause of damage.

Treatment of seizures is best achieved by rectal paraldehyde, parenteral phenobarbitone or phenytoin. Diazepam is often used, but it may depress respiration and thus aggravate cerebral oedema. Interactions may occur between antimicrobials and other drugs, especially between Chloramphenicol and the anticonvulsants phenobarbitone and phenytoin, the former reducing and the latter increasing the blood levels of the antibiotic (Krasinski et al 1982).

Haemophilus influenza Type b meningitis

This form of meningitis is primarily a disease of the pre-school child and is rare beyond the second decade of life. There is a higher incidence of the order of three times in the United States than the United Kingdom. An increased risk of infection is present in negroes, children in overcrowded low income families, individuals who lack a spleen and in children with immunoglobulin deficiency syndromes. Feigin & Dodge (1976) have drawn attention to an unexplained male predominance. Strains of this gram-negative bacillus other than type b occasionally cause infections and include the other encapsulated strains (a, c, and f) and Parainfluenzae as well as unencapsulated strains. The latter are more likely to be found in association with trauma to the skull or concurrent otitis media (Greene 1978).

Symptoms of a mild upper respiratory tract infection or anorexia and lethargy for several days not infrequently precede the onset of the obvious meningitic illness. Meningococcal or pneumococcal infections, on the other hand, have a more abrupt onset. It is often during this early period that antibiotics are administered without an awareness of the diagnosis of meningitis. However, these early symptoms are not necessarily always present and the onset can be abrupt. Very rarely a sparse petechial rash may also be seen.

In addition to the characteristic changes in the CSF the organism can be detected in blood cultures in a high proportion of cases. Currently the mortality rate is between 3 and 4%.

Approximately 15% of children will develop subdural effusions. They are most frequent over the fronto-parietal regions and are often bilateral. They occur most frequently following H. influenzae and are least frequent in meningococcal infection. The diagnosis should be suspected if the temperature fails to decline or recurs after 3 or 5 days treatment, if vomiting or irritability occur after a similar period or if generalised or focal convulsions occur. Focal neurological signs may also be present. Daily measurement of the skull circumference in younger children may reveal an increase in size, but even a large effusion can be present without any increase in skull size. Transillumination of the skull or examination by CT scan may be of help in the diagnosis. If subdural taps show fluid to be present up to 15–20 ml should be removed. There is usually clinical improvement following this procedure and tapping should continue until symptoms subside; neurosurgical intervention is seldom required.

Earlier reports of long term sequelae indicated an incidence of 20–40%. Feigin and his colleagues (1978) have reported that only 9% of patients had long term sequelae and Emmett and her colleagues (1980) claim that prompt diagnosis and adequate treatment of children results in no detectable residual effects. Hearing loss is probably underestimated (Lundberg 1977) and it is not yet clear if the disease itself is primarily responsible or the deafness may possibly be associated in some unexplained way with the use of ampicillin and chloramphenicol in combination. Later convulsive disorders, intellectual impairment and behaviour problems may require continued supervision.

Treatment of *H. influenzae* meningitis has undergone considerable change in the last two decades. For a number of years ampicillin in high doses (400 mg/kg per day) was the mainstay of treatment. The inevitable then occurred with the emergence of β-lactamase-producing strains of the organism. At present initial treatment should consist of ampicillin (400 mg/kg per day in 6 divided doses) and chloramphenicol (100 mg/kg per day in 4 divided doses) administered intravenously until sensitivity tests are available. If the bacteria are sensitive to ampicillin, chloramphenicol is discontinued and vice versa. Chloramphenicol alone can be used for the initial treatment but with caution since occasional strains have been found to be resistant to this drug. The isolation of a strain resistant to both ampicillin and chloramphenicol from a child with meningitis (Kenny et al 1980) is disturbing; cefotaxime or moxalactam could be used in such circumstances. The duration of treatment should be at least 10 days and should be given by the intravenous route, but chloramphenicol by the oral route is satisfactory in the last few days of treatment if the child is fully conscious, afebrile and is not vomiting.

Most children will become afebrile within 4–5 days of starting treatment, and persisting fever is an indication for re-examination of the CSF. Recurrence of fever may be due to intercurrent infection, 'drug fever' or neurological complications (Rutman & Wald 1981). A higher rate of neurological complications occurs in patients with persistent fever compared with those with recurrent fever. Other features which may be associated with lasting morbidity include persisting seizures, deep coma, shock, age less than 12 months and pretreatment symptoms for greater than 3 days (Herson & Todd 1977). Anaemia, which is due to increased red cell destruction, is frequently seen in bacterial meningitis, but is commoner and severer in *H. influenzae* infection; by contrast it is infrequent in aseptic meningitis (Kaplan & Oski 1980).

Unlike meningococcal infections *H. influenzae* infection has not been considered to be a communicable disease, but it has now been shown that the secondary attack rate in household contacts is some 800 times that of the endemic attack rate in children under five years of age (Ward et al 1979, Glode et al 1980). The secondary attack rate irrespective of age is 0.26% and in household contacts less than 2 years of age the risk is of the order of 3% (Granoff & Daum 1980).

As a result of these observations attempts have been made to eradicate the bacteria from the pharynx by various drugs such as ampicillin, chloramphenicol, co-trimoxazole, cefaclor and rifampicin. The latter is the only agent shown to have any significant degree of efficacy but further studies are needed before this drug can be recommended for widespread use. Wilson (1981) has recommended that consideration should be given to rifampicin chemoprophylaxis (20 mg/kg per day for 4 days) to the most susceptible age groups, namely those less than 2 years of age in the home or in a nursery.

Meningococcal meningitis

Neisseria meningitidis (meningococcus), a Gram-negative coccus, is the commonest cause of acute bacterial meningitis in the United Kingdom and Scandinavia, whereas in the United States and Australia it is second to *H. influenzae* in frequency. However, these differences may not be constant. Several types of the meningococcus are identified by agglutination tests for different capsular or cell wall antigens. The groups presently identified are A, B, C, D, X, Y, Z and W 135. These antigens can be found in the blood, CSF and urine during active infection. The bacteria are present in the nasopharynx in approximately 5% of apparently healthy individuals; however the conditions which result in the development of invasive disease are unknown.

Two important features of this infection are epidemic forms and the severe overwhelming disease which may be seen in some individuals with meningococcaemia.

Epidemics are most often caused by Group A and sometimes Group C organisms. Group B and the others are usually responsible for sporadic infections. Acute meningitis is a rapidly developing disease, symptoms sometimes being present for only a few hours. In addition to the usual features of meningitis, petechiae or purpuric lesions in the skin are seen in about 50% of patients (Swartz & Dodge 1965). However, petechiae are occasionally observed in children with pneumococcal meningitis and in some enteroviral infections. Another exanthem may occur in the early stages of meningococcal infection consisting of pale reddish macules or papules without a purpuric element (Christie 1980a). The bacteria can be identified in these and in the petechial lesions. A rapid progression of the skin purpura may herald an impending catastrophic illness with disseminated intravascular coagulation and shock. In addition to endotoxaemia there is often bacterial embolization which may be prominent in the lungs. High concentrations of bacterial antigen can frequently be detected in the circulation of these patients by countercurrent electrophoresis.

Persisting fever may be a problem in these patients. Pericarditis and arthritis are other complications and may be the cause, but the commonest cause is probably drugs.

As with all forms of meningitis, a major factor in the prognosis is the early recognition of the infection and treatment with penicillin by the intravenous route. Careful monitoring is important to detect the occurrence of shock and to introduce measures to maintain an adequate circulation, but excess fluids may aggravate cerebral oedema; corticosteroids are of unproven value. The benefit of sulphonamides has been greatly diminished by the emergence of sulphonamide-resistant strains but these vary according to the type. For example in the United Kingdom in 1977 only 5% of Group B were resistant compared with 50% of Group A and 20% of Group C strains but in 1980 20% of Group B and 66% and 15% of serotypes B and C were resistant (CDR 1981).

Resistance to sulphonamides has created problems in the management of close contacts such as other members of the family or other intimate contacts, in whom the attack rate is approximately 1000 times the endemic attack rate (McCormick & Bennett 1975). The secondary attack rate may reach 15 000 times the endemic rate during epidemics. The object of chemoprophylaxis is to eliminate the organism from the nasopharynx before it causes disease or before transmission to others occurs (Wilson 1981).

Penicillin is not effective in preventing invasive disease and sulphonamide resistance has made it necessary to use other agents such as minocycline or rifampicin. The high incidence of side-effects precludes the use of the former and thus rifampicin is now recommended for household contacts but not for classmates, unless there are additional cases in the school.

Pneumococcal meningitis

Streptococcus pneumoniae are Gram-positive cocci with over 80 serotypes. The organism is the commonest cause of bacterial meningitis in the adult but occurs at all ages in childhood beyond the neonatal period. Most cases of meningitis are due to bacteraemia, but direct extension from a septic focus in the ears or after a skull fracture with CSF leak also occurs with this organism. In the latter situation it may cause recurrent meningitis.

Other groups of patients at special risk from pneumococcal meningitis are those in whom the spleen has been removed and children with sickle cell syndromes especially during the first 3–5 years of life. Fraser and colleagues (1973) as a result of their community study in South Carolina calculated that by 4 years of age one in twenty-four children with sickle cell disease will develop pneumococcal meningitis.

This infection has the highest mortality of the three common bacterial meningitides even in countries where adequate facilities for medical care are available (Table 22.5).

The progression of the illness is usually rapid, especially in the very young, and coma is frequent.

Table 22.5 Mortality from pneumococcal meningitis in different countries (Baird et al 1976)

Country	Mortality (%)	Country	Mortality (%)
UK	13	Malawi	43
Denmark	17	Zambia	45
USA — Los Angeles	22	Uganda	51
USA — Boston	29	Nigeria	51
USA — Philadephia	37[a]	Ghana	55
USA — Harlem	47[a]	Upper Volta	60
India	45		
Egypt	33		

[a] High proportion of Negro patients

Penicillin remains the antibiotic of choice but chloramphenicol should be used in patients who are allergic to penicillin. Treatment should continue for 10–14 days. The recent emergence of penicillin-resistant strains of these bacteria (Ahronheim et al 1979) is disturbing especially as some are multiply resistant (Jacobs et al 1978, Radetsky et al 1981). Sensitivity tests should therefore be performed on all isolates of *S. pneumoniae* from the CSF and blood.

Neonatal meningitis

Two of the major features of bacterial meningitis in this age group are the great variability and often non-specific nature of the symptoms and signs and a wider spectrum of infecting organisms. Although the most frequent bacteria are Gram-negative bacilli, usually *E. coli*, infections with group B β-haemolytic streptococci (GBS) have become increasingly frequent and in some areas in the United States are now the commonest single cause of neonatal meningitis (Anthony & Okada 1977).

A notable feature of the strains of *E. coli* causing meningitis at this age is that bacteria containing K1 capsular polysaccharide antigen are both the commonest and most virulent (Table 22.6). A similar feature has been observed in group B streptococci in which the type III strain appears to be the most virulent, and it is interesting that these capsular antigens are immunologically similar.

Other causes include *Pseudomonas aeruginosa*, proteus, klebsiella-aerobacter, and citrobacter species; salmonellae, *Listeria monocytogenes* and *Flavobacterium meningosepticum*. *H. influenzae type b*

Table 22.6 Outcome of neonatal meningitis due to K1 and non-K1 strains of *E. coli* (McCracken et al 1974)

Outcome	Number and % of infants	
	K1 *E. coli*	Non-K1 *E. coli*
Died	15 (31%)	0 (–)
Survived		
neurological defect	14 (29%)	1 (11%)
normal at 6 mths	19 (40%)	8 (89%)
Total	48 (100%)	9 (100%)

infection is occasionally seen in the newborn. Staphylococcal infections are infrequent but predominate in infections of ventricular shunts used for treating hydrocephalus.

In most cases of neonatal meningitis there is little difficulty in identifying the bacteria. However, in the presence of CSF changes consistent with bacterial meningitis and negative cultures unusual organisms such as *Mycoplasma hominis* should be considered (Gerwitz et al 1979).

The emergence of GBS as an important cause of infections in the neonate has drawn attention to syndromes associated with 'early onset' and 'late onset' bacterial sepsis. This also occurs in *Listeria monocytogenes* infection (Larsson et al 1979) and with *E. coli*. 'Early onset' disease shows itself within 48 hours of birth, often within a few hours in cases of GBS infections. The infant is frequently premature and in most the signs are those of generalised sepsis and/or respiratory disease. The signs of meningitis are often absent. 'Late onset' disease, on the other hand, takes the form of more easily recognisable meningitis and occurs towards the end of the first week of life. Many of these infants are not premature. Whereas these infections may be acquired from the mother, as in all cases of early onset disease, some are acquired from other individuals in the nursery. Other causes of 'late onset' disease include *Pseudomonas aeruginosa, staphylococcus aureus*, citrobacter species and salmonellae.

One of the major problems in the management of Gram-negative meningitis is the failure of parenterally administered aminoglycoside antibiotics to achieve adequate levels in the CSF. The unidirectional flow of CSF prevents the effective use of the lumbar route for administration (McCracken & Mize 1976). Encouraging responses were obtained following the administration of parenteral together with intraventricular gentamicin combined with ampicillin (Lee et al 1976) but an unexplained higher mortality on this regime in a more recent study (McCracken et al 1980) has indicated the need to consider other approaches; these include the use of chloramphenicol in doses known not to cause the 'grey syndrome' (25 mg/kg per day) or newer cephalosporins such as moxalactam and cefotaxime. However, because of the considerable differences in the pharmacokinetics of chloramphenicol in individual infants monitoring of blood levels should be carried out (Black et al 1978).

Treatment of neonatal meningitis should be continued for 21–28 days after sterilisation of the CSF. Intermittent drainage by means of a ventricular reservoir may be useful for both the management of acute hydrocephalus and access to CSF for assessment of levels of antimicrobials as well as bacteriological studies. However, it may not be possible to insert a reservoir in the early stages of the infection because of compression of the ventricles by generalised brain swelling.

Cerebrospinal fluid (CSF) shunt infections

One of the major advances in neurosurgery has been the development of methods to bypass obstruction to the flow of CSF. This may be achieved by means of ventricular bypass internally or by drainage from the lateral ventricles to an extracranial site, either the peritoneal cavity or into the right atrium.

Table 22.7 Organisms isolated from first shunt infections Hospital for Sick Children, Great Ormond Street, 1969–1979

Bacteria	No. of isolates:
Staphylococcus epidermidis	65
Staphylococcus aureus	15
Pseudomonas aeruginosa	5
Escherichia coli	2
Enterococcus	1
Klebsiella	1
Citrobacter	1
Gram-negative bacilli (unidentified)	3
Total	93

One of the most serious and frequent complications of these shunts is infection with or without ventriculitis. This necessitates appropriate antimicrobial treatment and replacement of the shunt. Infection rates have been reported to be as high as 20–27% (Schoenbaum et al 1975) and are probably the same in both types of shunt (O'Brien et al 1979). The organisms responsible are mainly strains of staphylococci especially those which colonise the skin (Bayston & Lari 1974). This is illustrated by the types of bacteria isolated from first shunt infections at The Hospital for Sick Children in the period from 1969–1979 (Table 22.7). The low incidence of Gram-negative infections has been stressed by Sells and his colleagues (1977).

Attempts have been made to reduce colonisation by greater attention to surgical techniques, particularly skin sterilization, and this can be effective in reducing the numbers of infections. Antibiotic prophylaxis has not been shown to be very effective. This may be due to failure to use the intrathecal route of administration; when given by this route aminoglycosides have been shown to be effective (Welch et al 1979).

The symptoms and signs of infection usually develop within 2 to 3 months of surgery. 'Late' infections are also observed but these may in reality have been unrecognised 'early' infections. (Bayston 1980). The symptoms and signs of ventriculo-atrial shunt infections include fever, chills and sometimes rigors, anaemia, splenomegaly, rashes and arthralgia; shunt 'nephritis' may occur if infection has persisted for some time.

Ventriculo-peritoneal shunt infections more often present insidiously with fever, abdominal pain, shoulder tip pain, a palpable swelling at the end of the abdominal catheter, or only a blockage of the shunt.

The treatment of shunt infection is difficult. Parenteral antimicrobial therapy alone is not effective and this probably stems from the unpredictable penetration into the ventricles of the agents which have been used. Similarly co-incident administration of agents into the CSF has not been successful. Removal of the infected shunt and its replacement is the only satisfactory method. The most effective management appears to be removal of the shunt and administration of both intraventricular and intravenous antimicrobials for a period of one week before insertion of a new shunt (James et al 1980).

However, if earlier recognition of infection were possible, for example by serial measurement of C-reactive protein (CRP) and *Staph. epidermidis* antibodies (Bayston 1975) treatment with drugs such as rifampicin and co-trimoxazole might result in eradication of the infection without the need for removal of the shunt.

Tuberculous meningitis

Communities in which there has been a marked decline in the incidence of tuberculosis have a disadvantage; a decrease in the awareness of the possibility of the diagnosis of this form of intracranial infection, either in the form of meningitis, or the much rarer tuberculoma. The latter is commoner in some parts of the world than others, such as the Indian subcontinent (Sinh et al 1968, Udani & Dastur 1970). Involvement of the calvarium is very rare, but is more common in children and young adults. The bone infection, which is usually an expanding osteolytic lesion in the fronto-temporal region, may be confused with histiocytosis (Danziger et al 1976).

The mortality rate and incidence of sequelae in tuberculous meningitis is higher with delayed diagnosis, in the younger children or if coma or focal neurological signs are present when treatment is commenced (Idriss et al 1976, Delage & Dusseault 1979, Kennedy & Fallon 1979). Even though there are advances in the availability of anti-tuberculous drugs which enter the cerebrospinal fluid (Fallon & Kennedy 1981), the cornerstone of successful management is early diagnosis.

Meningitis occurs following rupture into the ventricles or subarachnoid space of a tubercle on the meninges or in the brain or spinal cord. However, progression is not invariable. Emond and McKendrick (1973) have described 'transient aseptic meningitis' and recovery without treatment. In many children with tuberculous meningitis miliary disease is also present and may be recognised on chest X-ray or on fundoscopy. Tuberculin sensitivity is usually present even in the very ill child. However, anergy may be the consequence of severe malnutrition, malaria, recent measles or rubella or following the administration of measles or rubella vaccines.

The early symptoms of infection are vague; irritability or apathy, headache, vomiting and constipation may be present. Low grade fever and loss of weight are common but signs of meningeal irritation may not be obvious. Drowsiness then begins to dominate the clinical picture and may be accompanied by generalised or focal seizures. Papilloedema is not infrequent and careful search may reveal choroidal tubercles. Progression to frank meningitis with increasing stupor and cranial nerve involvement, usually the 3rd, 4th, 6th and 8th nerves, then occurs. It is probably at this stage that vasculitis, one of the major pathological features of the disorder, starts to exert its effect.

Fallon & Kennedy (1981) have suggested several possible reasons for the delay in diagnosis of tuberculous meningitis. The disease may not be suspected because it may be thought to be a manifestation of an already diagnosed condition or some other disorder is suspected, for example viral meningitis, partially treated bacterial meningitis or a space-occupying lesion. Focal signs or papilloedema are rare in the above meningitides. Mumps meningitis and herpes encephalitis may be other possible causes of confusion but these illnesses are usually of very short duration.

Another important cause of delay is misinterpretation of the laboratory findings. The protein content of CSF is almost always raised. Lymphocytosis of up to 400 per cu mm is usual but a preponderance of polymorphonuclear cells may be found (Smith 1975). The CSF glucose is often normal in the early stages but lowish levels of glucose may not be followed up with sufficient persistence to exclude tuberculosis. This leads to another reason, namely a failure to search diligently for the bacteria. The bacteriologist should be aware of the suspicion of the diagnosis and must examine all CSF specimens which contain cells and raised protein if no other diagnosis has been made. The examination requires skill and experience in preparation of the CSF. The search for the tubercle bacillus is a very demanding, time-consuming and sometimes tedious procedure. However, the use of the technique of fluorescent microscopy may hasten the speed of the search. If the infection is strongly suspected further specimens of CSF should be examined. If the patient is of Asian origin this is an additional feature to raise the suspicion of tuberculosis (Swart et al 1981).

Institution of therapy before the CSF is obtained does not preclude the identification of the organisms by microcopy; the bacilli can often be found in the CSF even after treatment has started. Cultures may also provide the diagnosis but only after several weeks. Sensitivity tests can be performed when the organism has been obtained. In some instances treatment may be justified where a microbiological diagnosis of tuberculous meningitis has not been established.

The optimal treatment of tuberculous meningitis has not yet been determined and the clinician who is called upon to treat the occasional patient, even in centres where excellent facilities are available, can be at a disadvantage. It is appropriate to use rifampicin, streptomycin and isoniazid as the initial drugs, but it should be stressed that serious hepatotoxicity may follow high doses of rifampicin and isoniazid especially in children (Linna & Uhari 1980). The benefit of intrathecal streptomycin in combination with the newer anti-tuberculous drugs has not been established. Both ethambutol and ethionamide penetrate the inflamed meninges and the latter will also penetrate normal meninges. Optic neuritis may follow the use of ethambutol and the early signs of this may be difficult to detect in a young child.

Dexamethasone is of unproven value in the presence of cerebral oedema and the role of corticosteroids in reducing the meningeal inflammatory reaction is debatable. Still less is known of their benefit in either the prevention or the treatment of

arteritis, one of the most important lesions produced by this infection. However, Escobar and colleagues (1975) have found them to be of benefit. The CT scan can be very helpful in the early stages of management. Neurosurgery has an important role in treatment including the early stages of the disease. Ventricular drainage, externally or by shunt for acute hydrocephalus, may result in a dramatic improvement in the neurological state of the patient. The treatment should be carried out with optimism for quite unpredictable recoveries occur.

Tuberculomas are usually multiple and may also be found in the infratentorial region. The symptoms may be indistinguishable from other space occupying lesions. Most are rounded or oval, and calcification is an uncommon and a late feature. The appearance of tuberculomata in the CT scan is illustrated in Figure 22.2, but Shiga and colleagues (1979) have stressed the variations in the radiographic findings; the density on the precontrast scan can be high or low, but increased density occurs following the injection of contrast.

The role of BCG vaccine in prevention of tuberculous meningitis or miliary tuberculosis has been well established in the United Kingdom but the same cannot be said for all countries in which it is used. Both in Singapore and Burma tuberculous meningitis has been described in children who have received BCG vaccination in the newborn period (Paul 1961, Myint 1980). Thus the presence of a BCG scar should not preclude the search for the bacillus if tuberculous meningitis is suspected.

Aseptic meningitis syndrome

Aseptic meningitis can be defined as a syndrome with inflammatory cells in the cerebrospinal fluid in the absence of bacteria as shown by examination of Gram's stain, by culture and failure to detect bacterial antigens by immunological methods. Thus some cases of bacterial meningitis will fall into this group, for example, those in which previous antimicrobial therapy has rendered the CSF sterile.

However the vast majority will be caused by viruses to which the cellular response is predominantly lymphocytic at some stage of the infection. There is a tendency to equate viral meningitis or

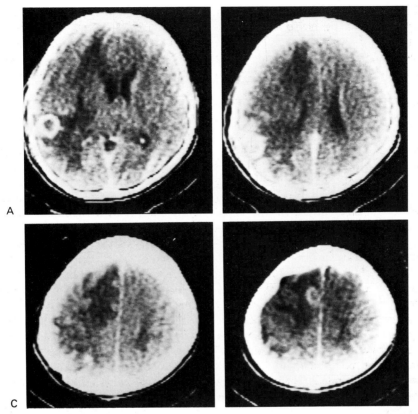

Fig. 22.2 Multiple tuberculomata in a 12-year-old girl who presented with headache, fever and vomiting. She showed bilateral papilloedema, flaccid weakness of right arm and bilateral extensor plantar responses. CT scan (A–D) shows extensive oedema with mass effect in the left cerebral hemisphere. In (A) and (B) a lesion which appeared isodense on the pre-contrast scans shows thick rim enchancement. A second lesion is present in the medial and posterior part of the frontal lobe in (D). The rim is somewhat thinner. The left parietal lesion was removed but follow-up scans showed some reduction in size of the frontal lesion but also revealed a third lesion in the right parietal lobe.

meningoencephalitis with aseptic meningitis, but whilst most patients who have a CSF lymphocytic pleocytosis have a viral infection the terms are not synonymous.

Infection in the region of the meninges may produce an inflammatory cell response, for example cerebral or epidural abscess, mastoiditis or osteomyelitis of the skull. Such cases may also be included in the aseptic meningitis syndrome as well as those infections of the meninges in which Gram's stain will not detect the organism which yet may be detected by other staining techniques or methods. Such infections include *Mycobacterium tuberculosis*, brucellosis, mycoplasma, leptospirosis, toxoplasmosis, syphilis, amoebae or one of a variety of fungal infections. In this group of causes very special attention should be paid to tuberculosis. Causes of a non-infectious nature are also included in the syndrome; these include neoplastic disorders, various collagen diseases and intrathecal injections of chemical and other substances.

The major problem with aseptic meningitis is to determine if it is caused by an infection for which specific therapy is necessary. This can often be difficult and there are many children who receive antimicrobials unnecessarily because bacterial infection cannot be excluded with confidence. Although the introduction of methods for rapid detection of bacterial antigens is an important advance, these can only detect the infection for which the corresponding antibody is used. Other methods,

Table 22.8 Laboratory tests reported to distinguish bacterial meningitis from other agents

Test	Reference
Creatine kinase	Katz & Liebman (1970)
Isocritic dehydrogenase	Van Rymenant et al (1966)
Glutamic oxaloacetic transaminase	Lending (1964)
Lactic dehydrogenase and specific isoenzyme pattern	Feldman (1975)
Lactic acid	Beatty & Oppenheim (1968)
	Controni et al (1977)
Limulus (endotoxin)	Berman (1976)
Nitroblue tetrazolium	Fikrig (1973)
C-reactive protein	Corrall et al (1981)

such as measurement of lactic acid and other substances in the CSF (Table 22.8) may be available but these cannot be guaranteed to differentiate bacterial from viral infections in all patients.

Intracranial abscess

Intracranial suppuration may occur in several sites; between the skull and dura (extradural), between the dura and arachnoid (subdural) or at any site within the substance of the brain. Infection can arise from the blood stream, as an extension from adjacent sites such as the middle ear, mastoid or paranasal sinuses, following penetrating injuries to the skull, or through a midline congenital dermal sinus. These infections may result in the development of a localised collection of pus which may be more prone to occur in the brain if there is preceding damage, either from trauma or hypoxia. The pus becomes encapsulated and the surrounding brain may be compressed by the space occupying lesion, or affected by an inflammatory reaction.

Brain abscesses are seen at all ages. In a series of 66 children seen at The Hospital for Sick Children, 11 were less than 6 months of age, and six of these had suffered from bacterial meningitis or septicaemia in the neonatal period (Eggerding 1981). Thirty-nine of the children were boys. The

most common symptoms in these children were headache and vomiting, which occurred in half the patients. The next most frequent clinical manifestations were lethargy and fever which occurred in only 25 and 24 patients respectively. Nineteen presented with fits and fourteen children had focal signs such as plegias and abnormalities of the cranial nerves; the most common was facial palsy. Symptoms were usually present for 1–3 weeks but occasionally were of 2–3 months' duration. Papilloedema was common (54%) and neck stiffness was not infrequent. Five children had a normal neurological examination and over one-third had normal mental status on admission. Peripheral white cell numbers were either normal or elevated with an increase in polymorphonuclear leucocytes. The CSF, on the other hand, was very rarely normal. A lymphocytic response with normal levels of glucose and mild elevation of protein was the most frequent abnormality. Large numbers of polymorphs with low levels of glucose were found in some children and probably reflected rupture or leakage of the abscess into the subarachnoid space. However, if a cerebral abscess is strongly suspected, lumbar puncture should be avoided and is contraindicated if papilloedema is present.

The use of the CT scan has enabled the diagnosis of cerebral abscess to be made with greater ease and with less risk than the older techniques of arteriography and pneumography. Thus the scan has probably been a major contributing factor in decline in mortality of patients seen in this hospital and the increase in the proportion of survivors without apparent sequelae (Table 22.9). A similar suggestion has been made by Fischer and his colleagues (1981).

The largest single group of children were those in whom there was no detectable underlying disorder (Table 22.10). Cyanotic congenital heart disease was the most frequent predisposing factor but ear and sinus infections were numerically impor-

Table 22.9 Mortality and clinical status of patients with cerebral abscess before and after the introduction of the CT scanner at the Hospital for Sick Children

	Mortality	Patients without sequelae
Prior to use of CT scan	10/42 (24%)	11/42 (26%)
Following use of CT scan	1/24 (4%)	13/24 (54%)

Table 22.10 Predisposing factors in 66 children with cerebral abscess

Condition	Number of patients
Congenital heart disease	19
Otitis media/mastoiditis	6
Sinusitis	3
Facial/orbital cellulitis	3
Trauma	3
Neonatal meningitis	3
Neonatal septicaemia	2
Caries	2
Chronic subdural haematoma	2
Occipital dermal sinus	2
Meningitis (*H. influenzae* type b)	1
No predisposing factor	20

Table 22.12 Bacteria isolated from 64 children with cerebral abscess

Organisms	Number
Microaerophilic streptococci	20
S. pneumoniae	8
Staph. epidermidis	7
Staph. aureus	6
E. coli	5
Proteus	5
Bacteroides	5
Klebsiella	3

tant. The former was less common in older children in this group but this probably reflects the effect of early corrective surgery. In both the children with an occipital dermal sinus the abscess was situated in the posterior fossa. A careful search may be needed to detect the midline skin lesions but a characteristic 'key hole' defect on the skull may be visible on the X-rays (Till 1975). Cerebral abscess is rare in children with immunodeficiences and extremely rare in children with chronic suppurative lung disease such as cystic fibrosis (Fischer et al 1979).

The sites of the abscesses are shown in Table 22.11. The most frequent bacteria isolated were micro-aerophilic streptococci (31%) which were usually sensitive to both penicillin and chloramphenicol. Other bacteria which were isolated are shown in Table 22.12.

Mixed infections occurred in 24% of the patients. The wide variety of organisms which are found underlines the importance of immediate microscopic examination of the pus and special attention to the culture techniques used; many of the organisms require special conditions for growth. The fungi and other organisms which may cause cerebral abscess are *Nocardia asteroides*, candida and aspergillus species and amoebae.

Treatment of cerebral abscess is based on surgical drainage or aspiration and the use of appropriate antimicrobial agents. Pending the results of sensitivity tests the most appropriate drugs to use are penicillin and chloramphenicol by the intravenous route; consideration may be given to the addition of metronidazole. It has been suggested that surgery may not be necessary in some instances, especially when the diagnosis has been made early in the illness (Berg et al 1978).

Spinal, epidural and subdural abscess

Abscesses adjacent to the spinal cord, which may be subdural or epidural, are rare in children. Infection may arise from a haematogenous source, adjacent osteomyelitis of the vertebrae, penetrating injury or from infection of dermoid cysts from a persistent dermal sinus. The symptoms and signs are those of infection and those referrable to disease of the spine; fever, irritability, neck and back stiffness, pain and spinal tenderness and signs of spinal cord compression. The signs may be those of transverse myelitis. In almost all instances of epidural abscesses, the infection is caused by *Staphylococcus aureus* (Baker 1971), but various streptococci, *Pseudomonas aeruginosa* and *E. coli* may be isolated.

The CSF is often sterile but an acute inflammatory response is usually present. Investigations should include myelography and the disorder must be treated urgently by surgical exploration and drainage. The myelographic features of a child with an epidural abscess are shown in Figure 22.3.

Table 22.11 Sites of intracranial abscess

Frontal	15	
Fronto-parietal	13	
Parietal	7	
Temporal	8	
Temporo-parietal	6	
Occipital	2	
Ponto-medullary	1	
Cerebellar	5	
Deep hemisphere	2	
Diffuse multiple	5	
Subdural	11	(bilateral 4)
Extra-dural	2	

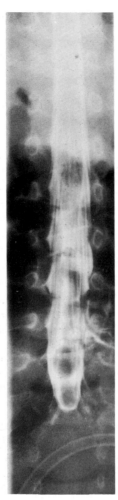

Fig. 22.3 Lumbar dermoid cyst with epidural abscess. A 10-month-old boy with fever, irritability, marked stiffness of the neck and spine. CSF showed polymorphonuclear leucocytosis, elevated protein, reduced glucose level and was sterile prior to onset of treatment. Lumbar myelogram performed following drainage of the epidural abscess. The theca is displaced to the left from the lower thoracic region to S1 indicating that there is still fluid in the epidural space. There are multiple intra-arachnoid filling defects caused by the lobulated dermoid cyst. The tip of the conus is at the level of L2/3 disc space, being tethered by a dermal sinus track related to the intrathecal dermoid.

VIRUS INFECTIONS

The wide spectrum of clinical disease of the nervous system associated wth virus infection includes many illnesses so mild and so brief that medical assistance is not sought and their cause is not known. One reason for the lack of identification of the cause is that on rapid recovery investigations are understandably not pursued. Thus, there is a paucity of accurate data on both the incidence of CNS involvement in individual virus infections and the overall incidence of virus infections in the causation of CNS disease. Most figures probably underestimate the problem for several reasons. With a few exceptions the symptoms and signs of CNS disease caused by individual infections are not specific for that infection. The lack of simple or rapid methods of diagnosis is a major factor and one of the most neglected features of investigation is the study of immunological or other responses in CSF.

There are, however, a number of features which are often overlooked but may be very helpful. Many virus infections occur in epidemic form or possess some geographical features to their epidemiology; inferences can sometimes be drawn from these features. In the evaluation of the patient precise information on the previous immunisation status, of contact with known infections or of illness of a similar type in the home, in the school or nursery, or in the neighbourhood is of special importance. Enquiry into recent travel is essential.

Chun (1976) has classified these infections into those in which the disease is only clinically significant when there is involvement of the CNS; polioviruses and some arboviruses are examples. Another group are those in which the infection usually causes a systemic disease, for example measles, mumps, herpes simplex and varicella-zoster virus, but may occasionally cause CNS disease which can be very severe. This is a useful classification but the mechanisms involved in the second group are variable and complex. On the other hand, a classification based on the clinical syndromes of aseptic meningitis, paralytic poliomyelitis, acute polyneuritis and encephalitis (acute, subacute, or chronic) has merit in that many instances of an aetiological agent cannot be ascribed.

Aseptic meningitis

Aseptic meningitis of viral aetiology is usually of acute onset and exhibits the symptoms and signs of fever, headache, vomiting, neck stiffness and predominantly lymphocytic pleocytosis with little or no elevation in protein and normal levels of glucose. It is most often caused by mumps virus and several of the enteroviruses.

Mumps is the most frequently identified virus causing aseptic meningitis and occurs in 0.5–2% of patients with mumps. Rarely encephalitis, transverse myelitis and even cerebellar ataxia may be caused by this virus. In some series parotitis was absent in one third or more of patients (Meyer 1962) and in the absence of epidemiological evidence to suggest mumps infection the diagnosis can only be made serologically or by isolation of virus from the CSF. Fortunately this is common in the early stages of the disease (McLean et al 1967). Mumps meningitis can also be diagnosed by electromicroscopic examination of the CSF (Doane et al 1967).

Most cases of aseptic meningitis occur in the week following the onset of parotitis. A very high fever is often also present in addition to the signs of meningitis. The leucocyte count in the CSF can be very high and the fluid may even be opalescent; lymphocytes predominate, but early in the disease there may also be polymorphonuclear leucocytes present. On occasions glucose levels may be low, thus presenting a CSF which could be interpreted as indicating a 'partially treated' bacterial meningitis.

The predominance of polymorphonuclear leucocytes in mumps and in all forms of viral meningitis in the early hours or days of the meningeal infection is a frequent cause for concern. When this occurs without a significant depression of glucose (less than 40 mg/100 ml or less than two thirds of simultaneously obtained blood glucose levels) it may not be possible to exclude bacterial meningitis with confidence even when bacteria are not visible on Gram's stain. Appropriate antimicrobial treatment should then be instituted. However, Feigin & Shackleford (1973) suggest that if the child is not ill, close observation and examination of another specimen of CSF in 6–12 hours may allow a distinction to be made in most patients. In viral meningitis a rapid shift in the cells to a predominant lymphocyte response occurs in 80 to 90% of cases.

A number of other techniques have been described (Table 22.8) to provide rapid differentiation between viral and bacterial meningitis but most are non-specific and not completely reliable. Diagnosis by means of electron microscopy, the use of rapid methods to detect viral antigen or investigation of specific immune response in CSF has not been widely investigated.

Recovery is usually rapid but the most frequent complication is nerve deafness which is often unilateral. Thus these and indeed all children with aseptic meningitis should have careful audiometric examination carried out after recovery.

The picorna viruses which are commonly associated with aseptic meningitis are Coxsackie B1–5 and Coxsackie A7, 9 and 25, ECHO viruses 4, 6, 9, 11, 14, 16, 18, 20 and 30, as well as polioviruses in areas where vaccination programmes have not been introduced. These enterovirus infections usually occur in the summer months whereas mumps is usually most frequent in late winter and early spring months of the year in temperate regions. Recently a 'new' picorna virus, Enterovirus 71 has been identified and may cause both aseptic meningitis and paralytic disease (Schmidt et al 1974).

Gastrointestinal symptoms are infrequent and usually mild in these enteroviral infections but sore throat, fever and rashes may be present. A maculopapular rash is sometimes seen in Coxsackie A9 or 23, and ECHO viruses 4, 9 and 16 infections and may be helpful in arriving at a clinical diagnosis. In epidemics, which are most frequently caused by Coxsackie B5 and ECHO viruses 6 and 9, illness in other members of the family may be suggestive of an enterovirus infection. Because of the many types of enterovirus sero-diagnosis is cumbersome and rarely indicated. Isolation of the virus from stool, urine, pharyngeal washings or CSF is the most practical approach to diagnosis.

The true frequency of sequelae following enteroviral meningitis is not known. There is little doubt that severe neonatal disease not infrequently results in brain damage. Infections beyond that age particularly in the first year of life, although mild, may cause permanent sequelae. It has been suggested that some of the effects may be caused by retardation of brain growth (Sells et al 1975). Insufficient attention has been paid to the long term evaluation of patients with these infections, particularly in those under one year (Lepow 1978).

Paralytic poliomyelitis

Paralytic poliomyelitis is caused by one of the three strains of poliovirus but is rarely seen in countries with adequate immunisation programmes. Thus the infection may not be suspected until paralysis is obvious. In others, usually tropical countries, infection is often endemic and primarily affects infants and very young children.

The neurological illness is usually preceded by sore throat and fever; thus there may be a biphasic illness, the second component starting 3 to 7 days after the first with recurrence of fever, together with headache, vomiting, neck and spine stiffness and muscle pain or spasm. These rapidly progress to the signs of paralysis with loss of deep tendon reflexes. The asymmetrical nature will give a clue to the diagnosis. In the younger patient, involvement of the lower limbs is more frequent than upper limbs. Bulbar involvement is more frequent in the older child. However, signs of aseptic meningitis together with weakness and flaccidity, sometimes associated with spasm and tenderness occur albeit rarely in some Coxsackie B and ECHO virus infections. Sabin (1981) has stressed that the presence of somnolence, disorientation and coma, the absence of fever or neck stiffness at the time of onset of paralysis and complete recovery of weakness within 7 to 10 days should make the diagnosis of poliovirus infection very doubtful. Paralytic disease may occur in recipients of oral polio vaccine or even in close contacts of vaccinees, but this is an extremely rare complication (Nightingale et al 1977).

Adenoviruses of various types have been infrequent causes of meningitis or encephalitis (Kelsey 1978). Rarely dual virus infections may occur and even mixed enteroviral and bacterial infections have been observed. It has usually been *H. influenzae* in these circumstances. This latter phenomenon may be more common than is realised because once bacterial meningitis is diagnosed, viral studies are rarely performed.

Acute polyneuritis

Acute polyneuritis, with symmetrical flaccid paralysis, is sometimes associated with virus and other infections and is discussed later in this chapter and in Chapter 4. There is also a temporal association with some types of influenza vaccines (Schonberger et al 1979).

Encephalitis

Encephalitis, in contrast to the other syndromes caused by viruses, is a much more complex disorder both in clinical features and in its causation. There may also be meningeal involvement and thus in many instances the term 'meningo-encephalitis' would be more correct. Fever is often high, the level of consciousness is depressed from drowsiness, confusion to deep coma. Seizures, which are usually generalised but may be focal, can dominate the disease. It is in this group of patients that aetiologies of a non-infectious nature have to be considered. This includes toxins such as lead, and accidental overdose with drugs including medications as well as metabolic and cerebrovascular diseases.

The viral causes include agents which cause disease by direct invasion and an associated inflammatory response. The virus may be isolated from the nervous system in such cases. The major causes of this type of disease are the arboviruses, herpes simplex, varicella-zoster, mumps, the enteroviruses and rabies.

The second group comprises those viruses which are associated with the so-called 'post-infectious' encephalitis. This usually follows a number of common infections or the use of certain live virus vaccines. The 'characteristic' pathology of post-infectious encephalitis consists of perivascular infiltration with lymphocytes and perivenous demyelination, the latter being the most important distinguishing feature. In this group, vascular disease may play a greater role in the process than hitherto believed.

The term 'para-infectious' CNS disease has been used by Ray (1976) for those forms of acute CNS diseases without either evidence of viral invasion or a post-infectious inflammatory process which may have a close temporal relationship to a presumed 'viral' illness. Cerebral oedema is often a prominent feature in these cases.

The arboviruses

These are a very large and heterogeneous group of RNA viruses which are 'maintained in nature principally or to an important extent, through biological transmission between susceptible vertebrate hosts by hematophagous arthropods' (WHO 1967). The principal clinical syndromes caused by the viruses are fever/arthralgia, haemorrhagic fever with or without hepatitis or nephritis and encephalitis. Arboviruses causing encephalitis are shown in Table 22.13.

There is often a prodromal illness followed by neurological symptoms which vary from a mild aseptic meningitis syndrome to encephalitis of varying severity. Focal neurological signs may be present in some infections. Sequelae are usually more common in younger patients.

Rabies

This is an acute, fatal encephalitis, the incubation period of which can extend beyond a year; the mean period is about 6 weeks but it may be as short as 10 days. Infection is almost always acquired by the bite of a rabid animal. Death usually occurs within 1 to 2 weeks of the onset of coma which follows a prodromal period of about 1 week. The characteristic pathological finding in the nervous system is a cytoplasmic inclusion, the Negri body. A great advance has been the recent development of a vaccine produced in human diploid cells. It has far greater immunogenicity than the vaccine produced in duck embryo cell cultures and side effects are minimal (Plotkin 1981).

Herpesvirus hominis (herpes simplex)

Encephalitis caused by herpes simplex virus (HSV) occurs sporadically and causes either focal or diffuse haemorrhagic lesions with a predilection for the temporal or temporo-parietal regions although probably no area of the brain is immune; for example it has been observed as brain stem encephalitis (Fenton et al 1977). Most infections are caused by the type 1 strain of the virus whereas type 2 or 'genital' strains predominate in the more generalised encephalitis occurring in disseminated neonatal infections. Isolation of the virus from the CSF is extremely rare in HSV encephalitis whereas it is not infrequent in neonatal infections involving the brain. The CSF may show a mild lymphocytosis and red cells may be present in patients who have had neurological symptoms for several days. Protein is moderately elevated but levels of glucose are rarely decreased.

The role of primary infection or reactivation of latent virus in the nervous system in HSV encephalitis is not clear. The bimodal age distribution reported by Whitley et al (1977) may indicate more than one mechanism; it could be argued that primary infections predominate in children and young adults, disease in the older age groups being caused by reactivation of latent virus. Although entry to the nervous system by the blood stream is likely, the frequent localisation of the necrotising encephalitis to the temporal lobe could reflect entry to the

Table 22.13 Principal arboviruses associated with encephalitis (after Fenner & White 1976)

Virus/disease	Distribution	Vector	Reservoir
Eastern equine encephalitis (EEE)	Americas	Mosquito	Birds
Western equine encephalitis (WEE)	Americas	Mosquito	Birds, reptiles?
Venezuelan equine encephalitis (VEE)	Americas	Mosquito	Rodents
St. Louis encephalitis (SLE)	Americas	Mosquito	Birds
Japanese encephalitis (JE)	East Asia	Mosquito	Birds
Australian encephalitis	Australia	Mosquito	Birds
West Nile encephalitis (WN)	Africa, Europe	Mosquito	Birds
Tick-borne encephalitis (TBE)	Eastern Europe	Tick	Mammals
Russian spring-summer encephalitis (RSSE)	USSR, Europe	Tick	Rodents
Louping ill	Britain	Tick	Sheep
Powassan	North America	Tick	Rodents
California encephalitis (CE)	North America	Mosquito	Rodents, rabbits

nervous system via the olfactory nerve fibres through the cribriform plate with spread to the interior frontal and medial frontal regions in primary infections; in cases of reactivation the trigeminal ganglia could be the source of the virus (Bastian et al 1972).

The pathology consists of haemorrhage, necrosis and oedema with inflammatory cell infiltration. Characteristic intranuclear inclusion bearing cells may be seen on light microscopy and herpesvirus particles are visible on electron-microscopy. Antigen can be detected by immunofluorescent techniques (McIntosh et al 1978) and the virus can often be detected in cell culture within 48–72 hours of inoculation of cerebral tissue.

The serum antibody responses may take up to 7–10 days to occur and antibody is absent from the CSF in the early stages of the infection with the currently used antibody tests. They are, therefore, unhelpful in the acute stages of the disease. However, local antibody production in the CSF which takes up to 14 days to appear is useful for retrospective diagnosis (MacCallum 1974). A diagnostic pattern consists of a CSF: serum HSV antibody ratio equal to or greater than 1 : 20 (Levine et al 1978, McKendrick 1979). More sensitive tests for antibody will enable the diagnosis to be made earlier than 10 days in a proportion of individuals (Klapper et al 1981).

Brain biopsy is advocated by many but virological confirmation is made in about 50% of clinically suspected cases (Whitley et al 1977). It can be argued that the biopsy may allow other causes, for which specific treatments are available, to be identified. An additional advantage of brain biopsy which is cited is the potential therapeutic effect achieved by its decompression mechanism. (Lauter 1980). In contrast the procedure may not be as innocuous as has been claimed; it may for example produce a focus for seizures (Caplan 1977). Since the lesions are patchy, it is possible to biopsy a normal area, giving a false negative result.

Both the CT and radionucleide brain scans and the EEG may be helpful in the investigation of the child suspected of having HSV encephalitis. The most common abnormality in the CT scan is an area of low attenuation involving at least one temporal lobe and sometimes other areas (Fig. 22.4); a mass effect may be detected and in about half the cases enhancement with contrast will be visible (Davis et al 1978). However it must be stressed that scans performed within 24–48 hours of onset of the neurological illness are sometimes normal. The EEG may show periodic complexes and focal abnormalities. The periodic complexes occur most commonly between the second and fifteenth day of the disease (Upton & Gumpert 1970) and are rarely seen after the second week (Schauseil-

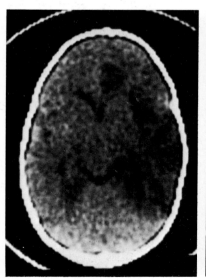

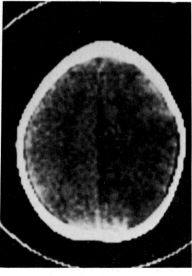

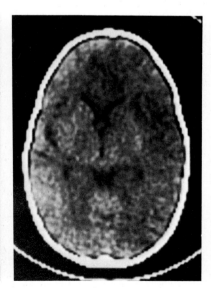

A   B   C

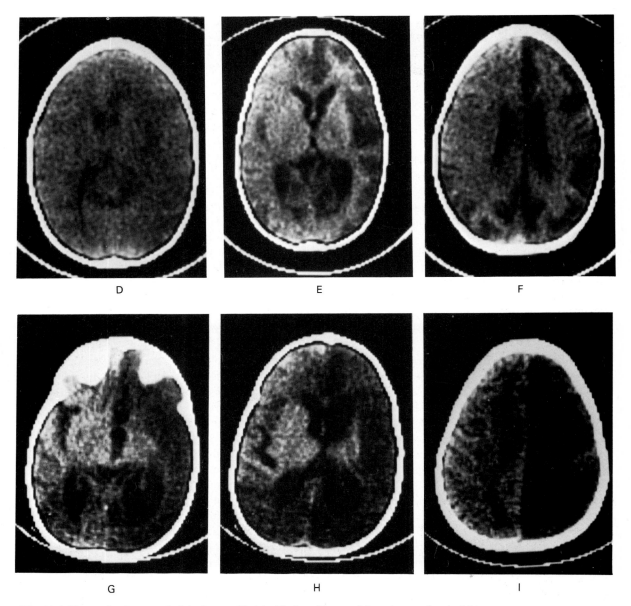

Fig. 22.4 Herpes simplex encephalitis. 2-year-old girl with short history of drowsiness and convulsions.
A, B. Scans made 3 days after onset of illness. There is swelling of the right hemisphere with compression of the lateral ventricle and displacement of the septum pellucidum to the left. There are (A) areas of low attenuation extending up from the temporal lobe across the insula into the frontal and parietal lobes, in medial part of the frontal lobe and (B) in the upper half of the hemisphere. There is also abnormality of the left hemisphere in the posterior temporal region and in the deep white matter. In (B) high density in the posterior parietal region indicates haemorrhage.
C, D. 7 days later. There is less swelling of the right hemisphere and the lateral ventricles are larger. Low attenuation in the right hemisphere is more confluent but abnormality of the left is more extensive.
E, F. 7 weeks following; there is no longer any swelling and the lateral ventricles are much larger and the Sylvian fissures wide indicating atrophy. The circumscribed areas of low attenuation in the cortex and white matter indicate areas of necrotic brain.
G, H, I. 16 weeks later. There is even more extensive necrosis of the right hemisphere and atrophy of the left with a large area of necrosis in the parieto-occipital region. Contrast medium had been injected at the time of the second and third examinations and had shown enhancement of the margins of the affected tissue (not reproduced).

Zipf et al 1982).

In most children there is a short prodromal period with non-specific features such as vomiting, lethargy, poor feeding, or symptoms referrable to a mild infection of the upper respiratory tract. Fever is not common and headache more likely to be apparent in the older child. Focal or generalised seizures may then occur and the level of consciousness becomes depressed.

Hemiplegia or cranial nerve palsies are not infrequent but rapid development of deep coma can mask these focal features. Personality changes and memory loss are rarely observed in children. Thus an acute neurological disorder with focal features should lead to suspicion of HSV encephalitis and the patient should be referred to a centre where appropriate investigation and treatment facilities are available.

Adenine-arabinoside has been shown to confer some benefit in a disease which carries a 70–80% mortality in the first 30 days and a 90% mortality by 4 to 6 months (Hirsch 1979); there was a significant reduction in mortality as well as morbidity in biopsy-proven cases in the patients reported by Whitley et al (1977). It is possible that the more recently developed drug Acylovir (Hirsch & Swartz 1980) may be still more effective. But the key to successful treatment is early suspicion of the infection and the institution of treatment before coma ensues. The beneficial effect of early treatment is illustrated in 23 patients under 30 years of age who were lethargic at the start of treatment with adenine arabinoside; 16 returned to normal and there were only two deaths (Whitley et al 1981). An important feature of these patients was that the final outcome could not be predicted immediately after completion of therapy; neurological improvement occurred for several months and in children even for a year or more. Rarely a post-infectious encephalopathy, not associated with viral replication, occurs in some patients who are treated with adenine arabinoside (Koenig et al 1979).

Supportive treatment, which includes restriction of fluids and control of fits, is important. Surgical decompression may be life-saving when other methods of controlling raised intracranial pressure have failed. It is not clear whether dexamethasone has a beneficial or an adverse effect. Intracranial pressure monitoring may be helpful in controlling raised intracranial pressure and as experience develops may become standard practice in the management of this and many other causes of severe increase in intracranial pressure in childhood.

Measles virus

Measles is commonly associated with disturbances of the nervous system. Febrile convulsions are common but usually benign. The rate is of the order of 5–6 per 1000 cases and ranges from 7–8 per 1000 in the second year of life to 2 per 1000 in 5–6 year old children.

The most serious complication is 'post infectious' encephalitis and measles is usually cited as the paradigm of this form of encephalitis. It is an acute disseminated encephalomyelitis which may represent an immunological cell-mediated injury to brain cells and possibly blood vessels containing viral antigen. It is one of the major reasons for the use of measles vaccine in industrialised countries where measles is an otherwise mild infection.

Measles encephalitis occurs in 1 to 2 per 1000 children and usually develops during the 7–10 days after the onset of the rash but may occur within 48 hours or up to two weeks later. The onset is usually abrupt with high fever, generalised or focal convulsions and coma may be present. Recovery may be rapid but complete recovery can still occur in children with signs of severe disease for 3–4 weeks; it is a very unpredictable disorder. The CSF may be normal or contain up to 100 lymphocytes. EEG changes of a generalised disturbance of cerebral function are usual and changes of a similar but less severe type may also be seen in many children without clinical evidence of encephalitis (Pampiglione 1964). The mortality is high (10–15%) and permanent sequelae occur in approximately 20% of survivors (Greenberg et al 1955).

Treatment with dexamethasone is usually recommended but steroids have not been subjected to a controlled trial in this disorder. Fits should be treated with anticonvulsants and electrolyte disturbances such as those which result from the syndrome of inappropriate antidiuretic hormone activity should be managed by fluid restriction.

Encephalitis was very rarely observed following the earlier live measles vaccines used in this country, but the vaccines currently in use have not been reported to cause measles encephalitis. Another important but rare association with measles virus is subacute sclerosing panencephalitis (SSPE) which is discussed elsewhere.

A few children with acute leukaemia have been reported to develop fatal encephalitis in which very high levels of measles antibody are present in the serum and CSF (Pullan et al 1976, Smyth et al 1976). However, neither the clinical features nor the EEG resemble those seen in SSPE. Catatonia has been a striking feature in some of the patients with this form of measles encephalitis.

Rubella

This has also rarely been associated with the post-infectious encephalitis syndrome. It has been reported to occur in less than 1 in 5000 cases (Sherman et al 1965). Death is very rare and most patients recover without sequelae. In contrast, infection acquired in utero may cause extensive disease of the CNS, the features of which are discussed later in this chapter.

Varicella zoster

Chicken pox and shingles are caused by the same virus; the former is the disease resulting from primary infection, and the latter occurs when there is reactivation of the latent virus in dorsal root ganglia.

Encephalitis, which is probably of the 'post-infectious' type, may appear at the onset of chickenpox or follow at any time in the subsequent 14 days. However, it should not be confused with the acute encephalopathy of Reye's syndrome, which may also be associated with chickenpox. Chickenpox encephalitis is usually mild and cerebellar dysfunction is frequent. The incidence is not precisely known but it is probably less common than measles encephalitis. An incidence of 31.7–55.8 per 100 000 cases has been reported in the United States (CDC 1978) and those at greatest risk are adults and children below five years of age (Preblud 1981). Recovery, particularly in those patients with cerebellar involvement, is usually complete, but may be delayed for several months. Transverse myelitis without encephalitis is rare but complete recovery within a few weeks is usual (McCarthy & Amer 1978).

Zoster has a frequency of the order of 0.74 per 1000 in the first decade, and 1.38 in the second decade of life (Hope-Simpson 1965). The disease, however, is more frequently seen in children with malignancy, especially lymphoma and leukaemia. But, unlike the adult, infants and children with shingles rarely suffer much discomfort or pain, and post-herpetic neuralgia is very rare. Within a few days of the onset of shingles a generalised vesicular rash may develop called zoster-varicellosis.

If an infant or a child develops shingles without a previous history of chickenpox, it is possible that his mother may have had chickenpox during pregnancy; in these circumstances it has been suggested by Brunell & Kotchmar (1981) that latency cannot be maintained as effectively as following post-natal infection.

Epstein-Barr virus

This is a herpesvirus and is the causal organism in infectious mononucleosis. Infection is common in the first decade of life but there is also a period of increased prevalence in the latter part of the second decade. Most infections in early childhood are subclinical or occur with mild non-specific symptoms. The infection can be suspected from the appearance of atypical lymphocytes in the peripheral blood and good evidence of EBV infection is obtained by the detection of heterophile antibody though a proportion of children and young adults fail to develop these antibodies. However, specific antibody tests for EBV virus which detect both IgM and IgG antibody overcome this deficiency. Neurological disease is rare but the infection has been shown to be associated with ascending polyneuritis, encephalitis and Bell's palsy (Gross et al 1975). Acute cerebellar ataxia has also been reported (Bergen & Grossman 1976). The prognosis of these complications is said to be good.

Lymphocytic choriomeningitis virus (LCM)

LCM is an RNA virus of the arena virus group. It is usually an infection of small rodents including mice and hamsters. Infection of man is rare, but occurs when there is very close contact with infected animals (Hirsch et al 1974). Subclinical infection is probably more common than is realised.

The commonest clinical manifestation, aseptic meningitis, is infrequent. The lymphocytic pleocytosis may persist for several weeks and the diagnosis can be established serologically. Severe CNS involvement is extremely rare (Green et al 1974). Ataxia and tremors may be present. The fundi are usually normal but mild degrees of papilloedema can be seen. Stiffness of the neck and spine become prominent when there is associated meningeal involvement.

Cat scratch disease

This is a presumed viral infection in which there is regional lymphadenitis and fever which follows the development of an erythematous lesion at the site of the cat scratch, occurring one or several weeks beforehand. Rarely an abrupt encephalitic illness, usually of short duration, has developed in such a patient but the majority of patients have made a complete recovery (Steiner et al 1963).

CHRONIC VIRUS INFECTIONS

The vast majority of virus infections involving the nervous system consist of an acute process but there are a few in which the infection is chronic; these include subacute sclerosing panencephalitis (SSPE), progressive multifocal leucoencephalopathy (PML). Kuru, Jakob-Creutzfeldt disease and rubella subacute panencephalitis. An encephalitis associated with measles virus occurring in children undergoing treatment for haematogenous malignancies can be considered in this category. In each the incubation period, which is conventionally defined as the interval between the acquisition of infection and the onset of symptoms, is measured in months or years. The term 'slow virus disease' is also used to describe these conditions, some of the features of which are summarised in Table 22.14. Subacute sclerosing-panencephalitis together with congenital rubella panencephalitis primarily affect children whereas the child, if affected by the remainder, represents the lower end of an age range in which adults bear the brunt of the infections.

Subacute sclerosing panencephalitis

SSPE is the commonest of the chronic virus infections to affect children and has been known for sev-

Table 22.14 Some features of chronic virus infections of man (from Brody & Gibbs 1976)

Disease	Agent	Distribution	M:F ratio	Incubation period	Other features	Animal transmission
Transmissable spongiform encephalopathies						
Kuru		New Guinea Highlands	1:3	? years	Associated with ritual cannibalism	Chimpanzees, old and new world monkeys, mink
Creutzfeldt-Jacob		Worldwide	1:1	4–18 mths	Organ/tissue transplantation neurosurgery	Chimpanzees, old and new world monkeys, guinea pigs.
Subacute sclerosing panencephalitis	Measles	Worldwide	3:1	6 years	? rural exposure	Hamsters, dogs, lambs, calves
Chronic progressive rubella panencephalitis	Rubella	? Worldwide	?	10–15 yrs	Follows prenatal infection	–
Progressive multifocal encephalitis	Papova-virus	Many countries	15:1	?	Occurs in patients with lymphoid malignancies	–

eral decades as a clinical disorder in which measles virus plays a role. Death occurs in the vast majority of patients. The onset has been as early as 3 months and rarely later than 20 years but is most often between 5 and 15 years. In most series boys outnumber girls by 3 or 2 to one. Among many descriptions of the clinical features are those of Dawson (1934), Van Bogaert (1945), Foley & Williams (1953) and Metz et al (1964).

Four stages of the disease are recognised. The first stage, usually of several months' duration, is marked by an insidious deterioration in behaviour and intellectual performance but the exact time of onset may be difficult to determine. This may be more obvious on retrospective enquiry, especially in children of school age, and may be first noted by teachers. Study of the previous written school work will often show deterioration starting some months before there was any concern. The writing may become smaller and less neat, with spelling mistakes and a decline in the quality of the content. At this stage there is a risk, as with other slowly progressive neurological disorders of childhood, that the organic nature of the disease may be overlooked and a diagnosis of behaviour disorder or psychological disturbance made, with reference to a psychiatric clinic.

The involuntary movements are a striking feature; at an early stage the child may have periodic episodes of falling backwards or of staggering backwards without falling as if pulled back by an invisible string. These episodes may cause great puzzlement and a cerebellar tumour may be suspected. In the second stage mental deterioration becomes progressively more obvious and the characteristic periodic abnormal movements develop. These are often described as myoclonic but this term scarcely does justice to their peculiar character. They differ from the classical myoclonic jerks with their explosive, momentary character. In 1964 Sandifer emphasised the repetitive, stereotyped character of the involuntary movements which are pathognomonic of the disease (Metz et al 1964). An important feature is their tempo. Each spasm starts with the instantaneous shock-like abruptness typical of the myoclonic jerk, but does not end as abruptly as it begins.

Instead it ceases gradually, taking much longer to fade away than to appear and usually persisting for at least one second. The movement produced is thus arrested, 'frozen' or 'hung-up' for several moments before it gently melts away.

The spasms are usually bilateral and symmetrical but may be unilateral or asymmetrical and may affect whole limbs or parts of limbs, such as some or all of the fingers and toes or even the lower jaw or tongue. When gross and frequent they are obvious, but in some cases they are only detected by careful observation over several minutes. They may be provoked or increased by excitement or a loud noise. A typical feature is their repetitiveness usually with a regular periodicity at between four and twenty seconds while awake, but absent during sleep. In the early stages of the disease the movements may not show obvious periodicity and in their later stages they may be obscured by increasing hypertonia. They may also be hidden when embedded in the general restlessness of the dementing child, a restlessness which is sometimes repetitive, recurring at intervals several times a minute.

Rarely the movements are more highly organised and repetitive yawning or whistling may occur. Similar grosser movements of the trunk may be seen with flexion or rotation, so that, if walking, the child will periodically bow from the waist or sink towards the ground, usually recovering himself, but sometimes falling. Repetitive postural lapses of the outstretched arms may be seen. It is helpful to look for these, encouraging the child with the promise of a sweet balanced on the dorsum of his hand as it is held extended in front. Stereotyped periodic high-voltage slow waves (Radermecker complexes) are seen in the EEG (Ch. 24) coinciding with the movements described above (Pampiglione 1964) though on occasions the clinical features may not accompany all the electrical discharges but only a proportion of them. The spasms may be extremely distressing, both to the child and his family (and indeed to his doctors and nurses). Their treatment is difficult but in some cases they are reduced by chlorpromazine.

Apart from the periodic spasms, seizures of more conventional type may also occur, particularly grand mal convulsions. However, they are less frequent and of no pathognomonic significance.

Focal neurological deficits are common in SSPE. Spastic hemiplegia was an early feature in 7 of the 17 children reported by Metz et al (1964). One mode of presentation is with cortical blindness or hemianopia. Rarely specific learning difficulties arise as a result of parietal lobe dysfunction. These features may cause great diagnostic difficulty if the possibility of SSPE is overlooked.

The ophthalmic manifestations were reviewed by Robb & Watters (1970). Cortical blindness and focal chorioretinitis was observed. The chorioretinitis may be most marked at the maculae where scars are seen with 'splinters' of pigment and with adjacent blood vessels drawn towards the scar (Fig. 22.5). Nystagmus and optic atrophy were also seen. Raised intracranial pressure can occur transiently and the finding of papilloedema may suggest a space-occupying lesion. Attacks of sudden transient blindness have been described. Neurophysiological investigations are helpful in elucidating cortical blindness, the electroretinogram (ERG) usually being normal and the cortical visual evoked responses (VER) impaired.

In the third stage of the disease there is evidence of extrapyramidal and/or pyramidal dysfunction, often with a rather Parkinsonian stance and gait, hypertonia of rigid type, sometimes with a cogwheel element, and an expressionless facies. Spasticity may also be present and the tendon reflexes are often increased with extensor plantar responses. Dementia is severe and the child becomes bedridden. The periodic spasms may continue and may show a ballismic flinging character in the limbs, while convulsions may also occur.

The fourth and final stage with decerebrate rigidity and coma is reached one or more years from onset and may last for a few months to a few years. Frontal lobe features such as a palmar grasp and oral rooting reactions may be seen. Dysphagia makes feeding more and more difficult with aspiration pneumonia a common problem which is often the cause of death.

The tempo of the illness is variable. In general it tends to be more rapid in older than in younger children. (Table 22.15.) Rare cases of spontaneous 'arrest' of the disease in the second stage are seen (this lasted for 8 years in one personal case). There are reported cases of complete remission of the disease with full recovery e.g. Cobb & Morgan-Hughes (1968) but for practical purposes the disease leads to death and treatment has yet to be shown to be effective.

The association of measles virus with SSPE is well established, although the precise role of the virus is still not understood. The electron microscopic appearances of the measles virus involved in SSPE are indentical to those of the ordinary virus. The intranuclear and intracytoplasmic inclusions seen in SSPE show bright fluorescence when stained with labelled measles antibody. Only by co-cultivation techniques can measles virus be isolated from explants of brain with cell cultures which

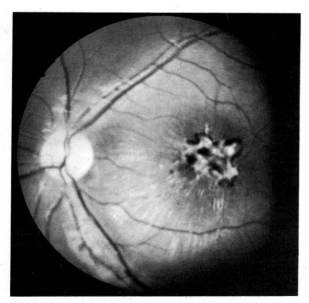

Fig. 22.5 Eight-year-old boy with fits, behaviour problems and visual loss. There is a raised pigmented scar at the macula with elevated retinal ridges radiating from it (courtesy Mr David Taylor)

Table 22.15 Age of onset of SSPE and survival*

Age of onset (years)	Mean survival (months)
4	29.9 (SD 30.3)
5–9	28.6 (SD 29.5)
10–14	16.9 (SD 15.3)
15	9.1 (SD 9.3)

* Data from Modlin et al 1979

normally support the growth of 'conventional' measles virus. Virus strains isolated in this way did not seem to differ significantly from those of 'wild' measles virus but Hall & Choppin (1981) have shown a defect in one of the several proteins known as M. protein which plays an essential part in the assembly of the virus at the cell membrane. This observation would not be inconsistent with the hypothesis that there is a defect in the measles virus of SSPE which is not spontaneous but may be induced by the host cell of the affected patient. 'Defective virus' consists of large amounts of viral nucleoprotein which cannot be released in the normal way and accumulation of which causes formation of characteristic inclusion bodies.

Measles has been noted to have occurred at an early age in an abnormally high proportion of patients with SSPE. In the report of the United Kingdom SSPE Register (Bellman & Dick 1980) of the 110 patients in whom the age of occurrence of natural measles was known, it was reported under the age of 2 years in 40. Similar findings have been noted in the United States (Table 22.16).

The period from the known measles infection to the onset of SSPE in the United Kingdom showed a range from 9 months to 18 years with an average of 6.8 years: 69% of them were between 4 and 9 years of age.

Many interesting but puzzling epidemiological aspects of the disease have been noted from various parts of the world. These have been reviewed by Modlin et al (1979).

Clustering of cases in an urban area of Ulster was noted by Connolly et al (1967), yet it is very rare for more than one child in a family to fall victim to the disease. Geographical clustering on a wider scale has been noted in many parts of the world;

Table 22.16 Age of onset of measles infection in 261 patients with SSPE (Modlin et al 1979)

Age of onset of measles (years)	Number of cases
< 1	24%
1	22%
2	10%
3	14%
4, 5, 6, 7,	9%, 6%, 4%, 5%,
8, 9, 10, 12,	2%, 2%, 0.4%, 1.1%

Table 22.17 Racial differences in SSPE in the United States[†]

Race	Incidence rate[*] Males	Females	Total
White	5.1	2.4	3.8
Black	1.4	0.6	0.9

[*] Per 10^7 population less than 20 years of age
[†] Data from Modlin et al 1979

in the northern and western counties of Belgium, in the Cape Province of South Africa, in the northern counties of England and in the Ohio River Valley and the South Eastern United States. Ten American states contributed 48% of all reported cases though containing only 19% of the United States population under 20 years of age. This does not appear to be due to artefacts of reporting.

A tendency has been noted in some parts of the world for patients to live in rural areas and this has caused speculation that some additional factor such as a zoonosis may be needed for SSPE to develop (Brody & Detels 1970).

Racial differences have been noted in the United States with an incidence four times higher in whites than in negroes (Table 22.17). How far this may be due to racial differences in rural and urban distribution is uncertain.

A common genetic background shared by many children with SSPE could be a factor in their developing the disease due to an altered host response to infection with measles virus. A small but significant increase in the expected frequency of HL-A antigen W-29 was found by Kurent et al (1975) but this has not been confirmed by others (Kreth et al 1975).

The decline in the number of cases of SSPE in the United States which has been noted since 1970 is impressive. This shows a close temporal relationship to the decline in the incidence of measles which has followed the use of measles vaccine (Fig. 22.6). During the same period there have been a number of children with SSPE and a history of vaccination against measles but not of measles infection. It is possible that the attenuated strain of measles virus used in the vaccine may have the same association with SSPE as does wild measles virus. If this is so, the incidence of SSPE after measles vaccination is much lower, by a factor of ten times, than after natural measles.

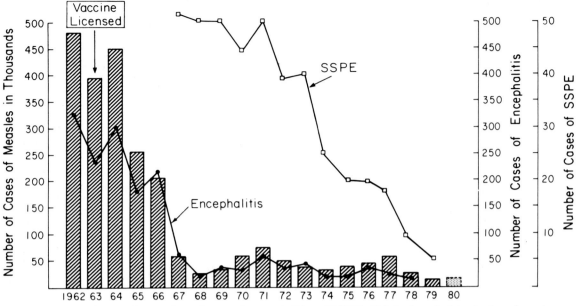

Fig. 22.6 Numbers of reported cases of measles, measles encephalitis and SSPE in U.S.A. since the introduction of measles vaccine (courtesy Dr Saul Krugman)

The EEG features with the pathognomonic periodic complexes occurring simultaneously with the involuntary movements have been described. Polymyographic studies of these spasms have shown periodic EMG changes simultaneous with the clinical and EEG features (Fig. 24.11). These often take the form of groups of muscle action potentials lasting more than a quarter of a second (Pampiglione 1964). A common phenomenon, especially in the early stages of the disease, is a complex sequence of fluctuating activity in the EMG from various groups of muscles during each involuntary movement. After an initial group of muscle action potentials, at about the start of the complex wave form in the EEG, there may be either a period of complete electrical 'silence' or a period of marked diminution of muscle action potentials. The visual evoked cortical responses are helpful in children with blindness of cortical origin.

Serological studies have shown abnormally high titres of measles antibody of both complement-fixing (CF) and haemagglutination-inhibiting (HI) type, in the serum of patients with SSPE, the level of CF antibody being generally higher than those of HI (Legg 1967), but the most striking feature

is the presence of high levels of antibody in the CSF (Fig. 22.7).

The CSF may show a normal or slightly raised protein level. The gamma globulin, mainly IgG, is invariably increased and this is associated with a 'paretic' or first zone colloidal gold curve, a typical finding in SSPE. The CSF cell count may be normal or slightly increased with mononuclear cells predominating. Brain biopsy is quite unnecessary and totally unjustified with EEG and serological investigations giving clearly diagnostic results.

Rarely, signs of raised intracranial pressure may be seen in the skull X-rays. In some children with raised intracranial pressure the lateral ventricles may appear as small and slit-like and may be almost invisible on the CT scan.

The changes in the brain are variable and depend on the stage of the disease. There are both inflammatory and degenerative features consisting of perivascular mononuclear cell infiltration, astrocytic proliferation and destruction of myelin, particularly in the subcortical white matter of the cerebral hemispheres.

The cardinal feature, first described by Dawson in 1933, is the presence of acidophilic intranuclear and intracytoplasmic inclusion bodies in neurons

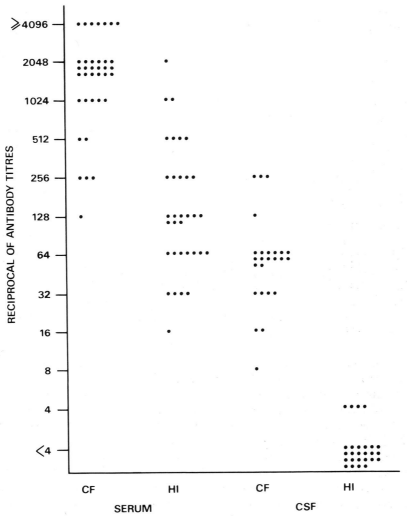

Fig. 22.7 Comparison of titres of measles CF and HI antibody in serum and cerebrospinal fluid in a series of cases of SSPE

and glial cells, (whence the earlier name 'subacute inclusion body encephalitis'). Electron-microscopic examination of these inclusions shows structures identical to that of measles virus. The distribution of the inclusion bodies may be patchy and sometimes a prolonged search is needed before they are found.

The variable natural history of SSPE with occasional prolonged remissions makes assessment of the results of treatment difficult. Many therapeutic agents have been tried, including cortical steroids, Interferon, transfer factor and antiviral agents, all of which have failed to show a convincing beneficial effect. A few patients have been treated by plas-mapheresis and exchange of CSF, also without any improvement.

The antiviral agent Isoprinosine has also been used in small numbers of children (Huttenlocher 1976, Silverberg et al 1979, McGrath & Rosen-bloom 1980) but the results reported have not been impressive. Silverberg and his colleagues concluded that in their six patients the course of the disease was not dissimilar from that usually seen in SSPE.

Progressive rubella panencephalitis

Several children with congenital rubella have been

reported to develop a fatal panencephalitis at the end of the first decade of life, or during the second decade (Weil et al 1975, Townsend et al 1975). The major clinical features of this illness have been a progressive dementia with signs of both pyramidal and extrapyramidal involvement. Myoclonic seizures and choreiform movements have occurred and signs of cerebellar disease have also been reported.

The serological findings consist of greatly elevated levels of rubella antibody in both serum and cerebrospinal fluid; hence the original description of an 'SSPE-like' disorder, but clinically the tempo of the illness is slower than SSPE. Some elevation of CSF protein and an oligoclonal pattern of the globulins is found (Wolinsky et al 1976). Rubella virus has been isolated from the brain by means of co-cultivation techniques. The EEG does not show any characteristic features.

Progressive multifocal leuco-encephalopathy (PML)

This is an extremely rare virus infection caused by a polyomavirus, usually of the strain designated JC (Coleman 1980). Most patients have serious underlying disease, frequently malignancy of the lymphoreticular system, and have usually been adults. However, this disorder has been described in a child with severe combined immunodeficiency (ZuRhein et al 1978).

There are multifocal areas of demyelination in the cerebral cortex and the virus, identified as the JC strain, can be seen in the nuclei of oligodendrocytes. The CT scan shows varying circular areas of low attenuation which do not show enhancement. Clinically the disease, which is usually fatal within twelve months, may resemble progressive multiple sclerosis with bizarre clinical symptoms and signs.

MISCELLANEOUS INFECTIONS

Mycoplasma pneumoniae

This usually causes a self-limited infection of the respiratory tract but severe infections may be associated with a wide range of non-respiratory manifestations. These include rashes, involvement of

Table 22.18 CNS disease associated with mycoplasma pneumoniae infection

Encephalitis	Ascending polyneuritis
Meningoencephalitis	Transverse myelitis
Aseptic meningitis	Cerebral infarction
Brain stem encephalitis	Polyradiculitis
Acute cerebellar ataxia	

the haemopoietic system, heart, musculo-skeletal, gastro-intestinal and renal tract and the nervous system (Cassell & Cole 1981). The various neurological disorders which have been reported are shown in Table 22.18. It has been suggested that 0.1% of all patients have involvement of the nervous system and this is probably the commonest non-respiratory complication. Lerer & Kalavsky (1973) observed the high frequency of preceding respiratory symptoms occurring 3–23 days previously and drew attention to some children with combinations of various neurological syndromes. These included radiculitis together with cranial nerve involvement, non-focal encephalitis and nerve root involvement, cerebral involvement and cerebellar dysfunction as well as transverse myelitis and signs of non-focal encephalitis.

The CSF often shows a lymphocytosis and elevated protein but normal levels of glucose. Long-term sequelae are not infrequent. The organism has been isolated from the CSF on only one occasion (Ponka 1980) and the mechanism of the neurological disease is not known. The case of a cerebral infarct causing hemiplegia in an 8-year-old girl (Parker et al 1981) suggests that a vasculitis may play a role in some forms of the neurological disease. The detection of cold agglutinins may aid in the diagnosis but specific serological tests are available.

Leptospirosis

Infection of man by leptospiral organisms has long been held to be principally an occupational disease and the clinical syndromes of Weil's disease and Canicola fever form the basis of the descriptions in text books. There is a tendency to associate particular serotypes with these syndromes; *Leptospira icterohaemorrhagica* with the former and *L. canicola* with the latter. There are very large numbers of serotypes of this slender tightly spiralled organism and a wide range of animals can be infected. Dogs are a particularly common source of infection in children (Wong et al 1972).

The spectrum of disease caused by these organisms is wide and subclinical infection is common. Infection causes a biphasic illness with the well known hepatic and renal involvement together with neurological involvement, if it occurs, manifest in the second phase. The most striking manifestations of neurological disease are severe headaches which may be associated with signs of meningeal irritation. Photophobia may be present together with conjunctivitis, and muscle pain and tenderness may also occur.

The CSF often contains up to 300–400 WBC per cu mm with a predominance of polymorphonuclear leucocytes in the early stages. Increased concentration of protein and normal levels of glucose accompany these changes. The abnormalities in the CSF can persist for several weeks (Heath et al 1965). The organisms may be present in the blood and CSF within the first few days of the onset of symptoms and for 7–10 days thereafter, following which they are then to be found in urine during the period of the second phase of the disease. Two to three weeks may elapse before a diagnostic antibody response can be detected.

Guillain-Barré syndrome (GBS)

The ascending polyneuritis syndrome remains a disorder of unknown aetiology and obscure pathogenesis. The clinical features of the syndrome are described in Chapter 4. A temporal association with a number of common infections such as infectious mononucleosis, herpes simplex, chickenpox, measles, mumps, rubella and myocoplasma pneumoniae has been described. However, in many cases no preceding recognisable specific infection is present. Schmitz & Enders (1977) have drawn attention to a high incidence of cytomegalovirus infection in these patients but the higher than expected incidence of GBS following the recent use of an influenza vaccine in the United States emphasises that it is a complex disorder of multiple aetiologies (Schonberger et al 1978).

The usual absence of an inflammatory response in the cerebrospinal fluid and the rather slow progression have led to the suggestion that a neuro-allergic process of some type underlies the disorder. Insufficient attention has been paid in the examination of the CSF later in the illness, for example 4 to 6 weeks after the onset of symptoms, for antibody and possible immunological abnormalities. It has already been shown that later examination of CSF may reveal mononuclear pleocytosis which is usually absent in the acute stage of the clinical illness (Link et al 1979).

Eosinophilic meningitis

Eosinophils are rarely observed in CSF. The majority of the causes of eosinophilic pleocytosis are also associated with an eosinophilia in the peripheral blood. The phenomenon has been known to occur in neurosyphilis and other rare causes warrant brief mention. Less than 4% eosinophilia in CSF is considered to lack diagnostic specificity (Fishman 1980). The most common causes of 5 to 10% or greater eosinophils are parasitic infections. The most striking of these is caused by the rat lungworm, *Angiostrongylus cantonensis*, an infection occurring in South East Asia and the Pacific Islands. The disease is usually benign in man, who is an accidental host who becomes infected by eating terrestrial snails. The larvae are often visible in the CSF (Yii 1976).

Other infections which have been reported to be associated with eosinophils in the CSF are shown in Table 22.19. However, in a number of these the evidence is only circumstantial. Recently Chesney and colleagues (1979) have drawn attention to eosinophilia in the CSF in a child with chronic lymphocytic choriomeningitis. The report of the presence of eosinophils in the CSF of a child with Coxsackie B4 viral meningitis (Chesney & Hodgson 1980) emphasises the importance of considering the use of Wright's or Giemsa's stains in examination

Table 22.19 Infections associated with eosinophils in the CSF

Helminths	Others
Angiostrongylus cantonensis	*Coccidioides immitis*
Taenia solium	*Candida albicans*
Gnathostroma spinigerum	*Toxoplasma gondii*
Toxocara (Visceral larva migrans)	*Treponema pallidum*
Paragonimus westermani	*Mycobacterium tuberculosis*
Echinococcus	*Lymphocytic choriomeningitis*

of the CSF; eosinophilia may be more common than is realised.

CONGENITAL INFECTIONS

Infections during pregnancy are common but most are of no great significance either to the mother or the fetus. In addition to infection of the fetus it is not clear whether fetal damage may be a consequence of some other process such as fever (Pleet et al 1981), 'toxins', damage to the placenta, or the result of medication used to treat the infection in the mother (Karkeinen-Jaaskelainen & Saxen 1974).

The infections can be divided into those in which fetal infection is known to occur and a second group which are suspected of causing infection or damage though conclusive proof is lacking (Table 22.20). Micro-organisms may reach the fetus by several routes: from the maternal blood stream when there will be a placentitis, from the genital tract, either ascending before birth (cervical-amniotic route) or during the process of delivery or by direct inoculation during intra-uterine transfusions or during procedures such as amniocentesis or fetal blood sampling.

Two important consequences of fetal or perinatal infections are:

Table 22.20 Agents proven or suspected of causing fetal infection and damage

Proven	Suspected
Rubella virus	Mumps virus
Rubella vaccine virus	Influenza viruses
Cytomegalovirus	Hepatitis A, non A/non B viruses
Herpes simplex	Coxsackie viruses
Varicella-zoster virus	Echoviruses
Epstein-Barr virus	Measles virus
Vaccinia virus	
Variola virus	
Hepatitis B virus	
Poliovirus	
Listeria monocytogenes	
Treponema pallidum	
Mycobacterium tuberculosis	
Toxoplasma gondii	
Plasmodia	
Trypanosomes	
Filaria	

1. Immune responsiveness of the fetus or newborn

There is premature synthesis of immunoglobulins so that there are increased levels of IgM and sometimes IgA at birth and a 'specific' response in which antibody to the agent can be detected in the IgM fraction in cord blood. This immune responsiveness of the fetus and the neonate has led to screening programmes for the more common infections which Nahmias and his colleagues (1971) have designated by the acronym TORCH: TO (Toxoplasmosis) R (rubella) C (cytomegalovirus) H (herpes simplex). However, it should be stressed that these infections are not a major problem in numerical terms (Table 22.21).

2. Persistence of the infection

One of the major ways in which prenatal infections differ from those acquired post-natally is that the infection persists for considerably longer, in some instances for weeks or even years after birth. This may allow the infecting organism to be identified long after infection has occurred. Its continued presence may cause further damage.

Agents which infect the fetus should not be considered to be teratogens, for in addition to those defects caused by defective organogenesis, much of the damage is the consequence of infection in tissues that have undergone normal development. Another important feature is that some infections can cause damage at some time after the original infection which may extend to weeks, months or even years after birth, the so-called 'late onset disease' (Marshall 1973). In a few infections there may be characteristic clinical manifestations but in most the symptoms and signs are non-specific and are common to many of them (Table 22.22). Involve-

Table 22.21 Estimated frequency of fetal infections (per 1000 live births)

Agent	U.K.	U.S.A. (Alford)[†]
Rubella	0.5*	0.5*
CMV	5–10	5–15
Toxoplasmosis	0.05	0.75–1.3
Syphilis	0.1	0.1
HVH	Rare	Rare

[†] Alford et al (1974)
* 4–30 in an epidemic year

Table 22.22 Summary of the defects caused by intrauterine infections of major clinical importance

	Rubella	CMV	Herpesvirus hominis	Toxoplasma gondii	Treponema pallidum
Microcephaly	++	+++	+	+	-
Hydrocephalus	-	±	-	++	±
Meningoencephalitis	++	+	+	+++	++
Psychomotor retardation	++	++	±	++	±
Cerebral palsy	+	+	±	±	-
Seizures	-	+	++	++	+
Intracranial calcification	±	+	±	++	-
Deafness	+++	++	+	±	+
Retinopathy	+++	+	-	-	-
Retinitis	-	-	±	++	-
Cataract	++	-	-	-	-
Microphthalmos	++	±	-	±	-
Keratitis	±	-	+	-	+
Glaucoma	+	-	-	-	-
Congential heart defects	++	-	-	-	-
Myocarditis	++	?	±	±	-
Arterial stenosis	+	-	-	-	-
Pneumonitis	±	++	++	±	-
Anaemia	++	±	+	+	++
Hepatosplenomegaly	++	+++	++	+	+++
Hepatitis	++	++	++	+	++
Jaundice	++	++	+	+	++
Adenopathy	++	-	-	++	+
Thrombocytopenia ± purpura	±	++	++	±	-
Skin rashes	++	-	-	-	++
Radiological changes of the skeleton	-	±	?	-	+
Prematurity	++	±	-	+	-
Intrauterine growth retardation		±	-	?	-

Key: +++ → ±, relative frequency of defects caused by individual agents; ?, doubtful occurrence; -, not present.

ment of the nervous system may occur in almost all of the known infections.

Rubella

Fetal infection results from primary infection in pregnancy, and although reinfection may occur as a subclinical phenomenon, there is no convincing evidence that the fetus is at risk in these circumstances. The types and risks of damage caused by rubella are related to fetal age at the time of infection. It is estimated that the risk is of the order of 40–60% for infection up to 8 weeks, 30–35% for the third month and approximately 10% for the fourth month of gestation (Dudgeon 1967). A small risk extends up to 20–24 weeks. The earlier the infection, the more likely there is to be multiple organ involvement. Infection after the tenth week is more likely to result in involvement of only a single organ, which is usually the organ of Corti, leading to perceptive deafness. Fetal infection may occur at any stage of gestation without evidence of damage at birth.

Virus can be detected in urine and throat washings for up to twelve months after birth and transmission of infection to susceptible contacts is well documented. IgM rubella antibody is present in cord blood and can be detected for several months after birth; persistence of antibody beyond six months of age is another method of serodiagnosis.

The 'rubella syndrome', the combination of congenital heart defects, cataracts, deafness and mental retardation is only part of the spectrum of disorders caused by the virus. Additional multisystem involvement can occur with hepatitis, splenomegaly, thrombocytopenic purpura and glaucoma (Rubella Symposium 1965).

The results of infection on the nervous system are very complex. They may be due either to damage to the brain or to the visual and auditory defects, but most children show a combination of these.

Microcephaly and mental retardation are well known and assumed to be common. It has been stated that up to 30% of children may have intellectual impairment (Cooper & Krugman 1967). It might be inferred that small head size is closely related to mental retardation but this is not nec-

essarily the case. These children should be considered to be small children rather than children with small heads (MacFarlane et al 1975) and thus the tendency to overestimate the degree of intellectual impairment can be avoided.

Meningoencephalitis is often present at birth and in early infancy. There may be irritability and increased tension of the anterior fontanelle which is usually enlarged. Convulsions are rare. The CSF frequently shows some increase in protein and a mild pleocytosis and it is often possible to isolate the virus from CSF (Desmond et al 1976). These CSF abnormalities may be present in infants who appear neurologically normal and Desmond and his collegues (1978) believe that some degree of damage can be detected in such children when assessed towards the end of the first decade of life.

At this age the defects are remarkably diverse and include disorders of intelligence, behaviour, tactile perception, gait and posture. Hearing loss may become more severe or develop with the passage of time. On the other hand, the incidence of abnormal tone and reflexes decreases. Infants who have been considered to have cerebral palsy in infancy may no longer exhibit signs of such a disorder (Desmond et al 1978).

Visual defects result mainly from cataracts which are usually present at birth but may occasionally appear at several weeks of age. These are unilateral in about 50% of affected children. The eye containing the cataract is often small but mild degrees of microphthalmia are difficult to assess if bilateral cataracts are present. Microcornea may also be present. The importance of surgery before three months of age is stressed but success depends on a careful surgical technique. The virus is very often isolated from cataractous material even at several years of age. A few children also have raised intraocular pressure (buphthalmos) which may be associated with cloudiness of the cornea (Wolf 1973). Strabismus is common in children with these various eye disorders.

A useful clinical marker of congenital rubella is the retinal disorder; a diffuse disturbance of pigment is very common and consists of patchy dark pigmentation interspersed with patchy depigmentation. It may be extensive but does not affect vision (Kresky & Nauheim 1967). Very rarely

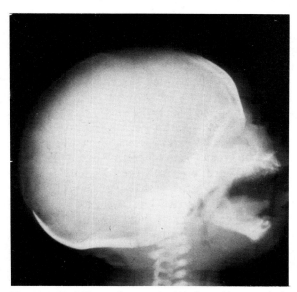

Fig. 22.8 Skull X-ray of a 6-week-old infant with congenital rubella showing poor mineralisation of the vault

severe visual disturbance may result from a so-called disciform degeneration of the macula which occurs in childhood in patients with rubella retinopathy (Deutman & Grizzard 1978).

X-rays of the skull often show poor mineralisation of the vault in early infancy (Fig. 22.8). Intracranial calcification is extremely rare in congenital rubella and it is probably the result of small haemorrhages caused by severe neonatal thrombocytopenia.

Deafness is one of the most frequent consequences and the most common defect, sensorineural deafness being caused by damage to the organ of Corti. It may be unilateral and may not be detected for some years. The frequency of unilateral deafness is not known. It is important to realise that sensorineural deafness may develop several months or even years after birth (Peckham 1972). A less common defect of hearing is central auditory imperception. (Ames et al 1970).

Hearing defects, unless recognised and treated, lead to impaired speech, but disturbance of speech with normal hearing has also been observed in children with congenital rubella. In the second decade of life, a few children known to have congenital rubella have developed a fatal progressive panencephalitis. Very high titres of rubella antibody are present in serum and CSF and rubella virus has been isolated from the brain by co-cultivation technique (Weil et al 1975, Townsend et al 1975).

The assessment of the child with congenital rubella can be extremely difficult as much of the handicap may be due to defects of hearing and vision but direct damage to the brain can be an important contributory factor. The hyperactivity and easy distractability of these children may be striking and a serious handicap to learning. Autistic features are not infrequently present (Chess 1971). The defects in other systems necessitate a multi-discipline approach to the care of these children.

Although some of the attenuated strains of the virus used in the rubella vaccines have been isolated from the products of conception and fetal tissues in a number of instances (Modlin et al 1975) there is as yet no evidence that this virus causes damage. The risk of fetal infection is of the order of 20% (Hayden et al 1980) but the numbers of infants born to mothers who were inadvertently given vaccine when pregnant are far too small to conclude that damage does not occur.

Cytomegalovirus (CMV)

This virus is a member of the herpes group and is also responsible for a disseminated fetal infection. Damage to many organs and tissues may occur and involvement of the central nervous system is common.

Infection may occur during pregnancy or at the time of delivery either as a result of primary maternal infection or from reactivation of latent maternal infections (Stagno et al 1977a). But it is probable that infections of the fetus which result from a primary infection are those which case fetal damage. The risks of infection and damage have not been clearly established, but MacDonald & Tobin (1978) have proposed the scheme shown in Figure 22.9.

Fetal infection can be diagnosed by two methods; by identification of IgM CMV antibody in cord blood or in blood within a few days of birth or by isolation of virus from the urine at or within seven to ten days of birth. Virus isolation, although expensive and time-consuming, is to be preferred

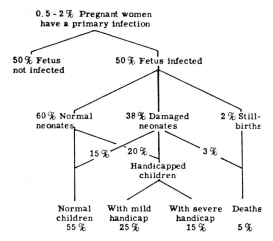

Fig. 22.9 Predicted outcome of congenital CMV infection (MacDonald & Tobin 1978)

because of technical difficulties associated with the antibody tests at this age. Identification of characteristic CMV inclusion bearing cells in urine is of little value in diagnosis as the proportion of positive results in proven congenital infections is low.

In the newborn infant three major clinical forms of congenital CMV can be recognised.

1. Approximately 1% of infected children show severe multisystem disease at birth which was previously described as congenital cytomegalic inclusion disease (Table 22.23). These infants have a high mortality, and the survivors are usually microcephalic and have severe mental retardation.

2. Some infants present with enlargement of the liver and spleen with or without mild to moderate thrombocytopenic purpura. Jaundice due to neonatal hepatitis may be striking and persist for several weeks. The fate of these, who comprise approximately 5% of the total number of infected infants, is not accurately known, but at least one third or even one half have some permanent sequelae of which microcephaly and deafness are prominent (Hanshaw et al 1976, Pass et al 1980).

Table 22.23 Congenital cytomegalic inclusion disease: features of severe multisystem involvement present at birth

Hepatomegaly	Microcephaly
Jaundice	Chorioretinitis
Splenomegaly	Convulsions
Thrombocytopenia	Intracranial calcification
Purpura	Pneumonitis
Lymphadenopathy	Intrauterine growth retardation

3. The majority of infants do not exhibit symptoms and signs at birth and the diagnosis can only be established by virological tests. Far less is known of the fate of these infants, but it is thought that up to 20% may have defects in later life; low IQ and hearing loss are probably the major problems. (Reynolds et al 1974).

Infants with congenital CMV may show CSF abnormalities with mild elevation of protein or increase in cells. These changes may be present in the absence of any signs of congenital infection (Hanshaw et al 1976). Eye defects are infrequent in congenital CMV: severe microcephaly may be associated with optic atrophy, and chorioretinitis of a type similar to that seen in congenital toxoplasmosis is described; a squint may draw attention to the retinal lesions. Intracranial calcification is not infrequent and is characteristically periventricular in distribution; it may be progressive.

In infancy the CT scan may show areas of low attenuation in the periventricular areas and can be very useful to detect calcification which is not visible on X-rays (Anders et al 1980). Virus persistence is a feature of the infection and viruria may be detected for several years after birth. Similar virological findings occur in infants who acquire infection at the time of delivery or soon after but these infections are not believed to cause damage in later life (Alford et al 1980). In those infants with perinatal infection virus shedding does not commence until after seven to ten days of age.

Treatment of congenital CMV infection with antiviral agents or immunological means such as transfer factor have not been successful. Cessation of virus excretion has been observed during some of these treatments but recurrence has taken place on stopping them.

Herpesvirus hominis (HVH) (Herpes simplex)

Primary HVH infection in early pregnancy is rare and the few reported cases have involved the birth of a microcephalic infant with intracranial calcification. Atrophy of the cerebral hemispheres and retinal dysplasia have also been present.

The major clinical impact of this virus is the result of genital tract infection at or near the time of delivery. Clinical disease need not be present in the mother. In most instances type 2 or 'genital' strain of the virus is involved. The illness in the infant may take the form of a generalised 'septicaemic' illness, usually with vesicles on the skin, and sometimes involvement of the conjunctivae and cornea. An encephalitic illness may be present. In both forms there is a very high mortality rate particularly in premature infants and a very high incidence of sequelae in survivors (Nahmias & Visintine 1976). Treatment with antiviral agents has not been as successful as had been hoped but the use of new agents such as adenine arabinoside (Whitley et al 1980) or acyclovir may be beneficial. It has been suggested that the risk of infection may be reduced if infants are delivered by Caesarian section provided this is performed less than four hours after rupture of the membranes.

Varicella-zoster (VZ) virus

Primary infection with VZ virus causes chickenpox or reactivation of latent infection manifest as shingles. Shingles in pregnancy is not recognised as being hazardous to the fetus but when a pregnant woman develops chickenpox the effect on the fetus depends on the time of maternal infection. Early gestational chickenpox may have no observable effect but fetal loss may occur and very rarely the congenital varicella syndrome (Hanshaw & Dudgeon 1978) (Table 22.24). The two most characteristic features are the cicatricial skin lesions and hypoplasia of bone; the latter may cause shortening of part of a limb.

Infection in mid- and late pregnancy may result in the birth of an infant with healed chickenpox scars. The infant may develop shingles within a few months or years of birth. (Brunell & Kotchmar 1981). Infection near to term may result in perinatal or neonatal chickenpox. This can range from a mild illness to severe multisystem disease with involvement of the brain and death. The mortality is confined to infants born to mothers who develop

Table 22.24 Clinical manifestations of congenital varicella syndrome

Cutaneous scars
Low birth weight
Hypoplasia of a limb
Rudimentary digits
Paralysis with muscular atrophy of a limb
Convulsions and/or psychomotor retardation
Chorioretinitis
Cataracts, microphthalmia
Cortical atrophy

chickenpox within five days of delivery (de Nicola & Hanshaw 1979). These infants develop the disease ten or more days after birth (Table 22.25). This group should be given immunoprophylaxis in the form of zoster immune globulin (ZIG) at birth.

Poliovirus

Poliovirus infection in adults is now extremely rare because of the development of highly effective vaccines. Nevertheless, maternal infection and the birth of an infant with congenital poliomyelitis is well documented.

Treponema pallidum

Antenatal screening and treatment in pregnancy has made a major contribution to the reduction in the incidence of congenital syphilis.

Fetal infection is extremely rare before the fourth month of gestation. Intra-uterine death is common but the infection lacks pathognomonic symptoms and signs. Lymphadenopathy, hepatosplenomegaly, anaemia, fever, vomiting and failure to thrive may be prominent. The skin and mucous membrane manifestations, if present, frequently provide the clue to the infection; mucopurulent or haemorrhagic nasal discharge, vesicular and papulosquamous rashes especially affecting the palms and soles occur. Osteochondritis and periostitis are

Table 22.25 Relationship between onset of perinatal varicella and outcome

Maternal onset before delivery	Infant onset	Total	Numbers Survived	Fatal	Fatality rate
≥ 5 days	0–4 days	27	27	0	0
≤ 4 days	5–10 days	23	16	7	30.4%

Adapted from De Nicola & Hanshaw (1979)

important features of congenital syphilis.

The CSF is often abnormal, with raised levels of protein and a pleocytosis and these changes may be present in the absence of any clinical manifestations of the infection in the infant.

In later infancy and childhood the well known classical manifestations of congenital syphilis evolve. The early features of the disease are primarily meningitic, while in later infancy vomiting, seizures and progressive hydrocephalus may occur. Juvenile paresis does not appear until later in childhood or early adolescence. Tabes dorsalis is rarer, but involvement of the cerebral cortex and the spinal cord become evident. There may be optic atrophy, multiple cranial nerve lesions and deafness.

The non-CNS manifestations consist of interstitial keratitis, abnormalities of the second dentition, deafness and skull bone and cartilage disease.

Treatment in pregnancy with benzathine penicillin is effective, but in congenital infection, intramuscular aqueous crystalline penicillin G (50 000 units per kg/day) should be given for 14 days (McCracken & Kaplan 1974).

Toxoplasmosis

The protozoon toxoplasma gondii may cause an easily recognisable syndrome of congenital infection consisting of chorioretinitis, hydrocephalus and irregular calcification scattered throughout the cerebral hemispheres. As with many of the intra-uterine infections, this is but one part of a spectrum of severity ranging from subclinical infection to the above. Hepatosplenomegaly, jaundice,

Table 22.26 Incidence of congenital toxoplasmosis (per 1000 live births)

Vienna	6.0–7.0	Mexico City	2.0
Gottingen	5.0	Birmingham, Ala	1.3
Paris	3.0	New York	1.3
		U.K.	0.05

anaemia and lymphadenopathy may also occur. Increase in cells and protein in the CSF may be seen in all the clinical forms as well as in subclinical infection.

The major features of the disease in the survivors are chorioretinitis (Fig. 22.10), cerebral palsy, mental retardation and seizures, but significant defects can occur later in infants who do not show disease in the newborn period or early infancy (Wilson et al 1980).

There is a wide variation in the incidence of congenital infection (Table 22.26). Unlike rubella, the risk of infection is less likely and damage extends throughout pregnancy. Early gestational infection is less likely to result in fetal infection, but the infected infants are more likely to show signs of the disease. Infections later in pregnancy result in a higher rate of congenital infection but there are more mildly affected infants and infants with subclinical infection (Fig. 22.11). There is no evidence to show that there is a risk to a fetus during a subsequent pregnancy.

The diagnosis of congenital toxoplasmosis is usually established by serological means using the IgM toxoplasma fluorescent antibody test. Careful examination of the CSF may show the presence of

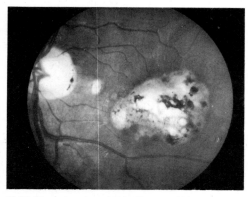

Fig. 22.10 Toxoplasmic retinitis (Courtesy Mr D. Taylor)

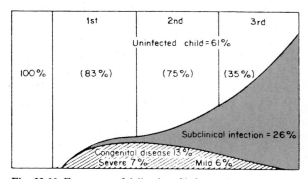

Fig. 22.11 Frequency of deliveries of infants with clinical congenital toxoplasmosis (hatched area), subclinical infection (stippled area), and with no infection (unshaded area), following acquisition either before or during the three trimesters of pregnancy (Desmonts & Couvreur 1975)

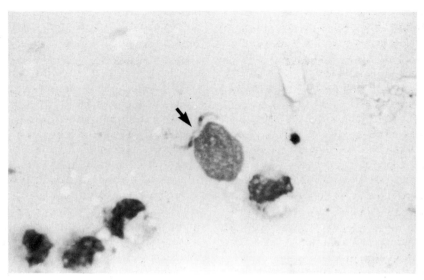

Fig. 22.12 Sporozoites present in CSF of a 6-week-old infant with congenital toxoplasmosis. Giemsa stain of CSF deposit after centrifugation of CSF at 1000 rpm (Courtesy W. Hamilton)

the organism (Fig. 22.12). Treatment of maternal infection with spiramycin has been disappointing in its results (Couvreur 1979). The same drug or sulphadiazine and pyrimethamine can be used in the affected infant and should also be considered when subclinical infection has been diagnosed.

Susceptible women can reduce the risk of infection by not eating uncooked or partially cooked meat and by avoiding exposure to the faeces of infected cats during pregnancy.

Other infections in pregnancy include vaccinia virus. The risks of infection with this and with other live vaccines can be avoided by observing the rule that no live vaccines should be used in pregnancy (Marshall 1981).

Infections in which there is inconclusive evidence of fetal infection are shown in Table 22.20. Influenza A virus has been suggested as a causative factor in abnormality including anencephaly and spina bifida, but as there is very rarely a viraemia in influenza and indeed in most respiratory virus infections, any adverse effect on the fetus is more likely to be due to some other factor such as toxin, fever or possibly medications. Mumps virus which had been thought to cause cardiac defects may play a role in defects of the central nervous system by virtue of its propensity to infect the nervous system after birth.

A similar statement can be made for the enteroviruses, Coxsackie and ECHO virus infections. However infections with some of these viruses in the neonatal period may produce a devastating multisystem disease (Nagington et al 1978).

In endemic areas, malaria in pregnancy causes intra-uterine growth retardation because of the heavy infection of the placenta, but rarely congenital malaria. However, in the susceptible individual congenital malaria may result from infection during pregnancy.

Congenital tuberculosis is rare, but the neonatal disorder usually takes the form of multisystem disease with the liver and lungs affected; involvement of the nervous system may be present and choroid tubercles may be seen.

INFECTIONS ASSOCIATED WITH DEFECTS IN HOST DEFENCE MECHANISMS

Individuals with defects in host defence mechanisms have an increased risk of various infections including those which can involve the nervous system. Anatomical defects, either congenital or secondary to trauma, are discussed earlier in this chapter. The organisms which infect these patients are usually bacteria of which *S. aureus* and Gram-negative bacteria are the most common. But where there is a leak of CSF in the region of the nose and pharynx meningitis can be caused by *S. pneumoniae* and *H. influenzae*; because of the risk of recurrence prophylactic antibiotics are indicated for such patients (Lancet 1966).

Infections of ventriculo-atrial or ventriculo-peritoneal shunts are discussed earlier. Bacteria may be introduced into the CSF during instillation of drugs in the treatment of malignant diseases. Insertion of CSF pressure monitoring devices is an additional hazard and may become increasingly important in the future. The most frequent organisms are *Staph. aureus, Staph. epidermidis* and *Pseudomonas aeruginosa*. Candida species may sometimes be encountered.

In patients with defects of the specific or non-specific immune system, infections of the nervous system are not numerically important. However, they are sometimes caused by unusual organisms and the symptoms and signs can be masked by underlying disease or the immunosuppressive drugs used for treatment.

Defects in granulocyte numbers and/or function are usually secondary to treatment of acute leukaemia and other malignancies. Bacterial meningitis in patients with malignancy is usually caused by *Listeria monocytogenes, Staph. aureus* and *Pseudomonas aeruginosa* (Chernik et al 1977). Candida or aspergillus species are the most frequent fungal infections. Autopsy studies have shown that unrecognised cerebral abscess may be present in patients with candidaemia (Edwards et al 1978). Septicaemia may occur in patients with the inherited granulocytic defect in bacterial killing and the commonest organisms to cause septicaemia and meningitis in these patients are the salmonellae (Johnston & Newman 1977).

Individuals with defects in antibody and cell mediated immunity are at increased risk of infection from viruses and fungi as well as bacteria. When these defects are congenital in origin infections often become troublesome in early or late infancy. *S. pneumoniae* and *H. influenzae* are the most common bacteria to cause infection and recurrent meningitis may be the clue to an underlying congenital immunoglobulin defect. Although patients with such defects tolerate common virus infections without apparent difficulty, there is an unexplained hazard from some enteroviruses. Wild or attenuated vaccine strains of polio-viruses may be persistently excreted and have been reported to cause progressive disease (Davis et al 1977). A number of children with hypogammoglobulinaemia of the X–linked variety have been recognised as having a slowly progressive encephalitis caused by several echoviruses; polymyositis has also been present in some of these children (Webster et al 1978, Mease et al 1981).

Defects in cell-mediated immunity are most commonly the result of malignancy, especially of the lymphoreticular system and the treatments of these diseases. Congenital defects of cell-mediated immunity alone are rare; most are seen in combined immunodeficiency syndromes. The pattern of immunodeficiency in severe malnutrition, especially protein calorie malnutrition, is variable but includes degrees of deficiency in cell-mediated immunity.

The most common bacterial infections to affect the nervous system in patients with defects in cell-mediated immunity are *Listeria monocytogenes* and *Nocardia asteroides*. These are most frequently seen following organ transplantation and in lymphoreticular malignancies. Tuberculosis is more likely to occur in adult patients and is frequently unrecognised.

Listeria monocytogenes is a Gram-positive motile bacillus which stains poorly; it may fail to be recognised as a pathogen by an inexperienced laboratory worker. It is becoming increasingly observed in adults (Chernik et al 1977) and has very rarely been recognised in children other than infection in the neonatal period. Most patients have a bacteraemic illness and maningitis is the most frequent complication. The CSF contains increased numbers of leucocytes, elevation of protein and low levels of glucose but frequently there are red blood cells as well.

Infection with the Gram-positive and weakly acid fast bacillus *Nocardia asteroides* usually involves the lungs. Disseminated infections, which may include nodular skin lesions, are frequent and cerebral involvement consists of multiple or single abscesses; most patients with cerebral abscesses have pulmonary infection.

Cryptococcal meningitis, caused by the ubiquitous fungus, *Cryptococcus neoformans*, also occurs in immunologically normal hosts and is discussed later. Infection appears to be infrequent in the United Kingdom. Other fungal infections are caused by aspergillus species which occur either as meningitis or multiple or single cerebral abscesses. Zygomycosis in its form of rhinocerebral zygomycosis is a rapidly progressive and usually fatal infection and is most commonly seen in diabetic patients who are poorly controlled. Infection in children is rare.

Invasion of the nervous system by herpes simplex virus is also rare and is most likely to occur in children with lymphomas or leukaemia in relapse who have clinically obvious infection elsewhere; the most common site is the lips or area around the nose. Chickenpox in children with malignancy is often very severe especially if the lymphocyte count is less than 500 per cu mm. Encephalitis may occur in these patients and permanent brain damage seems more likely than following varicella encephalitis in normal children. Shingles is usually a less painful and distressing illness in the child than in adults. Encephalitis may complicate shingles.

Cytomegalovirus is a common infection in the immunocompromised host but involvement of the nervous system is exceedingly rare, unlike the very high frequency of encephalitis which occurs in congenital infections. CMV meningoencephalitis has rarely been described in post-natal infections in adults (Perham et al 1971). However, retinal lesions causing blindness have been observed and retinal biopsy has proved useful in establishing the diagnosis (Taylor et al 1981). Progressive multifocal leucoencephalopathy caused by papovaviruses is rare in children and is most frequently observed in patients with lymphoreticular malignancies. Toxoplasma gondii can be reactivated by immunosuppressive drugs. The infection manifests as meningoencephalitis, encephalitis or cerebral mass lesions. The neurological manifestations, which lack specificity, occur in more than half these individuals (Ruskin & Remington 1976). Changes in the CSF are usually mild with only moderate elevation of protein and increase in lymphocytes. Infections of this type have been very rarely recognised in the United Kingdom. This may be due to the very low frequency of infection in most areas of the country. *Strongyloides stercoralis* infection may disseminate in the immunosuppressed host and has caused a 'hyperinfestation' syndrome (Igra-Siegman et al 1981) consisting of diarrhoea, abdominal pain, lung infiltrates and encephalopathy. Micro-infarcts of the CNS and meningitis occur and the larvae may be visible in the CSF.

Other defects in host defences include congenital abnormalities of the complement system. Defective synthesis of C6, C7 and C8 (Peterson et al 1979) and more recently C5 (Peter et al 1981) have been associated with bacteraemic diseases due to neisseria species including *N. meningiditis*. However, these infections tend to occur towards the end of the first and during the second decade. An unexplained preponderance of infections with the Group Y strains of *N. meningitidis* has been reported.

Absence of the spleen increases the susceptibility to bacterial infections, especially *S. pneumoniae*. Meningitis may occur in these circumstances, but the severity and speed of progress of the infection may allow little time for the symptoms and signs of meningitis to evolve. Included in this group of patients are those with sickle cell disease. A measure of prevention can be achieved by means of penicillin prophylaxis. The results of pneumonococcal vaccines, especially in young children and in patients with Hodgkin's disease have so far not been encouraging.

TOXIN DISEASES

Bacterial cells produce two principal types of toxin, endotoxins and exotoxins. Exotoxins are released by viable organisms or on death of the cell, whereas endotoxins are produced when bacteria undergo autolysis. The former are proteins and generally affect specific tissue whereas the latter are composed of a lipopolysaccharide and protein complex derived from the bacterial cell wall which have a non-specific effect on the host.

Toxin diseases affecting the nervous system are tetanus, diphtheria, botulism and pertussis.

Tetanus

Clinical disease may follow infection of man with

the spore-forming gram-positive bacterium *Clostridium tetani* when spores germinate in suitable anaerobic conditions in tissues and release a powerful neurotoxin, tetanospasmin. Detoxification of tetanospasmin with formaldehyde produces the highly antigenic toxoid which is used for active immunisation.

The classical wounds which may lead to circumstances in which tetanus spores are introduced and can germinate are penetrating ones but tetanus can follow any wound including injection sites and surgical wounds. However, it is usually only possible to recover tetanus bacilli from about 30% of cases. The umbilical stump of newborns is of particular importance as a site of infection in some countries. In rare instances no apparent portal of entry is found or the wound was so mild as to have been forgotten or so trivial as not to have come to medical attention. Auto-infection is also known to occur particularly following surgery of the lower limbs in circumstances where the circulation is compromised.

The toxin is believed to spread from the site of production along motor nerves and up the spinal cord. It then becomes fixed to the neuromuscular end plates and anterior horn cells where it is believed to act by inhibiting release of acetycholine. Once fixed it is unaffected by antitoxin. In addition the sympathetic nervous system may be involved and a central action of the toxin is also postulated.

Tetanus usually has an incubation period of 5–14 days but this can range from 24 hours to 3 weeks. Short incubation cases usually have severe disease, but a long interval does not necessarily exclude severe disease. The earliest manifestations may be pain and stiffness of the neck and back but are usually trismus and dysphagia. Rarely cranial nerve palsies (cephalic tetanus) may be the initial feature, but these patients together with those who have local tetanus in the region of the infected wound usually develop trismus and generalised tetanus.

Spasms leading to abdominal rigidity, extension of limbs and opisthotonus may be spontaneous or induced by the most trivial of stimuli such as noise, sudden movement or bright light. They increase in frequency and duration to cause impairment of respiratory function. Death may occur from respiratory obstruction or as a consequence of impaired respiratory function caused by secretions. Fever is not common but indicates a poor prognosis if present. If the initial spasms are generalised the prognosis is also poor.

The more severe cases develop problems arising from the syndrome of sympathetic over-activity. Profuse sweating and salivation, fever, hypertension and tachycardia or arrhythmias together with peripheral vasoconstriction are the principal features.

Neonatal tetanus

The disease has its onset within 14 days of birth and may commence as early as 4 days. The early signs are difficulty in taking the breast or swallowing or the mother may state that the infant does not cry properly or has difficulty in opening his mouth. Convulsions or cyanotic attacks may be prominent. Soon the more easily recognised generalised spasms develop which are readily provoked by noise, light or handling. The highest mortality occurs in premature infants and those of low birth weight. If symptoms start within seven days of birth or if autonomic nervous system disturbance is prominent, the duration of the illness can be up to 4 weeks. Seizures due to intracranial birth trauma, hypoglycaemia, meningitis and generalised sepsis may need to be considered in the differential diagnosis. Neonatal tetanus commonly occurs in areas where neonatal jaundice is also common and kernicterus has to be considered in the differential diagnosis. The use of tetanus vaccine in pregnancy has been shown to have a profound effect in reducing the frequency of neonatal tetanus (Berggren & Berggren 1971).

Management of tetanus

In addition to the control of the spasms the management includes the administration of antitoxin and penicillin together with surgical treatment of the infected wound. The increased availability of human anti-tetanus immunoglobulin has removed the hazards of antitoxin of equine origin. The dose is not precisely known but should be of the order of 30–300 units per kg given by intramuscular injection. Equine antitoxin is given in doses of up

Table 22.27 Outline of management procedures in tetanus

Stage of tetanus	Management
Mild: no dysphagia or respiratory difficulty	Sedatives, diazepam, opiates
Moderate: more pronounced spasticity and some interference with swallowing and respiration	Sedatives, tracheostomy
Severe: gross spasticity and major spasms	Paralysis with curare and artificial ventilation
Very severe: severe spasms and sympathetic over-activity	Paralysis with curare, artificial ventilation with very heavy sedation, anaesthesia, adrenergic blocking agents

to 100 000 units intravenously divided equally into intravenous and intramuscular doses, but steps must be taken to manage 'hypersensitivity' to this product (Parish & Cannon 1962).

Intrathecal antitoxin has been used but its efficacy is still disputed (Sanders et al 1977, Lancet 1980).

Success in the management of tetanus depends on the skill and experience of the care team. It is experience which will enable the appropriate intervention to be taken at the optimal time, for full intensive care techniques may produce complications which cause death (Edmundson & Flowers 1979). Patients with mild disease, namely those in whom the incubation period exceeds 14 days and in whom the generalised spasms take a week to evolve, can usually be managed by sedation and careful nursing. More severe cases will require intubation or tracheostomy and the use of diazepam. Difficulty in coping with secretions in the upper airways is an indication for tracheostomy. More severe cases should be managed in centres with experience in treating this disease. For survival rates of over 75–80% the need for assisted ventilation has been stressed (Adams et al 1979). Pharmacologic α and β adrenergic blockade has been advocated for patients who exhibit the syndrome of sympathetic over-activity (Pry-Roberts et al 1969) but this treatment is not without danger. (Buchanan et al 1978) An outline of the management in tetanus of varying degrees of severity is shown in Table 22.27.

On recovery the patient should be given tetanus vaccine as the disease does not confer immunity.

Diphtheria

Immunisation has been the single most important factor in the control of diphtheria but it must be stressed that protection requires a full course of vaccine. Incomplete immunisation courses may leave the individual incompletely protected (Nelson et al 1978).

The diphtheria bacillus is a club-shaped Gram-positive rod, some strains of which produce an exotoxin which binds to specific cell receptors which are present on all human cells. The toxin causes tissue necrosis thus causing the local membrane formed at the site of multiplication in the upper respiratory tract; infection may also occur on other surfaces such as the skin, auditory canal, conjunctiva and vulvo-vaginal region. The toxin is poorly absorbed but is responsible for the myocardial injury.

The neurological disturbances in diphtheria are stated to be caused by a polyneuritis which results in muscle paralysis but the precise mechanism of paralysis is not known. It is seen in about 10% of patients and is usually symmetrical and occurs after the first week of the illness. The most frequent manifestation is palatal paralysis, but the extra-ocular muscles and muscles of accommodation may be involved. Less commonly the diaphragm and pharyngeal muscles may be affected and rarely limb paralysis occurs. These latter paralyses occur 6–8 weeks after the onset of infection. Some individuals may have a disorder closely resembling the Guillain-Barré syndrome. Most paralytic episodes resolve after 3–4 weeks, and it is a characteristic that recovery is complete (Christie 1980b). The treatment of diphtheria is described in standard texts, but there is no specific treatment of paralytic disease.

Botulism and infantile botulism

Botulism is a disease caused by the powerful exotoxins produced by the anaerobic Gram-positive bacterium *Clostridium botulinum*. In man, performed toxin, produced by bacteria of the types A, B, E and F, is consumed in food; the incubation period is measured in hours and the patient may succumb to rapidly progressive paralytic disease.

There is no convincing evidence that antitoxin is of benefit as the toxins rapidly fix to the myoneural junctions and are unaffected by antitoxin at that stage. The toxin interferes with release of acetylcholine from cholinergic nerve endings which results in neuromuscular paralysis. Management is based on support of a paralysed patient.

This well-known disorder has appeared in a 'new' form of infantile botulism as a subacute or acute condition. It differs from classical botulism as preformed toxin is not consumed, but is liberated in the gastrointestinal tract by multiplying bacteria under conditions which have not yet been defined.

The first description of the disorder by Pickett et al (1976) was of weakness and paralysis of cranial nerves and limbs which developed slowly over a period of several days. There was often a preceding history of constipation. The infants had difficulty in feeding and involvement of the chest muscles caused respiratory embarrassment. Mild forms of the disease consist of mild hypotonia, hyporeflexia, feeding difficulties and failure to thrive. In more severely affected infants there may be severe generalised weakness with ptosis, facial diplegia, extraocular palsies and a poor gag reflex. The hypotonia and ptosis are illustrated in Figure 22.13. In the severe forms deterioration may be rapid so that there may be a superficial resemblance to the 'sudden infant death syndrome'.

Recovery takes place over a period of several weeks, but some weakness may persist for months. The principal descriptions of the disease come from the United States where over one hundred cases have been reported. Only two cases have been described in Australia (Shield et al 1978, Murrell et al 1981) and only single cases in the United Kingdom (Turner et al 1978) and in Canada (McCurdy et al 1981). Most have been associated with type B organisms and the majority have been reported from western regions of the United States. Food sources have been sought, but the only food with which any correlation has been found is honey (Arnon et al 1979). The connection between honey and type B *Clostridium botulinum* is strong, but this is not true of type A bacteria. House dust and soil may be sources, but in the vast majority of cases no food or environmental source has been found. An unusual feature is that only infants under one year of age (1–8 months) have been affected and the mean age is of the order of 3–4 months. The sexes are equally

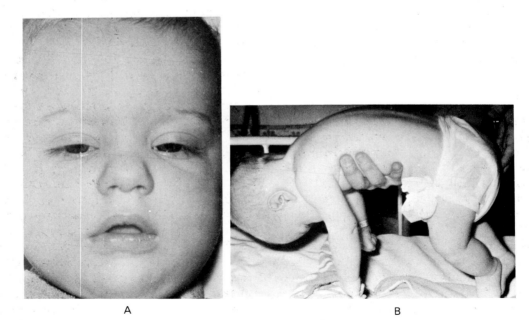

A   B

Fig. 22.13 Infant botulism:
(A) Ptosis and (B) marked hypotonia in a 24-week-old girl with infantile botulism described by Turner et al (1978)

affected. Ingested spores may be more likely to multiply in circumstances where there is an alteration in the ecology of the gut but in a recent survey most affected infants were breast-fed (Thompson et al 1980).

The diagnosis is established by demonstrating the specific toxin in stool and isolating the organisms. In contrast to the adult form of the disease, the toxin has not been detected in the circulation. Electromyographic changes which have been described consist of non-specific findings of brief small amplitude, abundant motor unit potentials, but augmentation of the amplitude by the evoked muscle action potential at stimulation frequency greater than 10 Hz; most cases show a positive incremental response, but this is also seen in other rare disorders, such as snake bite and antibiotic toxicity.

The role of infantile botulism in the 'sudden infant death syndrome' (SIDS) has not been firmly established, in spite of the interesting results of the survey of cases of SIDS for toxin or organisms in stools by Arnon & Chin (1979).

Recognition of the need supportive care is the essential first step in management. Careful monitoring and tube feeding will suffice in most infants, but respiratory ventilatory support may be required. There is no evidence that antibiotics are of help in the gastrointestinal infection but gentamicin is contra-indicated because of the risk of potentiating the paralysis (Santos et al 1981).

Pertussis

Pertussis is a very complex disease; less is known of its pathogenesis than of any other common disease of childhood. The infection is limited to the respiratory tract; invasion of tissues or blood does not occur. Although the bacteria can be eradicated by antibiotics yet the cough persists for many weeks. The multiple antigens of *Bordetella pertussis* and *B. parapertussis* have been shown to be responsible for responses such as lymphocytosis and increased sensitivity to histamine and both heat-labile and heat-stable toxins can be detected. Pittman (1979) considers that the harmful effects are caused by a complex macromolecule comprising at least two of the pertussis antigens with characteristics of an endotoxin. According to Pittman this endotoxin is islet-activating, lymphocyte-leucocyte promoting and histamine-sensitising. An antitoxin prepared from this substance may prove to be a more effective and probably less reactogenic vaccine than the present vaccine which is prepared from killed whole organisms.

Hypoxia is a frequent and visible event in pertussis. In the very young and particularly the premature infant, coughing may not be a feature of the early stages of infection. These infants not infrequently present with apnoeic attacks. A number of haemorrhagic events such as diffuse petechiae in the cerebral tissues, subdural or spinal epidural haematomata may cause damage to the nervous system. A very puzzling aspect of the disease is the ill-defined disorder termed pertussis encephalopathy which characteristically appears at the peak of the paroxymal cough. It is more frequent in the very young and is more common in females. There may be convulsions, coma and sometimes hemiplegia (Zellweger 1959). Although hypoxia or petechiae in the brain could account for these features there is no proof of this in all cases (Celemajer & Brown 1966). Hypoglycaemia is thought by Olson (1975) to contribute to some of the effects on the nervous system. Residual damage is well documented in patients with severe apnoea with convulsions in frank encephalopathy. There may also be an adverse effect on intellectual development (White et al 1964, Olson 1975).

The link between the neurological disorders of pertussis and the encephalopathic illness reported after pertussis vaccines is not clear; there is a greater lack of clarity as to the occurrence of an encephalopathic illness reported after pertussis vaccine. In a nationwide case-controlled study of children aged two months to their third birthday with acute severe neurological illness from July 1976 to June 1979 Miller and his colleagues (1981) found that there was a relatively higher risk of children suffering from acute severe neurological illness in the seven days following immunisation with Diptheria/Tetanus/Pertussis vaccines than in control cases. From this study a calculated attributable risk of serious neurological reaction was 1 per 110 000 immunisations and of persisting neurological damage in one year was 1 per 310 000 immunisations. However the study failed to identify a positive 'reaction' syndrome (Lancet 1981).

It is possible that in some infants receiving vaccine the effects of a coincidental virus infection may be worsened by the adjuvant effect of the vaccine and a similar phenomenon occurs and is related to the neurological illness in some natural infections (Cavanagh et al 1981). Febrile convulsion may also occur following Diptheria/Pertussis/Tetanus vaccines but they do not appear to be of any greater or more serious consequence than febrile convulsion in other children.

FUNGUS INFECTIONS

Infections with fungi are acquired from the environment and usually gain entry via the respiratory tract. Infection of the nervous system may occur in normal individuals but most involve patients with defects in host defence mechanisms.

Diagnosis of infection can be difficult and repeated examination of CSF may be necessary for culture or visualisation of the organism by direct microscopy. The use of methylene blue or India ink preparation is particularly useful in cryptococcal infections. Cryptococcal and coccidioidal antibody may be detected in CSF but a most useful development has been the latex agglutination test for cryptococcal polysaccharide antigen (Ellner & Bennett 1976).

Cryptococcus neoformans is the commonest cause of fungal meningitis. The other agent which is likely to affect children is candida albicans. Patients with cryptococcal meningitis often present with symptoms and signs similar to those which occur in tuberculous meningitis; however the levels of glucose in the CSF are usually not depressed. Rarely cystic cavities and intracranial calcification develop. Treatment with amphotericin B and flucytosine has been reported to be more successful than amphotericin alone (Bennett et al 1979).

The same combination of drugs probably provides optimal treatment for candida meningitis (Chesney et al 1978) which occurs most frequently in young infants, especially prematures. However, the imidazole, miconazole, has not been evaluated. The severely malnourished infant who is being fed by the intravenous route is especially vulnerable to candidaemia and meningitis. Some patients may present with acute meningitic illness. The organism is readily identified in the CSF which may otherwise be normal or show elevated protein levels and a wide range in the number of cells; glucose levels are usually depressed. In both cryptococcal and candida meningitis sterilisation of the CSF may take 7–14 days.

Cerebral abscesses may form in infections with both aspergillus and actinomyces species but a chronic low grade meningitis may be present in the latter.

Other fungal infections are rare in children. Fungal cerebral abscess is often the result of infection with blastomycosis but there is usually involvement of other organs and tissues. *Coccidioides immitis* and *Histoplasma capsulatum* can present as chronic meningitis but disseminated disease is more frequent. Mucormycoses in the form of rhino-cerebral or orbito-cerebral disease cause ischaemic infarction as a result of arterial thrombosis but are far less common in children than in adults.

PARASITIC INFECTIONS

A number of parasites may migrate to the brain causing diffuse involvement or the development of a space-occupying lesion. Eosinophilic meningitis can be a striking feature of some of these infections and has been discussed earlier in this chapter. The symptomatology of these infections can, at times, be very puzzling. In most instances the parasites are acquired in tropical environments but some, such as larval hookworms, strongyloides, hydatid disease, cysticerosis, may also be found in temperate regions.

Investigation by means of tests for antibody, using immunofluorescence, immuno-electrophoresis or gel precipitation in both serum and CSF may provide the diagnosis in some of these infections.

The use of improved neuro-radiological investigation has not been extended to all these various parasitic infections, hence it is not known whether there are any specific features for individual infections.

Infections of the nervous system with cestodes include hydatid disease and cysticerocosis, although fly maggots (tumbu fly and sheep and cattle bot flies) may even have to be considered in certain circumstances (Lancet 1976).

Hydatid disease

Man and sheep are intermediate hosts in the cycle of *Echinococcus granulosa* or *multilocularis* and are infected by ingestion of ova discharged from the intestine of the definitive host, usually the dog. The cystic stage of the parasites then evolves which causes a space-occupying lesion, unless it ruptures. In children cysts of the liver are more common than in the lung, the reverse to the situation in adults (Meyers 1960). Intracranial involvement is usually with a single cyst; the symptoms and signs are those of raised intracranial pressure, seizures or a focal neurological disorder. The appearance on CT scan of a cyst in a 4-year-old boy is shown in Figure 22.14. Calcification of hydatid cysts takes two or more decades to occur and unlike cysts of the liver and spleen, intracranial cysts rarely calcify.

The intermediate hypersensitivity (Casoni) test is now rarely performed because of the frequency of non-specific reactions; complement-fixing, hae-magglutination and fluorescent antibody tests (Matossian 1977) can be performed and may be helpful, but the diagnosis should not be excluded on the basis of negative tests. High levels of serum IgE are present which decline after removal of cysts. Serial measurement of IgE can be useful to detect recurrence. The basis of successful treatment remains in the hands of an experienced surgeon. Drug therapy in the form of merbendazole (Bekhtia et al 1977) has yet to be evaluated in controlled trials.

Cysticercosis

Infection is acquired from ingestion of ova of the pork tapeworm, Taenia solium, which may be present in contaminated water as well as food, but autoinfection may also occur. The interval between ingestion and appearance of symptoms averages 5 years (Dixon & Hargreaves 1944) and thus the patient may reside outside an endemic area at the time of onset of symptoms. The most frequent sites of infection are muscles, eyes and brain and the latter manifests most commonly as seizures. However, the presentation may be as a space-occupying lesion or eosinophilic meningitis. Intracerebral calcification of degenerative larvae which vary in size

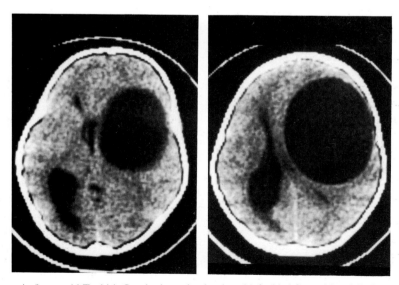

Fig. 22.14 Hydatid cyst in 5-year-old Turkish-Cypriot boy who developed left-sided fits and hemiplegia 2 months previously. CT shows a large, very clearly demarcated lesion of low attenuation in the right frontal lobe which causes expansion of the right hemicranium with thinning of the overlying frontal bone, compression of the right lateral ventricle and marked displacement of the midline structures towards the left side.

up to 1–2 cm, may occur after several years; at this stage antibody which is sometimes detectable in CSF could have disappeared (Biagi & Willms 1974). The CT scan reveals single or multiple calcified areas which may not be visible on standard X-rays (Carbajal et al 1977). The detection of calcification of skeletal muscles may be a useful clue to the diagnosis. There is no specific treatment but control of seizures by anticonvulsants appear to be achieved without undue difficulty (Percy et al 1980).

The nematodes which may invade the nervous system include toxocara, trichinella, strongyloides, and the rat lungworm (angiostrongylus cantonensis). *Toxocara* infections, acquired either from dogs or cats, have a worldwide distribution. Although liver disease, wheezing and eosinophilia are the most common manifestations of infection in children, involvement of the eye is a serious complication. The infection is usually confined to children of the toddler age group. Meningoencephalitis and convulsions may also occur (Huntley et al 1965). Granulomata of the cerebellum have also been reported (Mok 1968). *Trichinella spiralis*, which is acquired from consumption of raw or partially cooked pork, is usually manifest as a disease of skeletal muscles. However, in rare instances, encephalitis or meningitis may be present in the acute stage of the infection (Kramer et al 1972). *Strongyloides stercoralis* may produce disseminated disease and involve the nervous system in immunosuppressed individuals. There can be long periods of dormancy, and the original infection may occur in childhood. Meningitis occurs and the larvae can be seen in wet preparations of the CSF. However, meningeal disease is but part of a 'hyper-infestation' syndrome which has been discussed elsewhere in this chapter. The intense eosinophilic meningitis caused by *angiostrongylus cantonensis* has been described previously.

The trematode infections include schistosomiasis and *Paragonimus westermani* (lung fluke). Many millions of individuals in Africa, South America and Asia are affected by Schistosomiasis and invasion of the portal and caval circulation with *S. Japonicum* and *S. Mansoni* may result in central nervous system disease of which there are two forms; granulomata and a diffuse pathology of the white and grey matter (Marcail-Rojas & Fiol 1963).

The lung fluke, *Paragonimus westermani*, occurs primarily in the Orient. The lung infection is of little consequence. The fluke causes not only meningitis, but often space-ocupying lesions from which seizures are common (Oh 1968). Most patients have abnormal chest X-rays and peripheral blood eosinophilia is common.

Other parasites which may have a serious impact on the nervous system include *plasmodium falciparum* and the trypanosomes. Cerebral malaria occurs mainly in children under 3–4 years of age and in 'non-immune' adults. There is usually a very high parasitaemia. The cerebral disturbance is due to obstruction of cerebral capillaries with red cells containing developing forms of *P. falciparum* (Bruce-Chwatt 1978). Cerebral hypoxia and oedema develop and convulsions and coma are the most frequent manifestations. Cerebral malaria has been found to be more frequent in the well-nourished child (Hendrickse et al 1971) and rarely there may be signs of meningeal irritation. The CSF is usually normal but a mild pleocytosis and mild to moderate elevation of protein is sometimes present.

Both American and African trypanosomiasis cause neurological disease. In South America the acute forms of infection with *Trypanosoma cruzi* are more frequent in children, especially in the very young. The primary lesion of the skin (Chagoma) is often present. There is fever with a generalised lymphadenopathy and local oedema, which can become generalised. Hepatosplenomegaly and myocarditis are other features which may develop. Rarely, meningoencephalitis can occur in the acute stage, and can be associated with focal or generalised seizures, The chronic focus of Chagas' disease is usually seen in adults. Treatment in the acute stage with nitrofuran compound, nifurtiniox, has been claimed to be effective. Congenital Chagas' disease may resemble the multisystem involvement which can occur in congenital toxoplasma gondii, cytomegalovirus or neonatal herpes simplex infections (Bittencourt 1976). Trypanosomes can be seen in the CSF in such infections.

African Trypanosomiasis, the result of infection with *Trypanosoma rhodesiense* or *gambiense*, does not behave differently in the child. The former is a more acute and may be a fulminating infection. Both can have a short incubation period of 1 to 2 weeks, but *T. gambiense* may be considerably longer. A nodule develops at the site of the infected bite and then a recurrent febrile illness occurs. In *T. gambiense* infection, severe headaches can be followed by deterioration in the mental state. Tremors and fits are late manifestations, then coma ensues. If the course of the illness in *T. rhodesiense* infection is rapid, as in epidemic disease, there may be little evidence of involvement of the nervous system, but mild pleocytosis and elevated protein are usually present in the CSF. Endemic disease is stated to be more prolonged and tremors of the limbs more common (Robertson 1978) Treatment early in these infections with metarsolprol and antrypol (suramin) is often curative but re-treatment may be required.

Primary amoebic meningoencephalitis

Infection with the amoebae of the genus Naegleriae is acquired from exposure to fresh waters contaminated with these free-living amoebae. The amoeba *Naegleria fowleri* grows rapidly as water temperature rises to 37–45°C, but the risk of infection from infected water is remote. Entry to the nervous system is thought to occur via the olfactory epithelium. The disease, which usually affects children and young adults (CDC 1980), presents as an acute fulminating meningoencephalitis which is usually fatal within seven days. There is usually a history of swimming in fresh warm water 1–2 weeks previously. The CSF contains several hundred white cells which are mainly polymorphs; the protein is usually increased and the glucose decreased. Motile amoebae may be seen in, or cultured from, the CFS. The organism may be identified in brain tissue at post-mortem by immunohistological techniques. Treatment has rarely been effective but success has been achieved using intravenous and intrathecal amphotericin B and miconazole, together with oral rifampicin. The infection is very rare in the United Kingdom (Cain et al 1981) but should be suspected in children who are severely ill with 'pyogenic' meningitis, in whom no bacteria are visible on staining.

In immunosuppressed patients, a chronic form of amoebic meningitis is caused by the genus *Acanthanoeba* and is presumed to be caused by spread to the nervous system from another site in the body, rather than being acquired from an environmental source such as infected water.

Rarely, disseminated disease is caused by *Entamoeba histolytica* with multiple abscesses of the liver and lung predominantly; cerebral abscesses and meningoencephalitis may complicate the infection in patients of this type.

The protozoon *Toxoplasma gondii* causes extensive disease of the nervous system when acquired prenatally as a primary infection during pregnancy. One of the hallmarks of infection is chorioretinitis. It is generally accepted that eye disease is always the result of prenatal infection even though it may make it appearance several years after birth. Post-natal infection very rarely causes disease of the nervous system, but takes the form of acute meningoencephalitis with some elevation of the protein and mild lymphocytic pleocytis (Keoze 1964). Reactivation of infection in the immunosuppressed host is discussed elsewhere in this chapter.

Reye's syndrome

Reye's syndrome is a severe disorder of unknown aetiology in which there is fatty infiltration of the liver and acute non-inflammatory encephalopathy without evidence of meningeal inflammation (Reye et al 1963).There are no pathognomonic features and no specific laboratory tests to confirm the diagnosis. Thus it is possible only to document the principal features which allow recognition of the disorder in order to institute measures which may influence its course.

Death is due to the cerebral disorder. The mortality is of the order of 40% and is highest in the younger age groups. Severe permanent sequelae occur in about 10% of survivors and are also higher in younger children (Crocker 1979) but follow-up studies have also shown neuropsychological disturbances which are not always apparent on clinical examination (Brunner et al 1979).

The syndrome is essentially a disorder of childhood, but very rarely young adults have been affected. Most cases are seen in the first decade of life from as young as three months. The sexes are equally affected. There is not infrequently a prodromal illness, often of viral aetiology (de Vito & Keating 1976), but the link between these and the subsequent events is obscure. These illnesses have included influenza B and less commonly influenza A, as well as other infections with upper respiratory symptoms. Chicken pox or other exanthemata have also preceded the disorder and in a few instances a temporal relationship with the administration of live viral vaccines has been reported (Morens et al 1979). Clustering has been observed in influenza B-associated cases (Corey et al 1976), and the risk is stated to be four times higher in rural than in urban areas in the United States (Corey et al 1977a).

A similar disorder is also been in Thailand, where it is associated with aflatoxin, a product of the fungus *Aspergillus larvus*. It also closely resembles the Jamaican vomiting sickness caused by a powerful toxin, hypoglycin A, which is present in the ackee apple. There is little evidence of association with toxins in the majority of cases, but a search should be made for these, including insecticides. An additional factor in the causation of Reye's syndrome is thought to be salicylates, the effect of which may be potentiated by fever (Starko et al 1980). Thus the disorder may be the consequence of a synergistic effect between an infective agent and a toxin. The role of genetic factors, in spite of occasional reports of the syndrome in twins and siblings, is far from clear.

Within 3 to 6 days of the 'prodrome' of 'gastro-enteritis' in younger children and signs of an upper respiratory tract infection in the older child vomiting commences which can be copious or protracted. Very soon after, even within a few hours, disturbances in the level of consciousness develop. Either lethargy or a hyperexcitable state of delirium may be present in this early stage; the behaviour of the patient has been described as combative, and hyperventilation may be a feature. There may then be progression to a comatose state. Generalised convulsion occur in about 30% of patients. The whole neurological illness can reach a climax in as little as three to four hours, but some patients show a slower evolution over one or two days. The more rapid the progression, the worse the prognosis and when death occurs it is most often within 24 hours, and usually within three days of onset of symptoms. Meningism and focal neurological signs are rare and the changes of raised intracranial pressure caused by diffuse oedema of the brain can be observed on fundoscopic examination. Cerebral oedema may be shown on the CT scan (Fig. 22.15). During the phase when the neurological features are established, the liver may enlarge to a moderate degree. High to extremely high levels of serum aminotransferases are present. It is possible to suspect that Reye's syndrome is the cause of an acute encephalopathic illness from the presence of abnormal liver function tests. Hyperammonaemia is found in the early stages, but may not be detected in all children as ammonia levels fall to normal 2–4 days after the onset of symptoms. Jaundice is most unusual but hypoglycaemia is not infrequent, and hypoglycorrhacia is sometimes found in otherwise normal CSF. The prothrombin time is usually prolonged and deficiencies of other clotting factors may be present.

There are several metabolic abnormalities from which attempts have been made to define the pathogenesis of Reye's syndrome. Increased amounts of ammonia, lactate, pyruvate, amino acids, uric and fatty acids, creatine kinase and amylase are present and decreases in glucose, cholesterol and total lipids have been observed in serum. A complex disturbance of acid-base balance occurs; $PaCO_2$ is depressed, but without a severe disturb-

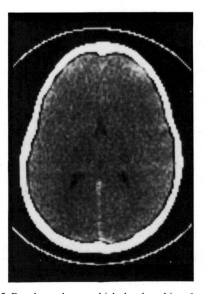

Fig. 22.15 Reye's syndrome which developed in a 6-year-old girl following chicken pox; she was in stage 3 at the time CT scan was performed. CT scan at the level of the lateral ventricles. Both lateral ventricles are very small but not displaced. There is diffuse low attenuation in the cerebral hemisphere due to oedema.

ance in pH in the early stages. In spite of these many abnormalities none are pathognomonic. The diagnosis can only be made by means of a needle liver biopsy which shows characteristic microvesicular fat in every liver cell. There is no displacement of the nucleus of the hepatocyte and no inflammatory cell response. Vitamin K and an infusion with fresh frozen plasma may be needed before the biopsy can be performed. Swelling of mitochondria is also seen in the liver and in the brain, but these changes are known to be reversible. The basic defect in Reye's syndrome may involve the mitochondria.

If a liver biopsy is not performed, Corey and colleagues (1977b) have suggested the following criteria for the diagnosis of Reye's syndrome:

1. A clinical history of a preceding viral-like prodrome and a biphasic illness

2. Fewer than 10 cells per cu mm in CSF

3. At least a 200% increase in serum transaminase and 150% increase in blood ammonia

4. Exclusion of other causes of encephalopathic illness with hepatocellular dysfunction.

The use of a staging system, of which there are several, is important since it allows a clinical estimation of the patient to be made so that appropriate treatment measures can be adopted and provides information for the evaluation of treatment.

The system developed by Lovejoy et al (1974) contained five stages of the neurological status. A modification of the Lovejoy staging is shown in Table 22.28.

The differential diagnosis of Reye's syndrome includes viral encephalitis, bacterial meningitis, acute viral hepatitis with encephalopathy, endotoxic and hypovolaemic shock, intoxications and metabolic diseases. Examination of the CSF is needed to exclude bacterial meningitis but carries a risk of herniation of the brain if the patient is suffering from brain swelling; the physician may be in a dilemma (Byers 1973). If papilloedema is present or if the patient is in deep coma, a lumbar puncture should not be performed.

Treatment of Reye's syndrome is based on the need to maintain adequate cerebral blood flow. The early stages I and II require only intravenous glucose and correction of fluid and electrolyte in balance, but patients should be treated whenever possible in a centre with facilities for intensive care including ventilatory support and the monitoring and treatment of raised intracranial pressure by means of hyperventilation and osmotherapy (Boutros et al 1980). The various treatments tried have included exchange transfusion, total body washout and peritoneal dialysis. No one system has proved greatly superior but survival rates are better in cen-

Table 22.28 Modification of clinical staging of severity of encephalopathy in Reye's syndrome of Lovejoy et al 1974 (after Mowat 1979)

Stages:	I Mild	II Moderate	III Severe	IV Very severe	V Brain death
Mental state	Quiet, normal response to verbal commands	Lethargic, slow mental processes such as difficulty in counting	Agitated delirium, out of contact with environment but responds to pain	Coma, decerebrate rigidity, pain produces exacerbation of decerebrate posture	Coma, spinal reflexes preserved
Muscular activity	Wishes to lie down but no other abnormality	Clumsy	Poorly controlled gross movements, intermittent clonus	Opisthotonos, extensor spasms of arms and legs	Flaccid paralysis
Respiration	Normal	Normal or increased rate	Normal or increased rate	Increased rate and depth	None
Pupillary responses	Normal	Normal	Dilated, but rapidly responsive	Dilated, but slowly responsive	Dilated and unresponsive
Fundi	Normal	Normal	Venous engorgement	Marked venous engorgement, discs blurred, papilloedema	Variable

tres which have experience in the management of this disorder (Nelson 1975). In the event of a second attack of a Reye's-like illness, congenital defects of branched chain amino acids or urea cycle enzymes should be suspected (Ch. 7).

Acute febrile mucocutaneous lymph node syndrome (MLCS) — (Kawasaki disease)

This bizarre disease, first described in Japan, is an acute exanthematous disease with a unique susceptibility for children; there is persistent fever for more than a week, hyperaemia of mucous membranes, particularly of the conjunctivae, non-purulent cervical lymphadenopathy, and periungual desquamation. Dryness and fissuring of the lips, erythema of the tongue and oedema of the hands and feet with a purple-red erythema of the palms and soles are often prominent.

Myocardial disease and aneurysms of the coronary arteries may be associated with sudden death in the second week onwards and there is a mortality of between 1 and 2% (Yamagawa 1976). Nearly 20 000 cases have been reported to the Japanese surveillance programme and it has now been described in almost all countries in the world but in much smaller numbers. There is no specific test for the disease; a marked polymorphonuclear leucocytosis, thrombocytosis and raised levels of serum IgE are usually present. High levels of circulating immune complexes are present during the first 6 to 8 weeks (Levin & Marshall 1981). There is a most striking irritability and emotional lability which may be present for many weeks. The CSF has been reported to show a mild pleocytosis with normal levels of protein and glucose. Retinal disease in the form of extensive 'cotton wool' exudates on the retina which progressed to a thick membrane covering the disc were described by Verghote et al (1981). Segmental venous thromboses were also visible. Steroids did not affect the lesions.

Because of the extensive vascular disease which affects the blood vessels of the heart, and which has also been described in medium-sized arteries such as the renal and splenic vessels, it is not inconceivable in an occasional patient that cerebral vessels may be involved in the process.

Much attention has been paid to a possible infectious aetiology of Kawasaki disease. Earlier evidence suggested that it may be caused by a rickettsial infection (Hamashima et al 1973). It does resemble scarlet fever in some respects but evidence of streptococcal infection has not been found. Extensive bacterial, viral and other microbiological studies have been negative (Yanagihara & Todd 1980). It may, on the other hand, represent a host response to an infection similar to the post-streptococcal disease, rheumatic fever and acute glomerulonephritis, or some other post-infectious immunologically mediated disorder (Melish 1981).

REFERENCES

Adams J M, Kenny J D, Rudolph A J 1979 Modern management of tetanus neonatorum. Pediatrics 64: 472–477

Ahronheim G A, Reich B, Marks M I 1979 Penicillin-insensitive pneumococci. American Journal of Diseases of Children 133: 187–191

Alford C A, Reynolds D M, Stagno S 1974 Current concepts of chronic perinatal infections. In: Gluck L (ed Modern perinatal medicine. Year book Medical Publishers, Chicago

Alford C A, Stagno S, Pass R 1980 Natural history of perinatal cytomegaloviral infection. In: Perinatal infections. Ciba Symposium 77, p 125–147

Ames M D, Plotkin S A, Winchester R A, Atkins T E 1970 Central auditory imperception: a significant factor in congenital rubella deafness. Journal of the American Medical Association 1970: 419–421

Anders B J, Lauer B A, Foley L C 1980 Computerised tomography to define CNS involvement in congenital cytomegalovirus infection. American Journal of Diseases of Children 134: 795–797

Anthony B F, Okada D M 1977 The emergence of Group B streptococci in infections of the newborn infant. Annual Review of Medicine 28: 355–369

American Acadamy of Pediatrics 1977 Report of the Committee on Infectious Diseases 18: 140

Armenguad M, Auvergnat J-CH, Le Net R, Massip P, Tho T C 1979 Des concentrations des antibiotiques dans le LCR au cours des traitements des meningites bacteriennes aiguës. Medécine et hygiène 30: 410–413

Arnon S S, Chin J 1979 The clinical spectrum of infant botulism. Reviews of Infectious Diseases 1: 614–621

Arnon S S, Midura T F, Damus K ,Thompson B, Word R W, Chin J 1979 Honey and other environmental risk factors for infant botulism. Journal of Pediatrics 94: 331–336

Baird D R, Whittle H C, Greenwood B M 1976 Mortality from pneumococcal meningitis. Lancet 2: 1344–1346

Baker C J 1971 Primary spinal epidural abscess. American Journal of Diseases of Children 121: 337–339

Barling R W A, Selkon J B 1978 The penetration of antibiotics with cerebrospinal fluid and brain tissue. Journal of Antimicrobial Chemotherapy 4: 205–227

Bastian F O, Rabson A S, Lee C Y, Tralka T S 1972 Herpes virus hominis: isolation from human trigeminal ganglion. Science 178: 306–307

Bayston R 1975 Serological surveillance of children with CSF shunting devices. Developmental Medicine & Child Neurology 17 (suppl. 35): 104–110

Bayston R 1980 Effect of antibiotic impregnation on the function of shunt valves used to control hydrocephalus. Zeitschrift für Kinderchirurgie 34: 353–358

Bayston R, Lari J 1974 A study of sources of infection in colonised shunts. Developmental Medicine and Child Neurology 16 (suppl. 22): 16–22

Beatty N H, Oppenheimer S 1968 Cerebrospinal fluid lactic dehydrogenase and its isoenzymes in infections of the central nervous system. New England Journal of Medicine 297: 1197–1202

Bekhtia A, Schaaps J P, Capron M, Dessaint J P, Santoro F, Capron A 1977 Treatment of hepatic hydatid disease with merbendazole; preliminary results in four cases. British Medical Journal 2: 1047–1051

Bellman M H, Dick G 1980 Surveillance of subacute sclerosing parencephalitis. British Medical Journal 2: 393–394

Bennett J E, Dismukes W E, Duma R J, Medcoff U, Sande M A, Gallis H et al 1979 A comparison of amphotericin alone and combined with flucytosine in the treatment of cryptococcal meningitis. New England Journal of Medicine 301: 126–131

Berg B, Franklin G, Cuneo R, Boldrey E, Strimling B 1978 Nonsurgical care of brain abscess: early diagnosis and follow-up with computerised tomography. Annals of Neurology 3: 474–478

Bergen D, Grossman H 1976 Infectious mononucleosis as a cause of acute cerebellar ataxia of childhood. Developmental Medicine and Child Neurology 18: 799–802

Berggren W L, Berggren G M 1971 Changing incidence of fatal tetanus in the newborn. American Journal of Tropical Medicine 20: 491–494

Berman N S, Siegil S E, Nachum R, Lipsey A, Leedom J 1976 Cerebrospinal fluid endotoxin concentration in gram-negative bacterial meningitis. Journal of Pediatrics 88: 553–556

Biagi F, Willms K 1974 Immunologic problems in the diagnosis of human cysticercosis. Annales de Parasitologie humaine et comparée 49: 509–513

Bittencourt A L 1976 Congenital Chagas disease. American Journal of Diseases of Children 130: 97–103

Black S B, Levine P, Shinefeld H R 1978 The necessity for monitoring chloramphenicol levels when treating neonatal meningitis. Journal of Pediatrics 92: 235–236

van Bogaert L 1945 Une leuco-encephalite sclerosante subaigue. Journal of Neurology, Neurosurgery and Psychiatry 8: 101–120

Brody J A, Gibbs C J 1976 Chronic neurological diseases. In: Evans A S (ed) Viral infections of humans, epidemiology and control. Plenum Medical Books, New York, p 519–537

Brody J A, Detels R 1970 Subacute sclerosing panencephalitis: a zoonosis following aberrant measles. Lancet 2: 500–501

Brook I, Bricknell K S, Overturf G D, Finegold S M 1978 Measurement of lactic acid in cerebrospinal fluid of patients with infections of the nervous system. Journal of Infectious Diseases 137: 384–390

Bruce-Chwatt L J 1978 Malaria. In: Jelliffe D B, Stanfield J P (ed) Disease of children in the subtropics and tropics, 3rd edn. Edward Arnold, London p 836

Brunell P A, Kotchmar G S 1981 Zoster in infancy: failure to maintain virus latency following intrauterine infection. Journal of Pediatrics 98: 71–73

Brunner R L, O'Grady D J, Partin J C, Partin J S, Schubert W K 1979 Neuropsychological consequences of Reye's Syndrome. Journal of Pediatrics 95: 706–711

Buchanan N, Smit L, Cane R D, de Andrade M 1978 Sympathetic overactivity in tetanus: fatality associated with propanolol. British Medical Journal 2: 254–255

Byers R K 1973 To tap or not to tap. Pediatrics 51: 561

Cain A R R, Wiley P F, Brownell B, Warhurst D C 1981 Primary amoebic meningoencephalitis. Archives of Disease in Childhood 56: 140–143

Caplan L R 1977 Ara-A for herpes encephalitis. New England Journal of Medicine 297: 1288–1289

Carbajal J R, Palacios E, Azar-Kia B, Churchill R 1977 Radiology of cysticercosis of the central nervous system including computed tomography. Radiology 125: 127–132

Cassell G H, Cole B C 1981 Mycoplasmas as agents of human disease. New England Journal of Medicine 304: 80–89

Cavanagh N P C, Brett E M, Marshall W C, Wilson J 1982 The possible adjuvant role of Bordetella pertussis and pertussis vaccine in causing severe encephalopathic illness: a presentation of three case histories. Neuropädiatrie 12: 374–381

Celermajer J M, Brown J 1966 The neurological complications of pertussis. Medical Journal of Australia 1: 1066–1069

Center for Disease Control 1978 Encephalitis surveillance: Annual Summary for 1976

Center for Disease Control 1980 Primary amebic meningoencephalitis — United States. Morbidity and Mortality Weekly Report. 29: 405–407

Chernik N L, Armstrong D, Posner J B 1977 Central nervous system infections in patients with cancer. Cancer 40: 268–274

Chesney J C, Hodgson G E 1980 CSF eosinophilia during acute Coxsackie B4 viral meningitis. American Journal of Diseases in Children 134: 703

Chesney P J, Justman R A, Bogdanowicz W M 1978 Candida meningitis in newborn infants: a review and report of combined amphotericin B-flucytosine therapy. John's Hopkins Medical Journal 142: 155–160

Chesney P J, Katcher M L, Nelson D B, Horowitz S D 1979 CSF eosinophilia and chronic lymphocytic choriomeningitis virus meningitis. Journal of Pediatrics 94: 750–752

Chess S 1971 Autism in children with congenital rubella. Journal of Autism and Childhood Schizophrenia 1: 33–47

Christie A B 1980a In: Infectious diseases: epidemiology and clinical practice Churchill Livingstone, Edinburgh, p 647

Christie A B 1980b In: Infectious diseases: epidemiology and clinical practice Churchill Livingstone, Edinburgh, p 876

Chun R W M 1975 Virus diseases of the nervous system. In: Swaiman K F, Wright F S (eds) The practice of pediatric neurology. C V Mosby, St Louis, p 572

Cobb W A, Morgan-Hughes J A 1968 Non-fatal subacute sclerosing leucoencephalitis. Journal of Neurology, Neurosurgery and Psychiatry 31: 115–123

Coleman D V 1980 Recent developments in papovaviruses: the human polyomaviruses (B K virus and J C virus). In: Waterson A P (ed) Recent advances in clinical virology, vol 2, p 89–110

Conner W T, Minielly J A 1980 Cerebral oedema in fatal meningococcaemia. Lancet 2: 967–969

Connolly J H, Allen I V, Hurwitz L J, Millar J H D 1967 Measles-virus antibody and antigen in subacute sclerosing panencephalitis. Lancet 1: 542–544

Controni C, Rodriguez W J, Hicks J M, Ficke M, Ross S, Friedman G et al 1977 Cerebrospinal fluid lactic acid levels in meningitis. Journal of Pediatrics 91: 379–384

Cooper L Z, Krugman S 1967 Clinical manifestations of postnatal and congenital rubella. Archives of Ophthalmology 77: 434–439

Corey L, Rubin R J, Bregman D, Gregg M D 1977b Diagnostic criteria for influenza B-associated Reye's Syndrome: clinical vs pathologic criteria. Pediatrics 60: 702–708

Corey L, Rubin R J, Hattwick M A W, Noble G R, Cassidy E 1976 A nationwide outbreak of Reye's syndrome: its epidemiologic relationship to influenza B. American Journal of Medicine 61: 615–625

Corey L, Rubin R J, Thompson T R, Noble G R, Cassidy E, Hattwick M A W et al 1977a Influenza B-associated Reye's syndrome: incidence in Michigan and potential for prevention. Journal of Infectious Diseases 135: 398–407

Corrall C J, Pepple J M, Moxon E R, Hughes W T 1981 C-reactive protein in spinal fluid of children with meningitis. Journal of Pediatrics 99: 365–369

Couvreur J 1980 In: Perinatal Infections. Ciba Foundation Symposium 77 (new series), Excerpta Medica, p 166–168

Crocker J (ed) 1979 Reye's syndrome: proceedings of a symposium. Grune and Stratton, New York

Danziger J, Bloch S, Cremin B J, Goldblatt M 1976 Cranial and intracranial tuberculosis. South African Medical Journal 50: 1403–1405

Davies P A 1977 Neonatal bacterial meningitis. Journal of Hospital Medicine November 1977, p 425

Davis J M, David K R, Kleinman G M, Kitchner H S, Taveras J M 1978 Computed tomography of herpes simplex encephalitis with clinicopathological correlation. Radiology 129: 409–417

Davis L E, Bodian D, Price D, Butler I J, Vickers J H 1977 Chronic progressive poliomyelitis secondary to vaccination of an immunodeficient child. New England Journal of Medicine 297: 241–245

Dawson J R 1934 Cellular inclusions in cerebral lesions of epidemic encephalitis. Archives of Neurology and Psychiatry 31: 685–700

Delage G, Dusseault M 1979 Tuberculous meningitis in children: retrospective study of 79 patients with an analysis of prognostic factors. Canadian Medical Association Journal 120: 305–309

DeLemos R A, Haggerty R J 1969 Corticosteroids as an adjunct to treatment in bacterial meningitis. Pediatrics 44: 30–34

DeNicola L K, Hanshaw J B 1979 Congenital and neonatal varicella. Journal of Pediatrics 94: 175–176

Desmond M M, Fisher E S, Vordeman A L, Schaffer H G, Andrew L P, Zion T E et al 1978 The longitudinal course of congenital rubella encephalitis in non-retarded children. Journal of Pediatrics 93: 584–591

Desmond M M, Wilson G S, Melnick J L, Singer D B, Zion T E, Rudolph A J et al 1976 Congenital rubella encephalitis. Journal of Pediatrics 71: 311–331

Desmonts G, Couvreur J 1975 Toxoplasmosis: epidemiologic and serologic aspects of perinatal infections. In: Krugman S, Gershon A A (eds) Infections of the fetus and the newborn infant. A R Liss, New York, vol 3, p 118

Deutman A F, Grizzard W S 1978 Rubella retinopathy and subretinal neovascularization. American Journal of Ophthamology 85: 82–87

De Vito D C, Keating J P 1976 Reye's syndrome. Advances in Pediatrics 22: 175–229

Dixon H B F, Hargreaves W H 1944 Cysticercosis (Taenia solium): further 10 years' clinical study, covering 284 cases. Quarterly Journal of Medicine 13: 107–121

Doane F W, Anderson N, Chatiyanonda K, Mclean D M, Balantyne R M, Rhodes A J 1967 Rapid laboratory diagnosis of paramyxovirus infections by electron microscopy. Lancet 2: 751–753

Dudgeon J A 1967 Maternal rubella and its effect on the foetus. Archives of Disease in Childhood 42: 110–125

Dworsky M, Whitley R, Alford C 1980 Herpes zoster in infancy. American Journal of Diseases of Children 174: 618–619

Edmondson R S, Flowers M W 1979 Intensive care in tetanus: management, complications and mortality in 100 cases. British Medical Journal 1: 1401–1404

Edwards J E 1978 Severe candida infections: clinical perspective, immune defense mechanisms and current concepts of therapy. Annals of Internal Medicine 89: 91–106

Eggerding C 1981 Personal communication

Ellner J J, Bennett J E 1976 Chronic meningitis. Medicine 55: 341–469

Emmett M, Jeffery H, Chandler D, Dugdale A E 1980 Sequelae of haemophilus influenzae meningitis. Australian Paediatric Journal 16: 90–93

Emond R T D, McKendrick G D W 1973 Tuberculosis as a cause of transient aseptic meningitis. Lancet 2: 234–236

Escobar J A, Belsey M A, Duenas A, Medina P 1975 Mortality from tuberculous meningitis reduced by steroid therapy. Pediatrics 56: 1050–1055

Fallon R J, Kennedy D H 1981 Treatment and prognosis in tuberculous meningitis. Journal of Infection 3 (suppl. 1): 39–44

Feigin R D 1981 Bacterial meningitis beyond the neonatal period. In: Feigin R D, Cherry J D (eds) Text book of pediatric infectious diseases. W B Saunders, Philadelphia, p 293–308

Feigin R D, Dodge P R 1976 Bacterial meningitis: newer concepts of pathophysiology and neurologic sequelae. Pediatric Clinics of North America 23: 541–556

Feigin R D, Shackleford P G 1973 Value of repeat lumbar puncture in the differential diagnosis of meningitis. New England Journal of Medicine 289: 571–574

Feigin R D, Stechenberg B W, Chang M J, Dunkle L M, Wong M L, Palkes H et al 1976 Prospective evaluation of treatment of hemophilus influenzae meningitis. Journal of Pediatrics 88: 542–548

Feigin R D, Wong M, Shackleford P G, Stechenberg B W, Dunkle L M, Kaplan S 1976 Countercurrent immunoelectrophoresis of urine as well as CSF and blood for diagnosis of bacterial meningitis. Journal of Pediatrics 89: 773–775

Feldman W E 1975 CSF lactic acid dehydrogenase activity. American Journal of Diseases of Children 129: 77–80

Feldman W E 1978, Effect of ampicillin and chloramphenicol against Haemophilus influenzae. Pediatrics 61: 406–409

Fenner F J, White D O 1976 In: Medical virology, 2nd edn. Academic Press, New York, p 364

Fenton T R, Marshall P C, Cavanagh N, Wilson J, Marshall

W C 1977 Herpes-simplex infection presenting as brainstem encephalitis. Lancet 2: 977

Fikrig S M, Berkovich S, Emmett S M, Gordon C 1973 Nitroblue tetrazolium dye test and differential diagnosis of meningitis. Journal of Pediatrics 82: 855–857

Fischer E G, McLennan J E, Suzuki Y 1981 Cerebral abscess in children. American Journal of Disease in Children 135: 746–749

Fischer E G, Schwachman H, Wepsic J G 1979 Brain abscess and cystic fibrosis. Journal of Pediatrics 95: 385–388

Fishman R A 1980 Cerebrospinal fluid. In: Diseases of the nervous system W B Saunders, Philadelphia, p 184

Fishman R A 1982 Steroids in the treatment of brain edema. New England Journal of Medicine 306: 359–360

Fraser D W, Darby C P, Koehler R E, Jacobs C F, Feldman R A 1973 Risk factors in bacterial meningitis: Charleston County, South Carolina. Journal of Infectious Diseases 127: 271–277

Friedman C A, Lovejoy F C, Smith A L 1979 Chloramphenicol disposition in infants and children. Journal of Pediatrics 95: 1071–1077

Foley J, Williams D 1953 Inclusion encephalitis and its relation to subacute sclerosing leucoencephalitis. A report of five cases. Quarterly Journal of Medicine 22: 157–194

Gewitz M, Dinwiddie R, Rees L, Volikas O, Yuille T, O'Connell B et al 1979 Mycoplasma hominis: a cause of neonatal meningitis. Archives of Disease in Childhood 54: 231–233

Glode M P, Daum R S, Goldman D H, Leclair J, Smith A 1980 Haemophilus influenzae type B meningitis. A contagious disease of children. British Medical Journal 280: 899–901

Goldachre M J 1976 Acute bacterial meningitis in childhood. Lancet 1: 28–31

Gotschlich E C 1978 Bacterial meningitis: the beginning of the end. American Journal of Medicine 65: 719–721

Gould I M, Irwin W J, Wadhwani R R 1980 The use of cerebrospinal fluid lactate determination in the diagnosis of meningitis. Scandanavian Journal of Infectious Disease 12: 185–188

Granoff D M, Daum R S 1980 Spread of Haemophilus influenzae type b: recent epidemiological and therapeutic considerations. Journal of Pediatrics 97: 854–860

Greene G R 1978 Meningitis due to Haemophilus influenzae other than type b: case report and review of the literature. Pediatrics 62: 1021–1025

Green W R, Sweet L K, Pritchard R W 1974 Acute lymphocytic choriomeningitis. Journal of Pediatrics 35: 688–701

Greenberg M, Pellitteri O, Eisenstein D T 1955 Measles encephalitis. I. Prophylactic effect of gamma globulin. Journal of Pediatrics 46: 462–467

Grose C, Henle W, Henle G, Feorino P M 1978 Primary Epstein-Barr virus infections in acute neurological diseases. New England Journal of Medicine 292: 392–395

Hall W W, Choppin P W 1981 Measles-virus proteins in brain tissue of patients with subacute sclerosing panencephalitis. New England Journal of Medicine 304: 1152–1155

Hamashima Y, Kishi K, Tasaka K 1973 Rickettsia-like bodies in infantile acute febrile mucocutaneous lymph node syndrome. Lancet 2: 42

Hanshaw J B, Dudgeon J A 1978 Varicella-zoster infections In: Viral diseases of the fetus and newborn. W B Saunders, Philadelphia, p 192–208

Hanshaw J B, Scheiner A P, Moxley A W, Gaev L, Abel V, Scheiner B 1976 School failure and deafness after 'silent' congenital cytomegalovirus infection. New England Journal of Medicine 295: 468–470

Hayden G F, Herremann K L, Buimovici-Klein E, Weiss K E, Nieburg P I, Mitchell J E 1980 Subclinical congenital rubella infection associated with maternal rubella vaccination in early pregnancy. Journal of Pediatrics 96: 869–872

Heath C W, Alexander A D, Gallon M 1965 Letospirosis in the United States. New England Journal of Medicine 273: 857–922

Hendrickse R G, Hasan A H, Olumide L O, Akinkunmi A 1971 Malaria in early childhood. Annals of Tropical Medicine and Parasitology 65: 1–20

Herson V C, Todd J K 1977 Prediction of morbidity in Hemophilus influenzae meningitis. Pediatrics 59: 35–39

Hirsch M S 1979 Discussion: In: Case Records of the Massachusetts General Hospital (case 44–1979). New England Journal of Medicine 301: 987–994

Hirsch M S, Moellering R C, Pope H G, Poskanzer D G 1974 Lymphocytic-choroemeningitis-virus infection traced to a pet hamster. New England Journal of Medicine 291: 610–612

Hirsch M S, Swartz M N 1980 Antiviral agents. New England Journal of Medicine 302: 949–953

Hope-Simpson R E 1965 The nature of herpes zoster. A long-term study and a new hypothesis. Proceedings of the Royal Society of Medicine 58: 9–20

Huntley C C, Costas M C, Lyverly B S 1965 Visceral larva migrans syndrome: clinical characteristics and immunologic studies in 51 patients. Pediatrics 36: 523–563

Huttenlocher P R 1976 Isoprinosine therapy in subacute sclerosing panencephalitis. (abstract) Neurology 26: 364

Idriss Z H, Sinno A A, Kronfol N M 1976 Tuberculous meningitis in childhood. American Journal of Diseases of Children 130: 364–367

Igra-Siegman Y, Kapila R, Sen P, Kaminski Z C, Louria D B 1981 Syndrome of hyperinfection with Strongyloides stercoralis. Reviews of Infectious Diseases 3: 397–407

Jacobs M J, Koornhof H J, Robins-Browne R M, Stevenson C M, Zermaak Z A Freiman I et al 1978 Emergence of multiply resistant pneumonocci. New England Journal of Medicine OO: 735–740

James H E, Walsh J W, Wilson H D, Connor J D, Bean J R Tibbs P A 1980 Prospective randomised study of therapy in cerebrospinal fluid shunt infection. Neurosurgery 7: 459–463

Johnston R B, Newman S L 1977 Chronic granulomatous disease. Pediatric Clinics of North America 24: 365–376

Kaiser A B, McGee Z A 1975 Aminoglyoside therapy of Gram-negative bacillary meningitis. New England Journal of Medicine 293: 1215–1220

Kaplan S L, Feigin R D, 1978 The syndrome of inappropriate secretion of antidiuretic hormone in children with bacterial meningitis. Journal of Pediatrics 92: 758–761

Kaplan K M, Oski F A 1980 Anemia with Haemophilus influenzae meningitis. Pediatrics 65: 1101–1104

Karkinen-Jääskelainen M, Saxen L 1974 Maternal influenza, drug consumption and congenital defects of the central nervous system. American Journal of Obstetrics and Gynaecology 118: 815

Katz R M, Liebman W 1970 Creatine phosphokinase activity in central nervous system disorders and infections. American Journal of Disease in Children 120: 543–546

Kelsey D S 1978 Adenovirus meningoencephalitis. Pediatrics 61: 291–293

Kennedy D H, Fallon R J 1979 Tuberculous meningtitis. Journal of the American Medical Association 241: 264–268

Kenny J F, Isburg C D, Michaels R H 1980 Meningitis due to haemophilus influenzae type b resistant to both ampicillin and chloramphenicol. Pediatries 66: 14–21

Klapper P E, Laing I, Longson M 1981 Rapid non-invasive diagnosis of herpes encephalitis. Lancet 2: 607–608

Klein J C, Marcy S M 1976 Bacterial infections. In: Remington J S, Klein J O (eds) Infectious diseases of the fetus and newborn infant. W B Saunders Philadelphia, p. 770

Koenig H, Rabinowitz S G, Day E, Miller V 1979 Post-infectious encephalomyelitis after successful treatment of herpes simplex encephalitis with adenine arabinoside. New England Journal of Medicine 300: 1089–1093

Koeze T H, Klingon G H 1964 Acquired toxoplasmosis. Archives of Neurology 11: 191–197

Kramer M D, Aita J F 1972 Trichinosis with central nervous system involvement. Neurology 22: 485–491

Krasinski K, Kusmiesz H, Nelson J D 1982 Pharmacologic interactions among chloramphenicol, phenytoin and phenobarbitone. Pediatric Infectious Disease 1: 322–324

Kresky B, Nauheim J S 1967 Rubella retinitis. American Journal of Diseases of Children 113: 305–310

Kreth H W, Ter Meulen V, Eckert G 1975 HL-A and subacute sclerosing panencephalitis. Lancet 2: 415–416

Kurent J E, Sever J L, Terasaki P I 1975 HL-A W29 and subacute sclerosing panencephalitis. Lancet 2: 927

Lancet 1966 Recurrent meningitis. Lancet 2: 379

Lancet 1976 Parasites which migrate to the brain. Lancet 1: 1116–1117

Lancet 1980 Tetanus immune globulin: the intrathecal route. Lancet 2: 464

Lancet 1981 Vaccination against whooping cough. Lancet 1: 1138–1139

Landesman S H, Corrado M L, Shah P M, Armengard M, Barza M, Cherubin C E 1981 Past and present roles of cephalosporin antibiotics in treatment of meningitis. American Journal of Medicine 71: 693–703

Larsson S, Cronberg S, Winblad S 1979 Listeriosis during pregnancy and neonatal period in Sweden 1958-1974. Acta paediatrica scandanavica 68: 485–493

Lauter C B 1980 Herpes simplex encephalitis: a great clinical challenge. Annals of Internal Medicine 93: 696–698

Lee E L, Robinson J J, Tjong M L, Ong T H, Ng K K 1977 Intraventricular Chemotherapy in Neonatal Meningitis. Journal of Pediatrics 91: 991–995

Legg N J 1967 Virus antibodies in subacute sclerosing panencephalitis: a study of 22 patients. British Medical Journal 3: 350–352

Lending M, Spohody L B, Mastern J 1964 CSF glutamic oxalacetic transaminase and lactic dehydrogenase activities in children with neurological disorders. Journal of Pediatrics 65: 415–421

Lepow M L 1978 Enteroviral meningitis: a reappraisal. Pediatrics 62: 267–269

Lever R J, Kalavsky S M 1973 Central nervous system disease associated with Mycoplasma pneumonia infection; a report of five cases and review of the literature. Pediatrics 52: 658–668

Levin M, Marshall W C 1981 unpublished observations

Levine D P, Lauter C B, Lerner A M 1978 Simultaneous serum and CSF antibodies in herpes simplex encephalitis. Journal of the American Medical Association 240: 356–360

Lietman P S 1978 In: Ehrlichman R J (ed) Clinical conferences at the Johns Hopkins Hospital. Johns Hopkins Medical Journal 143: 60–63

Lindberg J, Rosenhall U, Nylen O, Ringmer A 1977 Long-term outcome of Hemophilus influenzae meningitis related to antibiotic treatment. Pediatrics 60: 1–6

Link H, Wahren B, Norrby E 1979 Pleocytosis and immunoglobulin changes in cerebrospinal fluid and herpesvirus serology in patients with Guillain-Barré syndrome. Journal of Clinical Microbiology 9: 305–316

Linnemann C C, May D B, Schubert W K, Caraway C T, Schiff G M 1973 Fatal viral encephalitis in children with X-linked hypogammaglobulinaemia. American Journal of Disease in Children 126: 100–103

Lovejoy F R, Smith A L, Bresnan M J, Word J N, Victor D I, Adams P C 1974 Clinical staging in Reye's syndrome. American Journal of Diseases of Children 128: 36–41

MacCallum F O, Chin I J, Gostling J V T 1974 Antibodies to herpes simplex virus in the cerebrospinal fluid of patients with herpetic encephalitis. Journal of Medical Microbiology 7: 325–331

McCarthy J I, Amer J 1978 Post varicella acute transverse myelitis: a case presentation and review of the literature. Pediatrics 62: 202–204

McCormick J B, Bennett J V 1975 Public health consideration in the management of meningococeal disease. Annals of Internal Medicine 83: 883–886

McCracken G H, Mize S G, Threlkeld N 1980 Intraventricular Gentamicin therapy in Gram-negative bacillary meningitis of infancy. Lancet 1: 787–791

McCracken G H, Kaplan J M 1974 Penicillin treatment for congenital syphilis. Journal of the American Medical Association 228: 855–858

McCracken G H, Mize S G 1976 A controlled study of intrathecal antibiotic therapy in Gram negative enteric meningitis in infancy. Journal of Pediatrics 89: 66–72

McCracken G H, Sarff L D, Glode M P, Mize S G 1974 Relationship between Escherichia coli Kl capsular polysaccharide antigen and clinical outcome in neonatal meningitis. Lancet 2: 246–250

McCurdy D M, Krishnan C, Hauschild A H W 1981 Infant botulism in Canada. Canadian Medical Association Journal 125: 741–743

MacDonald H, Tobin J O H 1978 Congenital cytomegalovirus infection: a collaborative study on epidemiological clinical and laboratory findings. Developmental Medicine and Child Neurology 20: 471–482

Macfarlane D W, Boyd R D, Dodrill C B, Tufts E 1975 Intrauterine rubella, head size and intellect. Pediatrics 55: 797–801

McGrath E, Rosenbloom L 1980 Use of isoprinosine in subacute sclerosing panencephalitis. Archives of Disease in Childhood 55: 829–830

McIntosh K, Wilfrert K, Chernesky M, Plotkin S, Mattheis M J 1978 Summary of a workshop on new and useful methods in viral diagnosis. Journal of Infectious Diseases 138: 414–419

McKendrick G D W 1979 Diagnosis of herpes simplex encephalitis. Lancet 2: 1181–1182

McLean D M, Larke R P B, Cobb C, Griffis E D, Hackett S M R 1967 Mumps and enteroviral meningitis in Toronto 1966. Canadian Medical Association Journal 96: 1355–1361

Marcial-Rojas R A, Fiol R E 1963 Neurologic complications of Schistosomiasis: review of the literature and report of two cases of transverse myelitis. Annals of Internal Medicine 59: 215–230

Marshall W C 1981 Damage to the fetus and newborn from prophylactic procedures. In: Lambert H P, Wood C B S (eds) Immunological aspects of infection in the fetus and newborn Academic Press, p. 217–222

Marshall W C 1973 The clinical impact of intrauterine rubella in: Intrauterine infections. Ciba Foundation Symposium 10 (new series), Elsevier-Excerpta Medica, North Holland, p. 3–12

Matossian R M 1977 The immunological diagnosis of human hydatid disease. Transactions of the Royal Society of Tropical Medicine and Hygiene 71: 101–104

Matson D J, Ingraham F D 1951 Intracranial complications of congenital dermal sinuses. Pediatrics 8: 463–474

Mease P T, Ochs H D, Wedgewood R J 1981 Successful treatment of Echovirus meningoencephalitis and myositis fasciitis with intravenous immune globulin in a patient with X-linked agammoglobulinaemia. New England Journal of Medicine 304: 1278–1281

Melish M E 1981 Kawasaki syndrome: a new infectious disease. Journal of Infectious Diseases 143: 317–324

Menkes J H 1979 Improving the long-term outlook in bacterial meningitis. Lancet 2: 559–560

Metz H, Gregoriou M, Sandifer P 1964 Subacute sclerosing pan-encephalitis. Archives of Disease in Childhood 39: 554–557

Meyer H B 1962 An epidemiologic study of mumps: its spread in schools and families. American Journal of Hygiene 75: 259–281

Meyers N A 1960 Hydatid disease in a children's hospital. Medical Journal of Australia 1: 806–808

Miller D L, Ross E M, Alderslade R, Bellman M H, Rawson N S B 1981 Pertussis immunisation and serious neurological illness in children. British Medical Journal 282: 1595–1599

Modlin J F, Brandling-Bennett D, Witte J J, Campbell C C, Meyers J D 1975 A review of five years experience with rubella vaccine in the United States. Pediatrics 55: 20–29

Modlin J F, Halsey N A, Eddins D L, Conrad J L, Jabbour J T, Chien L et al 1979 Epidemiology of subacute sclerosing panencephalitis. Journal of Pediatrics 94: 231–236

Mok C H 1968 Visceral larva migrans. Clinical Pediatrics 7: 565–573

Morens D M, Halsey N A, Schonberger L B, Baublis J V 1979 Reye syndrome associated with vaccination with live virus vaccines: an exploration of possible etiologic relationships. Clinical Pediatrics 18: 42–4

Mortimer E A 1973 Immunization against Hemophilus influenzae. Pediatrics 52: 633–635

Murray P R, Hampton C M 1980 Recovery of pathogenic bacteria from cerebrospinal fluid. Journal of Clinical Microbiology 12: 554–557

Murrell W G, Ouvrier R A, Stewart B J, Dorman D C 1981 Infant botulism in a breast-fed infant from rural New outh Wales. Medical Journal of Australia 1: 583–585

Myint T T 1980 Tuberculous meningitis and BCG vaccination in Burmese children. Journal of Tropical Pediatrics 26: 227–231

Nagington J, Wreghitt J G, Gondy G, Roberton N R C, Berry P J 1978 Fatal echovirus 11 infections in outbreak in special care baby unit. Lancet 2: 725–728

Nahmias A J, Visintine 1976 In: Remington J S, Klein J O (eds) Injections of the fetus and newborn. W B Saunders, Philadelphia, p. 164

Nahmias A J, Walls K W, Stewart J A, Herremann K L, Flynt W 1971 The TORCH complex-perinatal infections associated with toxoplasma and rubella, cytomegalo-and herpes simplex viruses. Pediatric Research 5: 405–406

Nelson J D 1976 Odd creatures in the blood and cerebrospinal fluid. American Journal of Diseases of Children 130: 800–801

Nelson L A, Peri Reiger C H L, Newcomb R W, Rothberg R M 1978 Immunity to diphtheria in urban population. Paediatrics 61: 703–710

Nelson W E 1975 Commentary: the treatment of Reye's syndrome. Journal of Pediatrics 87: 868

Nightingale E O 1977 Recommendations for a national polic on poliomyelitis vaccination. New England Journal of Medicine 297: 249–253

O'Brien M, Parent A, Davis B 1979 Management of ventricular shunt infections. Child's Brain 5: 304–309

Oh S J 1968 Paragonimus meningitis. Journal of the Neurological Sciences 6: 419–433

Olson L C 1975 Pertussis. Medicine 54: 427–469

Olson L C, Bourgeois C H, Cotton R B, Harikul S, Grossma R A, Smith T J 1971 Encephalopathy and visceral fatty degeneration of the viscera in North Eastern Thailand: clinical syndrome and epidemiology. Pediatrics 47: 707–716

Overall J C 1970 Neonatal bacterial meningitis. Journal of Pediatrics 76: 499–51

Overturf G D, Powars D, Baraff L J 1977 Bacterial meningitis and septicaemia in sickle cell disease. American Journal of Diseases of Children 131: 784–787

Pampiglione G 1964 Polymyographic studies of some involuntary movement in subacute sclerosing pan-encephalitis. Archives of Disease in Childhood 39: 558–563

Parish H J, Cannon D A 1962 Antisera, toxoids, vaccines and tuberculins in prophylaxis and treatment. Livingstone' Edinburgh

Parker P, Puck J, Fernandez F 1981 Cerebral infarction associated with Mycoplasma pneumoniae. Pediatrics 67: 373–375

Pass R F, Stagno S, Myers G J, Alford C A 1980 Outcome of symptomatic congenital cytomegalovirus infection: results of long-term longitudinal follow-up. Pediatrics 66: 758–762

Paul F M 1961 Tuberculosis in BCG vaccinated children in Singapore. Archives of Disease in Childhood 36: 530–536

Pavlarkis S C, McCormick K L, Bromberg K, Peter G 1980 Cerebrospinal fluid anion gap in meningitis. Journal of Pediatrics 96: 874–876

Peckham C S 1972 A clinical and laboratory study of children exposed in utero to maternal rubella. Archives of Disease in Childhood 47: 571–577

Peraj A K, Byrd S E, Locke G E 1980 Cerebral cysticercosis. Pediatrics 66: 967–971

Perham T G M, Caul E O, Clarke S K P, Gibson A G F 1971 Cytomegalovirus meningo-encephalitis. British Medical Journal 2: 50

Peter G, Weigert M B, Bissel A R, Gold R, Kreutzer D, McLean R H 1981 Meningococcal meningitis in familial deficiency of the fifth component of complement. Pediatrics 67: 882–886

Peterson B H, Lee T J, Snyderman R, Brooks G F 1979 Neisseria meningitidis and Neisseria gonorrhoeae bacteremia associated with C6, C7 or C8 deficiency. Annals of Internal Medicine 90: 917–920

Pickett J, Berg B, Chaplin E, Brunsteller-Shafer M A 1976 Syndrome of botulism in infancy: clinical and electrophysiologic study. New England Journal of Medicine 295: 770–772

Pittman M 1979 Pertussis toxin: the cause of the harmful effects and prolonged immunity of whooping cough: a hypothesis. Reviews of Infectious Diseases 1: 407–412

Pleet H, Graham J M, Smith D W 1981 Central nervous system and facial defects associated with maternal hypothermia at 4 to 14 weeks gestation. Pediatrics 67: 785–789

Plotkin S A 1981 New rabies vaccine. Pediatrics 68: 131–132

Ponka A 1980 Central nervous system manifestations associated with serologically verified Mycoplasma pneumoniae infection. Scandanavian Journal of Infectious Disease 12: 175–184

Preblud S R 1981 Age-specific attack rates of varicella complications. Pediatrics 68: 14–17

Prys-Roberts C, Corbett J L, Kerr J H, Crampton-Smith A, Spalding J M K 1969 Treatment of sympathetic overactivity in tetanus. Lancet 1: 542–546

Pullan C R, Noble C T, Scott D J, Wisnienski K, Gardner P S 1976 Atypical measles infection in leukaemic children on immunosuppressive treatment. British Medical Journal 1: 1562–1565

Ratcliffe J C, Wolf S M 1977 Febrile convulsions caused by meningitis in young children. Annals of Neurology 1: 285–286

Radetsky M S, Johanses T L, Lauer B A, Istre G R, Parmelée S W, Wlesen Thal A M et al 1981 Multiply-resistant pneumococcus causing meningitis: its epidemiology within a day-care centre. Lancet 2: 771–773

Ray C G 1976 Virus infections of the central nervous system. In: Lawrence Drew W (ed) Virus infections: a clinical approach F A Davis Co, Philadelphia, p. 102

Reye R D K, Morgan G, Baral J 1963 Encephalopathy and fatty degeneration of the viscera; a disease entity in childhood. Lancet 2: 749–752

Robb R M, Waters G V 1970 Ophthalmic manifestations of subacute sclerosing panencephalitis. Archives of Ophthalmology 83: 426–435

Robertson H H 1978 In: Jelliffe D B, Paget Stanfield J (eds) Diseases of children in the tropica and subtropics Arnold, London, p 858

Rubella Symposium 1965 American Journal of Diseases of Children 110: 345–478

Ruskin J, Remington J S 1976 Toxoplasmosis in the compromised host. Annals of Internal Medicine 84: 193–199

Rutlidge J, Benjamin D, Hood L, Smith A 1981 Is the CSF lactate measurement useful in the management of children with suspected bacterial meningitis? Journal of Pediatrics 98: 20–24

Rutman D L, Wald E R 1981 Fever in Hemophilus influenzae type b. meningitis. Clinical Pediatrics 20: 192–195

Rutter N, Smales O R C 1977 Calcium magnesium and glucose levels in blood and CSF of children with febrile convulsions. Archives Diseases in Childhood 51: 141–143

Sanders R K M, Martyn B, Joseph R, Peacock M L 1977 Intrathecal antitetanus serum (horse) in the treatment of tetanus. Lancet 1: 974–977

Sabin A B 1981 Paralytic poliomyelitis: old dogmas and new perspectives. Reviews of Infectious Diseases 3: 543–564

Santos J I, Swenson P, Glasgow L A 1981 Potentiation of Clostridium botulinium toxin by aminoglycoside antibiotics: clinical and laboratory observations. Pediatrics 68: 50–54

Schaad U B, Nelson J D, McCracken G H 1981 Recrudescence and relapse in bacterial meningitis of children. Pediatrics 67: 188–195

Schauseil-Zipf U, Harden A, Hoare R, Lyen K, Lingam S, Marshall W C et al 1982 Early diagnosis of Herpes simplex encephalitis in childhood European Journal of Pediatrics 138: 154–161

Schmidt N J, Lennette E H, Ho H H 1974 An apparently new enterovirus isolated from patients with disease of the central nervous system. Journal of Infectious Diseases 129: 304–309

Schmitz H, Enders G 1977 Cytomegalovirus as a frequent cause of Guillain-Barré syndrome. Journal of Medical Virology 1: 21–27

Schoenbaum S C, Gardner P, Shillito J 1975 Infections of cerebrospinal fluid shunts; epidemiology, clinical manifestations and therapy. Journal of Infectious Diseases 131: 543–552

Schonberger L B, Bregman D J, Sullivan-Bolyai J Z, Keenlyside R A, Ziegler D W, Retailliaw H F et al 1979 Guillain-Barré syndrome following vaccination in the National Influenza Immunisation Program, United States 1976–1977. American Journal of Epidemiology 110: 105–123

Sells C J, Carpenter R L, Ray C G 1975 Sequelae of central nervous system enterovirus infections. New England Journal of Medicine 293: 1–4

Sells C T, Sturtleff D B, Loeser J D 1977 Gram-negative cerebrospinal fluid shunt infections. Pediatrics 59: 614–618

Sherman F E, Michaels R H, Kenny F M 1965 Acute encephalopathy (encephalitis) complicating rubella. Journal of the American Medical Association 192: 675–681

Shield L K, Wilkinson R G, Ritchie M 1978 Infant botulism in Australia. Medical Journal of Australia 2: 157

Shiga H, Yagishita A, Akiyama T 1979 The neuroradiological findings in a case of cerebral tuberuloma. Neuroradiology 17: 279–281

Silverberg R, Brenner T, Abramsky O 1979 Inosiplex in the treatment of subacute sclerosing panencephalitis. Archives of Neurology 36: 374–375

Sinh G, Pandya S K, Dastur D K 1968 Pathogenesis of unusual intracranial tuberculomas and tubeculous space-occupying lesions. Journal of Neurosurgery 29: 149–159

Smith A L 1975 Tuberculous meningitis in childhood. Medical Journal of Australia 1: 57–60

Smyth D, Tripp J H, Brett E M, Marshall W C, Almeida J, Dayan A D et al 1976 Atypical measles encephalitis in leukaemic children in remission. Lancet 2: 574

Starko K M, Ray C G, Dominquez L B, Stomberg W L, Woodall D F 1980 Reye's syndrome and salicylate use. Pediatrics 66: 859–864

Stagno S, Reynolds D W, Huang E S, Thams S D, Smith R J, Alford C A 1979 Congenital cytomegalovirus infection: occurrence in an immune population. New England Journal of Medicine 296: 1254–1258

Stagno S, Reynolds D W, Amos C S, Dahle A J, McCollister F P, Mohindra I et al 1977b Auditory and visual defects resulting from symptomatic and subclinical congenital cytomegaloviral and toxoplasma infections. Pediatrics 59: 669–678

Steiner M M, Vuckovitch D, Hadawi S A 1963 Cat-scratch

disease with encephalopathy. Journal of Pediatrics 62: 514–520

Stovring J, Synder R D 1980 Computed tomography in childhood bacterial meningitis. Journal of Pediatrics 96: 821–835

Swart S, Briggs R S, Millac P A 1981 Tuberculous meningitis in Asian patients. Lancet 2: 15–16

Swartz M N, Dodge P R 1965 Bacterial meningitis — a review of selected aspects. II. Special neurologic problems, postmeningitic complications and clinicopathological correlations. New England Journal of Medicine 272: 954–960

Taylor D, Day S, Tiedmann K, Chessells J, Marshall W C, Constable I J 1981 Chorioretinal biopsy in a patient with leukaemia. British Journal of Ophthalmology 65: 489–493

Thompson J A, Glasgow L A, Warpinski J R, Olson C 1980 Infant botulism: clinical spectrum and epidemiology. Pediatrics 66: 936–942

Thong M L, Puthucheary S D, Lee E H 1981 Flavobacterium meningosepticum infection: an epidemiological study in a newborn nursery. Journal of Clinical Pathology 34: 429–433

Till K 1975 Paediatric neurosurgery. Blackwell, London, p 61

Townsend J J, Baringer J R, Wolinksy J S, Malamud N, Mednick J P, Panitch H S et al 1975 Progressive rubella panencephalitis: late onset after congenital rubella. New England Journal of Medicine 292: 990–993

Turner H D, Brett E M, Gilbert R J, Ghosh A C, Liebeschuetz H 1978 Infant botulism in England. Lancet 1: 1277–1278

Udani P M, Dastur D K 1970 Tuberculous encephalopathy with and without meningitis. Clinical and pathological correlations. Journal of Neurological Science 10: 541–561

Upton A, Gumpert J 1970 Electroencephalography in herpes simplex encephalitis. Lancet 1: 650–652

Van Rymenant M, Robert J, Otten J 1966 Isocitric dehydrogenase in the CSF: clinical usefulness of its determination. Neurology 16: 351

Verghote M, Rousseau E, Jacob J L, Lapointe N 1981 An uncommon clinical sign in mucocutaneous lymphnode syndrome. Acta paediatrica scandanavica 70: 591–593

Ward J P, Fraser D W, Baratt L J, Plikeylis B P 1979 Haemophilus influenzae meningitis; a national study of secondary spread in household contacts. New England Journal of Medicine 301: 122–126

Webster A D B, Tripp J H, Hayward A R, Dyan A D, Dishi R, MacIntyre E H et al 1978 Echovirus encephalitis and myositis in primary immunoglobulin deficiency. Archives of Disease in Childhood 53: 33–37

Weil H L, Itabashi H H, Cremer N E, Oshiro L S, Lennette E H Carney L 1975 Chronic progressive panencephalitis due to rubella virus simulating subacute sclerosing panencephalitis. New England Journal of Medicine 292: 994–998

Welch L 1977 The prevention of shunt infection. Zeitschrift für Kinderchirurgie 22: 465–475

White R, Finberg L, Tramer A 1964 The modern morbidity of pertussis in infants. Pediatrics 33:705–710

Whitley R J, Nahmias A J, Soon S J, Galasso G G, Fleming C L, Alford C A 1980 Vidarabine treatment of neonatal herpes. Pediatrics 66: 495–501

Whitley R J, Soong Sen-Jaw, Dolin R, Galasso G J, Ch'ien L T, Alford C A, and the Collaborative Study Group 1977 Adenine arabinoside therapy of biopsy-proved herpes simplex encephalitis. 297: 289–294

Whitley R J, Soon S J, Hirsch M S, Karchmer A M, Dolin R, Galasso G et al 1981 Herpes simplex encephalitis: vidarabine therapy and diagnostic problems. New England Journal of Medicine 304: 313–318

Whittle H C, Tugwell P, Egler L J, Greenwood B M 1974 Rapid bacteriological diagnosis of pyogenic meningitis by latex agglutination. Lancet 2: 619–621

Wilson C B, Remington J S, Stagno S S, Reynolds D W 1980 Development of adverse sequlae in children born with subclinical congenital toxoplasma infection. Pediatrics 66: 767–774

Wilson H D 1981 Prophylaxis in bacterial meningitis. Archives of Disease in Childhood 56: 817–819

Wolf S M 1978 Laboratory evaluation of the child with a febrile convulsion. Pediatrics 62: 1074–1076

Wolf S M 1973 The ocular manifestations of congenital rubella. Journal of Pediatric Ophthalmology 10: 107–141

Wolinsky J S, Berg B O, Maitland C J 1976 Progressive rubella panencephalitis. Archives of Neurology 33: 722–723

Wong M L, Kaplan S, Dunkle L M, Stechenburg B W, Feigin R D 1977 Leptospirosis: a childhood disease. Journal of Pediatrics 90: 53d–537

World Health Organisation 1967 Arboviruses and human disease. Technical Report Series 369: 9

Yanagawa H 1976 Epidemiology of Kawasaki disease. Japanese Journal of Clinical Medicine 34: 275–283

Yanagihara R, Todd J K 1980 Acute febrile mucocutaneous lymph node syndrome. American Journal of Diseases of Children 134: 603–614

Yii C 1976 Clinical observations on eosinophilic meningitis and meningoencephalitis caused by Angiostrongylus cantonensis on Taiwan. American Journal of Tropical Medicine and Hygiene 25: 233–249

Zellweger H 1959 Pertussis encephalopathy. Archives of Pediatrics 76: 381–386

ZuRhein G M, Padgett B L, Walker D L, Chun R W M, Horowitz S D, Hong R 1978 Progressive multifocal leukoencephalopathy in a child with severe combined immunodeficiency. New England Journal of Medicine 299: 256–257

23

Neurological aspects of childhood reticuloses and some other medical diseases

E. M. Brett

'No man can be a pure specialist without being in the strict sense an idiot'.

George Bernard Shaw, *Man and Superman*.

The paediatric neurologist, even more than his adult counterpart, must be ever alert to the possibility of disease in other systems than the nervous system. Many neurological disorders presenting in childhood are associated with altered structure and function in other systems and can be regarded as multi-system diseases. Examples are provided by some of the neurocutaneous syndromes, especially tuberose sclerosis, and by the spinocerebellar syndromes and related disorders. Endocrinopathies, heart disease, renal insufficiency and arterial hypertension may also have profound implications for the nervous system. Some of these are discussed in other chapters.

In this chapter the impact of the reticuloses and certain other blood disorders on paediatric neurology will be considered.

Neurological problems are commonly seen in children with leukaemia and certain other haematological disorders. The neurology of leukaemia and of its treatment and the management of these problems have become increasingly important for the paediatrician and paediatric neurologist.

LEUKAEMIA

Neurological complications of leukaemia and of its tre~~ ~~ent

~~ge~~

bleeding is the commonest cause of
~~ ~~dren with acute lymphoblastic leukae-

mia (ALL) and is usually associated with severe thrombocytopenia. Blastic crises with very high white cell counts and infections with bacteria or fungi may also predispose to intracranial bleeding. The haemorrhages may be intracerebral or subdural. Chronic subdural haematoma results from petechial haemorrhages and repeated episodes of leukaemic infiltration.

In 2 series of 438 children with leukaemia or lymphoma (333 with ALL) seen at the Hospital for Sick Children, Great Ormond Street, between 1967 and 1977 (Campbell et al 1977), eight patients (3 with ALL and 5 with acute myeloblastic leukaemia AML) had intracranial haemorrhage. All 8 children developed this complication in the first days or weeks after diagnosis of leukaemia. All 8 died and these formed the majority of the 11 dying from neurological complications. Four of these patients had evidence of disseminated intravascular coagulation (DIC).

Leukaemic infiltration

Extramedullary leukaemia in children in haematological remission is common in the CNS and the testis.

Leukaemic infiltration of the CNS has been noted in increasing numbers of children with the improvements in treatment which have produced haematological remission of the disease in a very high proportion of cases of acute lymphoblastic leukaemia (Hardisty & Norman 1967, Evans et al, 1970). Pochedly (1977) has aptly described the CNS as a 'sanctuary' in which leukaemic cells are protected and may later give rise to haematological relapse.

CNS infiltration can occur at any stage of the

disease and eventually affects over 80% of children with ALL who do *not* receive prophylactic CNS therapy. Meningeal infiltration causes raised intracranial pressure with the classical clinical features of headache, vomiting and papilloedema. The diagnosis can be confirmed by lumbar puncture and examination of a cytocentrifuge preparation of CSF in which blast cells are normally seen. The cell count is often raised and the glucose level reduced. The CT scan is helpful, particularly in cases with normal CSF, in distinguishing leukaemic infiltration from the various iatrogenic syndromes related to therapy, and from unrelated disorders.

Types of leukaemic infiltration

Two main types of leukaemic lesions are found in the CNS in childhood ALL. Large nodules of leukaemic tissue surrounded by areas of haemorrhage within the brain ('ball disease') occur in untreated, less vigorously treated or fulminating cases. More common today are arachnoid infiltrates which were found in 70% of the brains of 126 children with ALL dying between 1962 and 1969 following intensive chemotherapy (Price & Johnson 1973). The leukaemic infiltration of the arachnoid follows a predictable anatomical pattern which has been well reviewed by Price & Johnson (1973) and Pochedly (1977). It starts with infiltration of the walls of superficial arachnoid veins, which goes on to destruction of the arachnoid trabeculae allowing the CSF to become contaminated with leukaemic cells, so that the diagnosis of CNS leukaemia can be made by CSF examination at this stage. Increasing leukaemic infiltration of the leptomeninges interferes both with the flow of CSF, causing raised intracranial pressure and communicating hydrocephalus and, by compression of cerebral arterioles and venules, with blood supply, causing hypoperfusion encephalopathy. The clinical effects of the perfusion defect depend on the area involved, the duration and extent of the infiltration, the vulnerability of the neurons affected and the collateral circulation. Direct effects of infiltration of the brain account for only a small proportion of leukaemic encephalopathy. Only 17 of the 126 brains examined at autopsy from children dying with ALL showed leukaemic cells in the parenchyma of the CNS (Price & Johnson 1973).

Raised intracranial pressure may result from defective CSF absorption due to infiltration of arachnoid granulations and also from infiltration of the choroid plexuses causing increased CSF secretion and from obstruction to the flow of CSF at the base of the brain or Sylvian aqueduct. Any or all of these three mechanisms may operate.

Leukaemic involvement of the dura mater was commoner in the past than it is in the present era of aggressive and effective treatment. Chronic subdural haematoma is found in about 10% of children with ALL (Pitner & Johnson 1973). The lesion probably starts with petechial haemorrhages from dural capillaries which, with repeated episodes of leukaemic infiltration, lead to the formation of space-occupying granulation tissue in the subdural space with haemorrhage and proliferation of capillaries and fibroblasts. During relapses leukaemic cells are found in these lesions at autopsy, but are absent during remissions.

The rôle of CNS prophylaxis

In a few children CNS involvement is already present when leukaemia is first diagnosed. This was the case in 5 of 74 children with ALL seen at the Hospital for Sick Children, London (Gribbin et al 1974). Only one of these 5 children survived for longer than one year, whereas the prognosis was much better in the other cases. Once leukaemic infiltration of the CNS is established it is difficult to treat and tends to recur, causing chronic disability in patients whose leukaemia is otherwise well controlled.

In the management of ALL, therefore, 'CNS prophylaxis', treatment aimed at preventing overt leukaemic infiltration of the nervous system, has become an integral part.

The prophylactic options of radiotherapy in various doses and chemotherapy have been reviewed by workers at different centres. Aur et al (1975), in prospective trials from St. Jude Children's Research Hospital, showed that prophylactic craniospinal irradiation in a dose of 1200 R could not prevent leukaemic infiltration of the CNS in children with ALL. In most children a dose of 2400 R to the whole craniospinal axis, or cranial irradiation at this dose combined with a course of five intrathecal injections of methotrexate was effective.

The merits of various regimes were also assessed in the United Kingdom (Ukall I trial, Medical Research Council 1973, Ukall II trial 1978). The value of CNS prophylaxis was confirmed, but full-dose (2400 R) craniospinal irradiation was found to be associated with a higher risk of marrow relapse, especially in those with a high leucocyte count at presentation (MRC 1978). Doses of cranial irradiation intermediate between 1200 and 2400 R are now being investigated in the hope of finding a more satisfactory régime. The use of methotrexate alone by the intrathecal route seems inadequate for prophylaxis, but its administration by an Ommaya intraventricular reservoir may prove more effective. Another useful approach may be the use of intravenous infusions of methotrexate in high doses (Freeman et al 1977) to give therapeutic levels in the CSF.

At present it seems appropriate to recommend that all patients with ALL should be given CNS prophylaxis after haematological remission is obtained. In children undergoing prolonged 'induction' prophylaxis should start with intrathecal chemotherapy during induction. Cranial irradiation should be given in a dose of 2400 R [or possibly 1800 R, since it has been shown that the lower dose is not associated with a significant increase in the frequency of CNS or bone-marrow relapse or death (Nesbit et al 1981)] combined with a course of at least 5 injections of intrathecal methotrexate. An important exception should be made for very young children (those under one year, and possibly under two). The neurological and psychological complications of cranial irradiation (Eiser 1978) make it advisable to defer this treatment and to give regular intrathecal methotrexate alone initially.

The question of CNS prophylaxis in *acute myeloblastic leukaemia* (AML) is less clear. Craniospinal irradiation was unhelpful in one group of children with AML (Dahl et al 1978). Intrathecal cytosine arabinoside or methotrexate may be appropriate CNS prophylaxis for patients with AML in remission.

CNS disease in AML was remarkable for the frequency of early presentation (30%) and the very poor prognosis in the series of 134 patients seen at the Royal Marsden Hospital between 1972 and 1974 (McElwain et al 1979). All were dead within 11 weeks, suggesting that the only hope for this type of patient is early diagnosis and aggressive combined treatment. CNS leukaemia should be looked for early in patients with AML and routine diagnostic lumbar puncture should be done as soon as haematological remission has been achieved.

The management of overt CNS leukaemia

Despite the introduction of routine CNS prophylaxis in children with ALL, overt CNS leukaemia still occurs in 5 to 10% of cases at some stage of the disease, and the management of this complication remains difficult.

The problems involved are well illustrated by the survey by Gribbin et al (1977) of 74 children with ALL who had one or more episodes of CNS leukaemia. 5 children already had CNS involvement at the time of diagnosis, and only one of these survived longer than one year. The treatment of this complication is usually with weekly intrathecal methotrexate and, once complete remission is achieved, cranial irradiation and continuing intrathecal chemotherapy.

Those without CNS involvement at the time of diagnosis fared better. The CNS relapse which develops in 5 to 10% of patients despite prophylaxis can usually be successfully treated by weekly intrathecal injections of methotrexate. Long remissions may be achieved by regular use of methotrexate every 4 to 6 weeks for at least 2 or 3 years (Gribbin et al 1977). Still longer CNS remissions can be obtained by using an Ommaya reservoir or by further craniospinal irradiation, though there is a risk of leucoencephalopathy resulting from the latter. The combination of cranial irradiation and intraventricular methotrexate should be avoided because of the high risk of leucoencephalopathy (see below).

Infections

21 of the 438 children with acute leukaemia in the series of Campbell et al (1977) had complicating infections. Virus, or presumed virus, infections accounted for 12 and bacterial for 9 of these 21 cases. All but one patient were in remission at the time of the infection.

Mumps was the commonest virus infection and

affected 5 children, one of whom died, while the others recovered quickly and completely after a mild meningitic illness.

Encephalitis caused by measles virus affected one child together with a further 2 patients suffering from the recently described syndrome of 'atypical measles encephalitis' (Smyth et al 1976). In one of these 2 children the encephalitis followed 3 months after clinical measles with death 2 months after its onset. In the other case seroconversion to measles occurred without clinical measles, and measles antigen and virus were shown in a brain biopsy by immunofluorescence and electron microscopy. This patient remained alive but severely brain-damaged some 5 years after the onset of his neurological illness with large areas of low attenuation in his CT scan. Both these children had high measles complement-fixing (CF) antibody in the serum and CSF. This measles-related encephalitis in immunosuppressed patients is reviewed (British Medical Journal 1976). It has certain resemblances to subacute sclerosing panencephalitis (Ch. 22), but the EEG, though abnormal, does not show the typical periodic complexes seen in that disorder.

Three children suffered an acute CNS illness during or soon after typical chickenpox. One died and at necropsy showed visceral dissemination of varicella, though no virus was cultured from the brain. Of the 2 survivors, one recovered completely and one remains ataxic and dysarthric. Treatment with acyclovir has since proved helpful in such cases.

The 9 bacterial infections included 4 cases of meningitis associated with intraventricular reservoirs.

Herpes zoster is a common complication of leukaemia. It may be associated with various neurological disorders such as myelitis and encephalomyelitis (Ch. 22), and disseminated herpes zoster develops in a small proportion of cases.

Methotrexate-radiation encephalopathy

A severe disseminated leucoencephalopathy occurs in some patients with ALL treated by cranial irradiation and intraventricular methotrexate and other antimetabolites. (Bresnan et al 1972, Kay et al 1972, Rubinstein et al 1975, Price & Jamison 1975). The clinical features include dementia, confusion, tremor, ataxia and convulsions leading in some cases to coma and death. Symptoms began between 2 weeks and 8 months after completing irradiation in the cases of Kay et al (1972). CNS irradiation and prolonged treatment with methotrexate seem to be common factors in the development of the syndrome, though similar findings have been noted in some non-irradiated children (Peylan-Ramu et al 1977). Adolescence is also a predisposing factor, perhaps because brain size at this age is relatively less in relation to body size than in younger children. It has been suggested that the dose of methotrexate should be related to head circumference rather than to body surface area. The brain pathologically and radiologically shows widespread, bilateral, asymmetrical, largely juxtaventricular leucoencephalopathy. There are discrete multifocal necrotic lesions randomly disseminated in the cerebral white matter becoming confluent, with absence of an inflammatory cellular response (Rubinstein et al 1975). It is possible that cranial irradiation allows methotrexate to diffuse through the blood-brain barrier or that in children with some degree of ventricular obstruction there may be transependymal absorption of the drug. This form of leucoencephalopathy does not occur with treatment schedules using short-term intrathecal methotrexate and moderate later doses.

Intracerebral calcification has been noted during the course of ALL in some patients treated with methotrexate and irradiation (Fig. 23.1). In the case of Flament-Durand et al (1975) skull X-rays showed diffuse bilateral calcium deposits in both cerebral and cerebellar hemispheres. This was confirmed by a cerebral biopsy and also at autopsy when bilateral necrosis of the centrum semi-ovale with demyelination was found. Peylan-Ramu et al (1977) noted calcification on CT scan in 2 children with ALL who had received cranial irradiation and intrathecal or intraventricular methotrexate. The basal ganglia were calcified in both cases and the cortical grey matter in addition in one. Dense paraventricular calcification mimicking the Sturge-Weber syndrome was noted radiologically by Bornes & Rancier (1974) in similar cases. In 3 other children Mueller et al (1976) found paraventricular calcification on plain skull X-rays or CT

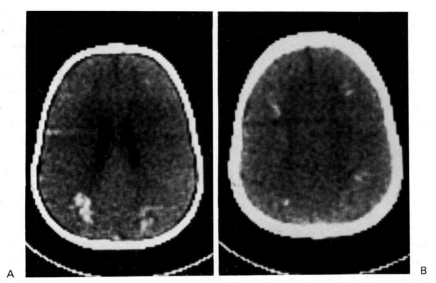

Fig. 23.1 A & B. Methotrexate leucoencephalopathy. 18-month-old boy with acute lymphoblastic leukaemia. Note almost symmetrical, patchy calcification in the white matter of both hemispheres, most marked in the parieto-occipital regions, also slight generalized low attenuation in the white matter.

scan. This calcification progressed despite the cessation of both radiation and methotrexate therapy.

This form of leucoencephalopathy is not limited to leukaemic patients but was seen in a boy with an orbital rhabdomyosarcoma and metastases treated with radiotherapy and chemotherapy (Fusner et al 1977). After intraventricular treatment with methotrexate and cytosine arabinoside he showed neurological deterioration and areas of low attenuation on CT scan. There was clinical and radiological improvement after all intraventicular treatment was stopped.

Iatrogenic complications of this kind may be much commoner than is recognised, judging from the report of Peylan-Ramu et al (1978). 32 asymptomatic children with ALL who had received prophylactic cranial irradiation (2400 rad) and either methotrexate or cytosine arabinoside by the intrathecal route, had CT scans between 19 and 67 months after the start of prophylaxis. 53% had one or more abnormal findings on the scan. Ventricular dilatation (8 cases) and widening of the subarachnoid spaces (9 cases) were equally distributed among those who had received methotrexate and cytosine arabinoside. Areas of decreased attenuation were found in 4 patients and intracerebral calcification in one, and these lesions were seen only in those who had been given intrathecal methotrexate. Mild CNS dysfunction was found in 7 patients, but did not correlate with the CT abnormalities, which may represent preclinical lesions. A control group of ALL patients who had not received CNS prophylaxis showed no abnormal CT findings.

Drug toxicity

Methotrexate. As mentioned above, encephalopathy has been noted in some children with ALL who have received intrathecal or intraventricular methotrexate, but have not been irradiated. Reversible dementia was temporally associated with intraventricular methotrexate therapy in a non-irradiated child with acute myelogenous leukaemia (Pizzo et al 1976). The symptoms did not recur with subsequent intraventricular cytosine arabinoside.

Drug toxicity may be seen with other anti-leukaemic drugs. In the series of Campbell et al (1977) the following problems were encountered.

Cytosine arabinoside. Intrathecal cytosine arabinoside was thought to cause arachnoiditis in 4 patients but all recovered fully. Paraparesis and convulsions have also been reported with this drug (Hanefeld & Riehm 1980).

Vincristine. Vincristine was thought to be the cause of convulsions which occurred in 6 children between 18 hours and 6 days after administration. Convulsions and inappropriate antidiuretic hormone secretion are also reported after vincristine.

L-asparaginase. This was associated with a convulsion in one patient with ALL, and a transient encephalopathy has also been reported.

Polyneuropathy. Polyneuropathy of mild or severe degree is common in children treated for ALL especially with vincristine. Loss of reflexes and muscle pain occur between 2 and 3 weeks after starting treatment and paraesthesiae affecting the feet develop soon after. In more severe cases, after repeated doses, distal weakness, hypotonia and gait disorder may develop. A myopathic effect of the drug has also been reported (Bradley et al 1970). Cranial nerve involvement may occur with ptosis, sixth nerve palsy causing diplopia, and dysphagia. Autonomic neuropathy may give rise to abdominal colic or ileus.

Post-irradiation somnolence syndrome

A transient post-irradiation somnolence or 'apathy' syndrome in children with ALL who have received prophylactic cranial irradiation has been reported by Freeman et al (1973). The symptoms develop 1 to 2 months after completion of irradiation, with malaise, lethargy, anorexia and vomiting, and resolve after 10 to 20 days. They may be due to a transient disturbance of myelin metabolism and to cerebral oedema. This syndrome occurred in 21 of the 73 patients with ALL reported by Hanefeld & Riehm (1980) but was deliberately excluded by Campbell et al (1977) from their series.

Possible effects of CNS prophylaxis on intellectual development

A retrospective study of 15 children previously treated for ALL was made by Eiser & Lansdown (1977). There were nine younger children (mean age 6.3 years) and 6 older (mean age 9.0 years). All had been treated by cranial irradiation and later by chemotherapy for 2 or 3 years. Their intellectual status was assessed and compared with that of carefully matched controls. All the children were found to function within the normal range, but, whereas the older group performed as well as their matched controls in all tasks, the younger group tended to perform somewhat below their controls, especially in tasks measuring quantitative, memory and motor skills, but not in language tasks. It seems advisable therefore to monitor the development of children treated for leukaemia, especially when diagnosed in the 2 to 5 year age range.

MALIGNANT LYMPHOMA

CNS involvement is well recognized in the malignant lymphomas, though relatively rare in childhood. The patterns of involvement in non-Hodgkin's lymphoma and in Hodgkin's disease were reviewed by Lister et al (1979).

Non-Hodgkin's lymphoma (NHL)

Thirty previously untreated cases were studied prospectively. Seven of these showed clinical evidence of CNS involvement. Four of the remaining 23 cases developed involvement during systemic relapse. There were 9 episodes of meningitis, with cranial nerve palsies in six, abnormal affect in two and papilloedema with headaches in one. There were three episodes of extradural spinal cord compression diagnosed clinically and confirmed by myelography. One intracerebral deposit was diagnosed clinically and confirmed with CT scan and EEG. A very close relationship was seen between bone marrow and CNS involvement.

In children with NHL CNS involvement and leukaemic transformation are common occurrences (Murphy & Davis 1974). The CNS features are similar to those seen in acute leukaemia in childhood with signs of increased intracranial pressure and malignant pleocytosis, as well as focal findings, such as cranial nerve palsies and paraplegia. Jenkin (1974) found evidence of CNS involvement in 30 of 102 children with lymphocytic or histiocytic lymphoma, being equally common with lymphoma in different sites.

Hodgkin's disease (HD)

Approximately 400 cases of HD were studied retrospectively. Twenty-four patients with neurological disease were found. Five patients had extradural deposits causing spinal cord compression, 4 had basal meningeal involvement with cranial nerve palsies and 3 had intracerebral deposits. Dementia was present in 7 patients. Five patients had direct extension of HD into the nervous system at various sites (brain-stem, brachial plexus, cauda equina, and pelvic nerve roots). Many of these neurological complications showed a good response to treatment with radiotherapy, while 4 of the 13 cases of meningeal involvement, in both NHL and HD, responded well to radiotherapy combined with intrathecal chemotherapy.

Hodgkin's disease, like leukaemia, has a well recognized association with herpes zoster, which may be complicated by neurological disorders such as myelitis and encephalomyelitis.

Acute polyneuropathy and auto-immune haemolytic anaemia developed in a 13 year old boy with Hodgkin's disease (Kurczynski et al 1980). Sural nerve biopsy and postmortem examination showed no metastases and no cellular inflammatory infiltration in the nervous system, but significant axonal degeneration was found in peripheral nerves and the dorsal funiculus. Paraneoplastic syndromes of this kind are well recognised in adults with lymphoma, but the authors' review of 15 cases from the literature suggests that they are rare in childhood since they found only one other case, a boy of 14.

NEUROLOGICAL COMPLICATIONS OF SICKLE CELL DISEASE AND THALASSAEMIA

More than a hundred haemoglobinopathies are now recognized but neurological dysfunction is limited to sickle cell disease and its variants and to thalassaemia.

Sickle cell disease

In sickle haemoglobin (HbS) the substitution of glutamic acid by valine in the beta-polypeptide chain alters the physical properties of the haemoglobin, allowing its molecules to become rigid and to aggregate under certain conditions, so that sickled cells result which in turn produce clinical changes by vascular effects on various organs.

Neurological dysfunction occurs in 17 to 29% of patients with sickle cell disease and are second only to painful crises and cardiomegaly in frequency. The subject is well reviewed by Boros & Weiner (1979).

Ninety-six Birmingham children with sickle cell disease were reported by Mann (1981) in a survey entitled 'Sickle cell haemoglobinopathies in England'. Five of these had neurological complications, three with hemiplegia with or without epilepsy and low IQ, and two with subarachnoid haemorrhage.

Pathological processes

Five pathological causes of neurological dysfunction are recognized, of which four are vascular.

Small vessel thrombosis

The commonest mechanism is thrombosis of small cerebral vessels with infarction and focal necrosis. Similar changes can occur in the spinal cord. Rigidity of the abnormal haemoglobin molecule makes transit of the affected red blood cells through the capillary bed slower and more difficult, and irreversible sickling of the cells occurs at a critical level of oxygen tension (less than 40 mmHg) with occlusion of the vessels. This is compounded at times by fibrin-platelet thrombi, though the role of coagulation defects in contributing to thrombosis and infarction is unclear.

Occlusion of major cerebral vessels (Fig. 23.2)

This is probably less common but occlusion of the supraclinoid portion of the internal carotid and middle and anterior cerebral arteries had been demonstrated angiographically in patients, including children, with sickle cell disease and acute neurological deficit such as hemiplegia. Thrombosis of the superior longitudinal sinus has also been reported. Angiography in sickle cell disease can be harmful and should not be undertaken lightly.

Massive intracranial haemorrhage

This is a rare but very serious complication of sickle cell anaemia not seen in thalassaemia. Sub-

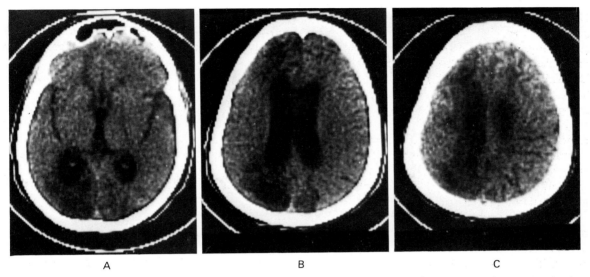

Fig. 23.2 A, B & C. Sickle cell anaemia with multiple infarcts in an African boy. There are multiple areas of low attenuation in the cerebral hemispheres. Posteriorly they are in the territory of the posterior cerebral arteries while the anterior lesions lie between the territories of the anterior and middle cerebral arteries and are watershed infarcts.

arachnoid haemorrhage may occur alone or in association with other intracranial haemorrhage. Subdural bleeding has also been reported.

Cerebral fat embolism

This is a very rare complication and a cause of coma and death in a few reported cases.

Meningitis

This is a common and often lethal complication, especially with the pneumococcus (see below). A functional asplenia is one factor predisposing to this, congestion, haemorrhage and infarction in the spleen producing a shrunken, fibrotic and immunologically functionally useless organ.

Clinical features

Vascular

Since these are mostly mediated by the vascular mechanisms described above, acute cerebrovascular episodes are common, with acute hemiplegia, aphasia, convulsions focal or generalized, subarachnoid and subdural haemorrhage. Portnoy & Herion (1972) in a series of 87 patients with sickle cell disease noted acute hemiplegia in 48%, convulsions in 43% and episodes of stupor and coma in 64%.

Sickling is predisposed to by hypoxia, infection, especially pneumonia, and fluid and electrolyte imbalance with acidosis, which can therefore provoke acute neurological episodes or aggravate deficits already present. Surgery, blood transfusion and intravascular procedures including angiography are further precipitating factors.

In some children a rapidly progressive course is seen with acute neurological episodes, particularly acute hemiplegia and convulsions, recurring over a period of months or years and leading to a state of dementia with spastic tetraplegia and bulbar palsy which is followed soon afterwards by death.

Meningitis

Sepsis is the commonest cause of death in sickle cell disease accounting for 60 to 70% of the mortality. Bacterial meningitis accounts for about 20% of the deaths from sepsis, and is about 300 times more common in patients with the disease than in the general population.

Most cases of meningitis occur in children under the age of three years with an unusually high proportion of pneumoccocal infection (normally only a common cause of meningitis after the age of five). A very rapid course with death within a few hours is often seen. In survivors recurrent attacks of pneumococcal meningitis may occur, as in other disorders with immunodeficiency.

Treatment

Management of the cerebrovascular complications of sickle cell disease is difficult. Avoidance and correction of predisposing factors such as infection and hypoxia are important. During acute episodes hydration, adequate oxygenation and blood transfusion to correct anaemia and reduce the proportion of sickled cells are helpful. Exchange transfusion has been used in some children with angiographically proved large cerebral vessel disease with apparent success. In the areas where sickle cell disease is common facilities for sophisticated treatment are unfortunately lacking.

The management of meningitis is along the usual lines. Prevention by means of antibiotics does not seem helpful, but the use of polyvalent pneumococcal immunization has given encouraging results.

THALASSAEMIA

Neurological problems are less common in this group of haemoglobinopathies than in the sickle cell diseases.

Three types of disorder are seen.

Meningitis

After splenectomy performed therapeutically for thalassaemia, meningitis, especially the pneumococcal type, is common, as in sickle cell disease. Prophylactic pneumococcal vaccination is helpful in these patients.

Spinal cord compression

Spinal cord compression by epidural accumulation of haemopoietic tissue has been reported in a few patients including one child. The lesions affect the thoracic region with incomplete cord involvement and seem to respond well to surgery and radiotherapy.

Muscular disorders

Myalgia, muscle wasting and a myopathic syndrome have been reported in thalassaemic patients.

SYSTEMIC (DISSEMINATED) LUPUS ERYTHEMATOSUS (SLE)

Since the time of Kaposi and Osler neuropsychiatric manifestations of SLE have been reported and are now known to occur in a high proportion (up to two thirds) of cases.

Clinical features

The neurological features of SLE were reviewed by Feinglass et al (1976) in 140 patients with mean age of onset of the disease 30 years (9–70). Fifty-two patients developed neuropsychiatric abnormalities secondary to SLE at some stage of their illness. Psychiatric disorders and seizures were the commonest symptoms. Sixteen patients developed pyramidal features and five had typical cerebrovascular accidents. Cranial nerve signs were found in 16 patients, the commonest being facial weakness, ptosis and diplopia. Optic neuritis occurred in one patient. Fifteen patients developed a peripheral neuropathy; in one case this resembled the Guillain-Barré syndrome.

The onset of neuropsychiatric illness in this series could occur at any time in the course of the SLE, but was early in many cases. In 63% neurological involvement either preceded the diagnosis or occurred within a year of diagnosis. In such cases there may be great diagnostic difficulty, since the possibility of SLE may not be considered until typical features emerge.

Reports of childhood cases of SLE with neurological complications are limited. The largest series is probably that of Gold & Yahr (1960) who described 14 children aged 3 to 15 years seen at Columbia-Presbyterian Medical Center over a 10-year period. 13 of these had involvement of the CNS. Most patients presented with constitutional symptoms but 5 had evidence of neurological dysfunction as their initial complaint. These features were convulsions in 3 cases, atypical migrainous headaches in one and polyneuritis in one. 8 others developed neurological manifestations later. In all

7 had convulsions. Other neurological features seen were progressive dementia, psychotic episodes of organic type, and spastic tetraplegia. Meningeal irritation occurred in two patients, with subarachnoid haemorrhage in one and aseptic meningitis in the other. Two children presented with papilloedema due in one case to raised intracranial pressure caused by widespread cerebrovascular lesions and aspergillus invasion of the CNS. Spinal cord involvement with complete transverse myelopathy occurred in one patient. The prognosis in this series was very bad, 11 of the 14 children having died. The mean interval from onset of SLE symptoms to death was 23 months, but that between the first neurological manifestations and death was much shorter at 13 months, over half the patients dying within 6 months.

Fulton & Dyken (1964) reported four patients in three of whom convulsions occurred in childhood, in one case 13 years before more classical features developed. The EEG showed focal abnormalities in two patients. One child died aged $10\frac{1}{2}$ years in coma after severe status epilepticus and at autopsy her brain showed a haemorrhagic infarct in the right frontal region. A similar lesion was shown angiographically in a 5 year old girl with SLE who had repeated cerebrovascular episodes, and autopsy in another child showed occlusion by thrombi of several branches of the right middle cerebral artery with old cerebral infarcts, and several old linear infarcts in the lateral and posterior columns of the spinal cord (Falko et al 1979).

Optic neuritis has been recorded in a few patients with SLE including an 11 year-old girl (Hackett et al 1974). In the three patients reported by these authors the onset of visual loss was sudden and unilateral with orbital pain in 3 of the 4 eyes affected. Initially all vision was lost but in most cases peripheral vision returned, leaving a central scotoma and permanent visual impairment. All patients later developed optic atrophy.

Investigation

The diagnosis of SLE by the finding of LE cells and antinuclear factor may be difficult. In one child neurological disease was present for $2\frac{1}{2}$ years before SLE could be confirmed serologically (Falko et al 1979). In two children, reported by these authors, with SLE and recurrent multifocal neurological

dysfunction, hyperlipoproteinaemia was present and deficiency of lipoprotein lipase was found. The authors suggest that this deficiency may be a marker for the endothelial disorder causing the cerebral vasculopathy in SLE.

Examination of the CSF may be helpful in some cases. It was examined in 37 patients during 44 episodes of neuropsychiatric illness in the series of Feinglass et al (1976) and was abnormal in 14 of these episodes. In 6 cases there was an isolated increase in protein, in 4 an increase in both protein and cells, and in 1 an isolated pleocytosis. The rise in protein level was generally modest. The increased cells found in the CSF were mononuclears in 4 of the 5 cases.

The EEG may assist by showing focal abnormality. Radiologically cerebral infarcts or atrophy may be shown by angiography or the CT scan. The scan is to be preferred as being less invasive. In one child calcification of the basal ganglia was shown with evidence of cerebral atrophy on the scan (Falko et al 1979).

Prognosis

Although death may occur in status epilepticus or coma or following an acute cerebrovascular incident in SLE, the immediate prognosis for improvement in neuropsychiatric function was found to be good in the experience of Feinglass et al (1976) with 84% of episodes showing complete or partial resolution. Corticosteroids appeared to be helpful in many patients, though their effect is difficult to assess. In only two of the 140 patients were steroids thought to have induced a psychosis. The better prognosis in more recent series such as that of Feinglass et al compared with earlier ones such as that of Gold & Yahr (1960) suggests that steroids are indeed valuable in treatment.

PERIARTERITIS NODOSA

This collagen vascular disease may also show neurological features, estimated to occur in at least 8% of cases. The various neurological manifestations depend on the varied types and patterns of involvement of the cerebral arteries and in some cases on the effects of cerebral oedema. Cerebral, cerebellar, brain stem, cranial nerve and peripheral nerve lesions occur and may be single or multiple.

Malamud (1945) reported a case of periarteritis nodosa (PAN) with decerebrate rigidity and extensive encephalomalacia in a 5-year-old child. The boy was convalescing from an upper respiratory infection and developed fleeting joint and abdominal pains with a systolic murmur and a leucocytosis. One week later, while these were starting to subside, he had a series of convulsions, became comatose and developed decerebrate rigidity and papilloedema. He died $2\frac{1}{2}$ months from the onset of the illness and necropsy showed massive necrosis of the cerebrum with complete destruction of its cytoarchitecture.

Ford & Siekert (1965) found that 46% of their patients with PAN had symptoms and signs referable to the CNS, and 68% had peripheral neuropathy. This took the form of polyneuropathy, mononeuritis or 'mononeuritis multiplex' or a mixture of the two. The commonest CNS sign was 'toxic retinopathy' in 36 patients, 11 of whom had papilloedema. Their patients included a 16 year old girl who developed generalized convulsions, incoordination of the left arm and multiple mononeuropathy with diffuse symmetrical polyneuropathy. At necropsy her brain showed cerebral oedema and petechial haemorrhages in the left occipital lobe. A 19-year-old boy with transient visual loss, convulsions, a confusional state and multiple mononeuropathy showed infarcts in the frontal and occipital lobes.

SARCOIDOSIS (BOECK'S SARCOID) IN CHILDHOOD

Sarcoidosis in childhood was first publicized by McGovern & Merritt (1956) whose survey of the world literature from 1875 to 1953 showed 104 cases in children under 15 years of age. They added 9 patients of their own to make a total of 113 cases. Jasper & Denny (1968) in their review added 86 more cases documented in 6 reports and added 25 personal cases seen at the North Carolina Memorial Hospital, the largest childhood series of the disease. In both series the age of onset was most often between 9 and 15 years, and the sexes were involved equally.

A high proportion of Negro children have been affected and this is reflected in the fact that 27% of the total reported children lived in the southeastern United States (Jasper & Denny 1968).

Multisystem involvement is common in childhood sarcoidosis, being present in 23 of the 25 North Carolina cases, most of whom had three systems involved. The nervous system was affected in 16% in this series and in 11% of the 113 cases collected by McGovern & Merritt (1956).

Neuropathies affecting cranial and peripheral nerves are common neurological features of sarcoidosis, and the central nervous system is much less often affected. In children facial palsy is a common symptom and is often associated with the so-called *uveo-parotid syndrome*. This is a triad of which the other features are ocular problems (uveitis, iridocyclitis, optic neuritis etc.) and swelling of the parotid glands, usually bilateral. There is usually intermittent low grade fever. Headache and drowsiness were present as an early symptom in four of the nine patients of McGovern and Merritt. Two others had signs of meningeal irritation. Cerebral symptoms, papilloedema, hemiplegia and aphasia were present in a 16-year-old patient reported by Douglas & Maloney (1973) in addition to left facial palsy.

Diagnostic tests in sarcoidosis include the Kveim test, the detection of hypercalcaemia, appropriate radiology and biopsy when indicated by the clinical situation. CSF examination may be helpful, though not diagnostic. The commonest finding is normal pressure and appearance, raised protein, with normal sugar and a variable number of cells, mainly lymphocytes. A low sugar is occasionally found.

Corticosteroid treatment in childhood sarcoid seemed effective in many cases (Jasper & Denny 1968) but it is difficult to comment on its value in children with neurological involvement. Steroids were effective in one young patient with facial palsy and other cranial nerve lesions (Delaney 1977) but were unhelpful in another with cerebral lesions and facial palsy who died after two years (Douglas & Maloney 1973). They should certainly be given a trial since no other treatment is available.

HISTIOCYTOSIS X

Histiocytosis X is a spectrum of diseases classified among the histiocytic disorders, in which there is proliferation of the mononuclear phagocyte system. These diseases are of unknown aetiology and are not genetically determined. Their earlier division into the groups eosinophilic granuloma of bone, Hand-Schüller-Christian disease and Letterer-Siwe disease seems to have little pathological justification. A preferable classification is one which divides them into:

1. Benign histiocytosis X
   a. solitary or multiple bone lesions
   b. benign disseminated histiocytosis X
2. Malignant histiocytosis X.

CNS involvement in histiocytosis X occurs in two different ways. The commoner is compression of the brain or spinal cord by subdural deposits of xanthomatous tissue. Less common is intracerebral or intraspinal infiltration by granulomatous xanthomata. Though often seen in the post-mortem room, subdural xanthomatous deposits rarely dominate the clinical picture (Elian et al 1969).

The clinical manifestations reflect the site of histiocytic proliferation and vary from a solitary bone lesion found by chance on X-rays to a disease with a rapidly fatal course affecting almost any organ (Bökkerink & De Vaan 1980). The commonest clinical features are bony skull defects, diabetes insipidus, and exophthalmos. These often occur together as a triad which is considered characteristic of the disease. Gingivitis and defective teeth are also common.

In a review of 49 cases in the literature Davison (1933) found that 33 patients had the onset of symptoms in the first decade. A later review of 22 cases (Elian et al 1969) showed only five cases with onset in childhood.

Neurological features appear relatively rare in most series of histiocytosis X (Bökkerink & De Vaan 1980) but were noted in 10 out of 42 children reported by Lucaya (1971). The symptoms included convulsions, mental retardation, deafness, intention tremor, optic atrophy and subdural haematoma. The triad of skull defects, diabetes insipidus and exophthalmos was rare in this series.

REFERENCES

Aur R J, Simone J V, Hustu H O, Versoza M S, Pinkel D 1975 Cessation of therapy during complete remission of childhood acute lymphocytic leukemia. New England Journal of Medicine 291: 1230–1234

Bökkerink J P M, De Vaan G A M 1980 Histiocytosis X. European Journal of Pediatrics 113: 129–146

Boros L, Weiner W J 1979 Sickle cell anemia and other hemoglobinopathies. In:Vinkin P J, Bruyn G W (eds) Neurological manifestations of systemic diseases, Part I. Handbook of Clinical Neurology vol 38. North Holland, Amsterdam

Bradley W G, Lassmann L, Pearce G W 1970 The neuromyopathy of vincristine in man: clinical, electrophysiological and pathological studies. Journal of the Neurological Sciences 10: 107

Bresnan M D, Gilles F H, Lorenzo A V, Watters G V, Barlow C F 1972 Leukoencephalopathy following combined irradiation and intraventricular methotrexate therapy of brain tumors in childhood. Transactions of the American Neurological Association 97: 204–206

British Medical Journal 1976 Measles encephalitis during immunosuppressive treatment. British Medical Journal 1: 1552

Campbell R H A, Marshall W C, Chessells J M 1977 Neurological complications of childhood leukaemia. Archives of Disease in Childhood 52: 850–858

Dahl G V, Simone J V, Husto O, Mason C, 1978 Preventive central nervous system irradiation in children with acute non-lymphocytic leukemia. Cancer 42: 2187–2192

Davison C 1933 Xanthomatosis of the central nervous system (Schuller-Christian syndrome). Archives of Neurology and Psychiatry 30: 75–98

Delaney P 1977 Neurologic manifestations in sarcoidosis. Review of the literature, with a report of 22 cases. Annals of Internal Medicine 87: 336–345

Douglas A C, Maloney A F J 1973 Sarcoidosis of the central nervous system. Journal of Neurology, Neurosurgery and Psychiatry 36: 1024–1033

Eiser C, Lansdown R G 1977 Retrospective study of intellectual development in children treated for acute lymphoblastic leukaemia. Archives of Disease in Childhood 52: 525–529

Eiser C 1978 Intellectual abilities among survivors of childhood leukaemia as a function of CNS irradiation. Archives of Disease in Childhood 53: 391–395

Elian M, Burnstein B, Matz S, Askenasy H M, Sandbank U 1969 Neurological manifestations of general xanthomatosis. Archives of Neurology 21: 115–120

Evans A E, Gilbert E S, Zandstra R 1970 The increasing incidence of central nervous system leukemia in children. Cancer 26: 404–409

Falko J M, Williams J C, Harvery D G, Weidman S W,

Schonfeld G, Dodson W E 1979 Hyperlipoproteinemia and multifocal neurological dysfunction in systemic lupus erythematosus. Journal of Pediatrics 95: 523–529

Feinglass E J, Arnett F C, Dorsch C A, Zizic T M, Stevens M B 1976 Neuropsychiatric manifestations of systemic lupus erythematosus: diagnosis, clinical spectrum and relationship to other features of the disease. Medicine 55: 323–339

Flament-Durand J, Ketelbant-Balasse P, Maurus R, Regnier R, Spehl M 1975 Intracerebral calcifications appearing during the course of acute lymphocytic leukaemia treated with methotrexate and X-rays. Cancer 35: 319–325

Ford R G, Siekert R G 1965 Central nervous system manifestations of periarteritis nodosa. Neurology 15: 114–122

Freeman J E, Johnston P G B, Voke J M 1973 Somnolence after prophylactic cranial irradiation in children with acute lymphoblastic leukaemia. British Medical Journal 4: 523–525

Fulton W H, Dyken P R 1964 Neurological syndromes of systemic lupus erythematosus. Neurology 14: 317–323

Fusner J E, Poplack D G, Pizzo P A, Di Chiro G 1977 Leukoencephalopathy following chemotherapy for rhabdomyosarcoma: reversibility of cerebral changes demonstrated by computer tomography. Journal of Pediatrics 91: 77–79

Gold A P, Yahr M D, 1960 Childhood lupus erythematosus. Transactions of the American Neurological Association 85: 96–102

Gribbin M, Hardisty R M, Chessells J M 1977 Long-term control of central nervous system leukaemia. Archives of Disease in Childhood 52: 673–678

Hackett E R, Martinez R D, Larson P F, Paddison R M 1974 Optic neuritis in systemic lupus erythematosus. Archives of Neurology 31: 9–11

Hanefeld F, Riehm H 1980 Therapy of acute lymphoblastic leukaemia in childhood: effects on the nervous system. Neuropädiatrie 11: 3–16

Hardisty R M, Norman P M 1967 Meningeal leukaemia. Archives of Disease in Childhood 42: 441–447

Jasper P L, Denny F W 1968 Sarcoidosis in children, with special emphasis on the natural history and treatment. Journal of Pediatrics 73: 499–512

Jenkin R D T 1974 The management of malignant lymphoma in childhood. In: Deeley T J (ed) Malignant diseases in children. Butterworths, London.

Kay H E M, Knapton P J, O'Sullivan J P, Wells D G, Harris R F, Innes E M et al 1972 Encephalopathy in acute leukaemia associated with methotrexate therapy. Archives of Disease in Childhood 47: 334–354

Keith H M, Baggenstoss A H 1941 Primary arteritis (periarteritis nodosa) among children. Journal of Pediatrics 18: 494–506

Kurczynski T W, Choudhury A A, Horwitz S J, Roessmann U, Gross S 1980 Remote effects of malignancy on the nervous system in children. Developmental Medicine and Child Neurology 22: 205–222

Lister T A, Sutcliffe S B J, Brearly R L, Cullen M H 1979 Patterns of CNS involvement in malignant lymphoma In: Whitehouse J M A, Kay H M (eds) CNS complications of malignant disease. Macmillan, London

Lucaya J 1971 Histiocytosis X. American Journal of Diseases of Children 121: 289–295

Malamud N 1945 A case of periarteritis nodosa with decerebrate rigidity and extensive encephalomalacia in a five-year-old child. Journal of Neuropathology and Experimental Neurology 4: 88–92

Mann J R 1981 Sickle cell haemoglobinopathies in England. Archives of Disease in Childhood 56: 676–683

McElwain T J, Clink H M, Jameson B, Kay H E M, Powles R L 1979 Central nervous system involvement in acute myelogenous leukaemia. In: Whitehouse J M A, Kay H E M (eds) CNS complications of malignant disease. Macmillan, London

McGovern J P, Merritt D H 1956 Sarcoidosis in childhood. Advances in Pediatrics 8: 97–135

Mueller S, Bell W, Seibert J 1978 Cerebral calcifications associated with intrathecal methotrexate therapy in acute lymphatic leukemia. Journal of Pediatrics 88: 650–653

Murphy S B, Davis L W 1974 Hodgkin's disease and the non-Hodgkin's lymphomas in childhood. Seminars in Oncology 1: 17–26

Nesbit M E, Sather H N, Robison L L, Ortega J, Littman P S, D'angio G J et al 1981 Presymptomatic central nervous system therapy in previously untreated childhood acute lymphoblastic leukaemia: comparison of 1800 rad and 2400 rad. A report for Children's Cancer Study Group, Lancet 1: 461–465

Peylan-Ramu N, Poplack D G, Blei C L, Herdt J R, Vermess M, Di Chiro G 1977 Computer assisted tomography in methotrexate encephalopathy. Journal of Computer Assisted Tomography 1(2): 216–221

Peylan-Ramu N, Poplack D G, Pizzo P A, Adornato B T, Di Chiro G, 1978 Abnormal CT scans of the brain in asymptomatic children with acute lymphoblastic leukemia after prophylactic treatment of the central nervous system with radiation and intrathecal chemotherapy. New England Journal of Medicine 298: 815–818

Pitner S E, Johnson W W 1973 Chronic subdural hematomata in childhood acute leukemia. Cancer 32: 185–190

Pizzo P A, Bleyer W A, Poplack D G, Leventhal B G 1976 Reversible dementia temporally associated with intraventricular therapy with methotrexate in a child with acute myelogenous leukemia. Journal of Pediatrics 88: 131–133

Pochedly C 1977 Leukemia and lymphoma in the nervous system. C. Thomas, Springfield, Illinois

Portnoy B A, Herion J C 1972 Neurological manifestations in sickle cell disease with a review of the literature and emphasis on the prevalence of hemiplegia. Annals of Internal Medicine 76: 643–652

Price R A, Johnson W W 1973 The central nervous system in childhood leukemia. I. The arachnoid. Cancer 31: 520–533

Price R A, Jamieson P A 1975 The central nervous system in childhood leukemia. II. Subacute leukoencephalophaty. Cancer 35: 306–318

Rubinstein L J, Herman M M, Long T, Wilbur J R 1975 Disseminated necrotizing leuko-encephalopathy: a complication of treated central nervous system leukaemia and lymphoma. Cancer 35: 291–305

Slyter H, Liwnicz B, Herrick M K, Mason R 1980 Fatal myeloencephalopathy caused by intrathecal vincristine. Neurology 30: 867–871

Smyth D, Tripp J H, Brett E M, Marshall W C, Almeida J, Dayan A D et al 1976 Atypical measles encephalitis in leukaemic children in remission. Lancet 2: 574

UKALL I 1973 Treatment of acute lymphoblastic leukaemia: effect of 'prophylactic' therapy against central nervous system leukaemia. Report to the Medical Research Council by the Leukaemia Committee and the Working Party on Leukaemia in Childhood. British Medical Journal 2: 381–384

UKALL II 1978 Effects of varying radiation schedule, cyclophosphamide treatment, and duration of treatment in acute lymphoblastic leukaemia. Report to the Medical Research Council by the Working Party on Leukaemia in Childhood. British Medical Journal 2: 787–791

24

I. Clinical neurophysiology in paediatric neurology

R. Harris

INTRODUCTION

There are a number of neurophysiological techniques which may be used to investigate certain aspects of the functions of the nervous system. Application of these procedures is of special value in the assessment of neurological problems in infancy and childhood, particularly when the clinical evaluation is difficult because of the child's age or unco-operative state. Apart from minor modifications, the methods of the various tests are the same as for adults. There are some special considerations of management particularly in very young, retarded or disturbed children who are unable to cooperate and, although the skill of those handling the patient is an extremely important factor (Cornish 1967), it may still be necessary to use some form of sedation in order to obtain satisfactory results.

The electroencephalograph (EEG) is the most widely used test and some of the problems of interpretation and application of the EEG in neurological disorders of childhood will be discussed, in addition to cerebral evoked potentials, electromyography (EMG), nerve conduction studies and polygraphic recording.

ELECTROENCEPHALOGRAPHY

Technique

It is usually best to use some form of 'stick-on' electrode in babies and children, such as a small silver/silver chloride disc applied with collodion. Once in place these are comfortable and are less likely than pad electrodes to cause artefacts if the child is restive. The method of electrode placement described by Pampiglione (1956) using measurements from bony landmarks is helpful, as this gives a comparable electrode location from one time to another in babies and children, particularly during the period of rapidly increasing head size in the first year of life. Only a limited number of electrodes can be placed over the heads of newborn and young babies and it may be impossible to apply a full set in a restless one to two year old. Figures 24.1 and 24.5 are examples of useful montages which employ a total of 13 electrodes (one over each superior frontal, central, sylvian, mid and posterior temporal regions of either hemisphere, a vertex and mid-occipital electrode plus an earth electrode).

Maturation

The pattern of EEG activity shows a sequence of change throughout infancy and childhood in both the sleeping and waking states and a working knowledge of this aspect of cerebral maturation is essential in paediatric EEG assessment.

The EEG patterns during the neonatal period in premature and full-time babies have been described in a number of papers. (Dreyfus-Brisac & Monod 1957, Dreyfus-Brisac et al 1957, Prechtl et al 1968). Intermittent cerebral electrical activity is seen in records from very premature infants, but by about 32 weeks of gestational age, activity is present more or less continuously. Behavioural changes, appropriate to the rapid eye movement (REM) and non-rapid eye movement (NREM) sleep states, have been described in premature infants together with some subtle variations in EEG pattern (Goldie et al 1971), but it is not until the 36th week of gestational age that there is a clear distinction in the sleeping and waking state-related EEG features. Generalised bursts of theta (4–7 c/sec) and delta (3 c/sec and slower) activity appear at about 10 second intervals in the NREM state with small amplitude activity of mixed frequencies in the intervals. This latter pattern appears continuously in the waking and REM conditions. In the newborn, REM sleep precedes NREM sleep after a period of wakefulness but at about 46 weeks (i.e. six weeks after full term), there is a transition to the adult organization of sleep cycles with a period of NREM sleep following wakefulness before the REM state is entered. At the same time the trend towards the diurnal distribution of the waking and sleeping state begins and these behavioural changes are paralleled by the appearance of sleep spindles and more continuous slow wave activity in the NREM state. The details of the maturation of sleep behaviour and EEG patterns in the neonatal period are now so precise that they can provide valuable information relating to gestational age when this is in doubt.

At about the time of the transition in the sleep cycle organization, rhythmic theta and delta rhythms begin to appear in the EEG during quiet wakefulness. The further maturation of the EEG through childhood to adult life has been described in some detail by Eeg-Olofsson (1971). In the waking state there is a gradual reduction in the amplitude and increase in the frequency of the rhythmic activity seen in the EEG of young babies and towards the end of the first year of life rhythmic activity at about 6–7 c/sec appears over the posterior regions of the head which, like the alpha rhythm of older children and adults, is attenuated by eye opening and other alerting stimuli. Activity at a similar frequency is seen over the anterior regions of the head and is unaffected by eye opening but may disappear in relation to proprioceptive stimuli produced by hand movements and thus resembles the 7–11 c/sec sharply outlined waves seen over the central regions (Mu rhythms) in older age groups. Lambda waves associated with scanning eye movements may be seen in the EEG of very young babies (Fig. 24.1). The amount of theta and delta activity decreases with increasing age and the posterior and central rhythms become progressively faster in frequency and smaller in amplitude until the adult characteristics are attained. There are considerable individual variations in this process and slower rhythmic components may persist, particularly over the posterior temporal regions, into early adult life.

The maturation of the sleeping EEG patterns has been reviewed by Harris (1973). A particular feature in early childhood is the increase in the amplitude and amount of generalised theta and delta activity during drowsiness. This activity may

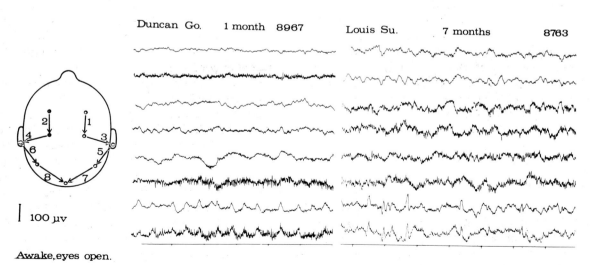

Duncan Go.   1 month   8967   Louis Su.   7 months   8763

100 µv

Awake, eyes open.

Fig. 24.1 EEGs from two young babies lying quietly, awake and making scanning eye movements. Lambda waves are seen in Channels 7 and 8 in both traces, but are of shorter duration in the record from the 7-month-old baby. The time marker in this, and other EEG figures, indicates 1 second intervals

Russel Wa.   2 years   16.9.76.   9022

Drowsy, Eyes open.

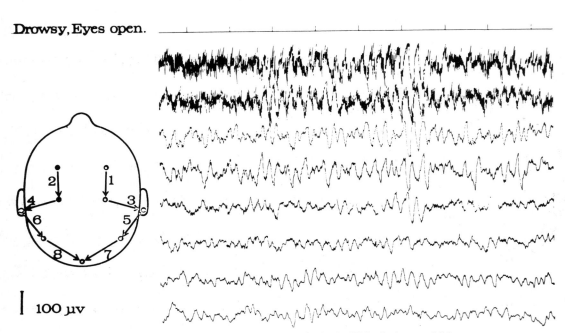

100 μv

Fig. 24.2 Diffuse theta activity, which is of largest amplitude anteriorly in the EEG of a drowsy child

appear up to about four years of age in children lying quietly and apparently alert and it sometimes precedes the eye closure of sleep for many minutes (Fig. 24.2). During childhood there is some reduction in the amplitude of the slow rhythms of the NREM sleep, and the sleep spindles, which appear independently over either hemisphere in early infancy, gradually become more synchronous. Vertex sharp waves, seen normally in sleep, are large in amplitude and short in duration in childhood and often have a spike like appearance. The 14 and 6 per second positive spike phenomenon of drowsiness and light sleep reaches its peak incidence in early adolescence but may be seen over a wide age range (Eeg-Olofsson 1971).

The activation procedure of hyperventilation can be carried out successfully in quite young children and is generally associated with a marked generalised increase in the amount and amplitude of delta activity which rapidly disappears when overbreathing stops. Such dramatic changes are unusual in adult EEGs. Similarly, the occipital cerebral evoked responses to flashing light in the on-going

EEG may be of much larger amplitude than those seen in adult recordings (Fig. 24.3).

Evaluation of the constantly changing pattern of the EEG through infancy and childhood has to be considered in the assessment of individual and serial records. In addition, a certain proportion of normal children will show undoubted abnormal EEG wave forms or a proportion of slow rhythms which is outside the mean values described in normal children by Eeg Olofsson (1971). This author found that only 68% of 743 children of 1 to 15 years and 77% of 185 adolescents of 16 to 21 years had totally 'normal' EEGs when those whose records showed paroxysmal and excess slow wave activity were excluded. The incidence of paroxysmal activity in this series of normal subjects was increased during hyperventilation, photic stimulation and sleep. Further problems of evaluation in paediatric EEG practice arise because of the ease with which the cerebral electrical rhythms may be disturbed during intercurrent illnesses (Pampiglione 1964c) and metabolic disturbances (Harden et al 1968).

The overall assessment of each EEG begins,

Melanie Gu.   3½ years   7.9.76.   8997.

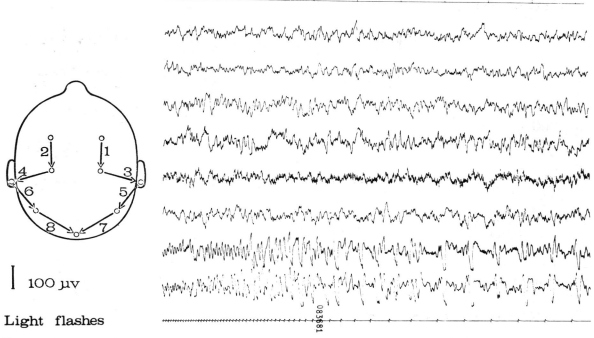

100 μv

Light flashes

Fig. 24.3 An example of the well-formed and large amplitude responses to photic stimulation commonly seen in records from young children

therefore, with consideration of the child's age and state at the time of the test and the possible effects that intercurrent disorders may have upon the ongoing EEG activity.

Epilepsy

Seizures are not an uncommon occurrence in babies and children during the course of some acute illness and, from the EEG point of view, the findings will be related to the cerebral effects of the underlying illness and are likely to be of a different kind from those seen in children with habitual epilepsy. There is an overlap, of course, for in some children repeated seizures will date from an initial acute episode and the EEG evolution in such instances will reflect the course of the cerebral involvement.

In general, the EEG abnormalities in epilepsy are similar to those found in adult patients and consist of spike and spike and slow wave complexes, often associated with some disturbance of the on-going EEG rhythms with excessive amounts of theta, delta and fast rhythms. The abnormalities tend to be more widespread in distribution and there is proportionally more disruption of the normal EEG patterns in children than in adults. The localisation of spike discharges is likely to vary over a period of time in children. Trojaborg (1968) found that in 85% of 242 children followed up for periods of from three to fifteen years, the distribution of spike discharges in their EEGs altered and in half of that percentage the change was from one hemisphere to the other. Spike discharges alone, therefore, have a limited value in indicating areas of abnormal brain.

Valuable information about the type of seizure may be obtained from EEG recordings during attacks and such opportunities commonly arise, particularly in babies and young children. The true petit mal absence is associated with generalised regularly repeating 3 per second spike and slow wave complexes, whereas other types of brief seizure, with short duration motor phenomena and possibly an associated brief lapse of consciousness, are accompanied by generalised irregular slow wave, spike and polyphasic spike discharges which may be asymmetrical in distribution. These attacks are not always clinically easy to distinguish from one another and, as this distinction may have important therapeutic implications, combined clinical and EEG observations are particularly helpful. Telemetered EEG recording, using radiotransmission of the cerebral potentials to operate a recorder, can be used to obtain EEGs from free moving subjects over long periods of time (Porter et al 1971, Ives et al 1976). The clinical changes and associated EEG phenomena may be obtained on film, as in the patient described by Ames (1974), or video-tape for subsequent detailed analysis and in this way a considerable variety of brief epileptic events may be studied. Focal theta and delta waves are commonly seen during the psychomotor attacks of temporal lobe epilepsy, the temporal spikes being an interictal EEG abnormality. Other types of focal epilepsy may show appropriately localised slow wave or repetitive spike discharges during attacks. During grand mal seizures the EEG traces are often masked by movement artefact and muscle action potentials, but preceding, or at the onset of the tonic phase of the attack, rapidly repeating spikes or fast rhythms may be seen, possibly located over a particular region of the head and subsequently delta and theta rhythms may be similarly localised. In minor epileptic status (Brett 1966), continuous, generalised slow wave and spike discharges accompany the abnormal clinical state, both of which may rapidly disappear after an intramuscular or intravenous dose of diazepam. There is a variable relationship between cerebral spikes and the large muscle action potentials found in patients with myoclonic epilepsy and this can be demonstrated by combined EEG and surface electrode muscle recording. The detail of the clinical and EEG phenomena of reflex epilepsy can be studied during recordings using the appropriate provocative stimulus. Jeavons & Harding (1975) have reviewed the literature on photic epilepsy, the commonest form

of reflex seizure, and have presented the findings from 460 patients of their own. Bursts of spike and slow wave discharges during photic stimulation may be found in normal children, particularly adolescent girls (Eeg-Olofsson 1971) and these should not be taken as evidence of photosensitive seizures, in the absence of a clinical history of attacks. The methods of testing for light sensitivity are important and these are discussed by Jeavons & Harding (1975). Children who induce seizures by hand flicking in front of their own eyes in bright light (Andermann et al 1962), usually show bursts of spike and wave discharges in their EEGs in response to various forms of light stimulus but are not often willing to induce seizures themselves in the laboratory setting.

In practice, classification of epilepsy in children is a difficult and rather unhelpful exercise, for both the clinical and EEG phenomena tend to vary over a period of time in any given child and several years may pass before a particular form of habitual seizure and EEG abnormality is established. The younger the child, the greater is the variability likely to be, but there are certain syndromes of infantile epilepsy, neonatal seizures, infantile spasms and convulsions, which may be associated with cerebral pathology leading to later habitual seizures and neurological impairment and which, for these reasons, deserve special consideration.

It has been known for many years that neonatal seizures may be associated with severe and sometimes bizarre EEG abnormalities (Dreyfus-Brisac & Monod 1964, Harris & Tizard 1960). The follow-up study reported by Monod et al (1972) demonstrated the more serious prognosis with regard to later development for those babies with EEG abnormalities appearing early in the neonatal period, as compared with those seen towards the end of the first and beginning of the second week of life. This corresponds with the bimodal incidence of neonatal seizures (Robinson 1974). The early seizures are more likely to be due to perinatal cerebral pathology, malformation or inborn metabolic error, whereas the late onset seizures tend to be associated with transient and reversible biochemical disturbances. The EEG abnormalities in both instances may be quite marked, but in the benign seizures usually due to hypocalcaemia there are peculiarly shaped repetitive discharges of variable location as a distinctive EEG phenomenon (Pampiglione et al 1970).

Infantile spasms have their peak incidence of onset at about six months of age and the severe EEG abnormality known as hypsarrhythmia is considered an integral part of the syndrome. This pattern was first described by Vasquez & Turner (1951) but the Gibbs' definition (1952) has become more widely quoted. The generalised large amplitude slow wave activity mixed with multifocal spikes and sharp waves, which are the characteristic features of hypsarrhythmia, may be modified according to the state of wakefulness or sleep (Harris 1964). A sleep recording may be needed to demonstrate hypsarrhythmia if the clinical and EEG aspects of a particular case are in doubt, as the typical abnormality may not be present in the waking state. The hypsarrhythmic trace, however, as Hess & Neuhaus pointed out in 1952, is not a diagnostic EEG abnormality as it may occur in babies suffering from other kinds of infantile epilepsy and cerebral diseases without seizures. What is certain is that the EEG pattern is associated with a poor prognosis for later development (Friedman & Pampiglione 1971), particularly in those babies suffering from the syndrome of infantile spasms who have undoubted evidence of an associated pathological condition (Jeavons & Bower 1964). The EEG abnormality itself gives no clue to any particular underlying cerebral disorder and brain biopsies, taken during the illness, show no uniform changes (Harris & Pampiglione 1962). Cerebral lesions may be suspected, however, if the EEG shows an asymmetry between the activities of the two hemispheres or if an asymmetry is revealed during ACTH therapy, when the severe global EEG disturbance tends to disappear (Harris 1964). This improvement may only be temporary, but unless the child continues to have other kinds of seizures, the EEG improvement is eventually maintained and the record may be virtually normal even though the child remains retarded. A porportion of patients merge into the 'Lennox-Gastaut syndrome', an electro-clinical concept which was reviewed in 1973 by Aicardi. This comprises a heterogeneous group of children who suffer from seizures, which are usually difficult to control, with

retardation and an inter-ictal EEG which shows generalised slow frequency spike and wave complexes, being often most prominent anteriorly. The boundaries for this syndrome are difficult to define. Focal spike discharges may appear several years after apparent EEG recovery from hypsarrhythmia and the variable sequence of the EEG evolution is not surprising in view of the wide range of conditions which may be associated with the syndrome of infantile spasms (Millichap et al 1962). There is a similar diverse EEG and clinical evolution in those babies with infantile spasms who prove to have tuberous sclerosis. This is an interesting, although unexplained association; no less than 69% of the patients with tuberous sclerosis reported by Pampiglione & Moynahan (1976), suffered from the syndrome of infantile spasms.

The EEG abnormalities seen in relation to febrile convulsions have been reviewed in a monograph by Lennox-Buchthal (1973). Up to 90 % of EEGs taken within a day of such a convulsion may be abnormal and about a third of the patients have excessive slow wave activity, particularly posteriorly, which is often asymmetrical in distribution in records taken during the first week after an episode. This slow activity disappears by about the seventh to tenth day but is said to increase the chance of a subsequent spike focus developing (Figs. 24.4 and 24.5). It is unusual to have the opportunity to record during an actual seizure but in prolonged attacks the EEG will show a combination of slow wave and spike discharges, usually of large amplitude. The aetiology of febrile convulsions is diverse and their precise definition contentious. Over half of the patients studied by Wallace & Zeally (1970) had evidence of a virus infection. The EEG disturbances found are in keeping with some form of acute encephalopathy but the combination of infection, fever, possible electrolyte disturbance and anoxia during the actual seizure, in addition to other associated cerebral pathology, often make it difficult to assign a single cause for the EEG abnormality in the acute phase or for the subsequent brain damage when this occurs. Generalised bursts of spike and wave may be seen in the follow up EEGs from one to two years of age, in about one third of patients (Lennox-Buchthal 1973) and spike foci may appear up

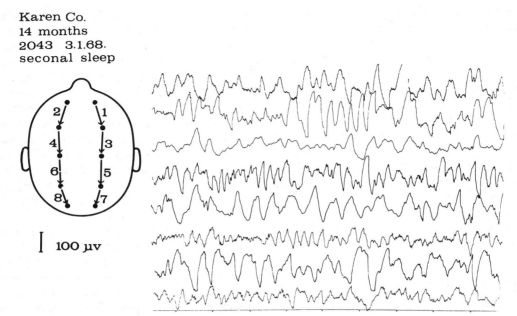

Karen Co.
14 months
2043 3.1.68.
seconal sleep

I 100 µv

Fig. 24.4 This child had repeated convulsions followed by transient weakness of the right arm and leg during a febrile illness. The seizures occurred 13 days before this EEG was obtained. There is an excess of large amplitude delta activity and, except for the frontal regions, it is most marked over the right hemisphere. Such apparent discrepancies between the clinical and EEG lateralisation are not unusual.

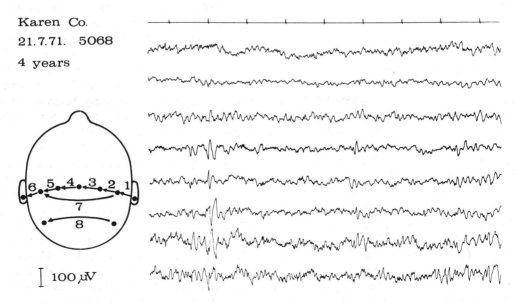

Karen Co.
21.7.71. 5068

4 years

I 100 µV

Fig. 24.5 A follow-up EEG from the same child as in Fig. 24.4. Several more febrile convulsions had occurred in spite of continuous anticonvulsant therapy. Serial EEGs in the interval had consistently shown slow waves and spikes over the left hemisphere. This record, taken 1 year after the last convulsion, still demonstrates persistent left-sided spikes and sharp waves

to nine years later. Although spike discharges do not necessarily indicate the development of later habitual epilepsy it is of interest to note that in Lennox-Bruchthal's own series, they were seen in all the patients who developed seizures in later childhood. Children who suffer repeated febrile convulsions commonly show a changing localisation to the EEG abnormality in each episode and this sort of documentation may be helpful in the subsequent assessment of the extent of possible brain damage. This is particularly relevant in the study of temporal lobe epilepsy, for as Ounsted et al (1966) have shown, febrile convulsions appear to be an important predisposing factor in the development of the psychomotor type of attack in later childhood.

Inborn errors of metabolism

These may be divided into three main groups.

1. Amino-acidurias, in which the metabolic defect may directly affect cerebral function and also lead to secondary brain damage. Examples are phenylketonuria, hyperglycinaemia and homocystinuria.

2. Other metabolic disorders with possible effects on brain function and maturation, including those with a risk of secondary brain damage such as galactosaemia, hypothyroidism and Wilson's disease.

3. The neurometabolic disorders which involve mainly neural tissues and which are associated with an accumulation of lipid or carbohydrate material. These include the lipidoses, leucodystrophies and mucopolysaccharidoses.

There are few specific EEG correlations with the various disorders in the first two groups, apart from those related to the age at which the metabolic defect has its greatest effect, its severity, the course of the disease and the possibility of treatment. In conditions such as ketotic hyperglycinaemia, maple syrup urine disease and galactosaemia, in which the clinical effects are manifest at birth and may even have begun to cause neural damage in utero, severe EEG abnormalities are commonly present in the neonatal period. There may be a complete disruption of the expected EEG patterns with excessive amounts of theta and delta activity, possibly mixed with multifocal spike discharges. The electrical

activity may only appear intermittently and the abnormalities are likely to be generalised but, as is common in the neonatal period, show inconsistent lateralising features. Similar EEG patterns may be found in other kinds of perinatal illness but the persistence of the EEG abnormality, together with the clinical features, will help to distinguish the inborn metabolic disorders from other conditions, especially the transient metabolic abnormalities associated with seizures (vide supra). If, as in phenylketonuria, the metabolic abnormality can be alleviated by treatment, the EEG abnormalities will tend to disappear and the expected maturation of the EEG rhythms will take place.

Failure of the maturation of the EEG rhythms may occur in those biochemical defects where, as in hypothyroidism, neural development is impaired (Harris et al 1965). Again satisfactory treatment will be reflected in the appropriate EEG improvement but in all the remediable metabolic defects there may be persistent EEG abnormalities if irreversible brain damage has already occurred. Inborn errors of metabolism, which have a variable cerebral effect and in which symptoms and signs become manifest in later infancy and childhood, will show a wide range of EEG abnormality, corresponding roughly in their type and severity to the degree of cerebral involvement. The on-going EEG rhythms may show an excess of theta, delta or beta rhythms of an entirely non-specific type and paroxysmal abnormalities of various kinds which are often appropriate to the seizure type when they occur, as in the patient with Type II hyperprolinaemia and petit mal epilepsy described by Emery et al (1968). In metabolic errors, in which the physical effects of the disorder are complex, the EEG abnormalities may be partly due to secondary cerebral complications such as the thrombo-embolic accidents in homocystinuria and sickle cell anaemia, liver failure in Wilson's disease and brain damage in conditions complicated by hypoglycaemic episodes.

In the third group, the neurometabolic disorders (Ch. 5) the EEG abnormalities, in addition to being related to the age of the child and evolution of the illness, are also partly distinguished by whether the abnormal storage of material is mainly in the cell bodies or in the myelin nerve sheaths. In the former conditions, i.e. the lipidoses, there is a gradual

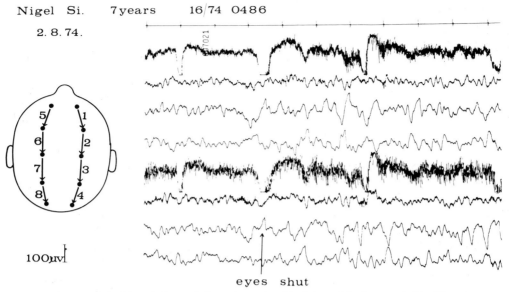

Fig. 24.6 An EEG from a child with metachromatic leucodystrophy. No alpha activity is recognisable. There is a generalised excess of delta and theta activities which increase in prominence after eye closure

disruption of the pattern of EEG activity with multifocal spike and slow wave and spike discharges in addition to increasing amounts of theta and delta activities. In the leucodystrophies there is a similar disorganisation of normal rhythmic activity and increase in the slower rhythms, but spike discharges tend to be rather uncommon (Fig. 24.6). The distinguishing EEG features of the various disorders have been described in a number of papers (Pampiglione 1968, Pampiglione & Harden 1973). The late infantile form of neuronal ceroid lipofuscinosis (Bielschowsky-Jansky or Batten's disease) is associated with characteristic spike discharges over the posterior regions of the head in response to single light flashes, and the wave form, and its relation to the normal visual evoked potential has been demonstrated by averaging techniques (Pampiglione & Harden 1973). The EEG evolution in these disorders may follow a particular course as in the group described by Santavuori et al (1974), in which the EEG eventually becomes isoelectric.

The rare metabolic disorders with cerebral degeneration show a relentless increase in the EEG abnormality which roughly parallels the clinical deterioration. The disruption of the normal EEG rhythms may precede the onset of the clinical features and this can be helpful in detecting affected, but symptomless, siblings.

Cerebral malformations

Gross cerebral malformations, which preclude normal development, may be associated with severe and often bizarre EEG abnormalities in the neonatal period and this investigation may be of great help in the management of babies who have multiple malformations. The absence of phasic electrical activity over large areas of the convexity of the skull will indicate the more severe degrees of porencephaly, hydrencephaly or other malformations (Fig. 24.7). The rhythms over the areas of developed cerebral tissue may be abnormal or relatively well preserved. An unusual location of cerebral evoked potentials may indicate distortion of cerebral structures. Thus, the EEG can quickly and easily provide information about major cerebral defects.

A localised excess of slow wave activity may be seen in the neonatal period in massive vascular malformations such as in the Sturge-Weber syndrome, but in this condition in later infancy the EEG may become almost equipotential over such

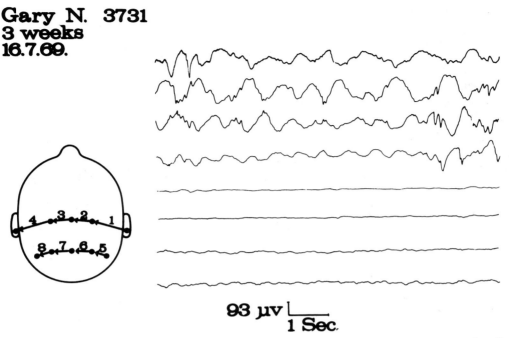

Gary N. 3731
3 weeks
16.7.69.

93 µv
1 Sec.

Fig. 24.7 This EEG was recorded from a baby with multiple malformations including hydrocephalus, a severe hare-lip and cleft palate. There is very little phasic activity present posteriorly, particularly over the right parietal and posterior temporal regions. Elsewhere, the EEG shows an excess of slow and sharp wave activity. At autopsy the Dandy-Walker malformation was found with a huge fourth ventricle cyst which filled a large part of the cranial vault posteriorly and displaced forwards, shrunken, but complete, cerebral hemispheres

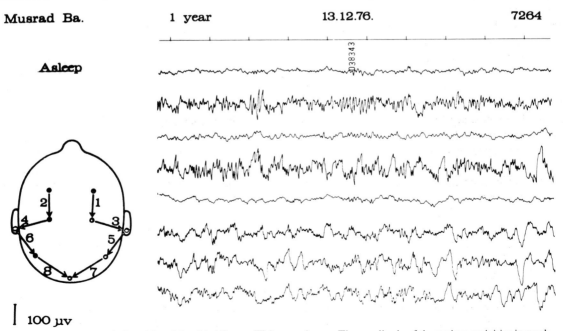

Musrad Ba.   1 year   13.12.76.   7264

Asleep

100 µv

Fig. 24.8 An EEG from a baby with a right-sided Sturge-Weber syndrome. The amplitude of the various activities is much smaller over the right than left fronto-central and temporal regions. In the neonatal period, EEGs had shown abnormal delta waves over a comparable region.

lesions (Fig. 24.8) and spike discharges may arise from the surrounding areas of brain.

The EEG in microcephaly may be within normal limits, but, as in other structural defects, the record will reflect the presence of coexisting localised brain damage.

Hydrocephalus, with of without spinal dysraphism, is the most common malformation presenting in early life which, with treatment, is compatible with a reasonable quality of life, although there is a high risk of some degree of retardation, and epilepsy occurs in one third of the surviving children (Hosking 1974). The EEG in the neonatal period is commonly normal even though the head is enlarged and the intra-cranial pressure high. Uncomplicated insertion of a valve is not necessarily associated with any post-operative or subsequent EEG abnormality. Many of these children, however, have some degree of brain damage and this, together with the possible recurrent problems associated with the presence of the valve, may cause diffuse or patchy EEG abnormalities. A rapid rise in intra-cranial pressure, due to a blocked valve, causes a dramatic increase in the amount and amplitude of diffuse slow wave activity, which soon disappears after satisfactory revision of the valve system (Figs. 24.9 and 24.10). Repeated infections

and biochemical disorders due to the renal problems arising in paraplegic children with spinal defects, add to the EEG abnormalities and, in some complex clinical situations, assessment of the cerebral component of a generally abnormal EEG can be extremely difficult.

Retardation and psychiatric disorders

The causes of retarded development in children are numerous but, excepting those patients with gross cerebral malformations or progressive cerebral diseases, there are unlikely to be any particular EEG features or trends in the EEG evolution which will give any diagnostic help. Changes in the pattern of sleep rhythms have been reported in mental retardation and some inborn errors of metabolism (Lenard 1970) and in infantile autism (Ornitz 1972), but such findings are non-specific and beyond the scope of routine electroencephalography. EEG surveys from groups of retarded children, however, have shown a relationship between the incidence of EEG abnormality and coexisting epilepsy (Gibbs & Gibbs 1965, Corbett et al 1975). A similar association was found in a group of children with unclassified retardation (Harris 1972). An epidemiological clinical and EEG survey of 155 severely retarded

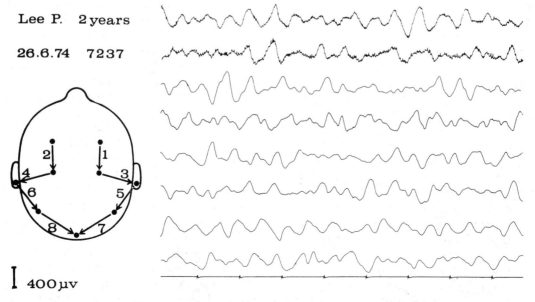

Fig. 24.9 This record was taken from a child with primary hydrocephalus at a time when the Spitz-Holter valve system had blocked. There is generalised huge amplitude delta and theta activity. (Note the calibration signal)

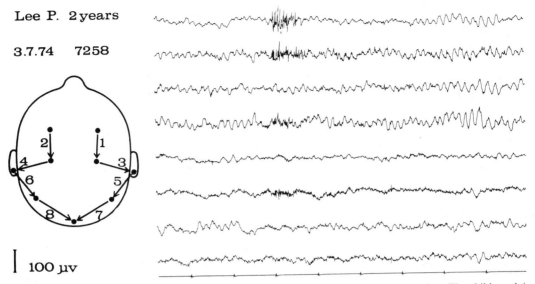

Lee P. 2 years

3.7.74   7258

100 μv

Fig. 24.10 An EEG from the same child as in Fig. 24.9 taken 7 days after revision of the valve system. The child was lying quietly with his eyes open. The previous severe EEG abnormality has disappeared

children described by Corbett et al (1975) reported an incidence of seizures at some time in 32% with 19% of the patients having had an attack within the year preceding the census date. The majority of abnormal EEGs in the survey were found in these epileptic children, three-quarters of whom had EEG abnormalities. The EEG has a useful role, therefore, in the management of epilepsy in these children and also in the detection of minor motor seizures, which may not always be easily apparent in the clinical setting of possible manneristic and bizarre behaviour (Harris 1972).

The EEG has a similar application in the assessment of children with psychiatric disorders. There is extensive literature on the subject, which has been reviewed by Harris (1976), but in general there is no convincing evidence that a particular kind of behaviour disorder or psychiatric illness is associated with characteristic EEG features (Ellingson 1954). A higher incidence of abnormal EEGs has been frequently reported amongst those children with added neurological handicaps, including epilepsy, and in addition it is known that behaviour disorders and psychiatric problems are commoner in retarded and epileptic children than in the general population (Graham & Rutter 1968). The main application of routine EEGs in psychiatric prob-

lems can, therefore, be directed towards the search for associated organic cerebral trouble.

Other cerebral disorders

The EEG abnormalities found in association with cerebral infections, trauma, tumours and systemic disorders with cerebral involvement will depend on the extent of that involvement and the course of the relevant condition. There is usually an excess of diffuse theta and delta activity in acute encephalopathies, often with a paradoxical increase in slow waves if a stuporose patient is aroused. The various acute infections (Ch. 22) do not produce distinctive EEG features except in herpes simplex encephalitis in which focal, usually temporal, repetitive slow wave complexes may appear transiently during the illness (Upton & Gumpert 1970). Regularly repetitive, stereotyped discharges are also found in subacute sclerosing panencephalitis (Cobb 1966), which is now thought to be an abnormal reaction to the measles virus. In the early phases of the disease it may be difficult to identify the recurrent EEG discharges which are not always generalised at that stage. Accompanying motor phenomena, of either a brief jerk or inhibition of movement, can be documented with simultaneous surface EMG

Andrew La   9 years   7145   28.5.74

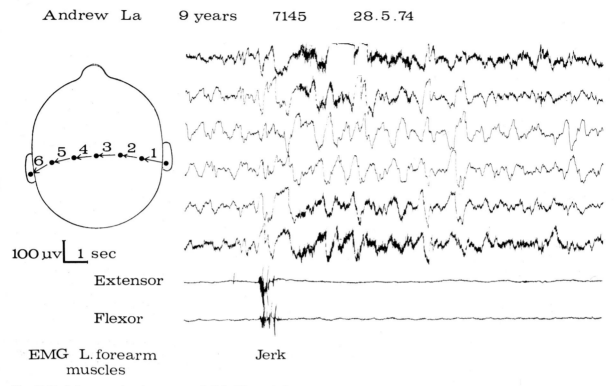

100 μv ⌐ 1 sec

Extensor

Flexor

EMG L. forearm   Jerk
      muscles

Fig. 24.11 Sub-acute sclerosing panencephalitis. The typical stereotyped repetitive discharges are not easy to recognise in this EEG. Simultaneous surface EMG recording shows a burst of muscle action potentials which accompanied a brief jerk and their association with a bilateral slow wave episode in the EEG

recording and this will demonstrate the relationship between the EEG and motor phenomena (Pampiglione 1964a) (Fig. 24.11). Localised cerebral infections leading to abscess formation will show appropriate focal slow wave EEG abnormalities.

Head injuries will be accompanied by EEG changes reflecting the extent and location of brain damage, but in the acute state in children, these abnormalities are likely to be increased by possible coexisting electrolyte disorders. During recovery from both infections and injuries there may be persistent EEG abnormalities relating to areas of brain damage.

Primary or metastatic supratentorial cerebral tumours will give rise to EEG changes which are appropriate to the extent and rapidity of tumour growth; slowly developing lesions are likely to show focal spike discharges as well as slow wave disturbances. In these, as well as other types of

focal brain pathology, there are more widespread abnormalities in the on-going cerebral rhythms than might occur with a comparable lesion in an adult. Posterior fossa tumours may only cause EEG abnormalities if there is coexisting distortion of the deep brain structures due to displacement, either by the tumour or through the effects of raised intracranial pressure (Fig. 24.12). A normal EEG in a child with clinical symptoms and signs of a posterior fossa lesion, certainly does not exclude the need for further investigation. As computer assisted X-ray tomographic systems (CT scan) become more widely available, the EEG is less likely to be used in these difficult problems of tumour diagnosis and location.

There may be cerebral involvement in many general systemic disorders leading to either focal or diffuse EEG abnormalities or both in combination, according to the proportion of direct brain damage and general metabolic disturbance concerned. In

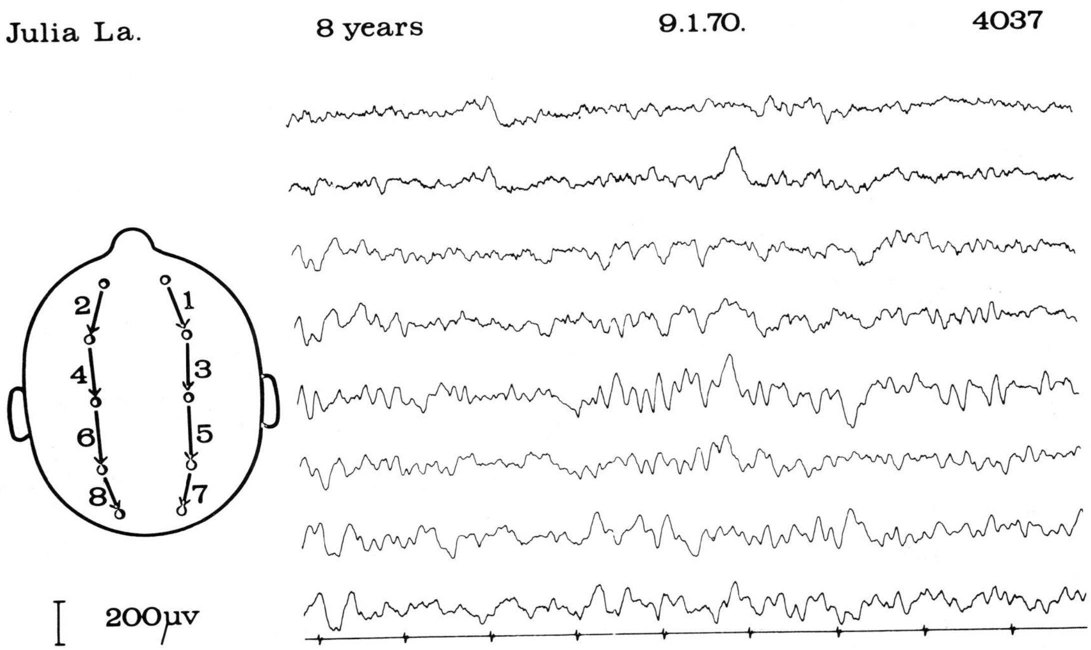

Julia La.　　　　8 years　　　　9.1.70.　　　　4037

Fig. 24.12 This child had vomited intermittently for several months. In the 4 weeks preceding this EEG she had vomited several times a day and developed headache and had had diplopia for 6 days at the time of recording. There is a generalised excess of large amplitude delta and theta activity which is most marked posteriorly. A medulloblastoma was subsequently confirmed

these situations the EEG may be of help in monitoring the progress of the brain disorder. Similarly, the extent of cerebral damage and likelihood of recovery after cardio-respiratory arrest may be assessed by serial EEG recordings (Pampiglione & Harden 1968), whatever underlying condition may be present.

EVOKED POTENTIALS

Now that small purpose-built computer systems are more generally available it has become possible to apply averaging techniques in the assessment of the integrity of specific nerve pathways on a routine basis. An appropriate sensory stimulus can be used to trigger a system which will average out the time-related evoked potentials from the random on-going cerebral electrical activity or be used, in a similar way, to study the small evoked end-organ potentials such as those arising in the retina and cochlea. The modalities commonly tested are sight, sound and tactile sensation.

Visual potentials

These can be sutdied at retinal and cerebral level in babies and small children, using the simple technique described by Harden & Pampiglione (1970). Silver/silver chloride disc electrodes are applied over the nasion to record the retinal responses to repeated light flash and over the occipital region for the cerebral potentials using a vertex reference electrode in each instance. Figure 24.13 shows a permanent record obtained in a few minutes from a restless baby, utilising the averaging device of an EMG machine. Impairment of the function of the retinal receptors as in retinitis pigmentosa can, in this way, be distinguished from defects in the visual pathway to the occipital cortex (Harden et al 1980). The latter groups will include optic nerve abnormalities such as retrobulbar neuritis and cerebral lesions including various degrees of agenesis where the potentials cannot be recorded or are in an abnormal location and the Bielschowsky-Jansky form of neuronal lipidosis where the potentials are abnormal and of large amplitude (Pampiglione &

Adrian Hi. 8 months   28.10.76.
55

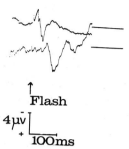

↑Flash

4μv

100ms

Fig. 24.13 A simultaneous recording of an electroretinogram (upper trace) and occipital visual evoked potential (lower trace). 64 responses to a light flash were averaged. (Low frequency setting equivalent to a cut of − 3 db at 1.6 Hz and high frequency, − 3 db at 160 Hz) These normal responses were from a severely retarded baby suffering from infantile spasms whose EEG showed hypsarrhythmia

Stephen Le. 11 years   8.2.77.

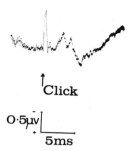

↑Click

0·5μv

5ms

Fig. 24.14 Cochlear and brain stem potentials recorded from surface electrodes (vertex to just above the ear). The responses to 512 clicks delivered to the ear were averaged. The early oscillations are the cochlear microphonic potentials and the main positive peak at about 6 msec. corresponds to the brain stem potential. (Low frequency setting equivalent to a cut of − 3db at 1.6 Hz and high frequency, − 3db at 16 Hz)

Harden 1973). The presence of an intact visual pathway can be demonstrated in babies with visual inattention due to severe mental retardation (Fig. 24.13). The application of moving pattern stimuli as a more subtle test of visual function, beyond the retinal level (Halliday et al 1972) is more difficult to apply in babies and very small children, because of problems of co-operation and fixation. These may be overcome by using a film cartoon superimposed upon the test pattern to hold the child's attention. Elaboration of these methods can be used to examine visual function in great detail, but many are outside the scope of routine testing.

Auditory potentials

The primary receiving cortical area for hearing is beyond the reach of recording from scalp electrodes, but the auditory pathway can be examined at three main levels; cochlea, the brain stem potentials and the non-specific vertex potentials. All the tests require meticulous attention to the type of sound stimulus used and recording techniques, the details of which may be found in the appropriate literature. The principles of the procedures are given clearly in the monograph by Davis (1976) and Gibson (1978). Cochlear action potentials can be

recorded from transtympanic electrodes or electrodes placed in the external auditory canal or on the nearby scalp or ear lobe. (Elberling & Salmon 1973, Sohmer & Pratt 1976). A complex wave-form of small amplitude and extremely short latency can be evoked by repetitive click stimuli with some variations in shape and size according to the method used. The brain stem potential, with slightly longer latency, can be recorded from the vertex using the ear lobes as the reference site (Fig. 24.14). A click type of stimulus is also required to study the post auricular ipsi- and contra-lateral myogenic response, which is a brain-stem reflex to sound. This is a useful screening test for demonstrating auditory reception but has been found to be absent or asymmetrical in about 10% of normally hearing subjects (Dus & Wilson 1975). The non-specific vertex potential can be evoked by a pure tone sound stimulus and is of relatively long duration and complex wave form. Threshold levels can be determined by decreasing the intensity of the sound stimulus applied to each ear in the various frequencies examined.

Conventional audiometry fails in very young, disturbed or retarded children and such patients are unlikely to be able to co-operate for the procedures described. The post-auricular myogenic response can be recorded in restless children

(Douek et al 1973) and the cochlear potentials are unaffected by anaesthesia (Davis 1976). The non-specific vertex response is altered by the state of alertness or anaesthesia, but nevertheless a combination of these tests may be able to show that the auditory pathway is intact or that there is a gross impairment of hearing. Comprehension of speech, however, cannot be assessed by these methods. In 1964 Walter et al demonstrated that there is a slow change in brain potential which is linked to some response by the subject. This state of 'expectancy' has been elaborated to test correct interpretation of speech, albeit at a simple level, by using words as one of the stimuli (Burian et al 1972).

Somato-sensory evoked potentials

Repetitive digital or peripheral nerve trunk stimulation will evoke potentials that can be recorded from surface electrodes placed over the spinal cord (Cracco 1973, Small 1976) and from those placed on the scalp over the appropriate sensory areas of the brain (Halliday 1967). Abnormalities of the cord potentials have been found in cord lesions and demyelinating disorders, but have so far found little practical application in neurological problems of infancy. The clinical applications of the cerebral potential have also been rather limited. Some patients suffering from myoclonic epilepsy have abnormally large potentials and the wave forms may be modified in gross unilateral cerebral lesions or severe unilateral peripheral nerve lesions (Halliday 1967). The author has made similar observations in the neonatal period in a baby with Erb's palsy. Desmedt et al (1976) have described the maturation of these potentials and have suggested that, combined with peripheral nerve conduction studies, much may be learnt about the development of the peripheral and central parts of the somato-sensory pathway in healthy and diseased children.

ELECTROMYOGRAPHY AND NERVE CONDUCTION TESTS

Peripheral neuromuscular disorders can be investigated by a combination of examination of muscle potentials and nerve conduction tests. Abnormali-ties in muscle function due to denervation can be distinguished from primary myopathic processes. In the former group of conditions, spontaneous small amplitude potentials arise from the denervated muscle at rest with some characteristic features. There is also a reduction in recruitment of motor units on volition and some of the potentials may be abnormally large in amplitude, polyphasic and of long duration, particularly in chronic denervating processes where re-innervation of muscle fibres from intact nearby motor units has occurred. Buchthal & Olsen (1970) have described the characteristics of the repetitive muscle action potentials arising from relaxed muscle in anterior horn cell disease in infancy (Werdnig-Hoffmann's disease). These potentials do not occur in other forms of denervation or in myopathies. There are fewer spontaneous small potentials recordable from the muscles at rest in myopathic disorders and the action potentials are of lower voltage and shorter duration than is normal. These myopathic potentials will be mixed with normal motor unit activity in the early phases of a myopathy and it is important to be able to measure the proportion of each. Problems of making such measurements in babies and young children arise, as they are often unable to co-operate for examination of the muscles at rest and during a series of graded voluntary effort. A combination of sedation, limb stimulation to produce active movements, and patience on the part of the examiner, will usually suffice for satisfactory recording of sufficient potentials for subsequent measurements to be made. Lack of co-operation also hampers the application of the computer analysis of motor unit potentials (Dowling et al 1968) which, in some instances, could possibly help in the early detection of a myopathy.

Nerve conduction studies do not present any particular difficulties in management, although it is helpful in some instances to give some preliminary sedation. It is important to evaluate the results with regard to age for the conduction time is related to the nerve length, the diameter of the nerve fibres, the thickness of the myelin sheath, internodal distance and the width of the nodes of Ranvier. There are considerable changes in these factors, not only in the neonatal period with regard to gestational age, but also over early infancy and childhood, and nerve conduction velocities within

Luke Bo.   9 months   18.11.76   249

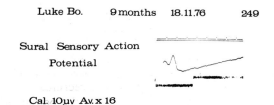

Sural Sensory Action
Potential

Cal. 10μv Av. x 16

Fig. 24.15 A normal sensory action potential evoked by a series of antidromic nerve stimuli and the responses averaged. The baby had suffered a rapid onset of a flaccid quadriplegia in the course of a febrile illness due to acute transverse myelitis. Normal nerve conduction studies excluded an associated peripheral neuropathy. (Time scale in 1 msec and 0.1 msec marks)

the adult range are not reached until about 3 to 4 years. The values for age-related nerve conduction velocities have been reviewed and discussed by Wagner & Buchthal (1972). Anterior horn cell diseases, myopathies and upper motor neuron disorders are accompanied by little, if any abnormality in peripheral nerve conduction. Acute and chronic polyneuropathies will be associated with delay in conduction and abnormalities of the evoked nerve and muscle potentials. It is possible to distinguish whether there is mainly demyelination, axonal degeneration or a combination of both. In many neuropathies the earliest abnormalities can be demonstrated in sensory conduction studies in the lower limb. The leg nerves should, therefore, be studied for preference (Fig. 24.15).

These tests can, therefore, provide rapid confirmatory evidence in such conditions as the Guillain-Barré syndrome, inborn errors of metabolism associated with peripheral as well as central nervous system demyelination (metachromatic leucodystrophy and Krabbe's disease) and local nerve lesions.

Myasthenic syndromes, as in adults, can be detected by the decrement in the amplitude of muscle action potentials in response to repeated nerve stimulation and the appropriate correct therapeutic response to intravenous edrophonium (Tensilon). Single muscle fibre recording techniques (Stalberg & Ekstedt 1973) are particularly helpful in myasthenia if the child can co-operate for the examination.

All these tests require meticulous attention to technical details including temperature control of the muscles and nerves under examination. By a judicious combination of muscle sampling and nerve conduction studies, including perhaps in the latter H-reflex times for afferent nerve function, it is possible to assess neuromuscular impairment in infancy and childhood, particularly when clinical testing of motor and sensory nerve function may be difficult.

POLYGRAPHIC RECORDING

Any number of physiological variables may be recorded simultaneously over short or long periods of time in order to study their inter-relationships in health and disease. The more commonly recorded activities are the EEG, respiratory, cardiac and skeletal muscle activity, psychogalvanic skin responses and gross body, limb and eye movement. These items may be processed in various ways. The EEG potentials, for example, may be expressed as units of 'power' combining changes in both frequency and amplitude in either a graphic or numerical form. Respiration and cardiac activity may be plotted as change in rate in unit time rather than actual rate. The possibilities are numerous and the particular application depends on the problem to be studied and method of presentation. It may be relatively simple, for instance by a polymyograph using surface electrodes, to record muscle potentials from different muscle groups, combined with EEG recording in order to demonstrate the characteristic pattern of movement during a bout of infantile spasms and the time-related EEG changes (Pampiglione 1964b). On the other hand, complex computer programmes may be employed to display, in compressed form, many physiological variables over several hours. This type of approach was used by Prechtl et al (1968) to examine the sleep and waking states in the neonatal period.

The link between central and peripheral events in neurological disorders in childhood requires further exploration. At a relatively simple level there is still much to be learnt in paediatric neurology from an open-minded application and combination of the various neurophysiological techniques which have been described in this chapter.

REFERENCES

Aicardi J 1973 The problem of the Lennox syndrome. Developmental Medicine and Child Neurology 15: 77–81

Ames F R 1974 Cinefilm and EEG recording during 'hand-waving' attacks of an epileptic, photosensitive child. Electroencephalography and Clinical Neurophysiology 37: 301–304

Andermann K, Berman S, Cooke P M, Dickson J, Gastaut H, Kennedy W A et al 1962 Self-induced epilepsy. A collection of self-induced epilepsy cases compared with some other photo-convulsive cases. Archives of Neurology 6: 49–65

Brett E M 1966 Minor epileptic status. Journal of the Neurological Sciences 3: 52–75

Buchthal F, Olsen P Z 1970 Electromyography and muscle biopsy in infantile spinal muscular atrophy. Brain 93: 15–30

Burian K, Gestring G F, Gloning K 1972 Objective examination of verbal discrimination and comprehension in aphasia using the contingent negative variation. Audiology 11: 410–316

Cobb W 1966 The periodic events of sub-acute sclerosing leucoencephalitis. Electroencephalography and Clinical Neurophysiology 21: 278–294

Corbett J A, Harris R, Robinson R G 1975 Epilepsy. In: Wortis J (ed) Mental retardation and developmental disabilities. Volume VII. Brunner/Mazel Inc, New York, p 79–111

Cornish R 1967 The child patient in the EEG department. Proceedings of the Electrophysiology Technologists' Association 14: 11–15

Cracco R Q 1973 Spinal evoked response: peripheral stimulation in man. Electroencephalography and Clinical Neurophysiology 35: 379–386

Davis H 1976 Principles of electric response audiometry. The Annals of Otology, Rhinology and Laryngology supplement 28: (85) no. 3.

Desmedt J E, Brunko E, Debecker J 1976 Maturation of the somato-sensory evoked potentials in normal infants and children, with special reference to the early N_1 component. Electroencephalography and Clinical Neurophysiology 40: 43–58

Douek E, Gibson W, Humphries K 1973 The crossed acoustic response. Journal of Laryngology 87: 711–726

Dowing M H, Fitch P, Willison R G 1968 A special purpose digital computer (Bromice 500) used in the analysis of the human electromyogram. Electroencephalography and Clinical Neurophysiology 25: 570–573

Dreyfus-Brisac C, Monod N 1957 Veille, sommeil et réactivité chez le nouveau-né à terme. In: Conditionnement et réactivité en electroencéphalographie. Electroencephalography and Clinical Neurophysiology supplement 6: 425–431

Dreyfus-Brisac C, Monod N 1964 Electroclinical studies of status epilepticus and convulsions in the newborn. In: Kellaway P, Petersen I (eds) Neurological and electroencephalographic correlative studies in infancy. Grune and Stratton, New York, p 250–271

Dreyfus-Brisac C, Samson-Dollfus D, Sainte-Anne-Dargassies S 1957 Veille, sommeil et réactivité sensorielle chez le prémature. In: Conditionnement et réactivité en electroencéphalographie. Electroencephalography and Clinical Neurophysiology supplement 6: 417–424

Dus V, Wilson S 1975 The click evoked post-auricular myogenic response in normal subjects. Electroencephalography and Clinical Neurophysiology 39: 523–525

Eeg-Olofsson O 1971 The development of the electroencephalogram in normal children and adolescents from the age of 1 through 21 years. Acta paediatrica scandinavica supplement 208

Elberling C, Salmon G 1973 Cochlear microphonics recorded from the ear canal in man. Acta otolaryngologica 75: 489–495

Ellingson R J 1954 The incidence of EEG abnormality among patients with mental disorders of apparently non-organic origin: a critical review. American Journal of Psychiatry 111: 263–275

Emery F A, Goldie L, Stern J 1968 Hyperprolinaemia type 2. Journal of Mental Deficiency Research 12: 187–195

Friedman E, Pampiglione G 1971 Prognostic implications of electroencephalographic findings of hypsarrhythmia in the first week of life. British Medical Journal 4: 323–325

Gibbs F A, Gibbs E L 1952 Atlas of electroencephalography, 2nd edn. Addison-Wesley Press, Cambridge, Massachusetts, vol 2, p 25

Gibbs F A, Gibbs E L 1965 The electroencephalogram in mental retardation. In: Carter C H (ed) Medical aspects of mental retardation. C Thomas Springfield, Illinois p 112–135

Gibson W P R 1978 Essentials of clinical electrical response audiometry. Churchill Livingstone, Edinburgh

Goldie L, Svedsen-Rhodes U, Easton J, Roberton N R C 1971 The development of innate sleep rhythms in short gestation infants. Developmental Medicine and Child Neurology 13: 40–50

Graham P, Rutter M 1968 Organic brain dysfunction and child psychiatric disorders. British Medical Journal 3: 695–700

Halliday A M 1967 Changes in the form of cerebral evoked responses in man associated with various lesions of the nervous system. In: Widen L (ed) Recent advances in clinical neurophysiology. Electroencephalography and Clinical Neurophysiology supplement 25: 178–192

Halliday A M, McDonald W I, Mushin J 1972 Delayed visual evoked response in optic neuritis. Lancet 1: 982–985

Harden A, Glaser G H, Pampiglione G 1968 Electroencephalographic and plasma electrolyte changes after cardiac surgery in children. British Medical Journal 4: 210–213

Harden A, Pampiglione G 1970 Neurophysiological approach to disorders of vision. Lancet 1: 805–809

Harden A, Pampiglione G 1977 Visual evoked potential, electroretinogram, and electroencephalogram studies in progressive neurometabolic 'storage' diseases of childhood. In: Desmedt J E (ed) Visual evoked potentials in man. Clarendon Press, Oxford, p 470–480

Harden A, Picton-Robinson N, Bradshaw K, Pempiglione G 1980 Ten years' experience of ERG VEP EEG studies on visual disorders in paediatrics. In: Barber C (ed) Evoked potentials. MTP Press Limited, Lancaster, England, p 257–266

Harris R 1964 Some EEG observations in children with infantile spasms treated with ACTH. Archives of Disease in childhood 39: 564–570

Harris R 1972 EEG aspects of unclassified mental retardation. In: Cavanagh J B (ed) The brain in unclassified mental retardation. Churchill Livingstone, Edinburgh, p 225–242

Harris R 1973 The maturation of sleep patterns. Proceedings of the Electrophysiology Technologists' Association 20: 70–83

Harris R 1976 The EEG. In: Rutter M, Hersov L (eds) Child psychiatry. Modern approaches. Blackwell Scientific Publications, Oxford, p 334–358

Harris R, Della Rovere M, Prior P F 1965 Electroencephalographic studies in infants and children with hypothyroidism. Archives of Disease in Childhood 40: 612–617

Harris R, Pampiglione G 1962 EEG and histopathology of 11 children with infantile spasms. Electroencephalography and Clinical Neurophysiology 14: 283

Harris R, Tizard J P M 1960 The electroencephalogram in neonatal convulsions. Journal of Pediatrics. 57: 501–520

Hess R, Neuhaus T 1952 Das elektroencephalogramm bei Blitz-Nick-, und Salaam Krampfen und bei andern anfallsformen des Kindesalters. Archiv für Psychiatrie und Nervenkrankheit 189: 37–58

Hosking G P 1974 Fits in hydrocephalic children. Archives of Disease in Childhood 49: 633–635

Ives J R, Thompson C J, Gloor P 1976 Seizure monitoring: a new tool in electroencephalography. Electroencephalography and Clinical Neurophysiology 41: 422–427

Jeavons P M, Bower B D 1964 Infantile spasms. Clinics in Developmental Medicine no. 15. Spastics Society/Heinemann, London

Jeavons P M Harding G F A 1975 Photosensitive epilepsy. Clinics in Developmental Medicine No. 56. Spastics International Medical Publications, Heinemann, London

Lenard H G 1970 Sleep studies in infancy. Acta paediatrica scandinavica 59: 572–581

Lennox-Buchthal M A 1973 Febrile convulsions. A reappraisal. Electroencephalography and Clinical Neurophysiology, supplement no. 32, Elsevier, Amsterdam

Millichap J G, Bickford R G, Klass D W, Backus R E 1962 Infantile spasms, hypsarrhythmia and mental retardation. A study of aetiologic factors in 61 patients. Epilepsia 3: 188–197

Monod N, Pajot N, Guidasci S 1972 The neonatal EEG: statistical studies and prognostic value in full term and pre-term babies. Electroencephalography and Clinical Neurophysiology 32: 529–544

Ornitz E M 1972 Development of sleep patterns in autistic children. In: Clemente C O, Purpura D P, Mayer F E (eds) Sleep and the maturing nervous system. Academic Press, New York, p 363–381

Ounsted C, Lindsay J, Norman R 1966 Biological factors in temporal lobe epilepsy. Clinics in Developmental Medicine 22, Heinemann, London

Pampiglione G 1956 Some anatomical considerations upon electrode placement in routine EEG. Proceedings of the Electrophysiology Technologists' Association 7: 1–20

Pampiglione G 1964a Polymyographic studies of some involuntary movements in subacute sclerosing pan-encephalities. Archives of Disease in Childhood 39: 558–563

Pampiglione G 1964b West's syndrome (infantile spasms) — a polymyographic study. Archives of Disease in Childhood 39: 571–575

Pampiglione G 1964c Prodromal phase of measles: some neurophysiological studies. British Medical Journal 2: 1296–1300

Pampiglione G 1968 Some inborn metabolic disorders affecting cerebral electrogenesis. In: Holt K S, Coffey V P (eds) Some recent advances in inborn errors of metabolism. Livingstone, Edinburgh

Pampiglione G, Harden A 1968 Resuscitation after cardio-circulatory arrest. Lancet 1: 1261–1265

Pampiglione G, Harden A, Chaloner J, Gumosz M 1970 Hypocalcaemia and seizures in young babies. Electroencephalography and Clinical Neurophysiology 28: 424

Pampiglione G, Harden A 1973 Neurophysiological identification of a late form of neuronal lipidosis. Journal of Neurology, Neurosurgery and Psychiatry 36: 68–74

Pampiglione G, Moynahan E J 1976 Tuberous sclerosis syndrome: clinical and EEG studies in 100 children. Journal of Neurology, Neurosurgery and Psychiatry 39: 666–673

Porter R J, Wolf A A Jr., Penry J K 1971 Human electroencephalographic telemetry. A review of systems and their applications and a new receiving system. The American Journal of EEG Technology 11: 145–159

Prechtl H F R 1968 Polygraphic studies of the full term newborn. 1. Computer analysis of recorded data. In: MacKeith R, Bax M (eds) Studies in infancy. Clinics in Developmental Medicine 27. Heinemann, London

Prechtl H F R, Akiyama Y, Zinkin P, Grant D K 1968 Polygraphic studies of the full term newborn. 2. Technical aspects and qualitative analysis. In: MacKeith R, Bax M (eds) Studies in infancy. Clinics in Developmental Medicine 27. Heinemann, London

Robinson R G 1974 Early childhood fits associated with mental deficits: a clinical view. In: Woodford F P (ed) Epilepsy and mental retardation. Institute for Research into Mental and Multiple Handicap. Symposium No. 16 p 1–26

Santavuori P, Haltia M, Rapola J 1974 Infantile type of so-called neuronal ceroid-lipofuscinosis. Developmental Medicine and Child Neurology 16: 664–667

Small D 1976 Peripherally evoked spinal cord potentials in neurological diagnosis. In: Nicholson J P (ed) Scientific aids in hospital diagnosis. Plenum Press, New York, p 155–163

Sohmer H, Pratt H 1976 Recording of the cochlear microphonic potential with surface electrodes. Electroencephalography and Clinical Neurophysiology 40: 253–260

Stålberg E, Ekstedt J 1973 Single fibre EMG and microphysiology of the motor unit in normal and diseased human muscle. In: New Developments in Electromyography and Clinical Neurophysiology. Karger, Basel, vol 1, p 113–129

Trojaborg W 1968 Changes in spike foci in children. In: Kellaway P, Petersen I (eds) Clinical electroencephalography in children. Grune and Stratton, New York, p 213–225

Upton A, Gumpert J 1970 Electroencephalography in herpes-simplex encephalitis. Lancet 1: 650–652

Vasquez, J H, Turner M 1951 Epilepsia en flexión generalizáda. Archivos Argentinos de Pediatria 35: 111–141

Wagner A L, Buchthal F 1972 Motor and sensory conduction in infancy and childhood: reappraisal. Developmental Medicine and Child Neurology 14: 189–216

Wallace S J, Zealley H 1970 Neurological, electroencephalographic and virological findings in febrile children. Archives of Disease in Childhood 45: 611–623

Walter W G, Cooper R, Aldridge V J, McCallum W C, Winter A L 1964 Contingent negative variation: an electric sign of sensorimotor association and expectancy in the human brain. Nature 203: 380–384

II. Recent advances in paediatric electromyography

D. P. L. Smyth

Most children on whom needle electromyography is requested can offer only limited co-operation, either because they are too young to understand the requirements of the test or because they are too fearful of the needle electrode in their muscle to move. Consequently the muscle contractions often occur in short bursts so that the EMG available for analysis may only be in portions of a few hundred milliseconds' duration making subjective assessment of the EMG by eye and ear poorly reproducible. Attempts to produce a reliable method of quantitative electromyography (QEMG) for children have included frequency analysis (Muller et al 1978) and measurement of features of the motor unit action potentials (Moosa & Brown 1972) but neither method has proved applicable or successful in practice. Surface electrodes are useless for diagnostic EMG because filtering and attenuation of the motor unit action potentials occurs in the tissues.

Recently a method of QEMG that is suitable for use in babies and young children has become available as a result of work by Smyth and Willison (Smyth & Willison 1975, 1982, Smyth 1980, 1982.) The method involves the conversion of the EMG to two trains of pulses using a modified analyser (now commercially available) of the type proposed by Fitch (1967). A ratio of the mean amplitude of the EMG signals to the number of changes in direction of the signals, known as turns, is derived and compared to findings from a group of children without neuromuscular disease. The method does not require measurement or control of the force of contraction and portions of EMG as short as 100 milliseconds are suitable for analysis. Between 15 and 20 portions of EMG are analysed in each patient to give a Mean Ratio of mean amplitude/turns per second. Only one needle puncture is required to do this.

Smyth & Willison (1982) and Smyth (1982) have presented the findings from 97 children aged 3 weeks to 15 years, suspected of having a neuromuscular disorder. Following full clinical examination and investigation the children were divided into four clinical groups without knowledge of the QEMG results. Twenty-two children had primary muscle disease, 21 a neurogenic disorder and 25 were considered to have no neuromuscular disease. Smyth and Willison called this last group the Apparent Control Group as it was not considered ethical to use needle electromyography in healthy children in order to obtain true control values. Support for placing the children in these groups was obtained from a 5-year follow-up study. There were 29 children in whom no definite diagnosis could be established, the evidence after investigation being inadequate or conflicting.

As no neuromuscular pathology occurred in the Apparent Control Group, Smyth and Willison considered the group to be homogeneous and derived an Apparent Control Group Mean Ratio of mean amplitude/turns per second with 95% confidence limits of 0.52 and 1.07. It was found that children with primary muscle disease had low Mean Ratios of mean amplitude/turns per second whereas children with neurogenic disease had high Mean Ratios. Furthermore the lowest and most abnormal ratios occurred in children with dystrophic muscle disease and Smyth concluded that this reflected the considerable loss of muscle fibres from the motor unit known to occur in dystrophic muscles, leading to the motor unit potentials becoming polyphasic and containing brief spikes of low amplitude. In contrast the children with metabolic myopathies where the structural changes are less, had results which were barely abnormal. Within the neurogenic group of patients the most abnormal Mean

Ratios occurred in children with anterior horn cell disease. These patients have a greater loss of axons with more collateral innervation and consequent enlargement of the motor unit than patients with peripheral neuropathy. None of the results were related to the severity or the duration of the symptoms or the child's sex. Smyth and Willison's findings represented concordance between the QEMG findings and clinical diagnosis in 68% of the children with primary muscle disease and 86% of the children with neurogenic disorders. Smyth concluded that whilst it cannot be assumed that children with results lying within the Apparent Control Group Range are necessarily normal, Mean Ratios outside of the range are highly likely to indicate myogenic or neurogenic disease. This method of QEMG overcomes the problems of limited co-operation and brevity of EMG activity that are commonly encountered in paediatric electromyography.

The problems of performing nerve conduction studies and electromyography in children have been referred to earlier in this chapter. The tests should be carried out with the child sitting on the lap of a parent or children's nurse, or lying on a couch with a familiar adult sitting close by to provide reassurance. Wherever possible personal contact should be established with the child before the visit to the laboratory. It is best to perform nerve conduction measurements using surface electrodes before EMG, because in many instances co-operation is lost after insertion of a needle electrode. The needle should be inserted quickly while the child's attention is diverted. Tickling of the sole of the foot can induce muscle activity in tibialis anterior whereas getting the child to kick towards a hand or a toy or posturing of the leg with the knee flexed usually results in enough spontaneous contraction in quadriceps femoris for observations to be made. Small children are frightened by close physical restraint and it is best to aim only at keeping the child reasonably still. Most children settle down during electromyography once a needle has been inserted but they may resist further sampling. It is therefore important to make a careful choice of muscles for examination before commencing the procedure. Thorough sampling of one or two muscles provides more information than inadequate sampling of a larger number. As with adults greatest information is obtained by sampling a muscle of only moderate weakness. Flexibility of approach and plenty of time and patience are required to obtain traces which are worth measuring.

REFERENCES

Fitch P 1967 An analyser for use in human electromyography. Electronic Engineering 39: 240–243

Moosa A, Brown B H 1972 Quantitative electromyography: a new analogue method for detecting changes in action potential duration. Journal of Neurology, Neurosurgery and Psychiatry 35: 216–220

Muller W, Hoffman W, Eulitz R, Muller I 1978 Klinische Anwendung der Quantitativen Beurteilung des kindlichen Elektromyogramms — charakteristiche Befunde bei neuromuskularen Erkrankunden. Paediatrie 15: 199–203

Smyth D P L 1980 The application of quantitative EMG to paediatrics. MD Thesis, University of London

Smyth D P L 1982 Quantitative electromyography in babies and young children with primary muscle disease and neurogenic lesions. Journal of the Neurological Sciences, in press

Smyth D P L, Willison R G 1975 The application of quantitative EMG to paediatrics. 5th International Congress of EMG, Rochester, Minn. 21–24 Sept.

Smyth D P L, Willison R G 1981 Quantitative electromyography in babies and young children with no evidence of neuromuscular disease. Journal of the Neurological Sciences, in press

Envoi

'The physician must never forget that medical art has a far higher range and aim than the prescription of drugs or even of food and hygienic means, and when neither of these avails it is still no small portion of his art to rid his patient's path of thorns if he cannot make it bloom with roses.'

Alfred Stillé (1813–1900)

Index

605